Annual Update in Intensive Care and Emergency Medicine 2017

The series *Annual Update in Intensive Care and Emergency Medicine* is the continuation of the series entitled *Yearbook of Intensive Care Medicine* in Europe and *Intensive Care Medicine: Annual Update* in the United States.

Jean-Louis Vincent
Editor

Annual Update in Intensive Care and Emergency Medicine 2017

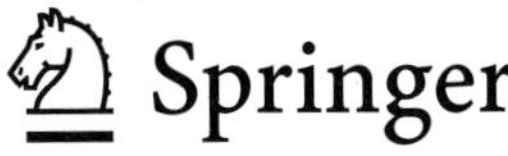

Springer

Editor

Prof. Jean-Louis Vincent
Dept. of Intensive Care
Erasme Hospital
Université libre de Bruxelles
Brussels, Belgium
jlvincent@intensive.org

ISSN 2191-5709 ISSN 2191-5717 (electronic)
Annual Update in Intensive Care and Emergency Medicine
ISBN 978-3-319-51907-4 ISBN 978-3-319-51908-1 (eBook)
DOI 10.1007/978-3-319-51908-1

Cover design: WMXDesign GmbH, Heidelberg

Printed on acid-free paper

This Springer imprint is published by Springer Nature
The registered company is Springer International Publishing AG
The registred company adress is: Gewerbestrasse 11, 6330 Cham, Switzerland

Contents

Part VII Cardiopulmonary Resuscitation

Part VIII Oxygenation and Respiratory Failure

Part IX Neurological Conditions

Common Abbreviations

AKI	Acute kidney injury
ARDS	Acute respiratory distress syndrome
AUC	Area under the curve
BMI	Body mass index
COPD	Chronic obstructive pulmonary disease
CPR	Cardiopulmonary resuscitation
CRP	C-reactive protein
CRRT	Continuous renal replacement therapy
CT	Computed tomography
CVP	Central venous pressure
ECMO	Extracorporeal membrane oxygenation
EKG	Electrocardiogram
ICU	Intensive care unit
IL	Interleukin
LPS	Lipopolysaccharide
LV	Left ventricular
MAP	Mean arterial pressure
MRI	Magnetic resonance imaging
OR	Odds ratio
PAOP	Pulmonary artery occlusion pressure
PCT	Procalcitonin
PEEP	Positive end-expiratory pressure
PPV	Pulse pressure variation
RCT	Randomized controlled trial
RRT	Renal replacement therapy
RV	Right ventricular
SIRS	Systematic inflammatory response syndrome
SOFA	Sequential organ failure assessment
SVV	Stroke volume variation
TLR	Toll-like receptor
TNF	Tumor necrosis factor

Part I
Infections

Severe Influenza Infection: Pathogenesis, Diagnosis, Management and Future Therapy

B. M. Tang and A. S. McLean

Introduction

Severe influenza infection is an important cause of acute lung injury. Although other respiratory viruses (e. g., respiratory syncytial virus, human metapneumovirus) can also cause considerable pulmonary damage, influenza virus remains the main cause of respiratory failure in patients with suspected viral respiratory tract infection. In addition, influenza virus is the only respiratory virus that has caused four pandemics over the last 100 years, making it one of the most transmissible and virulent viruses in the world. Here, we review the pathogenesis, diagnosis, current management and future therapy of severe influenza infection.

Pathogenesis

Understanding the pathogenesis of severe influenza infection is the key to developing new therapeutic strategies. Although the basic process of a mild influenza infection is well understood, our understanding of how a mild illness progresses to a potentially lethal pulmonary infection remains poor. In this section, we will review recent advances in the immunopathology of severe influenza infection.

Pulmonary epithelial cells are the first target of invasion by influenza virus. Like most cells, epithelial cells constitutionally upregulate the interferon pathway in response to infection by viruses. Types I and III interferon pathways are the natural

B. M. Tang (✉)
Department of Intensive Care Medicine, Level 2, North Block, Nepean Hospital
Derby Street, Kingswood, NSW 2747, Australia
Centre for Immunology and Allergy Research, Westmead Institute for Medical Research
Westmead, NSW 2145, Australia
e-mail: benjamin.tang@sydney.edu.au

A. S. McLean
Department of Intensive Care Medicine, Level 2, North Block, Nepean Hospital
Derby Street, Kingswood, NSW 2747, Australia

J.-L. Vincent (ed.), *Annual Update in Intensive Care and Emergency Medicine 2017*,
DOI 10.1007/978-3-319-51908-1_1

defense mechanism against influenza virus. Upon infection, epithelial cells upregulate interferon regulatory factors (IRF), such as IRF-3 and IRF-7. This leads to transcription and translation of a downstream interferon pathway, which in turn produces a family of interferon-stimulated genes/proteins. This vast family of interferon-stimulated genes/proteins (>300) provides a wide spectrum of anti-viral effects, ranging from inhibition of viral replication to sensing of influenza virus inside the host cells. This response is immediate and effective, making it a critical part of the innate immune response against influenza virus.

Whilst essential, the interferon response alone is not sufficient to prevent virus replication in severely infected cases. Multiple subsets of immune cells (e. g., macrophages, dendritic cells and neutrophils) are required to mount an effective immune response. The failure of this immune response is the hallmark of severe infection, which is characterized by multiple defects in immune cell recruitment, activation or proliferation, as described below.

Alveolar macrophages are among the early responders to influenza virus. They phagocytose infected cells containing influenza virus and initiate other cells of innate and adaptive immunity. Failure of alveolar macrophages to mount an effective early response is associated with increased viral dissemination and increased morbidity/mortality. Neutrophils are also early responders in severe influenza infection. Similar to alveolar macrophages, failure of this early neutrophil response is a prominent feature of severe influenza infection. Paradoxically, an exuberant or inappropriately exaggerated neutrophil response is also a feature of severe influenza infection. For example, in severe H1N1 and H5N1 infection, the large influx of neutrophils into the alveolar space is a classic feature [1]. During this massive neutrophil influx, the neutrophils release a large amount of cytokines, extracellular proteases and histones. This leads to a breakdown of the epithelial barrier, accumulation of reactive oxygen species (ROS), flooding of alveolar spaces by inflammatory fluid and increased barrier to oxygenation, all of which contribute to the clinical picture of acute lung injury commonly observed in patients with severe influenza infection.

Other immune cells are also involved in this early phase of infection (and contribute to pathogenesis). Monocytes, for example, traffic into the infected pulmonary tissue and participate in a pro-inflammatory response. Not surprisingly, inhibition of monocytes and preventing their subsequent participation in the pro-inflammatory response has been shown to decrease the extent of acute lung injury in animal models [2, 3]. Pulmonary dendritic cells are another important immune cell subset that contributes to pathogenesis. In a murine model of influenza infection, pulmonary dendritic depletion increased macrophage recruitment and enhanced pro-inflammatory responses (tumor necrosis factor [TNF]-α/interleukin [IL]-6 increased 5–35 fold) [4]. In another murine model, pulmonary dendritic cells induced T-regulatory cell responses that suppressed antigen-specific CD8 cells, thereby preventing an effective immune response [5]. Hence, the pathogenic role of dendritic cells seems to be to cause a dysregulated immune response, which either causes excessive lung injury (by causing increased inflammation) or impairs the effective clearance of influenza virus (by limiting CD8 cell response).

In the later phase of the host response, adaptive immunity becomes the dominant player. Here, activated CD8 T-lymphocytes cause lysis of the influenza-infected epithelial cells, which facilitates virus clearance. Impaired CD8 responses are a prominent feature of highly pathogenic influenza infection, such as the recently reported H7N9 outbreak in China [6]. In addition to cell lysis, CD8 cells also enhance the pro-inflammatory response, which could either contribute to host defense or, in some cases, worsen lung inflammation and cause further pulmonary damage.

Diagnosis

The detection of influenza virus is the first step in establishing a diagnosis. Rapid antigen detection assays offer a low-cost approach with a short turn-around time. However, a recent review demonstrated that such assays have an unacceptably low sensitivity [7]. Nucleic acid amplification (e. g., multiplex viral polymerase chain reaction [PCR]) has recently gained a much greater prominence due to its high sensitivity and specificity. Currently, this is the most accepted gold standard for virus detection in the initial evaluation of suspected influenza infection. However, there are three important caveats regarding the clinical utility of nucleic acid amplification assay:

(1) The reliability of such an assay is dependent on the fact that the viral genome is known. An unknown viral genome, mutant strain or new pandemic influenza virus will be difficult to detect.
(2) The sensitivity is affected by the way the sample is collected. Poor sample collection, inability to access lower airway or reduced virus shedding (due to prior anti-viral administration) all reduce detection sensitivity.
(3) Detection does not imply infection because the presence of influenza virus in the upper airway may be a co-incidental finding or active infection. In fact, 18% of exposed individuals show no clinical symptoms; therefore, the presence of the virus does not always imply that it is the causative agent. Furthermore, detection of an incomplete virus segment (by nucleic acid amplification) does not constitute sufficient proof that active viral replication is present.

In addition to virus detection, clinicians need to identify which patients are more likely to progress to severe disease or require admission to the intensive care unit (ICU). Table 1 summarizes virus-related and host factors that may contribute to progression to more severe disease. Some of these factors are clinically obvious (e. g., age, pre-existing medical conditions). Other factors (e. g., genetic susceptibility) require highly sophisticated laboratory testing (e. g., high-throughput genome sequencing), which are not yet available in the routine clinical setting.

Following the initial diagnostic work-up, the influenza infected patient needs to be continuously monitored for signs of bacterial co-infection. Several studies have shown that a significant proportion of influenza infected patients admitted to the

Table 1 Risk factors for progression to severe influenza infection

Viral factors	Host factors
Subtype of influenza virus (e. g., H7N9)	Genetic susceptibility (e. g., IFITM3)
Viral load (e. g., high viral load increases severity)	Pregnancy, obesity and extremes of age (elderly and neonates)
Mutation in viral genome (e. g., PB2 gene mutation enhances viral replication)	Pre-existing medical conditions (e. g., chronic lung diseases, cancer, chemotherapy)

IFITM3: interferon-induced transmembrane protein 3

ICU develop bacterial co-infection as a complication [8]. The causative bacterial co-pathogens are most likely to be *Streptococcus pneumoniae* or *Staphylococcus aureus*. The basis for increased susceptibility is thought to be due to production of type I interferon, which is increased initially in response to influenza virus infection, but also decreases the synthesis of IL-1B, IL-23, IL-17 and IL-22, which in turn inhibit the production of antimicrobial peptides [9]. Furthermore, the pro-inflammatory milieu caused by the influx of neutrophils also contributes towards increased susceptibility to bacterial super-infection. Other immune-related factors also contribute towards increased susceptibility including reduced type 17 immune response, impaired antimicrobial peptide (AMP) production by lung epithelia and reduced phagocyte function [9].

Host response biomarkers should form an important part of the diagnostic evaluation of an infected patient. Biomarkers assist clinical evaluation by providing additional information that is not available by conventional virus detection assay. This additional information includes an improved ability to distinguish between co-incidental 'bystander' virus and true infection, to predict clinical risk for further deterioration and to monitor treatment response. Table 2 summarizes the host response biomarkers that have been recently investigated in the literature.

Gene expression biomarkers are the most recent development in biomarker research. These biomarkers differ from conventional biomarkers (e. g., C-reactive protein [CRP] or procalcitonin [PCT]) in that they are much more influenza specific, due to the fact that many of them are interferon derived genes, which are upregulated in response to respiratory virus infection. A recently published landmark study

Table 2 Host response biomarkers for influenza infection

Biomarkers	Current evidence
Low antibody titer in serum	Could indicate increased risk of death
HLA-DR expression in monocytes	Suggests immune suppression
Procalcitonin (PCT) and C-reactive protein (CRP) in blood	May have some role in excluding bacterial co-infection
Mid-regional pro-adrenomedullin (MR-proADM)	May predict mortality or the need for mechanical ventilation
Gene expression biomarkers	May distinguish between virus detection and active infection

showed that these biomarkers could address several important clinical questions simultaneously (whereas conventional biomarkers could address only one question at a time) [10]. First, these biomarkers could assist clinicians to identify patients most likely to have infection (bacterial and viral) in a heterogeneous population of patients with undifferentiated respiratory illnesses. Second, among infected patients, the biomarkers could distinguish between bacterial and viral infection. Third, among infected patients, the biomarkers could prognosticate and predict clinical outcomes. In addition, the biomarkers could be easily measured in most clinical settings due to the ease of sampling (only 2.5 ml of whole blood is required) and the wide availability of PCR machines (to measure gene-expression). Importantly, because these biomarkers reflect changes in the immune pathway during influenza infection, they provide additional diagnostic information not offered by conventional pathogen detection assay (e. g., virus nucleic amplification). Although further validation studies are necessary before these biomarkers can be widely adopted in clinical practice, it is highly likely that they will be incorporated into the diagnostic armamentaria of modern laboratories in the future.

Management

The management of severe influenza infection is mainly supportive. Standard measures should include those used for the management of acute respiratory distress syndrome (ARDS). Therapeutic agents for severe influenza infection are limited, with oseltamivir being the most commonly used anti-viral agent. A recent meta-analysis showed that oseltamivir could reduce symptom duration and the risk of developing lower respiratory tract complications (e. g., viral pneumonia) [11]. However, its efficacy is dependent on oseltamivir being administered in the early phase of the illness. This may pose difficulty in the management of ICU patients, because these patients often present in the late phase of their illness. Regardless of the timing of presentation, oseltamivir should be considered in all high-risk patients. The current recommendation by the World Health Organization (WHO) indicates that it should be administered in immunocompromised patients, patients with severe comorbidities or underlying chronic lung diseases, age <2 or >65 years, morbid obesity, nursing home residents, women who are pregnant or post-partum, and patients with signs of severe respiratory disease.

Low-dose steroids are best avoided, as suggested by a recently published meta-analysis [12]. In this meta-analysis, the authors analyzed data from nine cohort studies (n = 1,405) and 14 case-control studies (n = 4,700). They found increased mortality associated with corticosteroid treatment in cohort studies (relative risk [RR] 1.85; 95% confidence interval [CI] 1.46–2.33; $p<0.0001$) and in case-control studies (odds ratio [OR] 4.22; 95% CI 3.10–5.76; $p<0.0001$). This increased mortality was consistent regardless of the quality of the included studies or the sample size of the individual studies. Other worrying findings are that corticosteroid use was associated with a higher incidence of hospital-acquired pneumonia, longer duration of mechanical ventilation and longer hospital stay. Therefore, the use of corticosteroids in severe influenza infection is not recommended in routine clinical care and should be restricted to patients in the setting of clinical trials.

Future Therapy

Although conventional treatment for severe influenza infection is limited, novel therapeutic agents have shown great promise. These novel agents consist of mainly two classes: immune agents that modulate host response and anti-viral agents that inhibit viral replication.

Immune Agents that Modulate Host Response

Host Factors that Control Viral RNA Replication

In order to replicate successfully, the influenza virus mRNA undergoes transcription. Initiation of primary viral RNA transcription depends on the activity of host RNA polymerase. Inhibition of this transcription process provides a therapeutic opportunity to halt the commencement of viral RNA replication. Inhibitors of this process, such as CDK9 inhibitor, have undergone preclinical evaluation.

Host Signaling Pathways Influenced by Redox Balance

The influenza virus hijacks the host cell signaling pathway to benefit its own propagation. Phosphorylation of the mitogen-activated protein kinase (MAPK) pathway has been shown to facilitate viral nucleoprotein trafficking [13]. Therefore, inhibition of the MAPK pathway could potentially reduce spread of the influenza virus. Of particular relevance to the intensivist is the fact that the activity of the MAPK pathway is determined by the oxidative-reductive state of the host cell. *N*-acetylcysteine, a well-established drug already commonly used in ICU patients, could modulate the oxidative-reductive state of the host cell, thereby affecting influenza virus propagation. A recent study has demonstrated the potential efficacy of this agent in treating severe influenza infection in an animal model [14]. Other antioxidant agents, such as p38 inhibitor or glutathione, are also potential new host-based therapeutic agents that modulate the redox balance within the host cell. In addition to the MAPK pathway, the PI3K pathway is also sensitive to the effect of redox balance. PI3K is a signaling pathway implicated in influenza infection [15]. An *in vitro* study showed that inhibition of this pathway could reduce influenza virus replication [16]. Importantly, PI3K inhibitors have already been approved as anticancer drugs. Therefore, the possibility of extending their use as anti-influenza agent offers a promising new avenue for future investigation.

Host Factors that Regulate Inflammation

Nuclear factor kappa B (NF-κB) is a family of transcription factors that initiate inflammation. Influenza virus benefits from the activation of the NF-κB pathway as the virus exploits the pathway machinery to facilitate viral replication. NF-κB pathway inhibitors, such as acetyl-salicylic acid, could block influenza virus replication and propagation. Other pathway inhibitors, such as SC75741, also decrease viral replication. This agent has the unique feature of having a low potential in selecting viral resistant variants, therefore making it unlikely to result in anti-viral resistance [17]. Furthermore, SC75741 has recently been shown to reduce viral replication and cytokine expression in highly pathogenic strains (e. g., H5N1 and H7N7), making it a potential candidate for further investigation in severe influenza infection [18].

The cyclooxygenase (COX) pathway is another pro-inflammatory pathway that has been implicated in influenza virus infection. Highly pathogenic influenza strains, such as H5N1, strongly upregulate COX-2 mediated pro-inflammatory signaling that causes hypercytokinemia during severe H5N1 infection. A non-steroidal COX-2 inhibitor has been shown to inhibit H5N1 infection in human macrophages, making it another potential agent for severe influenza infection [19].

Host Interferon Pathway

The interferon pathways (type I and type II) are the most potent defense of the host cell against influenza virus infection. Activation of interferon pathways leads to upregulation of more than 300 interferon-stimulated genes. Many of these interferon-stimulated genes have potent anti-influenza activity, such as *MX1* (anti-influenza), *ISG15* (inhibits influenza virus replication), *OAS1, OAS2, OAS3* (degrades viral RNA), *EIF2AK2* (inhibits viral replication), *HERC5* (positive regulator of anti-viral response) and *IFIT2* (inhibits expression of viral mRNA). In addition, these genes activate the adaptive immune response and induce programmed cell death of virally infected cells.

Novel therapeutic strategies take advantage of this endogenous anti-influenza defense by identifying trigger points that activate the interferon pathway. Several molecular pathways are known to trigger the interferon pathway. For example, Toll-like receptor (TLR) 3 and 7 are known to activate the interferon pathway in lung epithelium and immune cells. In plasmacytoid dendritic cells, TLR7 activation produces massive interferon release at 1,000 times that of any other immune cell in the human host. Ligands that selectively target TLR7 in plasmacytoid dendritic cells could be potential therapeutic targets. Other TLR ligands, such as CpG oligodeoxynucleotides (TLR9), have been shown to protect against lethal influenza infection in experimental settings [20]. In lung epithelium, TLR3 is the dominant pathway leading to interferon pathway activation. A large number of TLR3 and TLR9 agonists are currently in clinical trial phase for the treatment of autoimmune conditions, cancer and viruses. It is possible to extend the application of these agents to treat severe influenza infection. Further investigation on these promising new agents may open the door for developing new treatments in severe influenza infection.

Host Factors Implicated in Virus Entry into Human Cells

Before influenza virus replicates in human cells, it needs to gain entry successfully into the cells. The influenza virus harnesses host proteolytic enzymes to achieve this process. One example of such an enzyme is the transmembrane protease serine

S1 (TMPRSS) that belongs to the type II transmembrane serine protease family. This enzyme is located in the human airway epithelium and plays an important role in permitting influenza virus to gain entry into the host cell. Consequently, a protease inhibitor that binds to the TMPRSS molecule is a potential drug target in the treatment of influenza infection. Recent studies have identified three TMPRSS molecules, namely TMPRSS2, TMPRSS4 and TMPRSS11D, as potential drug targets [21]. These molecules have been detected in multiple locations within the human respiratory tract, including nasal mucosa, the trachea, the distal airway and the lung. Aprotinin, a drug familiar to most intensivists, is a protease inhibitor and has been shown to reduce influenza virus replication. In addition to reducing viral replication, aprotinin has also been shown to reduce inflammatory cytokines, suggesting a further benefit other than its impact on viral replication. So far, findings with the TMPRSS molecule have been derived mainly from *in vitro* models. Further studies in animal models and human clinical trials are needed in the future.

Anti-Viral Agents that Inhibit Viral Replication

Neuraminidase

Neuraminidase is a glycoside hydrolase that removes a sialic acid residue of the host cellular receptor recognized by influenza virus hemagglutinin. Therefore, it is an essential component of a process that allows virus penetration through mucosal barriers and subsequently to gain entry into the host cell. In addition, after virus replication, neuraminidase detaches the virion from the infected cells, thereby facilitating release and subsequent spread of the viral progeny. Consequently, neuraminidase is essential for viral infectivity to host cells. Therefore, inhibiting neuraminidase is the primary therapeutic strategy currently used in clinical practice. Most clinicians will be familiar with two neuraminidase inhibitors, zanamivir and oseltamivir.

Unfortunately, the true efficacy of these agents in treating patients with severe influenza infection in the ICU is yet to be established. The vast majority of the clinical trials on these drugs were performed in non-ICU patients. Furthermore, to be effective, these drugs need to be administered during the very early phase of the disease. Consequently, the clinical utility of current neuraminidase inhibitors is limited in ICU patients. To improve the clinical utility of these drugs, a recently developed strategy has been used to increase the efficacy of the approved neuraminidase inhibitors. This strategy involved use of multivalent inhibitors and conjugating the compounds to a biocompatible polymer. Using this innovative approach, recent studies have shown that neuraminidase inhibitors significantly increase their antiviral potency, to 1,000–10,000 times higher than their predecessors [22]. If proven in clinical trials, these newer formulations could become extremely valuable in treating patients with severe influenza infection.

Table 3 Drugs that block the two critical processes in hemagglutinin function

Virus interacting with cell surface	Virus fusion with cell membrane
Carbohydrate-binding agents that recognize glycosylation sites on hemagglutinin	Molecules that inhibit confirmation change in hemagglutinin
Peptides against hemagglutinin	Neutralizing antibodies directed against the stem region of hemagglutinin
Decoy receptor or sialic acid-containing inhibitors	
Neutralizing monoclonal antibodies directed against the globular head domain of hemagglutinin	

Hemagglutinin

Hemagglutinin is pivotal for the interaction between influenza virus and the sialic acid on the surface of the host cells. In addition, it is required for the fusion between the viral envelop and the endosomal membrane of the host cell, which is the final step in the virus's entry into the host cell. Inhibiting hemagglutinin could be achieved by two methods: (1) preventing the interaction between viral surface molecules and the host cell surface receptor; and (2) blocking the fusion of the viral envelop with the host cell membrane. Table 3 summarizes the recent development in the new drugs that utilize the above two strategies.

M2 Ion Channel

The M2 protein is a proton channel inside the influenza virus. After gaining entry into the host cell, the influenza virus activates the M2 protein by sensing a drop in the pH value inside the enveloped vesicle (the endosome). The activation of the M2 proton channel results in a proton flux from the endosome into the virion core. Acidification of the virus interior leads to dissociation of the viral ribonucleoprotein complexes. Subsequent membrane fusion releases the ribonucleoprotein into the cytoplasm. This release allows the virus to be imported into the nucleus to start viral replication. Other important functions of the M2 protein are: formation of the filamentous strains of the virus; release of the budding virion; and stabilization of the virion budding site. Due to these important functions, inhibition of M2 protein represents an ideal therapeutic target. A well-known licensed antiviral drug, amantadine, is an M2 blocker that binds the N-terminal channel lumen of the M2 pore resulting in repulsion of protons and subsequently prevent virus uncoating. Unfortunately, this class of drug is not active against all strains of influenza virus (e. g., influenza B). In addition, the emergence of drug-resistant virus variants has been reported. These drawbacks have significantly limited the use of M2 blockers.

Conclusion

Severe influenza infection remains an important clinical challenge for intensivists. The potentially high morbidity and mortality of this condition has remained unchanged over the last few decades, due mainly to a lack of effective new therapies with which to treat such patients.

However, we have gained a much better understanding of the mechanisms of the disease in recent years. This improved understanding points to the pivotal roles played by immune dysregulation in causing severe disease. Furthermore, our ability to diagnose influenza infection, to stratify high-risk patients and to prognosticate clinical outcomes has also improved thanks to recent advances in genomic science. Importantly, a large number of novel therapeutic agents are currently under investigation. These novel agents target multiple critical points of the host response pathway. Agents that modulate the host response hold particularly great promise since dysregulated immunity is the main driver towards more severe infection. In the future, clinical trials will be an important next step to demonstrate the efficacy of these novel agents.

References

1. Perrone LA, Plowden JK, Garcia-Sastre A, Katz JM, Tumpey TM (2008) H5N1 and 1918 pandemic influenza virus infection results in early and excessive infiltration of macrophages and neutrophils in the lung of mice. PLoS Pathog 4:e1000115
2. Peteranderl C, Morales-Nebreda L, Selvakumar B et al (2016) Macrophage-epithelial paracrine crosstalk inhibit lung edema clearance during influenza infection. J Clin Invest 126:1566–1580
3. Hogner K, Wolff T, Pleschka S et al (2013) Macrophage-expressed IFN-beta contributes to apoptotic alveolar epithelial cell injury in severe influenza virus pneumonia. PLoS Pathog 9:e1003188
4. Soloff A, Weirback H, Ross T, Barratt-Boyes SM (2012) Plasmacytoid dendritic cell depletion leads to an enhance mononuclear phagocyte response in lungs of mice with lethal influenza infection. Comp Immunol Microbiol Infect Dis 35:309–317
5. Moseman EA, Liang X, Dawson AJ et al (2004) Human plasmacytoid dendritic cells activated by CpG oligodeoxynucleotides induce the generation of CD4+CD25+regulatory T cells. J Immunol 173:4433–4442
6. Wang Z, Wan Y, Qiu C et al (2015) Recovery from severe H7N9 disease is associated with diverse response mechanisms dominated by CD8+ T cells. Nat Commun 6:6833
7. Chartrand C, Leeflang MM, Minion J, Brewer T, Pai M (2012) Accuracy of rapid influenza diagnostic tests: a meta-analysis. Ann Intern Med 156:500–511
8. Metersky ML, Masterton RG, Lode H et al (2012) Epidemiology, microbiology and treatment considerations for bacterial pneumonia complicating influenza. Int J Infect Dis 16:e321–e331
9. Robinson KM, Kolls JK, Alcorn J (2015) The immunology of influenza virus-associated bacterial pneumonia. Curr Opin Immunol 34:59–67
10. Sweeney TE, Wong HR, Khatri P (2016) Robust classification of bacterial and viral infections via integrated host gene expression diagnostics. Sci Transl Med 6:346ra91
11. Dobson J, Whitley RJ, Pocock S, Monto AS (2015) Oseltamivir treatment for influenza in adults: meta-analysis of randomised controlled trials. Lancet 385:1729–1737
12. Zhang Y, Sun W, Svendsen ER et al (2015) Do corticosteroids reduce the mortality of influenza A (H1N1) infection? A meta-analysis. Crit Care 19:46
13. Kujime K, Hashimoto S, Gon Y, Shimizu K, Horie T (2000) p38 mitogen-activated protein kinase and c-jun-NH2-terminal kinase regulate RANTES production by influenza virus-infected human bronchial epithelial cells. J Immunol 164:3222–3228

14. Geiler J, Michaelis M, Naczk P et al (2010) N-acetyl-L-cysteine (NAC) inhibits virus replication and expression of pro-inflammatory molecules in A549 cells infected with highly pathogenic H5N1 influenza A virus. Biochem Pharmacol 79:413–420
15. Ayllon J, Garcia-Sastre A, Hale BG (2012) Influenza A viruses and PI3K; are there time, place and manner restrictions? Virulence 3:411–414
16. Shin YK, Liu Q, Tikoo SK, Babiuk LA, Zhou Y (2007) Effect of the phosphatidylinositol 3-kinase/Akt pathway on influenza A virus propagaton. J Gen Virol 88:942–950
17. Ehrhardt C, Ruckle A, Hrincius ER et al (2013) The NF-kappaB inhibitor SC75741 efficiently blocks influenza virus propagation and confers a higher barrier for development of viral resistance. Cell Microbiol 15:1198–1211
18. Haasbach E, Reiling SJ, Ehrhardt C et al (2013) The NJ-kappaB inhibitor SC75741 protects mice against highly pathogenic avian influenza A virus. Antiviral Res 99:336–344
19. Lee SM, Gai WW, Cheung TK, Peiris JS (2011) Antiviral effect of a selective COX-2 inhibitor on H5N1 infection in vitro. Antiviral Res 91:330–334
20. Cheng WK, Plumb AW, Lai JCY, Abraham N, Dutz JP (2016) Topical CpG Oligodeoxynucleotide adjuvant enhances the adaptive immune response against influenza A infections. Font Immunol 7:284
21. Yamaya M, Shimotai Y, Hatachi Y, Homma M, Nishimura H (2016) Serine proteases and their inhibitors in human airway epithelial cells: effects on influenza virus replication and airway inflammation. Clin Microbiol 5:238
22. Weight AK, Haldar J, Alvarez de Cienfuegos L et al (2011) Attaching zanamivir to a polymer markedly enhances its activity against drug-resistant strains of influenza A virus. J Pharm Sci 100:831–835

Implementing Antimicrobial Stewardship in Critical Care: A Practical Guide

J. Schouten and J. J. De Waele

Introduction

Management of infections is an important issue in many health care settings, but severe infections are most prevalent and antimicrobial use is most abundant in the intensive care unit (ICU). Not surprisingly, antimicrobial resistance has emerged primarily in the intensive care setting, where multiple facilitators for the development of resistance are present: high antibiotic pressure, loss of physiological barriers and high transmission risk. 'Intensive care' had higher proportions of treated patients, combination therapy, hospital-acquired infections and parenteral administration of antibiotics in a point prevalence survey on antimicrobial prescription by the ESAC (European Surveillance of Antimicrobial Consumption) in 172 European hospitals across 25 countries [1].

Antimicrobial prescription is a complex process influenced by many factors. The appropriateness of antimicrobial use in hospitals varies among physicians, hospitals and countries due to differences in professional background, clinical experience, knowledge, attitudes, hospital antibiotic policies, collaboration and communication among professionals, care coordination and teamwork, care logistics, and differences in sociocultural and socioeconomic factors [2].

One can imagine that changing professional practice is a major challenge. The scientific literature is full of examples from which it would appear that patients are not given the care that, according to recent scientific or professional insight as summarized in guidelines, is desirable. A multitude of studies has shown that 30–

J. Schouten (✉)
Dept. of Intensive Care Medicine, Canisius Wilhelmina Ziekenhuis
Weg door Jonkerbos 100, 6532 SZ Nijmegen, Netherlands
IQ healthcare, Radboud University Medical Center
Nijmegen, Netherlands
e-mail: j.schouten@cwz.nl

J. J. De Waele
Dept. of Intensive Care Medicine, University Hospital Gent
9000 Gent, Belgium

J.-L. Vincent (ed.), *Annual Update in Intensive Care and Emergency Medicine 2017*,
DOI 10.1007/978-3-319-51908-1_2

40% of patients do not receive care according to guidelines and the findings for antimicrobial prescribing are similar [3]. This renders changing ICU antimicrobial use into a challenge of formidable complexity. Given that many influencing factors play a part, the measures or strategies undertaken to improve antimicrobial use need to be equally diverse.

Many interventions and programs have been designed to improve appropriate antimicrobial use in terms of choice of drugs, dosing, timing, de-escalation and discontinuation. Such interventions are collectively known as antimicrobial stewardship programs. An ICU antimicrobial stewardship program can be thought of as a menu of interventions that is adapted and customized to fit the infrastructure and organization of ICUs [4].

In this chapter, we will review the rationale for antimicrobial stewardship programs and take a step by step approach on how to implement such programs in the critical care setting and how to optimize compliance to relevant antibiotic stewardship recommendations in the ICU.

Rationale for Antibiotic Stewardship in Critical Care

Health care institutions have adopted antimicrobial stewardship programs as a mechanism to ensure more appropriate antimicrobial use. Antimicrobial stewardship programs can have a significant impact in the ICU, leading to improved antimicrobial use and resistance patterns and decreased infection rates and costs, due to the inherent nature of infections encountered and the high and often inappropriate antibiotic utilization in the ICU setting.

Stewardship programs are composed of two intrinsically different sets of interventions (Table 1). A first set of interventions describes recommended professional care interventions that define appropriate antimicrobial use in individual patients, regarding indication, choice of drug, dose, route or duration of treatment. For example, these may address 'de-escalation of therapy' in individual ICU patients. A second set of interventions describes recommended strategies to ensure that professionals apply these professional care interventions in daily practice. These include both restrictive (e. g., formulary restriction) and persuasive (e. g., education, feedback) strategies to improve appropriate antimicrobial use in patient care. The second set of interventions is therefore used to ensure that the first set of interventions is appropriately applied in patients [5]. These behavioral change interventions either directly or indirectly (through interventions targeting the system/organization) target the professional and, overall, restrict or guide towards the more effective professional use of antimicrobials.

The literature shows that in the ICU both restrictive and persuasive antimicrobial stewardship interventions – or improvement strategies – can ensure that professionals appropriately use antibiotics [6]. The evidence for antimicrobial stewardship programs in the ICU setting is, however, mostly based on quasi-experimental studies with or without times-series analysis and/or control groups and – with the exception of studies on procalcitonin (PCT) – there are no randomized controlled trials

Table 1 Antibiotic stewardship interventions: what are the recommendations and how can we ensure adherence?

What?	How?
Prescribe empirical antibiotics according to local guidelines	Audit and feedback
De-escalate broad-spectrum antibiotic therapy, once cultures become available	Reminders
Perform sequential PCT measurements and withdraw therapy if PCT < 0.5 µg/l	Daily review by clinical pharmacist and infectious disease physician
Administer antibiotics within an hour in sepsis and septic shock	Computerized decision support system
Perform TDM for selected antibiotics	Academic detailing
Perform appropriate cultures before start of therapy	Prior authorization from infectious disease physician for restricted antibiotics
...	...

PCT: procalcitonin; *TDM*: therapeutic drug monitoring

available. While the impact of antimicrobial stewardship programs on appropriateness of antibiotics, utilization and costs is fairly consistent across studies, there is no convincing evidence that there is an effect on individual patient outcomes. The absence of such direct evidence does not imply that antimicrobial stewardship strategies are not beneficial in the ICU setting: effects may especially affect future patients by reducing emergence of resistance [6, 7]. As an example of a persuasive intervention, audit and feedback by an antimicrobial stewardship program pharmacist to reduce broad-spectrum antibiotic prescribing was shown to be effective in an interrupted time interval analysis in a single center ICU, reducing both cost and development of Gram-negative resistance to carbapenems [8].

Restrictive strategies, such as formulary restrictions and prior authorization of rescue antibiotics by a pharmacist, infectious disease physician or clinical microbiologist, are considered effective at reducing antibiotic use and curbing development of resistance. However, there is a concern of a 'squeezing the balloon' phenomenon for this type of approach: restriction of certain classes of antibiotics may result in a reduction in their use and resistance rates, but it may also result in a shift to a higher usage of other antibiotics, thus negatively affecting the resistance rates for those alternative antibiotics. Restriction may be effective in an outbreak setting where there is a strong relationship between increased resistance and the use of a particular class of antibiotics, rather than a longterm solution [9].

Education, distributing evidence-based guidelines and using computer decision support systems or a combination of any of these interventions, generally have a positive impact on appropriate prescribing patterns. However, results on clinically relevant outcomes or resistance patterns are variable [10].

The ICU is – more than any department in the hospital – a meeting place where medical specialists need to work together to provide optimal patient care. This is especially a challenge in the treatment of patients with infections as infectious disease physicians, microbiologists and clinical pharmacists, relying on their own expertise, all advise the ICU physician on the optimal use of antibiotics. Recent evolution in the organization of ICUs, increasingly reverting from an open to a closed format (where intensivists are primarily responsible for patient care and provide 24/7 cover) may contribute to a reluctance of ICU physicians to accept outside interference.

An ICU antimicrobial stewardship program may exhibit some very ICU-specific goals and strategies, but an ICU is still located within the walls of a hospital and a large number of its admissions come through the wards. Resistance patterns in the ICU mimic those in the wards and antibiotic use patterns are usually similar. ICU physicians should thus be actively involved in hospital antibiotic stewardship teams and the responsibilities of infectious disease physicians, microbiologists and pharmacists within the ICU should be clearly defined in an antimicrobial stewardship program. Influencing the use of antibiotics in the ICU can be a challenging path for infectious disease physicians, clinical pharmacists and clinical microbiologists.

A Systematic Approach Towards Improving Antibiotic Prescribing in the ICU

Step 1. How Do You Measure Appropriate Antibiotic Prescribing in the ICU: Developing Quality Indicators for Your Unit

It is not only important to define what 'appropriate antimicrobial use in ICU patients' is but also how it can be validly and reliably measured. The development of so-called quality indicators can help to define and measure recommended professional performance in individual patients. A quality indicator is 'a measurable element of practice performance for which there is evidence or consensus that it can be used to assess the quality, and hence change the quality of care provided' [11]. While quality indicators for hospital stewardship programs have been well described, they may not all be so relevant for the ICU setting (e. g., antibiotic intravenous-oral switch therapy) or they may represent recommendations that are particularly relevant in an ICU setting (e. g., adequate measurement of antibiotic concentration levels: percentage of patients in whom a level was performed timely and for the correct indication)

As an example, a bundle of six quality indicators was developed to define and measure appropriate antimicrobial use in the ICU setting (Table 2; [12]). European experts specified – in a Rand modified Delphi procedure – that six professional performance interventions were crucial in antimicrobial use in ICU patients: (1) the clinical rationale of starting antibiotics should be documented in the chart; (2) appropriate microbiological cultures should be performed according to local and/or international guidelines; (3) the choice of empiric therapy should be in accordance with local and/or international guidelines; (4) diagnosis should be reviewed according to microbiological results; (5) de-escalation therapy should be considered in patients with microbiological diagnosis according to the susceptibility pattern of

Table 2 Evidence-based recommendations to increase the appropriate usage of antibiotics in ICU patients: a 5-day bundle

1st	The clinical rationale for antibiotic start should be documented in the medical chart at the start of therapy
	Appropriate microbiological culture according to local and/or international guidelines should be collected
	The choice of empirical antibiotic therapy should be performed according to local guidelines
2nd	Review of the diagnosis based on newly acquired microbiological cultures
	De-escalation therapy (the narrowest spectrum possible) according to available microbiological results
3rd–5th	Review of the diagnosis based on newly acquired microbiological cultures
	De-escalation therapy (the narrowest spectrum possible) according to available microbiological results
	Interruption of treatment should be considered according to local and/or international guidelines

From [21] with permission.

the isolate; and (6) short duration of therapy, according to international guidelines, should be considered in patients with a definitive diagnosis.

Comparable sets of quality indicators, oriented at national or local settings and culture, have been developed. To evaluate the effectiveness of an antimicrobial stewardship program, ideally, these qualitative data are reported together with quantitative data: antibiotic usage data and local patterns of resistance to the most relevant causative microorganisms, specific for the ICU. Regular (e. g., quarterly) feedback on the use of restricted (or rescue) antibiotics, such as carbapenems, glycopeptides, linezolid, colistin – expressed in defined daily dose (DDD)/100 patient days – may add to awareness of intensive care physicians and will facilitate discussions at ICU patient meetings.

Step 2. Stewardship Interventions

Stewardship interventions aim to improve antimicrobial prescribing so that patients receive the appropriate antibiotic for the indication, at the right time, with the appropriate dose and dosing interval, via the appropriate route and for the appropriate duration. These interventions intend to alter the behavior of individual prescribers and, as a final goal, to improve patient outcomes and ecological outcomes (curb the development of antimicrobial resistance).

Many studies have assessed strategies to improve professionals' prescribing practices, patient outcomes and microbial outcomes [6, 13–16]. They all conclude that *any* stewardship intervention – whether it is restrictive, persuasive or structural – can ensure that professionals appropriately use antimicrobials. Although the effects were overall positive, there were substantial differences in improvement between studies that compared similar stewardship interventions. If any behavioral stewardship intervention can improve antimicrobial use, how can you then choose – from the menu of potentially effective interventions – those that lead to improvement in a very specific setting (such as an ICU)?

Step 3. Understanding Key Drivers of Current Antibiotic Prescribing Behavior

Looking at change models and theories derived from various disciplines and scientific areas, the essential principle for successful behavior change is to link the choice of intervention as closely as possible to the results of an analysis of barriers [17]. Extensive assessment of an inventory of barriers and facilitators to change may lead to a tailored mix of interventions that is most likely to be effective.

So, to select those behavioral stewardship interventions that might work best in your own ICU from all the potentially effective interventions available in the literature, key drivers of current prescribing behavior must be understood: "It is not only microbes that we need to investigate: equally important is a better understanding of our own actions" [1].

Determinants of a prescribing practice are factors that may hinder or help improvements in that practice. The assessment of these determinants, both barriers and facilitators, should inform the choice of behavioral stewardship interventions, e. g., education should be chosen as a strategy to address a lack of knowledge with prescribers, or reminders if 'forgetting to apply the recommended prescribing practice' is the problem. An understanding of the determinants for change is crucial to the selection of effective interventions. In daily practice, however, the chosen interventions to improve health care are mostly based on implicit personal beliefs about human behavior and change [16]. For example, Charani et al. concluded, in their review on optimizing antimicrobial prescribing in acute care, that although qualitative research showed the influence of social norms, attitudes and beliefs on antimicrobial prescribing behavior, these behavioral determinants were not considered when developing improvement interventions [17].

For most changes in health care, a wide range of determinants influences whether appropriate care is provided or not. Flottorp et al. synthesized using a systematic review various frameworks and taxonomies of factors that help or hinder improvements in health care [18]. They developed an overview of 57 potential determinants categorized in seven domains. This can be a helpful stewardship tool to facilitate an inventory of factors that influence a specific prescribing practice in a specific hospital or ward. The following categories of determinants are distinguished:

1. guideline factors (e. g., the clarity of the recommendation, the evidence supporting the recommendation);
2. individual health professional factors (e. g., awareness and familiarity with the recommendation, or the skills needed to adhere);
3. patient factors (perceived demands of the patient, particular disease);

4. professional interactions (e. g., opinions and communication among professionals or referral processes);
5. incentives and resources (e. g., availability of necessary resources, or extent to which the information system influences adherence);
6. capacity for organizational change (e. g., capable leadership, or the relative priority given to making necessary changes); and
7. social, political, and legal factors (e. g., payer or funder policies).

There are various recommended antimicrobial prescribing practices, e. g., optimize antimicrobial dosing or de-escalation of antimicrobial therapy. The relevance and importance of determinants can vary across different recommendations. Therefore, when various prescribing practices need to be improved in daily practice, it is necessary to consider each determinant in relationship to each separate recommendation.

Flottorp et al. [18] developed various worksheets that can be used to help prioritize the prescribing practices that warrant stewardship team efforts and a worksheet to help measure determinants. Stewardship teams that aim to measure determinants of a specific antimicrobial prescribing practice can apply various methods to identify factors that help or hinder improvement of that practice: semi-structured interviews with individual professionals involved in the prescribing practice, group interviews, questionnaires, and observation.

Step 4. The Selection and Development of Effective Behavioral Stewardship Interventions: Intervention Mapping

To systematically link behavioral stewardship interventions to the various determinants, a structured approach should be followed. An important example of a theory-based approach is the Intervention Mapping approach [19]. Intervention mapping is a protocol for the design of intervention programs, which guides developers through a series of steps that assists them in theory-based and evidence-based program development. Following a needs assessment and a specification of determinants, theory-based methods are selected from the literature, translated into practical strategies, operationalized into plans, implemented and evaluated.

For a more pragmatic approach, Flottorp et al. also developed tools that can be used to support the selection of tailored behavioral stewardship interventions, i. e., a worksheet and a 'definitions questions examples' checklist to help the stewardship team to select and develop one or more tailored behavioral stewardship interventions in a pragmatic way [18].

Once one or more tailored behavioral stewardship interventions is selected, it is important to check whether the effectiveness of this intervention can be further enhanced. On the one hand, it is important to look at change theories relevant to the implementation of change in health care practice, as they should enable intervention developers in health care to design better interventions and programs to improve patient care. So, if, for example, an educational stewardship intervention was selected to address a lack of knowledge, educational theories would suggest that professionals should be involved in finding solutions for the prescribing practice problem, and that personal targets for improvement and individual learning plans related to the recommended practice should be defined.

On the other hand, it is important to determine whether systematic reviews of the effectiveness of the interventions chosen have been published, for example by checking the Prospero database or the Cochrane Effective Practice and Organization of Care (EPOC) website (http://epoc.cochrane.org/). EPOC focuses on state-of-the-art reviews of interventions (i. e., various forms of continuing education, quality assurance projects, financial, organizational, or regulatory interventions) designed to improve professional practice and the delivery of effective health services. Until now they have published over a hundred systematic reviews in the Cochrane Library. One of the reviews included is a review by Ivers et al. 'Audit and feedback: effects on professional practice and health care outcomes' [20]. They conclude that the effect of using audit and feedback varied widely across the included studies, ranging from little or no effect to a substantial effect on professional behavior and on patient outcomes. Multivariable meta-regression indicated that effectiveness could, among others, be augmented when it is delivered by a supervisor or colleague, it is delivered in both verbal and written formats, and when it includes both explicit targets and an action plan. All these success ingredients could be included in a feedback stewardship intervention if, of course, feedback was selected as a tailored intervention to address a lack of awareness and to make people conscious of problems in current care routines.

There is no behavioral change intervention – or magic bullet – that works in all circumstances: the challenge lies in systematically building an intervention on the careful assessment of determinants and on a coherent theoretical base, while linking determinants to interventions, taking the lessons regarding the effectiveness of various behavioral interventions into account.

Practical Application

In a single ICU setting, using relatively simple methods these challenges can be met. A point prevalence study in your ICU once a year will provide a good impression of which areas of care are most in need of improvement. A point prevalence study can be carried out together with infectious disease physicians/clinical microbiologists and the clinical pharmacy.

Once the stewardship recommendation that needs to be tackled most urgently is known, a well-structured group discussion focused on barriers and facilitators that influence appropriate performance of the recommendation can lead to surprising insights. Based on these insights and the supporting literature linking specific barriers to effective interventions, these can be selected and carried out.

It is clear that there is no one-size-fits-all approach possible here. Rather, a more tailored approach is advocated, sometimes leading to multifaceted interventions. Also, it is of importance to pace the work: Rome was not built in one day. PDSA

(Plan-Do-Study-Act) cycles can be used to target one relevant aspect of antibiotic care at a time, preferably going for the 'low hanging fruit' first.

A Practical Example

Until recently there has been little attention to the decision-making in the final phase of antibiotic therapy. As it is clear that the duration of antibiotic therapy is an important determinant of acquiring multidrug resistance (MDR), limiting antibiotic exposure at the end of the therapy is probably as important as making the correct empirical choice.

Although many guidelines recommend a duration of 7 days for many common ICU infections, in real life the duration of therapy is often longer. Therefore, duration of antibiotic therapy is certainly an attractive target if we want to reduce antibiotic exposure in critically ill patients. Multiple studies in different types of infections have demonstrated that prolonged duration – 10–14 days of antibiotic therapy or longer – is not necessary for most infections in the ICU, including hospital-acquired pneumonia.

A small audit on 40 patients in two ICUs (ICU A and ICU B) shows that the average duration of antibiotic therapy is > 10 days.

Barrier Analysis

In both ICUs a focus group session is performed with ICU physicians, their junior doctors, an infectious disease physician or clinical microbiologist and a clinical pharmacist.

In ICU A, ICU physicians indicate that they forget to discuss antibiotic therapy during ward rounds and do not feel it is an important part of their daily work.

In ICU B, ICU physicians indicate that often the patient may be improving but not yet fully recovered from organ dysfunction; traditional biomarkers do not offer much support to guide antibiotic therapy; and cultures from samples collected in the days after the start of antibiotic therapy may suggest persisting infection leading to prolongation of antibiotic therapy. Clinical criteria to discontinue antibiotic therapy are not helpful either so they feel left in the dark as to when to stop antibiotic therapy. They feel afraid that re-infection might occur if they withdraw antibiotic therapy early.

Choosing an Intervention

It is clear that in both ICUs a different strategy to reduce antibiotic duration is warranted. Whereas in ICU A an educational strategy may be used to fill the awareness/knowledge gap and provide reminders to change routine behavior, this is different in ICU 2. ICU 2 may benefit from using PCT, which has been shown to be of value in aiding antibiotic discontinuation decision-making. A recent pragmatic multicenter study from the Netherlands found that PCT-guided therapy can reduce antibiotic therapy in critically ill patients.

Pitfalls

Apart from choosing the intervention, it is important to optimize the delivery of the intervention. For ICU A, the literature suggests that education is more effective if personal targets for improvement and individual learning plans are established.

Other pitfalls in this context include failing to consider prior adequate antibiotic therapy after de-escalation in calculating the total duration of therapy, and ignoring the impact of exposure to small(er)-spectrum antibiotics. Predetermined duration of therapy upon initiation of the antibiotic, automatic stop orders and computerized physician order entry (CPOE) systems may provide easy tools to achieve this goal. Similarly, as antibiotics are often continued in the ward after a patient has been discharged from the ICU, clear instructions about the envisaged duration of therapy are mandatory.

Conclusion

In conclusion, antibiotic stewardship programs are an indispensable tool for improving antibiotic prescription in the critically ill patient. In the era of increasing antibiotic resistance the importance of this approach will only increase. Implementation of the different components of antibiotic stewardship programs is, however, very important, and often overlooked by critical care physicians. There is no superior behavioral change intervention – or magic bullet – that works in all circumstances: the challenge lies in systematically building an intervention based on the careful assessment of determinants and on a coherent theoretical base, while linking determinants to interventions, and taking the lessons regarding the effectiveness of various behavioral interventions into account.

References

1. European Academies Science Advisory Council (2016) Infectious diseases and the future: policies for Europe. A non-technical summary of an EASAC report. http://www.easac.eu/fileadmin/Reports/Infectious_Diseases/Easac_11_IDF.pdf. Accessed 1 November 2016
2. Hulscher ME, Grol RP, van der Meer JW (2010) Antibiotic prescribing in hospitals: a social and behavioural scientific approach. Lancet Infect Dis 10:167–175
3. Grimshaw JM, Thomas RE, MacLennan G et al (2004) Effectiveness and efficiency of guideline dissemination and implementation strategies. Health Technol Assess 8:iii–iv (1–72)
4. Bartlett JG (2011) Antimicrobial stewardship for the community hospital: Practical tools & techniques for implementation. Clin Infect Dis 53(suppl 1):S4–S7
5. De Waele JJ, Schouten J, Dimopoulos G (2015) Understanding antibiotic stewardship for the critically ill. Intensive Care Med 42:2063–2065
6. Kaki R, Elligsen M, Walker S, Simor A, Palmay L, Daneman N (2011) Impact of antimicrobial stewardship in critical care: a systematic review. J Antimicrob Chemother 66:1223–1230
7. Mertz D, Brooks A, Irfan N, Sung M (2015) Antimicrobial stewardship in the intensive care setting, a review and critical appraisal of the literature. Swiss Med Wkly 21:145
8. Elligsen M, Walker SA, Pinto R et al (2012) Audit and feedback to reduce broad-spectrum antibiotic use among intensive care unit patients: a controlled interrupted time series analysis. Infect Control Hosp Epidemiol 33:354–361

9. Burke JP (1998) Antibiotic resistance – squeezing the balloon? JAMA 280:1270–1271
10. Dellit TH, Owens RC, McGowan JE Jr et al (2007) Infectious Diseases Society of America and the Society for Healthcare Epidemiology of America guidelines for developing an institutional program to enhance antimicrobial stewardship. Clin Infect Dis 44:159–177
11. Lawrence M, Olesen F (1997) Indicators of quality in health care. Eur J Gen Pract 3:103–108
12. De Angelis G, De Santis P, Di Muzio F et al (2012) Evidence-based recommendations to increase the appropriate usage of antibiotics in ICU patients: a 5-day bundle. Poster presentation at 22nd European Congress of Clinical Microbiology and Infectious Diseases, London, 31/03–03/04/2012.
13. Wagner B, Filice GA, Drekonja D et al (2011) Antimicrobial stewardship programs in inpatient hospital settings: a systematic review. Infect Control Hosp Epidemiol 35:1209–1228
14. Patel D, Lawson W, Guglielmo BJ (2008) Antimicrobial stewardship programs: interventions and associated outcomes. Expert Rev Anti Infect Ther 6:209–222
15. Patel SJ, Larson EL, Kubin CJ, Saiman L (2007) A review of antimicrobial control strategies in hospitalized and ambulatory pediatric populations. Pediatr Infect Dis J 26:531–537
16. Grol R (1997) Beliefs and evidence in changing clinical practice. BMJ 315:518–521
17. Charani E, Edwards R, Sevdalis N et al (2011) Behavior change strategies to influence antimicrobial prescribing in acute care: a systematic review. Clin Infect Dis 53:651–662
18. Flottorp SA, Oxman AD, Krause J et al (2013) A checklist for identifying determinants of practice: a systematic review and synthesis of frameworks and taxonomies of factors that prevent or enable improvements in healthcare professional practice. Implement Sci 8:35
19. Bartholomew LK, Parcel GS, Kok G (1998) Intervention mapping: a process for developing theory- and evidence-based health education programs. Health Educ Behav 25:545–563
20. Ivers N, Jamtvedt G, Flottorp S et al (2012) Audit and feedback: effects on professional practice and healthcare outcomes. Cochrane Database Syst Rev CD000259
21. Schouten J, De Angelis G, van Groningen H et al (2012) Evidence-based recommendations to increase the appropriate usage of antibiotics in ICU patients: a 5-day bundle. Intensive Care Med 38(suppl 1):0878. http://www.esicm.org/events/webcast/lisbon-2012/3298?var=webcasts/lisbon-2012/3298. Accessed Nov 10, 2016

Part II
Sepsis

Microvesicles in Sepsis: Implications for the Activated Coagulation System

G. F. Lehner, A. K. Brandtner, and M. Joannidis

Introduction

The intimately linked inflammation and coagulation systems are considered to play a key role in the pathogenesis of the sepsis syndrome. The overwhelming systemic inflammatory host response to infection is frequently complicated by devastating coagulation disturbances leading to disseminated intravascular coagulation (DIC). A typical feature of sepsis is the release and elevated levels of different cytokines [1]. Several of these cytokines are capable of promoting the release of extracellular vesicles, such as microvesicles, from cells [2].

Microvesicles carry a wide range of receptors and signaling molecules on their surface. The composition and density of these molecules is dependent on the type and level of activation of the cells releasing the microvesicles. Levels of microvesicles are elevated in a broad range of diseases including malignancies, autoimmune diseases, metabolic and anaphylactic syndromes as well as in septic conditions [3]. The level of circulating microvesicles can reflect the extent of cellular stress or indicate progression of pathologies. Vesiculation induced by cellular stress and apoptosis creates a pool of bio-effectors, which likely mediate various transcellular communication mechanisms in homeostasis or orchestrate the observed host response in disease [4].

Microvesicles in Sepsis

Several studies have analyzed the amount of circulating microvesicles in sepsis to elucidate their role in the pathophysiology of this syndrome or to test them as potential biomarkers. A frequently used method to determine counts of distinct mi-

G. F. Lehner · A. K. Brandtner · M. Joannidis (✉)
Division of Intensive Care and Emergency Medicine, Department of Internal Medicine, Medical University Innsbruck
Anichstrasse 35, 6020 Innsbruck, Austria
e-mail: michael.joannidis@i-med.ac.at

J.-L. Vincent (ed.), *Annual Update in Intensive Care and Emergency Medicine 2017*,
DOI 10.1007/978-3-319-51908-1_3

crovesicle subtypes is quantification by flow cytometry. Techniques that use solid-phase capturing-assays or functional assays to determine levels and characteristics of microvesicles are also employed. The origin of the microvesicles can be determined by labeling microvesicles with antibodies directed against epitopes that are specific for the parental cell. The determination of a total microvesicle count is difficult, maybe even impossible at present. Some studies try to use exposed phosphatidylserine (e. g., annexin V+ or lactadherin+ microvesicle) as a surrogate for the total microvesicle amount. However, there is evidence that not all microvesicles carry phosphatidylserine on the surface [5, 6]. Thus, this approach might underestimate the actual microvesicle count. Nevertheless, it is a common measure used to approximate total microvesicle counts [7].

The following section provides an overview of the most relevant findings concerning counts of different microvesicle subtypes in septic populations compared to controls, i. e., mostly healthy volunteers or intensive care unit (ICU) patients without infection. Reflecting the fundamental difficulty of microvesicle quantification, published data on microvesicles in sepsis are often contradictory.

Total Amount of Microvesicles

With the intention of quantifying microvesicles in septic patients, two studies found higher counts of annexin V+ microvesicles in patients with severe sepsis compared to healthy controls [8, 9]. Similarly, Oehmcke et al. reported higher levels of phosphatidylserine equivalents (annexin V+ microvesicles) in septic patients, although the increase in annexin V+ microvesicle count was not statistically significant [10]. In contrast, Forest et al. reported a lower level of annexin V+ microvesicles in patients with infections fulfilling at least one of the systemic inflammatory response syndrome (SIRS) criteria compared to controls without infection [11].

No significant differences in annexin V+ microvesicles were detected in studies by Mostefai et al. [12]. These latter findings are in accordance with data from animal models in which there was no difference in annexin V+ microvesicles in septic rats [13] or in a mouse endotoxemia model [14]. Remarkably, Zhang et al. [15] reported increased counts of all microvesicle subtypes analyzed in a study in septic patients compared to healthy controls, using lactadherin positivity to determine phosphatidylserine harboring microvesicles, which is considered to be more sensitive in flow cytometry analysis [7].

Platelet-derived Microvesicles

Several studies have reported increased levels of platelet-derived microvesicles in patients with severe sepsis or septic shock [8, 9, 12, 16]. In contrast, three studies did not detect a significant difference in counts of platelet-derived microvesicles [11, 17, 18]. Joop et al. even reported decreased counts of CD61+ microvesicles [9] in septic patients, analogous to findings by Mortaza et al. in septic rats [13].

Interestingly, Woth et al. observed increased counts of one specific platelet-derived microvesicle subtype (CD42A+/annexin V+) only in patients with mixed fungal sepsis [8].

Erythrocyte-derived Microvesicles

Most studies did not report alterations in counts of erythrocyte-derived microvesicles (e. g., CD235a+ microvesicles) [11, 12, 16, 18, 19]. Intriguingly, only the subtype of annexin V negative erythrocyte-derived microvesicle (CD235a+/annexin V−) was increased in a study by Joop et al. [19]. Higher counts of erythrocyte-derived microvesicles were also detected in septic rats in a study by Mortaza et al. [13].

Leukocyte-derived Microvesicles

Overall, leukocyte-derived microvesicles can be analyzed using a common leukocyte marker (e. g., CD45). Two studies using this marker revealed opposite results – elevated levels in septic rats [13] and lower levels in humans when compared to ICU controls without infection [12]. However, in humans, Mostefai et al. reported elevated counts of CD62L+ microvesicles, a marker also known as L-selectin, which is considered a surrogate of leukocyte activation [12].

Two studies tried to measure counts of lymphocyte subsets (CD4+, CD8+, CD20 or CD38). Their numbers, however, were either not altered or below the detection limit [16, 19]. No differences were found in monocyte-derived microvesicles (i. e., CD14+ or CD11b+ microvesicles) [9, 12, 16]. Several studies detected increased counts of granulocyte-derived microvesicles, such as CD66b+ [16, 19], and neutrophil-derived [20, 21] microvesicles. Only Mostefai et al. found no significant differences in counts of granulocyte-derived microvesicles [12].

Endothelial-derived Microvesicles

The first study reporting counts of endothelium-derived microvesicles in septic patients was published in 2000 by Nieuwland et al. [16]. These authors reported a nonsignificantly increased number of endothelium-derived microvesicles (CD62E+) in patients with meningococcal sepsis compared to healthy controls [16]. In a study conducted in our lab, markedly increased levels of endothelium-derived microvesicles were only detected in a few patients, who were characterized by presence of liver injury, coagulation abnormalities and a highly proinflammatory state as well as increased levels of soluble markers of endothelial activation (i. e., soluble E-selectin) [17]. Joop et al. reported equal or even lower counts of endothelium-derived microvesicles (CD144+) compared to healthy controls in a population of septic patients with multiple organ dysfunction syndrome [19]. Similar results were found by Mortaza et al. investigating endothelium-derived microvesicle compositions in septic rats [13].

By contrast, several other studies have reported increased counts of endothelium-derived microvesicles [12, 15, 22, 23]. However, in these studies endothelium-derived microvesicles were defined with antibodies and combinations that are not specific for endothelial cells and therefore might also include, e. g., leukocyte-derived microvesicles [24].

Recently, we published a study in which the most comprehensive set of commonly used antibodies was applied [17]. We reported endothelium-derived microvesicle counts determined with sensitive but not endothelium-specific (e. g., CD31+/CD41−) and less sensitive but endothelium-specific (e. g., CD144+, CD62E+, CD106+) markers [17]. As mentioned above, counts of microvesicles labelled with endothelium specific markers were low in the general septic population, despite using high-sensitivity flow cytometry [17]. Conversely, in accordance with other earlier studies, a higher and significantly increased number of a not endothelium-specific microvesicle subtype (CD31+/CD41−) was identified [17]. However, our findings also indicate that a relevant number of these CD31+/CD41− microvesicles may not originate from endothelial cells but rather from leukocytes [17].

To summarize, markers chosen for analysis of microvesicles vary greatly from study to study. Despite that, the overall pattern found across several studies seems to suggest increased counts of granulocyte-derived microvesicles (e. g., CD66b+ microvesicles) and subtypes of platelet-derived microvesicles (e. g., CD41+ microvesicles). However, conclusive results cannot be obtained for all microvesicle subtypes from the aforementioned studies. This might, at least partially, be due to methodological differences and probably also to the heterogeneity of the analyzed populations as well as the heterogeneity of the sepsis syndrome itself. In particular, the findings regarding endothelium-derived microvesicle determinations with low levels are inconsistent. When it comes to endothelium-derived microvesicles, the difficulty selecting appropriate markers for microvesicle detection becomes evident. On the one hand, several studies that use sensitive but not endothelium-specific markers reported markedly increased endothelium-derived microvesicle counts in septic patients compared to healthy controls. On the other hand, in studies that defined endothelium-derived microvesicles with endothelium-specific markers, no or only moderate alterations in endothelium-derived microvesicle counts were detected in septic populations in general, although it seems that single patients with marked increases in such endothelium-derived microvesicle subtypes exhibited certain specific features, such as a pronounced activation of the coagulation system [16, 17].

In conclusion, despite these partly incongruent results concerning microvesicle counts in general septic populations, the investigation of microvesicles provides an additional perspective on the pathophysiology of this complex syndrome and might help to further stratify an overall sepsis syndrome into several distinct sepsis entities.

Interactions Between Microvesicles and the Coagulation System in Sepsis

In addition to the significant role of microvesicles in intercellular communication, their coagulation-active properties were one of the first observations in microvesicle research. Direct interaction of microvesicles with the coagulation system is predominantly mediated via two major mechanisms: i) the expression of tissue factor and ii) the exposure of anionic polyphosphates on their surface [25]. In 1999, Peter LA Giesen and colleagues first described a "blood-borne tissue-factor" which is expressed on circulating cells, but is also detectable on tissue factor-positive membrane vesicles, both facilitating intravascular thrombus formation without prior vascular injury [26]. The initial observation of granulocyte-derived, tissue factor-bearing microvesicles was particularized to monocytes and endothelial cells as the primary cellular sources [27]. In an *in vitro* experiment, platelet-derived microvesicles were able to activate monocytes and induce the release of tissue factor-expressing microvesicles. In homeostasis, the transcription of tissue factor in endothelial cells and hematopoietic cells is low. Small concentrations of this 'soluble' form of tissue factor are detectable in healthy individuals without initiating thrombus formation. This observation supports the assumption of an encrypted version of tissue factor and complementary inhibition of free tissue factor by circulating tissue-factor pathway inhibitors (TFPI) that can be activated upon specific local or systemic stimuli [27–29].

The second direct interaction of microvesicles with the coagulation system is conveyed by expression of polyanionic molecules, represented by phosphatidylserine exposure on the membrane of microvesicles, capacitating them to activate the coagulation cascade also via the intrinsic pathway by direct activation of prothrombinase [25]. On cellular membranes, the expression of phosphatidylserine is mainly coupled to phenotypical changes upon induction of apoptosis. These polyanionic molecules are recognized by neighboring cells as a stimulant for phagocytosis, a procedure required to maintain tissue homeostasis [30]. The initial paradigm, that phosphatidylserine expression on microvesicles is a result of vesiculation or apoptic processes, is opposed by the finding that the extent of phosphatidylserine exposure seems to be dependent on the primary stimulus for microvesicle release [31]. Proinflammatory agents stimulate the secretion of microvesicles by activated or injured cells. Exposure of procoagulant and simultaneously proinflammatory molecules is also enhanced [32, 33]. Thus microvesicles may have the potential to maintain pivotal roles in disease outcomes [15, 16, 34].

Endothelial cells were found to inherit a central role in regulating the pro- and anticoagulant balance in homeostasis. Aggressive secretion of proinflammatory cytokines in intensive host responses to infectious diseases alters the cellular structure as well as the composition of endothelial surface molecules. Responsive changes towards a proinflammatory and procoagulant phenotype of endothelial cells are associated with sepsis-induced vascular injury [35]. *In vitro* secretion of microvesicles by endothelial cells can be provoked by a number of cytokines and biological effectors such as tumor-necrosis factor alpha (TNF-α) [36], bacterial lipopolysac-

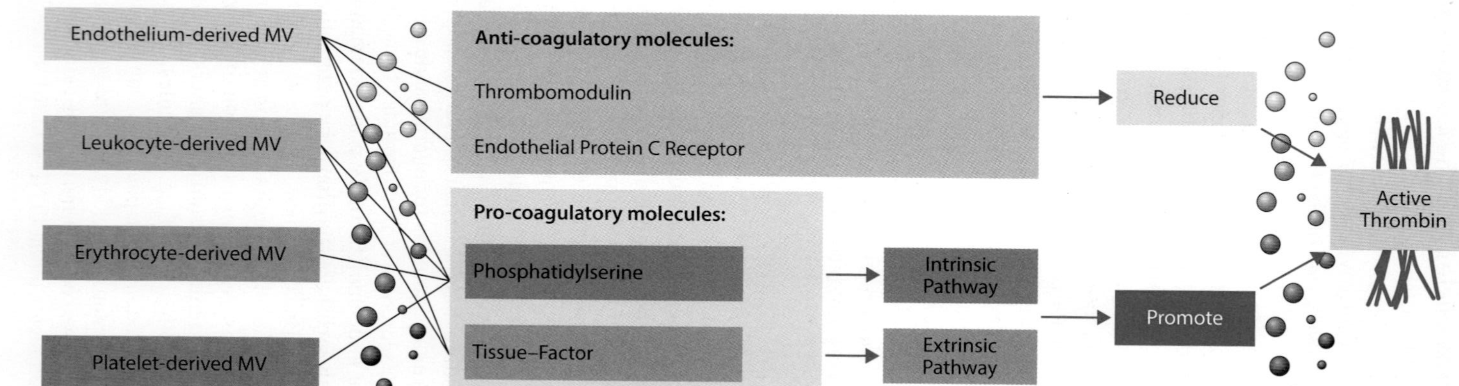

Fig. 1 Coagulation-active surface molecules on cell-derived microvesicles (MV). Molecules carried on the surface of microvesicles depend on the cell of origin. Endothelial-derived microvesicles carry both anti-coagulatory and procoagulatory molecules. Leukocyte-, erythrocyte- and platelet-derived microvesicles show predominantly procoagulatory molecules, such as phosphatidylserine, activating the intrinsic pathway, and tissue factor, activating the extrinsic pathway of the coagulation system

charides [37], thrombin [38], angiotensin II [39], uremic toxins [40] and other stimuli [32]. Microvesicles are able to foster the interplay between coagulation and inflammation via transmission of signaling molecules as biological vectors in a paracrine fashion. A central element of the microvesicle-transmitted signaling concept is that different stimuli induce the generation of different arrays of released vesicles [41].

As stated above, endothelial cells can be activated by thrombin, which may be generated by local coagulation processes. Thrombin induces the endothelial release of a soluble ligand of the TNF family, called TRAIL (TNF-related apoptosis-inducing ligand, ApoL2), which has the potential to induce apoptosis; TRAIL itself can bind to other endothelial cells, thus inducing the release of procoagulant, tissue factor-bearing endothelial microvesicles following activation of nuclear factor kappa B (NF-κB) [42].

Simultaneous to the enhanced pro-inflammatory and procoagulant signaling, natural anticoagulant mechanisms of endothelial cells, such as thrombomodulin, activated protein C and endothelial protein C receptor expression are downregulated by pro-inflammatory cytokines. Correspondingly, fewer microvesicles positive for these anticoagulant markers can be detected in acute sepsis [43]. Matsumoto et al. reported a significant negative correlation between the ratio of thrombomodulin-positive endothelial microvesicles to tissue factor-positive endothelial microvesicles and the overt diagnostic algorithm for DIC as defined by the International Society of Thrombosis and Hemostasis (ISTH-DIC score). This indicates the important protective effects of presumably endothelial-derived microvesicles positive for anticoagulant molecules ([23]; Fig. 1). Elevated levels of presumably endothelial-derived microvesicles were associated with early onset of septic shock-induced DIC and have been proposed as biomarkers [35]. Microvesicles exposing phosphatidylserine on their surface can also be generated by platelets, erythrocytes and leukocytes, thus potentially contributing to a prothrombotic state (Fig. 1). However, current evidence suggests that the expression of tissue factor on the microvesicle membrane seems to be limited to endothelial and monocytic vesicles [32].

Potential Diagnostic and Therapeutic Applications

As released microvesicles seem to be specific to the underlying stimulus, the idea of correlating microvesicles as biomarkers for diseases or their progression is appealing. To date, microvesicle compositions have been tested for their predictive value in a broad range of clinical disciplines. In the context of coagulation disorders, identification of patients prone to DIC by their microvesicle profile would be of high clinical relevance. A recently published observational study investigated the predictive value of a multi-parameter score to distinguish patients with septic shock disposed to develop DIC. The score, composed of counts of CD105+ microvesicles, platelet count and prothrombin time, enabled a 72.9% discrimination of the study population. The score reached a negative predictive value of 93.1% and a positive predictive value of 31% [44].

Therapeutic interventions targeting tissue factor-bearing microvesicles comprise intravenous administration of tissue factor antibodies [45], inactivated FVIIa [46] or recombinant TFPI. These approaches initially showed good results in rodent and avian studies, reducing overall mortality, systemic inflammation and fibrin deposition as well as attenuating sepsis-induced renal and respiratory failure [45–47]. However, in humans, inhibition of the tissue factor:factor VIIa complex with recombinant TFPI had no significant effect on overall mortality in a randomized phase III clinical study [48].

Recent research on microvesicles has focused on the identification of key players of the inflammation-mediated secretion process of vesicles. As such, the proinflammatory cytokine, interleukin (IL)-33 has been identified as inducing endothelial expression of tissue factor and release of tissue factor-bearing microvesicles, providing a potential new therapeutic target [49].

The concept of depletion of circulating endothelium-derived microvesicles by hemofiltration was tested by Abdelhafeez et al. in an *ex vivo* model in which a significant reduction of detectable endothelium-derived microvesicles was shown in a circuit model simulating continuous venovenous hemofiltration [50]. The clinical relevance of this interesting approach, however, has to be further investigated.

Conclusion

The functional importance of microvesicle properties on systemic regulation of hemostasis and their role in intercellular communication has been subject to basic research and clinical investigations since their discovery. Although publications on this topic have been increasing exponentially recently, no specific target amenable to therapeutic interventions in humans has yet been identified. A great challenge in sepsis research is to specify the functional properties of the involved variables and pathological mechanisms. Although direct measurement of microvesicles is feasible, precise characterization and quantification remains challenging and functional tests to define the effects of microvesicles in our patients are still to be developed.

References

1. Gogos CA, Drosou E, Bassaris HP, Skoutelis A (2000) Pro- versus anti-inflammatory cytokine profile in patients with severe sepsis: a marker for prognosis and future therapeutic options. J Infect Dis 181:176–180
2. Hellum M, Ovstebo R, Brusletto BS, Berg JP, Brandtzaeg P, Henriksson CE (2014) Microparticle-associated tissue factor activity correlates with plasma levels of bacterial lipopolysaccharides in meningococcal septic shock. Thromb Res 133:507–514
3. Reid VL, Webster NR (2012) Role of microparticles in sepsis. Br J Anaesth 109:503–513
4. Angelillo-Scherrer A (2012) Leukocyte-derived microparticles in vascular homeostasis. Circ Res 110:356–369
5. Dignat-George F, Boulanger CM (2011) The many faces of endothelial microparticles. Arterioscler Thromb Vasc Biol 31:27–33

6. Shet AS, Aras O, Gupta K et al (2003) Sickle blood contains tissue factor-positive microparticles derived from endothelial cells and monocytes. Blood 102:2678–2683
7. Latham SL, Tiberti N, Gokoolparsadh N et al (2015) Immuno-analysis of microparticles: probing at the limits of detection. Sci Rep 5:16314
8. Woth G, Tokes-Fuzesi M, Magyarlaki T, Kovacs GL, Vermes I, Muhl D (2012) Activated platelet-derived microparticle numbers are elevated in patients with severe fungal (Candida albicans) sepsis. Ann Clin Biochem 49:554–560
9. Tokes-Fuzesi M, Woth G, Ernyey B et al (2013) Microparticles and acute renal dysfunction in septic patients. J Crit Care 28:141–147
10. Oehmcke S, Morgelin M, Malmstrom J et al (2012) Stimulation of blood mononuclear cells with bacterial virulence factors leads to the release of pro-coagulant and pro-inflammatory microparticles. Cell Microbiol 14:107–119
11. Forest A, Pautas E, Ray P et al (2010) Circulating microparticles and procoagulant activity in elderly patients. J Gerontol A Biol Sci Med Sci 65:414–420
12. Mostefai HA, Meziani F, Mastronardi ML et al (2008) Circulating microparticles from patients with septic shock exert protective role in vascular function. Am J Respir Crit Care Med 178:1148–1155
13. Mortaza S, Martinez MC, Baron-Menguy C et al (2009) Detrimental hemodynamic and inflammatory effects of microparticles originating from septic rats. Crit Care Med 37:2045–2050
14. Wang JG, Manly D, Kirchhofer D, Pawlinski R, Mackman N (2009) Levels of microparticle tissue factor activity correlate with coagulation activation in endotoxemic mice. J Thromb Haemost 7:1092–1098
15. Zhang Y, Meng H, Ma R et al (2016) Circulating microparticles, blood cells, and endothelium induce procoagulant activity in sepsis through phosphatidylserine exposure. Shock 45:299–307
16. Nieuwland R, Berckmans RJ, McGregor S et al (2000) Cellular origin and procoagulant properties of microparticles in meningococcal sepsis. Blood 95:930–935
17. Lehner GF, Harler U, Haller VM et al (2016) Characterization of microvesicles in septic shock using high-sensitivity flow cytometry. Shock 46:373–381
18. Rank A, Nieuwland R, Toth B et al (2011) Microparticles for diagnosis of graft-versus-host disease after allogeneic stem transplantation. Transplantation 92:244–250
19. Joop K, Berckmans RJ, Nieuwland R et al (2001) Microparticles from patients with multiple organ dysfunction syndrome and sepsis support coagulation through multiple mechanisms. Thromb Haemost 85:810–820
20. Timar CI, Lorincz AM, Csepanyi-Komi R et al (2013) Antibacterial effect of microvesicles released from human neutrophilic granulocytes. Blood 121:510–518
21. Herrmann IK, Bertazzo S, O'Callaghan DJ et al (2015) Differentiating sepsis from non-infectious systemic inflammation based on microvesicle-bacteria aggregation. Nanoscale 7:13511–13520
22. Soriano AO, Jy W, Chirinos JA et al (2005) Levels of endothelial and platelet microparticles and their interactions with leukocytes negatively correlate with organ dysfunction and predict mortality in severe sepsis. Crit Care Med 33:2540–2546
23. Matsumoto H, Yamakawa K, Ogura H, Koh T, Matsumoto N, Shimazu T (2015) Enhanced expression of cell-specific surface antigens on endothelial microparticles in sepsis-induced disseminated intravascular coagulation. Shock 43:443–449
24. Lacroix R, Robert S, Poncelet P, Dignat-George F (2010) Overcoming limitations of microparticle measurement by flow cytometry. Semin Thromb Hemost 36:807–818
25. Owens AP 3rd, Mackman N (2011) Microparticles in hemostasis and thrombosis. Circ Res 108:1284–1297
26. Giesen PL, Rauch U, Bohrmann B et al (1999) Blood-borne tissue factor: another view of thrombosis. Proc Natl Acad Sci USA 96:2311–2315

27. Morel O, Morel N, Freyssinet JM, Toti F (2008) Platelet microparticles and vascular cells interactions: a checkpoint between the haemostatic and thrombotic responses. Platelets 19:9–23
28. Bach RR (2006) Tissue factor encryption. Arterioscler Thromb Vasc Biol 26:456–461
29. Puy C, Tucker EI, Matafonov A et al (2015) Activated factor XI increases the procoagulant activity of the extrinsic pathway by inactivating tissue factor pathway inhibitor. Blood 125:1488–1496
30. Hoffmann PR, deCathelineau AM, Ogden CA et al (2001) Phosphatidylserine (PS) induces PS receptor-mediated macropinocytosis and promotes clearance of apoptotic cells. J Cell Biol 155:649–659
31. Jimenez JJ, Jy W, Mauro LM, Soderland C, Horstman LL, Ahn YS (2003) Endothelial cells release phenotypically and quantitatively distinct microparticles in activation and apoptosis. Thromb Res 109:175–180
32. Curtis AM, Edelberg J, Jonas R et al (2013) Endothelial microparticles: sophisticated vesicles modulating vascular function. Vasc Med 18:204–214
33. Meziani F, Delabranche X, Asfar P, Toti F (2010) Bench-to-bedside review: circulating microparticles – a new player in sepsis? Crit Care 14:236
34. Zafrani L, Gerotziafas G, Byrnes C et al (2012) Calpastatin controls polymicrobial sepsis by limiting procoagulant microparticle release. Am J Respir Crit Care Med 185:744–755
35. Delabranche X, Boisrame-Helms J, Asfar P et al (2013) Microparticles are new biomarkers of septic shock-induced disseminated intravascular coagulopathy. Intensive Care Med 39:1695–1703
36. Combes V, Simon AC, Grau GE et al (1999) In vitro generation of endothelial microparticles and possible prothrombotic activity in patients with lupus anticoagulant. J Clin Invest 104:93–102
37. Kagawa H, Komiyama Y, Nakamura S et al (1998) Expression of functional tissue factor on small vesicles of lipopolysaccharide-stimulated human vascular endothelial cells. Thromb Res 91:297–304
38. Sapet C, Simoncini S, Loriod B et al (2006) Thrombin-induced endothelial microparticle generation: identification of a novel pathway involving ROCK-II activation by caspase-2. Blood 108:1868–1876
39. Burger D, Montezano AC, Nishigaki N, He Y, Carter A, Touyz RM (2011) Endothelial microparticle formation by angiotensin II is mediated via Ang II receptor type I/NADPH oxidase/Rho kinase pathways targeted to lipid rafts. Arterioscler Thromb Vasc Biol 31:1898–1907
40. Faure V, Dou L, Sabatier F et al (2006) Elevation of circulating endothelial microparticles in patients with chronic renal failure. J Thromb Haemost 4:566–573
41. Dignat-George F, Boulanger CM (2011) The many faces of endothelial microparticles. Arterioscler Thromb Vasc Biol 31:27–33
42. Simoncini S, Njock MS, Robert S et al (2009) TRAIL/Apo2L mediates the release of procoagulant endothelial microparticles induced by thrombin in vitro: a potential mechanism linking inflammation and coagulation. Circ Res 104:943–951
43. Perez-Casal M, Downey C, Cutillas-Moreno B, Zuzel M, Fukudome K, Toh CH (2009) Microparticle-associated endothelial protein C receptor and the induction of cytoprotective and anti-inflammatory effects. Haematologica 94:387–394
44. Delabranche X, Quenot JP, Lavigne T et al (2016) Early detection of disseminated intravascular coagulation during septic shock: a multicenter prospective study. Crit Care Med 44:e930–939
45. Welty-Wolf KE, Carraway MS, Ortel TL et al (2006) Blockade of tissue factor-factor X binding attenuates sepsis-induced respiratory and renal failure. Am J Physiol Lung Cell Mol Physiol 290:L21–31
46. Carraway MS, Welty-Wolf KE, Miller DL et al (2003) Blockade of tissue factor: treatment for organ injury in established sepsis. Am J Respir Crit Care Med 167:1200–1209
47. Xu H, Ploplis VA, Castellino FJ (2006) A coagulation factor VII deficiency protects against acute inflammatory responses in mice. J Pathol 210:488–496

48. Abraham E, Reinhart K, Opal S et al (2003) Efficacy and safety of tifacogin (recombinant tissue factor pathway inhibitor) in severe sepsis: a randomized controlled trial. JAMA 290:238–247
49. Stojkovic S, Kaun C, Basilio J et al (2016) Tissue factor is induced by interleukin-33 in human endothelial cells: a new link between coagulation and inflammation. Sci Rep 6:25171
50. Abdelhafeez AH, Jeziorczak PM, Schaid TR et al (2014) Clinical CVVH model removes endothelium-derived microparticles from circulation. J Extracell Vesicles 27:3

Mesenchymal Stem/Stromal Cells for Sepsis

C. Keane and J. G. Laffey

Introduction

Sepsis is a major public health concern, accounting for more than $20 billion (5.2%) of total US hospital costs in 2011 [1]. The reported incidence of sepsis is increasing [1], likely reflecting aging populations with more comorbidities that potentially impair immunity, and greater recognition of the condition. Conservative estimates indicate that sepsis is a leading cause of mortality and critical illness worldwide. Sepsis has a mortality of 40%, is responsible for more than 250,000 deaths in the United States annually, and has been implicated as a causative factor in up to 50% of all in-hospital deaths [2]. Furthermore, there is increasing awareness that patients who survive sepsis often have long-term physical, psychological, and cognitive disabilities with significant health care and social implications.

The most common sources of sepsis are, in descending order, pneumonia, intra-abdominal, urinary tract and soft tissue infections [3]. Blood cultures are positive in only one third of cases, and up to a third of cases are culture negative from all body sites. The most commonly isolated Gram-positive bacterial pathogens are *Staphylococcus aureus* and *Streptococcus pneumoniae*, and the most common Gram-negative pathogens are *Escherichia coli*, *Klebsiella spp*, and *Pseudomonas aeruginosa* [4]. While Gram-positive infections had been reported as surpassing Gram-negative infections in recent years, a recent study encompassing 14,000 ICU

C. Keane
Department of Anaesthesia, Galway University Hospitals and National University of Ireland Galway, Ireland

J. G. Laffey (✉)
Department of Anesthesia, Keenan Research Centre for Biomedical Sciences, St. Michael's Hospital
30 Bond Street, Toronto M5B 1W8, ON, Canada
Department of Anesthesia, Physiology and Interdepartmental Division of Critical Care Medicine, University of Toronto
Toronto, ON, Canada
e-mail: laffeyj@smh.ca

J.-L. Vincent (ed.), *Annual Update in Intensive Care and Emergency Medicine 2017*,
DOI 10.1007/978-3-319-51908-1_4

patients in 75 countries found that 62% of positive isolates were Gram-negative bacteria, *vs* 47% Gram-positive and 19% fungal [5].

Sepsis: A Therapeutic Failure

Despite extensive research, there is no direct treatment for sepsis, other than antimicrobial therapy, and new therapies are urgently needed. Most research on sepsis to date has focused on suppressing the initial hyper-inflammatory, cytokine-mediated phase of the disorder. Unfortunately, over 40 clinical trials of agents that block cytokines, pathogen recognition, or inflammation-signaling pathways have universally failed to improve outcomes, suggesting that inhibition of a single mediator is insufficient to restore a balanced and effective immune response. The timing of potential interventions is also important. Broad immunosuppressants, such as steroids, may reduce the early inflammatory response, but ultimately aggravated immune paralysis and worsened outcome [6].

The lack of success to date with standard 'pharmacologic' approaches suggests the need to consider more complex therapeutic approaches, aimed at reducing early injury while maintaining host immune competence, and facilitating tissue regeneration and repair. Mesenchymal stem/stromal cells (MSCs) might fit this new therapeutic paradigm for sepsis, and consequently are attracting considerable attention. MSCs are multipotent cells derived from adult tissues that are capable of self-renewal and differentiation into chondrocytes, osteocytes and adipocytes. The origin of MSCs in multiple adult tissues, coupled with their relative ease of isolation and expansion potential in culture make them attractive therapeutic candidates.

Rationale for Mesenchymal Stem/Stromal Cells in Sepsis

Sepsis is a syndrome of life-threatening physiologic, pathologic, and biochemical abnormalities resulting from a disordered immune response to microbial infection. MSCs offer substantial potential as a novel therapeutic approach to sepsis for several reasons. First, they possess several favorable biological characteristics, which make them potentially feasible as candidates for acute critical illnesses such as sepsis. These characteristics include their convenient isolation, ease of expansion in culture while maintaining genetic stability, minimal immunogenicity and feasibility for allogenic transplantation. MSCs are considered immune privileged as they constitutively express low levels of cell-surface HLA class I molecules and lack expression of HLA class II, CD40, CD80 and CD86. Consequently, MSCs cause relatively little activation of the innate and adaptive immune responses, and can therefore be used as an allogeneic therapy. Second, MSCs exert potent immune modulatory effects, which may be highly relevant given the role of the immune response in sepsis. While previous strategies to simply inhibit this response have been unsuccessful, the more complex, 'immunomodulatory' properties of MSCs may prove more effective. Importantly, MSCs may be able to 'reprogram' the immune response to reduce the destructive inflammatory elements while preserving the host response to pathogens. Third, MSCs may augment repair processes following sepsis. The resolution of sepsis is hindered by damage to the epithelial barrier. MSCs may restore epithelial and endothelial function, in part via secretion of paracrine factors to enhance injury resolution in these tissues. Fourth, sepsis frequently occurs in association with a generalized process resulting in dysfunction and failure of multiple organs. MSCs have been demonstrated to decrease injury and/or restore function in multiple organs. Fifth, MSCs may directly enhance bacterial killing, via a number of mechanisms, including enhancement of phagocytosis, increased bacterial clearance [7], and anti-microbial peptide secretion [8]. Sixth, MSCs have an encouraging safety record, and are being assessed in clinical studies for a wide range of disease processes, with a substantial body of evidence attesting to their safety in patients.

Efficacy of MSCs in Preclinical Sepsis Studies

The therapeutic potential of MSCs for sepsis has been established in multiple relevant models of early bacterial pneumonia [7, 9–12] and early abdominal sepsis [7, 11, 13, 14], the two most common causes of sepsis ([3]; Table 1). In early pulmonary sepsis, our group and others have demonstrated that human bone-marrow-derived MSCs decrease the severity of *E. coli* pneumonia, decreasing lung bacterial load, improving lung function and increasing survival [12, 15]. In early abdominal sepsis, bone-marrow-derived murine MSCs reduced inflammation and improved survival in a mouse model of sepsis induced by cecal ligation and puncture (CLP), a highly clinically relevant model of polymicrobial sepsis [11]. MSCs reduced inflammation and multiorgan injury, while decreasing bacterial load and improving survival in mice even when administered six hours after induction of polymicrobial sepsis in the CLP model [7]. In a mouse CLP model, mouse bone-marrow-derived MSCs attenuated sepsis-induced kidney injury through diminished inflammation and enhanced macrophage phagocytosis [13, 14]. In a genome-wide expression microarray analysis of animals post CLP, MSCs decreased transcription of genes relating to inflammation, upregulated genes relating to repair and microvasculature integrity and normalized transcriptional pathways responsible for maintaining mitochondrial function and cellular bioenergetics [16], which is consistent with the possibility of mitochondrial transfer between MSCs and cells of the host organs [17].

Mechanisms of Action of MSCs of Relevance to Sepsis

Effects on the Immune System

MSCs interact with a wide range of immune cells and exert multiple effects on the innate and adaptive immune responses. MSCs decrease the proinflammatory cytokine response [10, 18], while increasing concentrations of anti-inflammatory

Table 1 Key preclinical studies examining mechanisms of action of mesenchymal stem cells (MSCs) in sepsis

Study	Animal	Sepsis model	Cell therapy	MSC delivery route and timing of administration	Effect and mechanism of action
Nemeth et al. 2009 [11]	Mouse	CLP	BMSC	i. v., 24 hours pre/post injury	Prostaglandin E2-dependent reprogramming of macrophage to increase production of IL-10
Mei et al. 2010 [7]	Mouse	CLP	mMSC	i. v., 6 hours post injury	Modification of inflammatory gene transcriptional activity, downregulation of the acute inflammatory response and upregulation of pathways relevant to phagocytosis and bacterial clearance
dos Santos et al. 2012 [16]	Mouse	CLP	mMSC	i. v., 6 hours pre/post injury	On transcriptional analysis, MSCs i) attenuated sepsis-induced mitochondrial-related functional derangement, ii) decreased endotoxin/Toll-like receptor innate immune proinflammatory transcriptional responses, and iii) coordinated expression of transcriptional programs implicated in the preservation of endothelial/vascular integrity
Luo et al. 2014 [13]	Mouse	CLP	mMSC	i. v., 3 hours post injury	Improved survival and sepsis-related acute kidney injury, possibly by inhibition of IL-17 production and immunomodulation
Krasnodembskaya et al. 2010 [8]	Mouse	*E. coli* pneumonia	hMSC	i. t., 4/24 hours post injury	Secretion of the antimicrobial peptide, LL-37, resulting in increased bacterial clearance
Gupta et al. 2012 [9]	Mouse	*E. coli* pneumonia	mMSC	i. v., 4 hours post injury	mMSCs reduced the severity of *E. coli* pneumonia, in part via an antimicrobial peptide dependent mechanism
Krasnodembskaya et al. 2012 [15]	Mouse	GNPS	hMSC	i. v., 1 hour post injury	Increased animal survival and bacterial clearance secondary to enhanced monocyte phagocytosis
Elman et al. 2014 [19]	Mouse	LPS	hBM/AdMSC	i. p., at time of injury	BMMSC provide greater survival benefit and multi-organ protection versus AdMSC
Devaney et al. 2015 [12]	Rat	*E. coli* pneumonia	hBMMSC	i. v., 30 minutes post injury	Reduced lung injury and lung bacterial burden via enhanced macrophage phagocytosis and increased alveolar LL-37 concentrations

i. v.: intravenous; *IL*: interleukin; *TNF-α*: tumor necrosis factor alpha; *i. p.*: intra-peritoneal; *LPS*: lipopolysaccharide; *i. t.*: intra-tracheal; *m*: murine; *h*: human; *GNPS*: Gram-negative polymicrobial sepsis; *hBMMSCs*: human bone-marrow MSCs; *Ad*: adipose; *ROS*: reactive oxygen species; *CLP*: cecal ligation and puncture agents, including interleukin (IL)-1 receptor antagonist, IL-10, and prostaglandin E2 [11]. MSCs reduced the infiltration of neutrophils and monocyte/macrophages to target organs, including liver, lung, intestine and kidney, and improved the function of these organs in preclinical sepsis models [7, 11, 13, 14, 19, 20]. MSCs also suppressed T cell proliferation, natural killer cell function and inhibition of dendritic cell differentiation [21], although the implications of this in sepsis are not well understood. MSCs have been shown to prevent neutrophil apoptosis and degranulation in culture without inhibiting their phagocytic or chemotactic capabilities [22]. MSCs also regulate B cell [21] and monocyte function via poorly defined mechanisms.

Specific Antimicrobial Effects

MSCs may directly attenuate bacterial sepsis via a number of mechanisms. MSCs enhance macrophage phagocytosis, favoring maturation into a novel 'M2-like' macrophage phenotype [15], with enhanced anti-inflammatory properties and improved phagocytic activity [23]. MSCs also enhanced neutrophil phagocytosis and bacterial clearance in a murine CLP model, an effect abrogated by neutrophil depletion [14]. MSCs also exert direct antimicrobial effects via the secretion of antimicrobial peptides, such as LL-37 [8, 12].

Resolution and Reparative Effects

MSCs may augment repair processes following injury [24–26] via diverse mechanisms, which mainly appear to be paracrine. The resolution of sepsis is hindered by damage to the capillary endothelial barrier, which results in hypovolemia and tissue edema. MSCs can enhance endothelial function, in part via secretion of paracrine factors [27]. MSC production of specific resolution mediators, such as lipoxin A4, may play a key role in the injury resolution process [28].

How Do MSCs Exert Their Effects?

Contact-dependent Effects

Cell-cell contact appears to be an important mechanism by which MSCs modulate immune effector cells. In a mouse model of endotoxin-induced systemic sepsis, Xu et al. reported that the paracrine effect of MSCs in reducing lung inflammation, injury and edema was enhanced by direct cell-to-cell contact [29]. Islam et al. [17] demonstrated that MSCs can attach to alveolar epithelial cells via connexin-43-containing gap junctions, and transfer mitochondria to the endotoxin injured cells, thereby enhancing cellular ATP levels, restoring epithelial cell function and increasing animal survival [17]. CLP studies need to be conducted to assess these effects in more sepsis-related conditions.

MSC Secretome

The MSC 'secretome' contains multiple immunomodulatory mediators, including prostaglandin E2 [11], transforming growth factor (TGF)-β [30], indoleamine 2,3-dioxygenase [31], IL-1-receptor antagonist [32], tumor necrosis factor (TNF)-α-induced protein (TSG)-6 [18], and IL-10 [10]. Németh et al. reported that MSCs attenuated septic injury secondary to CLP, at least in part, through secretion of prostaglandin E2, which reprogrammed host macrophages to increase IL-10 production [11]. Endotoxin-induced stimulation of the Toll-like receptor (TLR)4 expressed by the MSCs resulted in increased production of cyclooxygenase-2 and prostaglandin E2. Krasnodembskaya et al. demonstrated that MSCs secrete the antimicrobial peptide LL-37, suggesting a direct role for MSCs in combating pathogen-mediated sepsis [8].

MSC-derived Microvesicles

MSCs, like most cell types, release small cellular particles, termed microvesicles, which carry with them cytoplasmic and membrane constituents, including mitochondria [17] and gene products (i. e., mRNA and miRNAs) [33]. MSC-derived microvesicles decreased injury in models of acute lung [33] and kidney [34] injury. MSC-derived microvesicles decreased the severity of *E. coli* induced severe pneumonia in a murine model [33].

Insights Regarding MSC Therapeutic Potential from Clinical Studies

Recently, MSCs have been tested in clinical trials in several conditions, taking advantage of their reparative, anti-inflammatory and immunoregulatory activities. The Cellular Immunotherapy for Septic Shock (CISS) trial was a dose escalation safety study utilizing allogeneic bone marrow MSCs for patients diagnosed with septic shock within 24 hours of critical care admission. Doses assessed for safety and tolerability were 0.3, 1.0, and 3.0 million cells/kg. A historical cohort that met CISS eligibility criteria was also enrolled to compare the incidence of adverse advents with the CISS interventional arm (NCT02421484). Preliminary results are due to be published at the time of writing. This key safety study should pave the way for later phase septic shock trials and ultimately to a large phase III randomized efficacy trial.

Of relevance to sepsis, a phase I trial of MSCs in acute respiratory distress syndrome (ARDS) has been completed [35] and a phase II study is underway in the US (NCT02097641). As MSCs contribute to tissue and immune system homeostasis under physiological conditions, their use in graft versus host disease (GVHD) is pertinent to sepsis due to the acute and chronic phases occurring in both pathologies. MSCs have been studied for the prevention [36] and treatment [37] of GVHD for over 15 years, with many additional completed [NCT01222039] and currently-enrolling trials [NCT01765634, NCT01765660], using specific MSC cell populations, varying dosage regimes, and evaluating the safety and efficacy of these cells, all of which is allowing us to better design future sepsis trials.

Translational Challenges and Knowledge Gaps

There is considerable enthusiasm for the translation of MSCs to clinical testing for patients with severe sepsis, based on a strong biologic rationale, an understanding of potentially key mechanisms of action, and an encouraging safety record for MSCs from clinical studies and use in other disease states. However, a number of barriers to translation exist, which will need to be addressed if we are to optimize the chances of successful clinical efficacy studies.

Mechanisms of Action

Our understanding of the key mechanisms of action of MSCs, particularly as they relate to sepsis, remains incomplete. A diverse array of paracrine mediators, such as prostaglandin E2 [11], keratinocyte growth factor [33], and LL-37 [8], have been demonstrated to possess therapeutic effects in preclinical sepsis models. In contrast, key effects of potential relevance in sepsis, such as modulation of macrophage phenotype and function, appear to be contact-dependent. The microvesicular fraction of the MSC secretome is effective in preclinical models of sepsis, via mechanisms involving mitochondrial and DNA transfer [33]. The precise micro-environmental conditions may profoundly influence MSC behavior [38]. Furthermore, there is growing evidence that MSCs represent a heterogeneous population of cells and that different MSC subtypes exist [39]. Dissecting out the relative importance of these different mechanisms of action, and determining which are of more importance in sepsis, is key to maximizing the therapeutic potential of these cells.

MSC Dosage Regimens

The intravenous route of MSC administration has been used in the majority of preclinical studies. The potential of local application, e. g., intra-peritoneal in the case of abdominal sepsis or intra-pulmonary, in the case of pneumonia, deserves further consideration. The optimal dose – or doses – of MSCs for critically ill patients with sepsis remains to be determined. Extrapolation from animal studies and from human studies of MSC administration in other disease states may be used as a guide, but is limited in terms of direct relevance to patients. In other studies in disease states, such as post-myocardial infarction, doses of 0.5–5 million cells/kg have been administered [40]. The CISS phase 1 study in sepsis tested the safety of doses up to 3 million cells/kg. Clearly, the optimal dose of stem cells may differ substantially in different disease states. In addition, the dose may be influenced by other factors, such as the stage of illness, type of MSCs, route of cell delivery, viability and purity of MSCs and condition of the patient. Timing of MSC delivery is also potentially important. Most preclinical studies have demonstrated that MSCs are effective when administered in the early phase of injury. However, recent data from our group suggest that MSCs may be effective after the injury has become established [24]. The demonstration that MSCs are effective when administered later in the course of the injury is important in terms of their clinical translation potential.

In vitro Cell Expansion

In vitro culture and passage of these cells is necessary, because the numbers of cells that can be directly isolated from tissues is insufficient to achieve a therapeutic effect. Repeated passaging can alter the MSC phenotype, and may give rise to more restricted self-renewing progenitors that lose their differentiation potential, and may result in loss of efficacy [41]. Repeated passage in culture may also give rise to chromosomal damage and even malignant transformation [42]. The demonstration that thawed cryopreserved banked MSCs (used in clinical studies) may be less effective than 'fresh' MSCs (used in preclinical studies) may explain inconsistencies in results between clinical and preclinical studies [43].

MSC Safety Concerns

There is a substantial and growing body of evidence attesting to the safety of MSC therapy in humans. Nevertheless, a number of potential concerns exist. An acute concern is the potential for acute infusional toxicity, due to the potential for clumping of the MSCs and their potential to act as microemboli. This has not been a significant issue in non-critically ill patients. Encouragingly, the recent phase I study of MSCs for critically ill patients with ARDS did not report any infusional toxicities [35]. A longer term concern is that MSCs could promote tumor formation either *via* direct malignant transformation of the MSCs themselves or *via* indirect effects that facilitate tumor formation by other cells. Reassuringly, there have been no reports of increased tumorigenesis in patients who have received MSCs in clinical trials to date.

Conclusion

The therapeutic potential of MSCs for sepsis is clear from preclinical studies. The mechanisms of action of MSCs are increasingly well understood and include stabilization of blood vessels, effective tissue and immune system homeostasis under physiological conditions and a more active role in tissue repair following injury.

Clinical evidence of MSC benefit in human sepsis is awaited, but early phase studies are in progress. Important knowledge gaps will need to be addressed if we are to truly realize the therapeutic potential of MSCs for our patients with sepsis.

References

1. Iwashyna TJ, Cooke CR, Wunsch H, Kahn JM (2012) Population burden of long-term survivorship after severe sepsis in older Americans. J Am Geriatr Soc 60:1070–1077
2. Liu V, Escobar GJ, Greene JD et al (2014) Hospital deaths in patients with sepsis from 2 independent cohorts. JAMA 312:90–92
3. Angus DC, van der Poll T (2013) Severe sepsis and septic shock. N Engl J Med 369:840–851
4. van der Poll T, Opal SM (2008) Host-pathogen interactions in sepsis. Lancet Infect Dis 8:32–43
5. Vincent JL, Rello J, Marshall J et al (2009) International study of the prevalence and outcomes of infection in intensive care units. JAMA 302:2323–2329
6. Cronin L, Cook DJ, Carlet J et al (1995) Corticosteroid treatment for sepsis: a critical appraisal and meta-analysis of the literature. Crit Care Med 23:1430–1439
7. Mei SH, Haitsma JJ, Dos Santos CC et al (2010) Mesenchymal stem cells reduce inflammation while enhancing bacterial clearance and improving survival in sepsis. Am J Respir Crit Care Med 182:1047–1057
8. Krasnodembskaya A, Song Y, Fang X et al (2010) Antibacterial effect of human mesenchymal stem cells is mediated in part from secretion of the antimicrobial peptide LL-37. Stem Cells 28:2229–2238
9. Gupta N, Krasnodembskaya A, Kapetanaki M et al (2012) Mesenchymal stem cells enhance survival and bacterial clearance in murine Escherichia coli pneumonia. Thorax 67:533–539
10. Gupta N, Su X, Popov B, Lee J, Serikov V, Matthay M (2007) Intrapulmonary delivery of bone marrow-derived mesenchymal stem cells improves survival and attenuates endotoxin-induced acute lung injury in mice. J Immunol 179:1855–1863
11. Németh K, Leelahavanichkul A, Yuen P et al (2009) Bone marrow stromal cells attenuate sepsis via prostaglandin E(2)-dependent reprogramming of host macrophages to increase their interleukin-10 production. Nat Med 15:42–49
12. Devaney J, Horie S, Masterson C et al (2015) Human mesenchymal stromal cells decrease the severity of acute lung injury induced by E.coli in the Rat. Thorax 70:625–635
13. Luo CJ, Zhang FJ, Zhang L et al (2014) Mesenchymal stem cells ameliorate sepsis-associated acute kidney injury in mice. Shock 41:123–129
14. Hall SR, Tsoyi K, Ith B et al (2013) Mesenchymal stromal cells improve survival during sepsis in the absence of heme oxygenase-1: the importance of neutrophils. Stem Cells 31:397–407
15. Krasnodembskaya A, Samarani G, Song Y et al (2012) Human mesenchymal stem cells reduce mortality and bacteremia in gram-negative sepsis in mice in part by enhancing the phagocytic activity of blood monocytes. Am J Physiol Lung Cell Mol Physiol 302:L1003–1013
16. dos Santos CC, Murthy S, Hu P et al (2012) Network analysis of transcriptional responses induced by mesenchymal stem cell treatment of experimental sepsis. Am J Pathol 181:1681–1692
17. Islam MN, Das SR, Emin MT et al (2012) Mitochondrial transfer from bone-marrow-derived stromal cells to pulmonary alveoli protects against acute lung injury. Nat Med 18:759–765
18. Danchuk S, Ylostalo JH, Hossain F et al (2011) Human multipotent stromal cells attenuate lipopolysaccharide-induced acute lung injury in mice via secretion of tumor necrosis factor-alpha-induced protein 6. Stem Cell Res Ther 2:27
19. Elman JS, Li M, Wang F, Gimble JM, Parekkadan B (2014) A comparison of adipose and bone marrow-derived mesenchymal stromal cell secreted factors in the treatment of systemic inflammation. J Inflamm (Lond) 11:1

20. Zhao X, Liu D, Gong W et al (2014) The toll-like receptor 3 ligand, poly(I:C), improves immunosuppressive function and therapeutic effect of mesenchymal stem cells on sepsis via inhibiting MiR-143. Stem Cells 32:521–533
21. Corcione A, Benvenuto F, Ferretti E et al (2006) Human mesenchymal stem cells modulate B-cell functions. Blood 107:367–372
22. Raffaghello L, Bianchi G, Bertolotto M et al (2008) Human mesenchymal stem cells inhibit neutrophil apoptosis: a model for neutrophil preservation in the bone marrow niche. Stem Cells 26:151–162
23. Kim J, Hematti P (2009) Mesenchymal stem cell-educated macrophages: a novel type of alternatively activated macrophages. Exp Hematol 37:1445–1453
24. Curley G, Hayes M, Ansari B et al (2012) Mesenchymal stem cells enhance recovery and repair following ventilator-induced lung injury in the rat. Thorax 67:496–501
25. Curley GF, Ansari B, Hayes M et al (2013) Effects of intratracheal mesenchymal stromal cell therapy during recovery and resolution after ventilator-induced lung injury. Anesthesiology 118:924–932
26. Hayes M, Masterson C, Devaney J (2015) Therapeutic efficacy of human mesenchymal stromal cells in the repair of established ventilator-induced lung injury in the rat. Anesthesiology 122:363–373
27. McAuley DF, Curley GF, Hamid UI et al (2014) Clinical grade allogeneic human mesenchymal stem cells restore alveolar fluid clearance in human lungs rejected for transplantation. Am J Physiol Lung Cell Mol Physiol 306(9):L809–815
28. Fang X, Abbott J, Cheng L et al (2015) Human mesenchymal stem (stromal) cells promote the resolution of acute lung injury in part through lipoxin A4. J Immunol 195:875–881
29. Xu G, Zhang L, Ren G et al (2007) Immunosuppressive properties of cloned bone marrow mesenchymal stem cells. Cell Res 17:240–248
30. Nemeth K, Keane-Myers A, Brown JM et al (2010) Bone marrow stromal cells use TGF-beta to suppress allergic responses in a mouse model of ragweed-induced asthma. Proc Natl Acad Sci USA 107:5652–5657
31. De Miguel MP, Fuentes-Julian S, Blazquez-Martinez A et al (2012) Immunosuppressive properties of mesenchymal stem cells: advances and applications. Curr Mol Med 12:574–591
32. Ortiz LA, Dutreil M, Fattman C et al (2007) Interleukin 1 receptor antagonist mediates the antiinflammatory and antifibrotic effect of mesenchymal stem cells during lung injury. Proc Natl Acad Sci USA 104:11002–11007
33. Monsel A, Zhu YG, Gennai S et al (2015) Therapeutic effects of human mesenchymal stem cell-derived microvesicles in severe pneumonia in mice. Am J Respir Crit Care Med 192:324–336
34. Bruno S, Grange C, Collino F et al (2012) Microvesicles derived from mesenchymal stem cells enhance survival in a lethal model of acute kidney injury. PLoS One 7:e33115
35. Wilson JG, Liu KD, Zhuo H et al (2015) Mesenchymal stem (stromal) cells for treatment of ARDS: a phase 1 clinical trial. Lancet Respir Med 3:24–32
36. Lee ST, Jang JH, Cheong JW et al (2002) Treatment of high-risk acute myelogenous leukaemia by myeloablative chemoradiotherapy followed by co-infusion of T cell-depleted haematopoietic stem cells and culture-expanded marrow mesenchymal stem cells from a related donor with one fully mismatched human leucocyte antigen haplotype. Br J Haematol 118:1128–1131
37. Le Blanc K, Rasmusson I, Sundberg B et al (2004) Treatment of severe acute graft-versus-host disease with third party haploidentical mesenchymal stem cells. Lancet 363:1439–1441
38. Gregory CA, Ylostalo J, Prockop DJ (2005) Adult bone marrow stem/progenitor cells (MSCs) are preconditioned by microenvironmental "niches" in culture: a two-stage hypothesis for regulation of MSC fate. Sci STKE 2005:pe37
39. Lee RH, Hsu SC, Munoz J et al (2006) A subset of human rapidly self-renewing marrow stromal cells preferentially engraft in mice. Blood 107:2153–2161

40. Hare JM, Traverse JH, Henry TD et al (2009) A randomized, double-blind, placebo-controlled, dose-escalation study of intravenous adult human mesenchymal stem cells (prochymal) after acute myocardial infarction. J Am Coll Cardiol 54:2277–2286
41. Sarugaser R, Hanoun L, Keating A, Stanford WL, Davies JE (2009) Human mesenchymal stem cells self-renew and differentiate according to a deterministic hierarchy. PLoS One 4:e6498
42. Rubio D, Garcia S, Paz MF et al (2008) Molecular characterization of spontaneous mesenchymal stem cell transformation. PLoS One 3:e1398
43. Francois M, Copland IB, Yuan S, Romieu-Mourez R, Waller EK, Galipeau J (2012) Cryopreserved mesenchymal stromal cells display impaired immunosuppressive properties as a result of heat-shock response and impaired interferon-gamma licensing. Cytotherapy 14:147–152

Part III
Fluids

Fluid Balance During Septic Shock: It's Time to Optimize

X. Chapalain, T. Gargadennec, and O. Huet

Introduction

During septic shock, acute circulatory failure results in an imbalance between cellular oxygen demand and delivery. Fluid infusion represents one of the cornerstones of resuscitation therapies and is a major tool to increase oxygen delivery during circulatory failure. However, a paradigm shift is currently occurring as concerns have been raised about the potential adverse effects of fluid therapy. Fluid overload is one of the major adverse effects reported. It is usually defined as a fluid accumulation $> 10\%$ of baseline weight and it is an independent factor of worse outcome in intensive care unit (ICU) patients [1]. It is now suggested that fluid administration should be conducted cautiously during resuscitation in order to avoid an unnecessary increase in fluid intake. To minimize unnecessary fluid resuscitation, use of factors predictive of volume responsiveness should be assessed before any fluid challenge [2, 3].

Fluid responsiveness depends on patient's preload status and does not have a constant linear relationship. The relationship between preload and changes in left ventricular stroke volume follows the Frank-Starling curve (Fig. 1). This curve can be divided into two sections: the ascending section can be considered as a linear relationship so that every fluid challenge is followed by an increase in cardiac output. The second section is nearly flat so that fluid challenges do not increase cardiac output and are responsible for unnecessary fluid intake. The precise shape of the curve depends on myocardial contractility properties.

In ICU patients, changes in hemodynamic status are often due to multiple causes: acute inflammatory states, hypovolemia, impaired cardiac function. Therefore, it is almost impossible to guide fluid resuscitation by only using the results of clinical examination (mottled skin, cyanosis, toe coloration time). It is now recommended

X. Chapalain · T. Gargadennec · O. Huet (✉)
Dept of Anesthesiology and Intensive Care, Hôpital de la Cavale Blanche, CHRU de Brest, University of Bretagne Occidental
Blvd Tanguy Prigent, 29609 Brest, France
e-mail: olivier.huet@chu-brest.fr

J.-L. Vincent (ed.), *Annual Update in Intensive Care and Emergency Medicine 2017*,
DOI 10.1007/978-3-319-51908-1_5

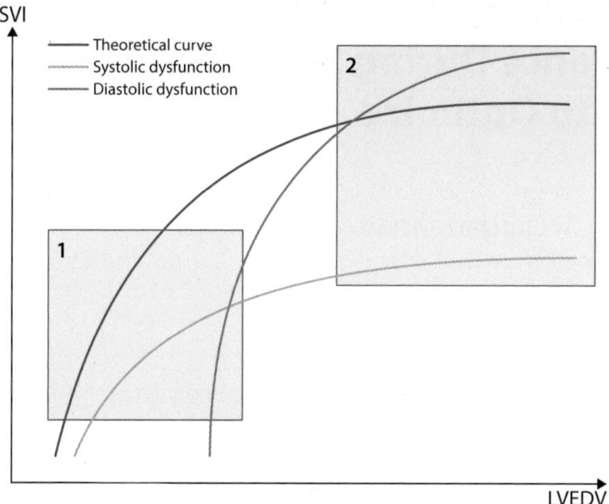

Fig. 1 Frank-Starling curve. This figure shows the theoretical relation between SVI (stroke volume index, ml/m^2) and LVEDV (left ventricular end-diastolic volume, ml). In the steep portion of the Frank-Starling curve (*square n°1*), an increase in LVEDV with fluid challenge will increase SVI and cardiac output. In the flat portion (*square n°2*), an increase in LVED will not influence SVI. Patients with left ventricular systolic dysfunction (*light blue curve*) have a limited increase in stroke volume in response to a fluid challenge. In patients with diastolic dysfunction (*mid-blue curve*), ventricular function is highly dependent upon preload: the Frank-Starling curve is shifted up and to the right

that hemodynamic parameters (especially cardiac output and stroke volume) be measured in order to assess a patient's hemodynamic status prior to fluid challenge. Among the hemodynamic parameters, 'static' parameters (e. g., blood pressure, central venous pressure [CVP], heart rate) or 'dynamic' parameters (e. g., pulse pressure variation [PPV] or stroke volume variation [SVV]) can be used. 'Dynamic' parameters are based on changes of cardiac preload in response to cyclic respiratory changes in pleural pressure during mechanical ventilation. Numerous parameters to assess fluid responsiveness have been studied [4–6], and 'dynamic' parameters are now considered as the gold standard in the decision making process for fluid resuscitation [7]. However, few clinicians actually use preload indicators to evaluate fluid responsiveness and to decide whether or not to perform a fluid challenge. A recent study reported that clinical practice in terms of assessment of fluid responsiveness is highly variable: 42.5% of fluid challenges were performed without evaluation of 'dynamic' markers and 35.5% using 'static' markers of preload [8].

A fluid optimization strategy during circulatory failure can be summarized as follows:

(i) before fluid challenge, assess dynamic parameters to evaluate a patient's likely fluid responsiveness,

(ii) if the patient is likely to be fluid responsive, perform a fluid challenge, usually with an infusion of 500 ml of crystalloids [8],
(iii) assess volume responsiveness (defined for example by an increase in left ventricular stroke volume of more than 10 or 15%).

Although this strategy seems to be obvious from a good clinical practice perspective there are currently no clinical data to confirm that it has a positive impact on patient prognosis. This may explain why this strategy has not been widely translated into clinical practice.

Impact of Increased Fluid Balance During Septic Shock

During sepsis, different phases of hemodynamic resuscitation have been described with different risks, goals and challenges: resuscitation, optimization, stabilization and de-escalation phases. During the resuscitation phase of septic shock, to respond to the inflammatory insult, current guidelines concerning fluid resuscitation suggest that aggressive fluid administration is the best initial therapy [3]. Then, in the optimization phase, the goal is to maintain tissue perfusion and avoid effects of fluid overload. During this phase, 'liberal' or uncontrolled fluid therapy can induce an increased positive fluid balance with tissue fluid overload.

Some pathophysiologic mechanisms can be identified to explain the harmful effect of fluid overload [9]. One of them can be outlined as follows: during sepsis, the increase in endothelial permeability induced by glycocalyx shedding and development of gaps between endothelial cells induces interstitial leakage. During the resuscitation phase after aggressive fluid therapy, the increase in the microcirculatory and macrocirculatory blood pressure induces a release of natriuretic peptides acting simultaneously with nitric oxide to cause an increase in vascular permeability and capillary leakage. The pathogenic effects of interstitial fluid overload are well described [1]. Theoretically, all organs can suffer from fluid overload in addition to ischemia and reperfusion insults, but adverse effects are particularly pronounced in encapsulated organs. In the kidneys, fluid overload increases interstitial edema and decreases glomerular filtration and renal blood flow. In the liver, fluid overload induces cholestasis and impairs liver synthetic functions. In the lung, pulmonary edema induced by fluid overload leads to impaired gas exchange.

These experimental data explain why a positive fluid balance may have a critical impact on prognosis in ICU patients. In a clinical setting, epidemiologic and experimental studies confirm these findings. An association between positive fluid balance in ICU patients and increased morbidity and mortality has been demonstrated in observational studies [6, 12], particularly for patients with acute respiratory distress syndrome (ARDS) [13]. It has, therefore, been suggested that a restrictive fluid therapy strategy should be considered in order to decrease fluid overload during the optimization phase in septic shock patients [14]. However, it is uncertain that such strategies will benefit every patient [15]. It seems obvious that fluid therapy has to be tailored to the patient's needs and a thoughtful approach can help to avoid the dele-

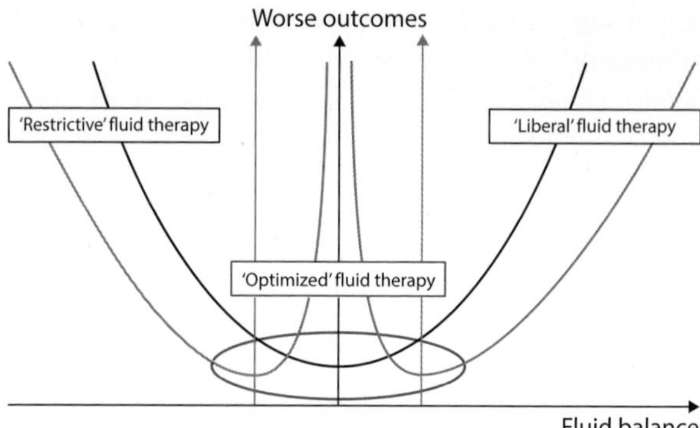

Fig. 2 The concept of "optimized" fluid therapy. This illustration shows theoretical (*black curve*) distribution of worse outcomes according to fluid balance in septic shock. "Optimized" fluid therapy (*dark blue circle*) is a theoretical state where optimized goal-directed therapy aims to optimize tissue perfusion. This distribution differs among patients according to their comorbidities, ages and organ dysfunction. Some patients may be more vulnerable to a liberal strategy (*gray curve*) others will be more vulnerable to restrictive strategies (*light blue curve*)

terious effects of an increased fluid balance [16]. This paradigm between 'liberal' or 'restrictive' strategies can be illustrated by the U-shaped curve shown in Fig. 2. Therefore, there seems to be a place for fluid optimization in clinical practice. Considering the four resuscitation phases described above, it is important to know when to start or stop giving fluids. This approach cannot be considered without accurate fluid responsiveness evaluation provided by hemodynamic monitoring.

Assessing Fluid Responsiveness with 'Dynamic' Parameters

It has recently been acknowledged that 'dynamic' hemodynamic parameters are more accurate than 'static' ones. Dynamic parameters are based on heart-lung interactions and cyclic changes in pleural pressure during mechanical ventilation [17]. During inspiratory cycles, the variations in intrathoracic pressure induce a decrease in systemic venous return and right ventricular (RV) filling pressure resulting in a diminution of the RV stroke volume. Due to the blood transit time through the pulmonary circulation, the consequences of decreased RV stroke volume occur in the left ventricle during the expiratory phase. These cyclic changes in left ventricular (LV) filling pressure induce changes in LV stroke volume and aortic blood flow. The aortic blood flow is proportional to the LV stroke volume and the magnitude of the cyclic changes in aortic blood flow is an indicator of preload dependency. At the bedside, the variations in aortic blood flow can be analyzed using the PPV and changes in LV stroke volume can be analyzed using the SVV.

The superiority of dynamic parameters (SVV, PPV) compared to static parameters has been demonstrated in the decision-making process of whether or not to perform a fluid challenge [5]. Their use is now recommended in clinical practice in order to decrease unnecessary fluid intake and decrease fluid overload [2]. In a study using invasive blood pressure monitoring, a 13% change in PPV was predictive of fluid responsiveness if the patient was in sinus rhythm and was not spontaneously breathing under conventional mechanical with a tidal volume > 8 ml/kg (sensitivity 94%, specificity 96%, area under the curve [AUC] 0.98) [4]. A recent meta-analysis pooled 22 studies about PPV in patients with sinus rhythm and without spontaneous breathing [18]. In this analysis, a 12% PPV cut-off was predictive of fluid responsiveness with a sensitivity of 88% and a specificity of 89%. These results were also validated using aortic blood flow variation. Use of beat-to-beat flow analysis by esophageal echocardiography showed that a respiratory variation in aortic blood flow peak velocity greater than 12% was able to predict fluid responsiveness with 100% sensitivity and 89% specificity [6].

SVV derived from pulse contour analysis can also predict fluid responsiveness. Using 29 studies (685 patients), Marik and coworkers [19] performed a pooled analysis of SVV accuracy. In this meta-analysis, SVV had good accuracy (AUC 0.84) for predicting volume responsiveness with a threshold variation at $11.6 \pm 1.9\%$. SVV had greater accuracy for predicting fluid responsiveness than the 'static' parameters analyzed (CVP, global end diastolic volume index, LV end-diastolic area index).

However all these 'dynamic' parameters have limitations that are frequently encountered in ICU patients: mechanical ventilation with a tidal volume < 8 ml/kg [20], spontaneous breathing, high heart rate/respiratory rate ratio (HR/RR < 3.6) and arrhythmia [20]. In 2011, among 12,000 patients undergoing surgery, only 39% met all the criteria (21% were ventilated with tidal volume < 8 ml/kg and 13% were spontaneously breathing) [21]. These data were confirmed in a study including 400 patients: 50% were ventilated with tidal volumes < 8 ml/kg and 9% had a heart rate/respiratory rate (HR/RR) < 3.6 [22]. Finally, there is a 'gray zone' where it is impossible to predict fluid responsiveness. The gray zone is the interval between PPV values of 9 and 13%; between these two values clinicians cannot predict fluid responsiveness. Among 413 ventilated surgical patients, Cannesson and coworkers demonstrated that such values were encountered in approximately 25% of patients [22]. These data were confirmed by two studies reporting a large proportion of patients (between 40 to 60%) considered to be in the gray zone [23, 24]. Thus, using only dynamic parameters in the decision making process whether or not to perform a fluid challenge seems to be insufficient, and new hemodynamic challenges have been developed in order to overcome these limitations.

Recent Advances in Fluid Responsiveness Assessment

To assess patient hemodynamic status, three methods have been described as alternatives to heart-lung interaction based parameters: the passive leg raising (PLR) maneuver, the mini-fluid challenge and end-expiratory occlusion [7]. The comparison between the accuracy of these methods and 'dynamic' parameters is summarized in Table 1.

Table 1 Sensitivity and specificity of 'dynamic' and alternative fluid responsiveness parameters

Indices	Monitoring methods	Cut-off (%)	AUC	Specificity (%)	Sensitivity (%)
PPV	Arterial waveform	PPV > 13	0.98	94	96
SVV	PCA, TTE, TEE, TT, PAC	SVV > 12	0.84	82	86
MFC	PCA, TTE, TEE, TPTD	ΔSV > 10 OR ΔVTI > 10	0.9	78	95
PLR	PCA, TPTD, EDM, PAC	CI > 10	0.95	91	85
EEO	PCA, TPTD	CI > 5	0.972	100	91

PPV: pulse pressure variation; *SVV*: stroke volume variation; *MFC*: mini-fluid challenge; *PLR*: passive leg raising; *EEO*: end-expiratory occlusion; *PCA*: pulse contour analysis; *TTE*: transthoracic echocardiography; *TEE*: transesophageal echocardiography; *TPTD*: transpulmonary thermodilution; *PAC*: pulmonary artery catheter; *EDM*: esophageal Doppler monitoring; *AUC*: area under the curve; *VTI*: velocity time integral

Passive Leg Raising

PLR was first described a decade ago [25], but since then the technique has been refined. PLR mimics rapid fluid infusion by mobilizing the non-stressed blood volume contained in the splanchnic circulation. By tilting the bed of a patient to a semi-recumbent position [26], about 300 ml of blood is mobilized and has a significant effect on cardiac preload. Measuring changes in cardiac output before, during and after PLR, with a device that can detect short-term and transient changes, enables assessment of fluid responsiveness. A 10% increase in cardiac output during the maneuver is predictive of a positive response to a fluid challenge [27]. PLR is reliable in patients with circulatory failure, under mechanical ventilation or spontaneously breathing, with arrhythmia or in sinus rhythm. Fluid responsiveness prediction performance is excellent with cited AUCs of between 0.84 and 1.00. A recent meta-analysis concluded that PLR has a good sensitivity/specificity ratio for identifying fluid responders (sensitivity 85%, specificity 91%, AUC 0.95) [28]. This meta-analysis confirmed that a 10% cardiac output increase was the cut-off to predict fluid responsiveness. Nevertheless, it seems important to stress that even though PLR seems to be a feasible method of assessing fluid responsiveness, it needs to be performed using a rigorous protocol otherwise the measures are biased by confounding factors [29].

Mini-fluid Challenge

The mini-fluid challenge consists of administering a bolus of a small colloid volume (100 ml in 1 minute) and comparing hemodynamic parameters before and after the bolus. Muller et al. showed that an increase in the velocity time index (VTI) greater than 10% after a mini-fluid challenge was predictive of fluid responsiveness with good reliability (AUC = 0.90) [30]. Likewise, Mallat et al. in a study enrolling 49 patients (mostly in septic shock) demonstrated that an increase in stroke volume assessed by transpulmonary thermodilution > 9.5% was predictive of fluid responsiveness [31]. These data are in agreement with previous data about perioperative hemodynamic optimization using stroke volume optimization with iterative fluid challenges [32–36]. The reliability of the mini-fluid challenge to predict fluid responsiveness is as good as that of SVV or PPV (AUC: SVV = 0.84 and PPV = 0.94 [19, 37] *versus* 0.90 for mini-fluid challenge [30, 31]). The mini-fluid challenge has fewer limitations than SVV and PPV. Guinot et al studied the mini-fluid challenge in spontaneously breathing patients under regional anesthesia and reported an AUC of 0.93 for prediction of fluid responsiveness [38]. Similar findings were reported in a study enrolling arrhythmic patients [39].

End-expiratory Occlusion

End-expiratory occlusion is based on heart-lung interactions and consists of a respiratory pause of 15 seconds at the end of the expiration phase during mechanical ventilation. As each insufflation sees intrathoracic pressure increase it is followed by a decrease in thoracic venous return. Therefore, when performing an end-expiratory occlusion, an increase in venous return and cardiac output is observed. A 5% increase in cardiac output for the last 5 seconds of the end-expiratory occlusion is predictive of a 500 ml fluid infusion responsiveness with 91% sensitivity, 100% specificity and an AUC of 0.97 [40, 41]. End-expiratory occlusion has also been validated in patients with arrhythmia and in spontaneously breathing patients and is also reliable in patients with altered pulmonary compliance [42].

Options for Hemodynamic Monitoring During Septic Shock

For many years, monitoring devices have evolved in operating rooms and the ICU. This evolution has been marked by decline in the use of the pulmonary artery catheter (PAC) and an increase in the use of less invasive monitoring devices. Bedside hemodynamic assessment helps clinicians to evaluate a patient's hemodynamic status and response to therapeutic interventions. Different monitoring devices are available and have their own limitations. These limitations must be appreciated in order to properly analyze the hemodynamic measurements provided by the device.

Pulse Contour Analysis and Transpulmonary Thermodilution

Transpulmonary thermodilution provides intermittent measurement of several hemodynamic parameters, including cardiac index, cardiac output, extravascular lung volume, and stroke volume. Transpulmonary thermodilution devices require a central venous catheter and a thermistor-tipped arterial catheter to obtain a thermodilution

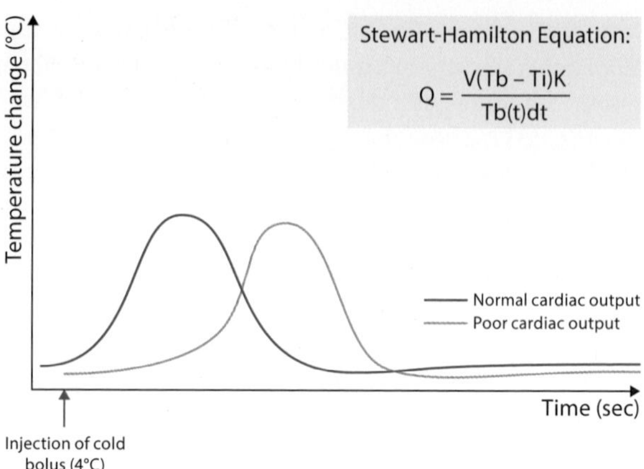

Fig. 3 Thermodilution curves representing changes in arterial blood temperature obtained after cold boluses according to the Stewart-Hamilton Equation. *Q*: cardiac output; *V*: injected volume; *Tb*: blood temperature; *Ti*: Temperature of injectate; *K*: correction coefficient; *Tb(t)dt*: change in blood temperature as a function of time

curve according to the Stewart-Hamilton equation (Fig. 3). Obtaining this curve needs three to five cold boluses (15 to 20 ml) and calibration should be performed at least four times daily and more frequently in very instable patients or in the presence of arrhythmia. Some monitoring devices combine transpulmonary thermodilution and pulse contour analysis (PCA) and continuously assess several parameters (especially cardiac index and stroke volume) using mathematic algorithms. Cardiac output measurements with transpulmonary thermodilution were compared to those obtained using a PAC [43], with acceptable agreement between the two monitoring devices. However, a recent analysis stressed that hemodynamic parameters (especially cardiac index) obtained by transpulmonary thermodilution without calibration poorly tracked cardiac index changes after therapeutic interventions [44] because of changes in arterial compliance. Transpulmonary thermodilution with PCA has been used to evaluate the response to hemodynamic 'challenges' (such as mini-fluid challenge, end-expiratory occlusion or PLR) in several studies [28, 31, 42].

Furthermore, transpulmonary thermodilution is the only technique that provides measurement of extravascular lung water (EVLW) and extravascular lung water index (EVLWI). EVLW is an estimation of the fluid accumulated in the extravascular space, especially in interstitial and alveolar spaces. An EVLW < 10 ml/kg is considered as a normal value. Some recent data stress that EVLWI may be an independent predictor for survival among septic patients [45]. However, these data remain descriptive and no interventional studies have yet shown that fluid therapy based on EVLWI improves outcomes.

Esophageal Doppler Monitoring and Echocardiography

Transthoracic echocardiography (TTE), transesophageal echocardiography (TEE) and esophageal Doppler monitoring (EDM) provide a beat-to-beat assessment of cardiac output according to aortic velocity measurements. Most perioperative studies use EDM or TEE to optimize patients during surgery and improve postoperative outcomes [46]. Among 46 ICU patients, EDM and PAC measurements showed good correlation [47]. EDM is able to track hemodynamic parameters induced by therapeutic interventions [48] like a fluid challenge. Aortic velocity analysis has already been used for bedside assessment of the 'hemodynamic' challenges cited above with good accuracy [28, 30].

Hemodynamic Management of ICU Patients: Time to Optimize

After the initial resuscitation phase, patients remaining unstable will need hemodynamic optimization to maintain tissue perfusion and improve organ dysfunction.

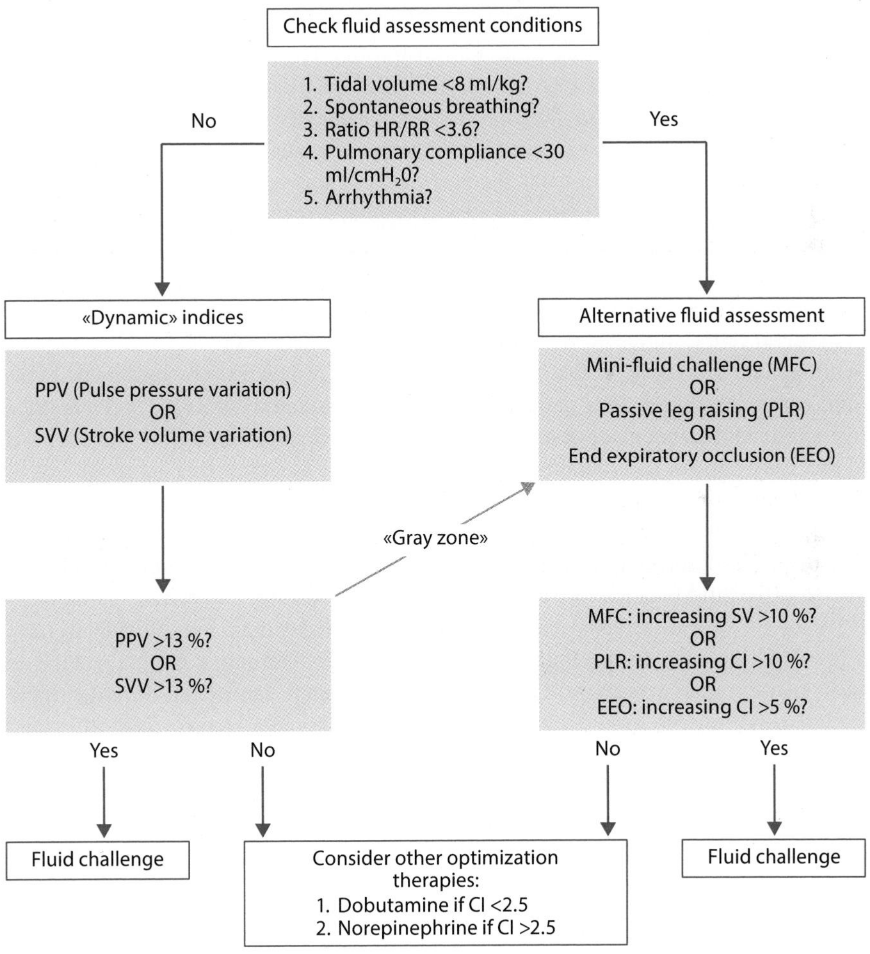

Fig. 4 Example of optimized goal-directed therapy protocol in septic shock. *CI*: cardiac index; *HR*: heart rate; *RR*: respiratory rate; *EEO*: end-expiratory occlusion; *PLR*: passive leg raising; *MFC*: mini-fluid challenge

Therefore, hemodynamic monitoring devices could be useful to detect whether or not a patient will require fluid infusion or a vasopressor to maintain a sufficient perfusion pressure to the organs. However, although this approach seems sound, the proportion of clinicians using hemodynamic devices and hemodynamic optimization protocols remains small. This can be explained by the constraint that goes along with the use of these devices, but also by the lack of belief in their usefulness at the bedside. Unlike perioperative fluid management, there is no clinical evidence demonstrating the efficiency of a hemodynamic goal-directed protocol in ICU patients. We believe that a goal-directed protocol could help clinicians to optimize tissue perfusion during sepsis, avoid fluid overload and therefore increase patient survival. In Fig. 4, we suggest an algorithm for bedside assessment of fluid responsiveness based on the most recent literature. This algorithm includes both the use of fluid challenge and the use of catecholamines. Indeed, optimizing a patient's hemodynamic status during acute circulatory failure, such as in septic shock, cannot be achieved by only considering fluid administration. Thus, combining vasopressors with fluid infusion is also key for optimal fluid balance management. Assessing a patient's requirements for fluid or vasopressor agents using a goal-directed approach with monitoring devices should be tested in a randomized controlled trial in order to demonstrate to clinicians the usefulness of this approach.

Conclusion

For several years, studies have highlighted an independent association between fluid overload and mortality. In the light of these studies, it has been recommended that fluid administration to ICU patients needs to be considered carefully, and a restrictive approach has been suggested to avoid fluid overload. Although it makes sense to precisely control ICU patients' fluid intake, the weakness of this approach lies in its generalization, as it is not tailored to the patients' individual fluid requirements. Instead of a general restrictive approach, an individual tailored approach should be considered in order to optimize patients' hemodynamics during circulatory failure. To optimize fluid balance, the clinician has several options. 'Dynamic' parameters (PPV or SVV) can be used but their limitations make their use reliable in only a few ICU patients. In the light of these limitations, alternative methods, such as PLR, end-expiratory occlusion and mini-fluid challenge have been developed and shown to be reliable in general ICU populations. The next step for hemodynamic management in the ICU should be to test a hemodynamic goal-directed approach in order to better control fluid management and eventually improve patient outcome.

References

1. Malbrain MLNG, Marik PE, Witters I et al (2014) Fluid overload, de-resuscitation, and outcomes in critically ill or injured patients: a systematic review with suggestions for clinical practice. Anaesthesiol Intensive Ther 46:361–380

2. Cecconi M, De Backer D, Antonelli M et al (2014) Consensus on circulatory shock and hemodynamic monitoring. Task force of the European Society of Intensive Care Medicine. Intensive Care Med 40:1795–1815
3. Dellinger RP, Levy MM, Rhodes A et al (2012) Surviving Sepsis Campaign: international guidelines for management of severe sepsis and septic shock, 2012. Intensive Care Med 39:165–228
4. Michard F, Boussat S, Chemla D et al (2000) Relation between respiratory changes in arterial pulse pressure and fluid responsiveness in septic patients with acute circulatory failure. Am J Respir Crit Care Med 162:134–138
5. Michard F, Teboul JL (2002) Predicting fluid responsiveness in ICU patients: a critical analysis of the evidence. Chest 121:2000–2008
6. Feissel M, Michard F, Mangin I, Ruyer O, Faller JP, Teboul JL (2001) Respiratory changes in aortic blood velocity as an indicator of fluid responsiveness in ventilated patients with septic shock. Chest 119:867–783
7. Monnet X, Teboul JL (2013) Assessment of volume responsiveness during mechanical ventilation: recent advances. Crit Care 17:217
8. Cecconi M, Hofer C, Teboul JL et al (2015) Fluid challenges in intensive care: the FENICE study: A global inception cohort study. Intensive Care Med 41:1529–1537
9. Marik PE (2014) Iatrogenic salt water drowning and the hazards of a high central venous pressure. Ann Intensive Care 4:21
10. Payen D, de Pont AC, Sakr Y et al (2008) A positive fluid balance is associated with a worse outcome in patients with acute renal failure. Crit Care 12:R74
11. Vincent JL, Sakr Y, Sprung CL et al (2006) Sepsis in European intensive care units: results of the SOAP study. Crit Care Med 34:344–353
12. Boyd JH, Forbes J, Nakada T, Walley KR, Russell JA (2011) Fluid resuscitation in septic shock: a positive fluid balance and elevated central venous pressure are associated with increased mortality. Crit Care Med 39:259–265
13. Wiedemann HP, Wheeler AP, Bernard GR et al (2006) Comparison of two fluid-management strategies in acute lung injury. N Engl J Med 354:2564–2575
14. Vincent JL (2011) Let's give some fluid and see what happens" versus the "mini-fluid challenge. Anesthesiology 115:455–456
15. Smith SH, Perner A (2012) Higher vs. lower fluid volume for septic shock: clinical characteristics and outcome in unselected patients in a prospective, multicenter cohort. Crit Care 16:R76
16. Bellamy MC (2006) Wet, dry or something else? Br J Anaesth 97:755–757
17. Jardin F, Delorme G, Hardy A, Auvert B, Beauchet A, Bourdarias JP (1990) Reevaluation of hemodynamic consequences of positive pressure ventilation: Emphasis on cyclic right ventricular afterloading by mechanical lung inflation. J Am Soc Anesthesiol 72:966–970
18. Yang X, Du B (2014) Does pulse pressure variation predict fluid responsiveness in critically ill patients? A systematic review and meta-analysis. Crit Care 18:650
19. Marik PE, Cavallazzi R, Vasu T, Hirani A (2009) Dynamic changes in arterial waveform derived variables and fluid responsiveness in mechanically ventilated patients: a systematic review of the literature. Crit Care Med 37:2642–2647
20. De Backer D, Taccone FS, Holsten R, Ibrahimi F, Vincent JL (2009) Influence of respiratory rate on stroke volume variation in mechanically ventilated patients. Anesthesiology 110:1092–1097
21. Maguire S, Rinehart J, Vakharia S, Cannesson M (2011) Technical communication: respiratory variation in pulse pressure and plethysmographic waveforms: intraoperative applicability in a North American academic center. Anesth Analg 112:94–96
22. Cannesson M, Le Manach Y, Hofer CK et al (2011) Assessing the diagnostic accuracy of pulse pressure variations for the prediction of fluid responsiveness: a "gray zone" approach. Anesthesiology 115:231–241

23. Vos JJ, Poterman M, Salm PP et al (2015) Noninvasive pulse pressure variation and stroke volume variation to predict fluid responsiveness at multiple thresholds: a prospective observational study. Can J Anaesth 62:1153–1160
24. Biais M, Ehrmann S, Mari A et al (2014) Clinical relevance of pulse pressure variations for predicting fluid responsiveness in mechanically ventilated intensive care unit patients: the grey zone approach. Crit Care 18:587
25. Lafanechère A, Pène F, Goulenok C et al (2006) Changes in aortic blood flow induced by passive leg raising predict fluid responsiveness in critically ill patients. Crit Care 10:R132
26. Jabot J, Teboul JL, Richard C, Monnet X (2009) Passive leg raising for predicting fluid responsiveness: importance of the postural change. Intensive Care Med 35:85–90
27. Monnet X, Rienzo M, Osman D et al (2006) Passive leg raising predicts fluid responsiveness in the critically ill. Crit Care Med 34:1402–1407
28. Monnet X, Cipriani F, Camous L et al (2016) The passive leg raising test to guide fluid removal in critically ill patients. Ann Intensive Care 6:46
29. Monnet X, Teboul JL (2015) Passive leg raising: five rules, not a drop of fluid! Crit Care 19:18
30. Muller L, Toumi M, Bousquet PJ et al (2011) An increase in aortic blood flow after an infusion of 100 ml colloid over 1 minute can predict fluid responsiveness: the mini-fluid challenge study. Anesthesiology 115:541–547
31. Mallat J, Meddour M, Durville E et al (2015) Decrease in pulse pressure and stroke volume variations after mini-fluid challenge accurately predicts fluid responsiveness. Br J Anaesth 6:222
32. Conway DH, Mayall R, Abdul-Latif MS, Gilligan S, Tackaberry C (2002) Randomised controlled trial investigating the influence of intravenous fluid titration using oesophageal Doppler monitoring during bowel surgery. Anaesthesia 57:845–849
33. Hamilton MA, Cecconi M, Rhodes A (2011) A systematic review and meta-analysis on the use of preemptive hemodynamic intervention to improve postoperative outcomes in moderate and high-risk surgical patients. Anesth Analg 112:1392–1402
34. Phan TD, Ismail H, Heriot AG, Ho KM (2008) Improving perioperative outcomes: fluid optimization with the esophageal Doppler monitor, a metaanalysis and review. J Am Coll Surg 207:935–941
35. Sinclair S, James S, Singer M (1997) Intraoperative intravascular volume optimisation and length of hospital stay after repair of proximal femoral fracture: randomised controlled trial. BMJ 315:909–912
36. Cecconi M, Corredor C, Arulkumaran N et al (2013) Clinical review: Goal-directed therapy – what is the evidence in surgical patients? The effect on different risk groups. Crit Care 17:209
37. Marik PE, Monnet X, Teboul JL (2011) Hemodynamic parameters to guide fluid therapy. Ann Intensive Care 1:1
38. Guinot P-G, Bernard E, Defrancq F et al (2015) Mini-fluid challenge predicts fluid responsiveness during spontaneous breathing under spinal anaesthesia: An observational study. Eur J Anaesthesiol 32:645–649
39. Vallet B, Blanloeil Y, Cholley B et al (2013) Guidelines for perioperative haemodynamic optimization. Ann Fr Anesthésie Réanimation 32:454–462
40. Silva S, Jozwiak M, Teboul JL, Persichini R, Richard C, Monnet X (2013) End-expiratory occlusion test predicts preload responsiveness independently of positive end-expiratory pressure during acute respiratory distress syndrome. Crit Care Med 41:1692–1701
41. Monnet X, Osman D, Ridel C, Lamia B, Richard C, Teboul JL (2009) Predicting volume responsiveness by using the end-expiratory occlusion in mechanically ventilated intensive care unit patients. Crit Care Med 37:951–956
42. Monnet X, Bleibtreu A, Ferré A et al (2012) Passive leg-raising and end-expiratory occlusion tests perform better than pulse pressure variation in patients with low respiratory system compliance. Crit Care Med 40:152–157

43. Biais M, Nouette-Gaulain K, Cottenceau V et al (2008) Cardiac output measurement in patients undergoing liver transplantation: pulmonary artery catheter versus uncalibrated arterial pressure waveform analysis. Anesth Analg 106:1480–1486
44. Monnet X, Anguel N, Naudin B, Jabot J, Richard C, Teboul JL (2010) Arterial pressure-based cardiac output in septic patients: different accuracy of pulse contour and uncalibrated pressure waveform devices. Crit Care 14:R109
45. Jozwiak M, Teboul JL, Monnet X (2015) Extravascular lung water in critical care: recent advances and clinical applications. Ann Intensive Care 5:38
46. Giglio MT, Marucci M, Testini M, Brienza N (2009) Goal-directed haemodynamic therapy and gastrointestinal complications in major surgery: a meta-analysis of randomized controlled trials. Br J Anaesth 103:637–646
47. Valtier B, Cholley BP, Belot JP, la de Coussaye JE, Mateo J, Payen DM (1998) Noninvasive monitoring of cardiac output in critically ill patients using transesophageal Doppler. Am J Respir Crit Care Med 158:77–83
48. Cariou A, Monchi M, Joly LM et al (1998) Noninvasive cardiac output monitoring by aortic blood flow determination: evaluation of the Sometec Dynemo-3000 system. Crit Care Med 26:2066–2072

How to Use Fluid Responsiveness in Sepsis

V. Mukherjee, S. B. Brosnahan, and J. Bakker

Introduction

Fluids in critically ill patients are mostly given to increase tissue perfusion. However, clinical practice shows that the administration of fluids is based on weak physiologic principles [1]. As a result, patients often receive large amounts of intravenous fluids in an effort to normalize their systemic hemodynamics. Careful titration is essential as both under-resuscitation and overtreatment can result in poor outcomes, including respiratory failure and increased mortality [2].

Fluid responsiveness is defined as an increase in stroke volume upon administration of intravenous fluids. As described by Starling over a century ago, increasing filling of the ventricle increases preload resulting in increased cardiac output but only until a certain tipping point where increasing any further can actually raise central venous pressure (CVP) rapidly resulting in a decrease in cardiac output (Fig. 1; [3]).

Frequently, static parameters of fluid status such as blood pressure and CVP have been used as indicators and predictors of successful fluid resuscitation. These measures, however, perform no better than chance in patients who are critically ill [4, 5]. Recently, functional hemodynamics with bedside maneuvers that rapidly change preload have been proposed to better assess fluid responsiveness. In this

V. Mukherjee · S. B. Brosnahan
Department of Pulmonary and Critical Care Medicine, Bellevue Hospital Center/New York University School of Medicine
New York, NY 10022, USA

J. Bakker (✉)
Department of Intensive Care Adults, Erasmus MC University Medical Center
3000 CA Rotterdam, Netherlands
Department of Pulmonary and Critical Care Medicine, New York University School of Medicine
New York, NY 10022, USA
Department of Pulmonary and Critical Care Medicine, Columbia University Medical Center
New York, NY 10032, USA
e-mail: jan.bakker@erasmusmc.nl

J.-L. Vincent (ed.), *Annual Update in Intensive Care and Emergency Medicine 2017*,
DOI 10.1007/978-3-319-51908-1_6

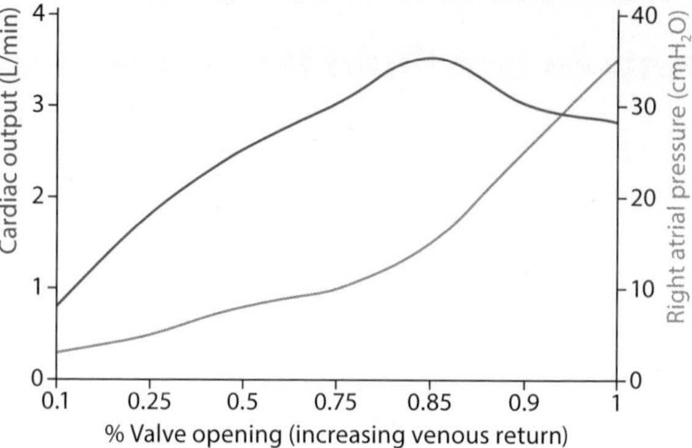

Fig. 1 Alternative presentation of the Frank-Starling curve with opening of the venous return valve (independent variable) on the X-axis and cardiac output and central venous pressure on the Y-axis. Reproduced from [3]

chapter, we will discuss the goals of fluid resuscitation in patients with sepsis, and the clinical use of the principles behind fluid responsiveness.

Goals of Fluid Resuscitation

The primary goal of fluid resuscitation is to increase the venous return, resulting in a global increase in blood flow and/or pressure so that tissue perfusion and thus oxygenation may improve [1].

This goal may be accomplished by:

1. the increase in cardiac output as a result of the increase in venous return results in better regional and finally microcirculatory perfusion;
2. an increase in blood pressure brought about by the increase in cardiac output so that perfusion pressure improves and thus results in optimization of microcirculatory perfusion.

The results of this fluid administration should not be limited to improvement in cardiac output, but should ultimately result in improvement of oxygen delivery to the tissues. This can be assessed by the following parameters:

a. Decrease in lactate levels: a decrease in lactate levels during treatment is universally associated with improved survival [6]. In addition, lactate-guided resuscitation has been shown to improve mortality in patients with septic shock [7]. However, there is emerging evidence that hyperlactatemia in sepsis may have a more complicated cause than simply tissue hypoperfusion [8]. For example, sepsis is often accompanied by a hypermetabolic state causing exaggerated skeletal muscle aerobic glycolysis that leads to lactate production even in the non-hypoperfused state [9]. Hence, in later stages of sepsis, caution should be taken before using fluid resuscitation to decrease lactate levels [8].
b. Recently, the venous-arterial carbon dioxide difference [$P_{v-a}CO_2$] has been studied as a marker for tissue hypoperfusion [10]. In addition, as a reflector of

increased CO_2 production from anaerobic metabolism, the ratio of $P_{v-a}CO_2$ and the arteriovenous oxygen content difference ($C_{a-v}O_2$) could predict the presence of anaerobic metabolism thus making the interpretation of increased lactate levels easier. Thus, increased lactate levels in the presence of an increased $P_{v-a}CO_2$ or increased $P_{v-a}CO_2/C_{a-v}O_2$ could make hypoperfusion as a cause more likely [10].

c. Peripheral perfusion can be used as a marker of regional and microcirculatory perfusion. Quick bedside clinical signs, such as increased capillary refill time and degree of skin mottling, can reflect peripheral and visceral organ hypoperfusion [11, 12].

Given that sepsis is a form of distributive shock, most critically ill, septic patients are hypovolemic at presentation and could benefit from an initial fluid bolus. On completion of this bolus, assessment should be made to see whether the hypoperfusion has resolved. If not, assessing fluid responsiveness helps to decide upon further fluid resuscitation. There are three categories of measurements that can be used to determine fluid responsiveness: static parameters, dynamic indices and peripheral perfusion parameters.

What Is Volume Responsiveness?

In general, as per the Frank-Starling principle, fluid infusion increases the stressed volume and hence venous return, which may increase cardiac output. While a specific value of CVP does not indicate fluid responsiveness, following these values over time can be a useful guide to estimating right ventricular (RV) filling pressures [13]. In addition very low or high values point to the likelihood of a positive response to a fluid bolus [14, 15].

It should be recognized that normal physiology places most mammals on the ascending limb of the Frank-Starling curve. Therefore, while a fluid bolus would increase preload and cardiac output, this does not necessarily mean that we are hypovolemic. It is important to acknowledge the difference between hypovolemia and fluid responsiveness in this context.

Of note, there is a close correlation between increases in cardiac output induced by altering preload and that obtained by volume expansion [4]. Thus, assessing the degree of cardiac output or stroke volume change with preload altering maneuvers may help identify patients who are severely hypovolemic and need fluid resuscitation.

Frequent reassessment is necessary; if fluid administration is excessive, the filling pressures increase resulting in pulmonary edema. Therefore, close attention must be paid to both filling pressures (left ventricular [LV] end-diastolic pressure) and cardiac output (heart rate and stroke volume).

What Is Volume Unresponsiveness?

Volume unresponsiveness is an abnormal state, and signifies that the patient's heart is operating on the flat part of the Frank-Starling curve [16]. Further fluid administration under these circumstances does not increase stroke volume, but could be detrimental and cause elevated filling pressures and result in tissue and pulmonary edema. This can be hazardous – patients with large amounts of extravascular lung water (EVLW > 15 ml/kg) have twice the mortality of those without (65% if EVLW > 15 ml/kg, 33% if EVLW < 10 ml/kg) [17]. Hence, close attention should be paid to such patients, and aggressive fluid administration should be avoided.

As shown in the FENICE study, global fluid challenge practices are highly variable and potentially dangerous. For example, the most common indication for fluid resuscitation was hypotension, which is an inaccurate marker of cardiac output. Additionally, predictors of fluid responsiveness and safety limits are rarely used [18].

Methods of Assessment of Fluid Responsiveness

There are multiple ways that a clinician can assess whether a patient is fluid responsive (Box 1). Numerous articles have proven that static measures of preload, filling pressures, pulmonary artery occlusion pressure (PAOP) are poor estimators of true volume responsiveness and only really provide information if they are extreme values [5, 19]. Perhaps the best known example of this is CVP, which is frequently used as a measure of intravascular volume. CVP has only been found to be useful at extremes. When a CVP is extremely low or high it probably represents a volume state; however anything in the middle has too many variables to adequately predict fluid status [14, 15].

Given these limitations of static pressures, we will review only dynamic measures of volume status in the hope of being able to predict and change fluid strategy earlier, prior to the patient moving to a maladaptive state. It should be noted that a dynamic measure, as the name suggests, involves an action and thus is not only more time intensive to measure but also subject to operator variability. Therefore, even though dynamic measures are a better predictor of volume status, the overall feasibility of using the measure, including the time needed to perform the measurement and the ease of preforming the measurement, makes use in clinical practice less accessible and often less frequent.

Mechanical ventilation and active breathing affect preload and filling pressures in the heart and so must be taken into account when interpreting these values. Additionally ventilator settings that cause overdistention of the lung can also impact volume responsiveness. These clinical parameters therefore can be used to help predict volume responsiveness but if not fully understood can confound values. This makes it important to note the context in which each dynamic parameter was validated so that its use is applied appropriately [20, 21].

To explore dynamic parameters, you must either actually increase blood volume or simulate the increase in venous return by using the internal volume. The most common techniques include simply giving a fluid bolus and a passive leg raise (PLR) maneuver. Other techniques can be used to predict fluid responsiveness, most of which use the differences in venous return during the respiratory cycle.

Box 1. Some methods of Assessing Whether a Patient Is Fluid Responsive

Static Macrocirculatory Hemodynamics:
- Mean arterial pressure (MAP)
- Central venous pressure (CVP)
- Pulmonary artery occlusion pressure (PAOP)

Dynamic parameters:
- Response to a fluid challenge
- Superior/inferior vena cava collapsibility
- Pulse pressure variation (PPV) and stroke volume variation (SVV)
- End-tidal CO_2 variation ($etCO_2$)
- End-expiratory occlusion test

Fluid Challenge

The most basic way to measure whether expanding blood volume improves hemodynamics is to expand the blood volume and then observe various clinical markers. This is most readily accomplished by giving crystalloid or colloid at a quick rate. Rates vary but most frequently a bolus of 500 ml in 30 min is used. The major issue with giving fluid is that the challenge is non-reversible and once fluids are given they cannot be readily ungiven. Therefore, if the fluid administration was in fact detrimental, there is no way to readily reverse this. Additionally, since fluid status should be almost continuously assessed as clinical pictures change, continuing to challenge with fluids can be detrimental.

Passive Leg Raise

A PLR maneuver may be the most widely accepted indicator of volume responsiveness. PLR is a dynamic test and similar to infusing a bolus of fluids. The PLR works by displacing approximately 300 ml of blood volume from the lower extremities to the thoracic compartment. By increasing thoracic blood volume, this directly increases preload, which makes this measure unique. The advantage of PLR over a fluid challenge is that the PLR is temporary, as there is no irreversibility. PLR use is limited by the operator's ability to correctly preform the test because clinically it is often implemented incorrectly [21, 22].

PLR responsiveness should be assessed by a direct measurement of cardiac output and not just monitoring of blood pressure. Simply using blood pressure greatly limits the reliability as even arterial pulse pressure measurement can be affected by compliance and pulse wave amplification. Direct measures of cardiac output such as arterial pulse contour analysis (PCA), end-tidal carbon dioxide (etCO_2), echocardiography, esophageal Doppler, or contour analysis of the volume clamp-derived arterial pressure are better measurements of volume status. All of these methods have fewer outside influences and, therefore, provide the most accurate assessment of the efficacy of PLR [22, 23]. PLR can accurately predict volume responsiveness even in the setting of cardiac arrhythmias and spontaneous, invasive and noninvasive ventilation modes.

Ultrasound Assessment of the Inferior (IVC) and Superior (SVC) Vena Cavae

There are several different methods that use the IVC to assess patient volume responsiveness, including IVC dispensibility, IVC collapsibility, and IVC diameter. The first two methods are dynamic, the other static. Each is affected by several factors that influence a patient's hemodynamics. There are currently studies looking at using SVC measurements over IVC measurements, as the SVC has fewer added variables and assumptions because it is the same body compartment as the heart [24, 25].

IVC Distensibility

IVC distensibility is best described in patients who are synchronous and passive on a mechanical ventilator. As the lungs are insufflated with positive pressure there is a reduction in preload. This reduction is enhanced when the pressure in the pulmonary veins is lower. The larger the reduction in preload the more the distention seen in IVC, meaning the more likely the patient is to be volume responsive [26].

The biggest limitation of IVC distensibility is the required use of a relatively high tidal volume with a relatively low positive end-expiratory pressure (PEEP). In addition, truly respiratory passive patients are relatively infrequent [27].

IVC Collapsibility

IVC collapsibility is a method similar to IVC distensibility but it assesses the amount of collapse observed in the IVC during active breaths. Basically, it is the physiologic opposite because the patient is now lowering intrathoracic pressure by making a respiratory effort, as opposed to increasing the thoracic pressure when receiving a positive pressure breath. The heart will partly fill from the IVC and the more volume it takes to support the augmentation of the preload, the more collapse will be seen in the IVC [28–30].

There are limitations to this measure including anything that would affect the balance of forces between the lungs and the right side of the heart as well as anything affecting abdominal pressures. Examples include cardiac remodeling, pulmonary hypertension, pericardial effusions, lung compliance and abdominal hypertension.

IVC Diameter

The measurement of IVC diameter is in essence a static measure and is roughly equivalent in its utility to CVP as they are physiologically similar. Both represent a reservoir that preload can either fill from or back up into. Therefore, almost all the same limitations of CVP should be applied to IVC diameter; however the IVC is additionally confounded by the abdominal pressures.

A meta-analysis of IVC diameter concluded that the maximal IVC diameter during expiration is lower in patients with hypovolemic states than those in euvolemic states, however it failed to establish clear cut-offs which could be used to distinguish these states [31, 32].

Stroke Volume Variation and Pulse Pressure Variation

Stroke volume variation (SVV) can be measured by a variety of methods including echocardiogram and continuous cardiac output monitors. SVV is the change between the maximal and minimal stroke volumes divided by the average value over a period of time. SVV occurs in normal patients who are breathing spontaneously, as the change in intrathoracic pressure causes arterial pulse pressure to decrease during inspiration and rises during expiration. This change is reversed when a patient is placed on positive pressure ventilation. Positive pressure ventilation increases the intrathoracic pressure causing arterial pressure to rise during inspiration and fall during expiration.

Pulse pressure variation (PPV) is obtained from the peripheral arterial pressure waveform. PPV and SVV are the same physiologically and only vary in the way they are measured and in their limitations from the ability to perform the measure and the technical differences in performing the measurements [33–35].

Given the way that both SVV and PPV are measured, neither are accurate in patients with arrhythmias. SVV is only validated with larger tidal volumes. Similarly the compliance of the lung can also affect SVV. Furthermore, increased RV pressure will minimize the effect of respiration on SVV so special consideration should be placed in patients with pulmonary hypertension or RV failure, and conversely the right ventricle can be more responsive with pericardial effusions or constrictive pericarditis [36, 37].

End-tidal CO_2 Variation

etCO_2 has been shown to correlate with cardiac output in patients. Physiologically, etCO_2 is a good surrogate for cardiac output because the lungs receive nearly all the cardiac output, therefor the efficiency in which the CO_2 is removed from the system correlates to the cardiac output. In a patient with a relatively stable metabolic rate this amount of CO_2 produced overtime does not change. Therefore, since the amount of CO_2 is stable, if the exhaled amount changes then it is the cardiac output that varied.

It should be remembered that the production of CO_2 can be affected by things such as fever, seizures, feeding, and infection to name a few. Additionally, the ability of a person to offload the CO_2 produced is related to their lung function meaning that a person with obstructive disease or low diffusing capacity may have a lower $etCO_2$ with each breath so that the $etCO_2$ cut-offs will not be an absolute number but rather a trend for each patient [38, 39]. Therefore, there will never be an equation that can take $etCO_2$ and relate it to cardiac output because it will vary by subject and by conditions.

End-Expiratory Occlusion Test

The end-expiration occlusion test can only be used in an intubated patient. The measurement works because when a mechanical ventilation breath is delivered, there is an increase in intrathoracic pressure, which decreases venous return. If the respiratory cycle is held at end-expiration, venous return is delayed and diminished. Once the hold is stopped, venous return is allowed and what is physiologically similar to a fluid bolus is experienced. The fluid bolus causes an increase in preload and if the patient is fluid responsive, stroke volume will increase.

The hemodynamic effects of an end-expiratory occlusion test can be monitored in various ways including arterial pulse pressure or the pulse contour-derived cardiac output. Because the maneuver occurs over 15 s it thus last for several cardiac cycles, which limits the impact of arrhythmias. The main limit of the end-expiratory occlusion test is the requirement for intubation and the ability to hold the patient's breath for 15 s. Although the test has been validated in patients with acute respiratory distress syndrome (ARDS) [40], more studies are needed to better define response cut-offs [40].

Microcirculatory Parameters

Even with normalization of macrocirculatory parameters, microcirculatory perfusion may remain impaired. This could be related to endothelial malfunction and glycocalyx rupture leading to microthrombi, endotoxin-mediated microvascular dysfunction, and dysregulation of vasomotor tone [41]. Fluid resuscitation can improve microcirculatory flow by increasing flow velocity in vessels that have sluggish flow, and by recruiting non-perfused vessels resulting in increased vascular density and improved oxygen delivery. Recent studies have shown promise with fluid administration targeting microcirculatory parameters and peripheral perfusion parameters, such as capillary refill time, peripheral perfusion index and tissue oxygenation saturation. This approach may lead to more appropriate fluid administration, a lower incidence of organ failure and shorter hospital length of stay, and serves as a complement to macro hemodynamic-targeted fluid resuscitation [41].

The final goal of fluid resuscitation is to improve tissue perfusion. While current guidelines aim for normalization of macro hemodynamic parameters to achieve this goal, this does not necessarily improve oxygen delivery and flow at the cellular level [42]. For example, studies have shown that microcirculatory indices of perfusion are not dependent on changes in cardiac output [43]. More importantly, fluid administration improved microcirculatory flow only in the early stages of sepsis [44]. Even in the volume responsive patient, increasing cardiac output with fluids may still be associated with reduction in oxygen delivery to the cells [42, 45].

Should Fluid Unresponsiveness Be an Endpoint When a Patient's Clinical Problem Persists

Fluid resuscitation is most frequently initiated in patients with hypotension and oliguria and the effectiveness of the response is most often assessed by the effect on blood pressure, urine output, heart rate, filling pressures and, in a few, the change in lactate [18]. Generally, it is believed that when the problem persists and the patient is still fluid responsive, additional fluids are indicated. There is however not much evidence for this. In the first place, following initial resuscitation the half-life of a fluid bolus is very short [46, 47]. Second, in patients with a clinical problem frequently treated with a fluid bolus, the fluid bolus did not improve microcirculatory perfusion even in the responders [43]. Only in patients with abnormal microcirculatory perfusion at baseline did fluid resuscitation result in improved microcirculation and resolution of the clinical problem [45]. Taken even further, Van Genderen et al. [48] showed that not using fluid resuscitation in patients with a clinical problem but normal peripheral circulation seemed to be safe and was associated with a decrease in organ failure when compared to the control group in whom fluid resuscitation was allowed. Also, the early use of norepinephrine instead of fluids to correct severe hypotension was associated with improved global blood flow and improved tissue oxygenation [49].

It could thus be that fluid resuscitation should only be used when a patient is fluid responsive *and* the microcirculation is abnormal. However, more studies are needed before this can be considered a sound clinical recommendation.

Conclusion

Fluid resuscitation should be initiated when the clinical problem one is trying to solve is likely to respond to an increase in cardiac output and, to some extent, blood pressure, brought about by an increase in venous return. Dynamic parameters of fluid responsiveness are more reliable to predict the increase in cardiac output following a fluid bolus then static parameters. Whether the patient should be fluid resuscitated to the un-physiologic state of fluid unresponsiveness while the clinical problem persists is not clear. Some evidence suggests that earlier use of vasopressors to correct hypotension improves tissue perfusion. Restricting fluid administration in septic shock patients with persisting clinical problems but with normal peripheral perfusion seems to be safe.

References

1. Coba V, Whitmill M, Mooney R et al (2011) Resuscitation bundle compliance in severe sepsis and septic shock: improves survival, is better late than never. J Intensive Care Med 26:304–313
2. Brotfain E, Koyfman L, Toledano R et al (2016) Positive fluid balance as a major predictor of clinical outcome of patients with sepsis/septic shock after discharge from intensive care unit. Am J Emerg Med 34:2122–2126
3. Berlin D, Bakker J (2015) Starling curves and central venous pressure. Crit Care 19:55
4. Boyd J, Sirounis D, Maizel J, Slama M (2016) Echocardiography as a guide for fluid management. Crit Care 20:274
5. Marik P, Baram M, Vahid B (2008) Does central venous pressure predict fluid responsiveness? A systematic review of the literature and the tale of seven mares. Chest 134:172–178
6. Vincent J, Quintairos E, Couto L, Taccone FS (2016) The value of blood lactate kinetics in critically ill patients: a systematic review. Crit Care 20:257
7. Jansen TC, van Bommel J, Schoonderbeek FJ et al (2010) Early lactate-guided therapy in intensive care unit patients: a multicenter, open-label, randomized controlled trial. Am J Respir Crit Care Med 182:752–761
8. Hernandez G, Luengo C, Bruhn A et al (2014) When to stop septic shock resuscitation: clues from a dynamic perfusion monitoring. Ann Intensive Care 4:30
9. Levy B (2006) Lactate and shock state: the metabolic view. Curr Opin Crit Care 12:315–321
10. Ospina-Tascon GA, Umana G, Bermudez W et al (2015) Combination of arterial lactate levels and venous-arterial CO2 to arterial-venous O 2 content difference ratio as markers of resuscitation in patients with septic shock. Intensive Care Med 41:796–805
11. Ait-Oufella H, Bourcier S, Alves M et al (2013) Alteration of skin perfusion in mottling area during septic shock. Ann Intensive Care 3:31
12. Brunauer A, Kokofer A, Bataar O et al (2016) Changes in peripheral perfusion relate to visceral organ perfusion in early septic shock: A pilot study. J Crit Care 35:105–109
13. Magder S (2015) Understanding central venous pressure: not a preload index? Curr Opin Crit Care 21:369–375
14. Magder S, Bafaqeeh F (2007) The clinical role of central venous pressure measurements. J Intensive Care Med 22:44–51
15. Heenen S, De Backer D, Vincent JL (2006) How can the response to volume expansion in patients with spontaneous respiratory movements be predicted? Crit Care 10:R102
16. Teboul JL, Monnet X (2009) Detecting volume responsiveness and unresponsiveness in intensive care unit patients: two different problems, only one solution. Crit Care 13:175
17. Sakka SG, Klein M, Reinhart K, Meier-Hellmann A (2002) Prognostic value of extravascular lung water in critically ill patients. Chest 122:2080–2086
18. Cecconi M, Hofer C, Teboul JL et al (2015) Fluid challenges in intensive care: the FENICE study: A global inception cohort study. Intensive Care Med 41:1529–1537
19. Michard F, Teboul JL (2002) Predicting fluid responsiveness in ICU patients: a critical analysis of the evidence. Chest 121:2000–2008
20. Cherpanath TG, Lagrand WK, Schultz MJ, Groeneveld AB (2013) Cardiopulmonary interactions during mechanical ventilation in critically ill patients. Neth Heart J 21:166–172
21. Bendjelid K, Romand JA (2003) Fluid responsiveness in mechanically ventilated patients: a review of indices used in intensive care. Intensive Care Med 29:352–360
22. Monnet X, Teboul JL (2015) Passive leg raising: five rules, not a drop of fluid! Crit Care 19:18

23. Monnet X, Rienzo M, Osman D et al (2006) Passive leg raising predicts fluid responsiveness in the critically ill. Crit Care Med 34:1402–1407
24. Vieillard-Baron A, Chergui K, Rabiller A et al (2004) Superior vena caval collapsibility as a gauge of volume status in ventilated septic patients. Intensive Care Med 30:1734–1739
25. Charbonneau H, Riu B, Faron M et al (2014) Predicting preload responsiveness using simultaneous recordings of inferior and superior vena cavae diameters. Crit Care 18:473
26. Barbier C, Loubieres Y, Schmit C et al (2004) Respiratory changes in inferior vena cava diameter are helpful in predicting fluid responsiveness in ventilated septic patients. Intensive Care Med 30:1740–1746
27. Corl K, Napoli AM, Gardiner F (2012) Bedside sonographic measurement of the inferior vena cava caval index is a poor predictor of fluid responsiveness in emergency department patients. Emerg Med Australas 24:534–539
28. Muller L, Bobbia X, Toumi M et al (2012) Respiratory variations of inferior vena cava diameter to predict fluid responsiveness in spontaneously breathing patients with acute circulatory failure: need for a cautious use. Crit Care 16:R188
29. Lanspa MJ, Grissom CK, Hirshberg EL, Jones JP, Brown SM (2013) Applying dynamic parameters to predict hemodynamic response to volume expansion in spontaneously breathing patients with septic shock: reply. Shock 39:462
30. Feissel M, Michard F, Faller JP, Teboul JL (2004) The respiratory variation in inferior vena cava diameter as a guide to fluid therapy. Intensive Care Med 30:1834–1837
31. Dipti A, Soucy Z, Surana A, Chandra S (2012) Role of inferior vena cava diameter in assessment of volume status: a meta-analysis. Am J Emerg Med 30:1414–1419.e1411
32. Brennan JM, Ronan A, Goonewardena S et al (2006) Handcarried ultrasound measurement of the inferior vena cava for assessment of intravascular volume status in the outpatient hemodialysis clinic. Clin J Am Soc Nephrol 1:749–753
33. De Backer D, Heenen S, Piagnerelli M, Koch M, Vincent JL (2005) Pulse pressure variations to predict fluid responsiveness: influence of tidal volume. Intensive Care Med 31:517–523
34. Lopes MR, Oliveira MA, Pereira VO et al (2007) Goal-directed fluid management based on pulse pressure variation monitoring during high-risk surgery: a pilot randomized controlled trial. Crit Care 11:R100
35. Mahjoub Y, Pila C, Friggeri A et al (2009) Assessing fluid responsiveness in critically ill patients: False-positive pulse pressure variation is detected by Doppler echocardiographic evaluation of the right ventricle. Crit Care Med 37:2570–2575
36. Feissel M, Michard F, Mangin I et al (2001) Respiratory changes in aortic blood velocity as an indicator of fluid responsiveness in ventilated patients with septic shock. Chest 119:867–873
37. Marik PE, Cavallazzi R, Vasu T, Hirani A (2009) Dynamic changes in arterial waveform derived variables and fluid responsiveness in mechanically ventilated patients: a systematic review of the literature. Crit Care Med 37:2642–2647
38. Ornato JP, Garnett AR, Glauser FL (1990) Relationship between cardiac output and the end-tidal carbon dioxide tension. Ann Emerg Med 19:1104–1106
39. Jacquet-Lagreze M, Baudin F, David JS et al (2016) End-tidal carbon dioxide variation after a 100- and a 500-ml fluid challenge to assess fluid responsiveness. Ann Intensive Care 6:37
40. Monnet X, Osman D, Ridel C et al (2009) Predicting volume responsiveness by using the end-expiratory occlusion in mechanically ventilated intensive care unit patients. Crit Care Med 37:951–956
41. Klijn E, Velzen MH, Lima AP et al (2015) Tissue perfusion and oxygenation to monitor fluid responsiveness in critically ill, septic patients after initial resuscitation: a prospective observational study. J Clin Monit Comput 29:707–712
42. Gruartmoner G, Mesquida J, Ince C (2015) Fluid therapy and the hypovolemic microcirculation. Curr Opin Crit Care 21:276–284
43. Pranskunas A, Koopmans M, Koetsier PM, Pilvinis V, Boerma EC (2013) Microcirculatory blood flow as a tool to select ICU patients eligible for fluid therapy. Intensive Care Med 39:612–619

44. Ospina-Tascon G, Neves A, Occhipinti G et al (2010) Effects of fluids on microvascular perfusion in patients with severe sepsis. Intensive Care Med 36:949–955
45. Vellinga NA, Ince C, Boerma EC (2013) Elevated central venous pressure is associated with impairment of microcirculatory blood flow in sepsis: a hypothesis generating post hoc analysis. BMC Anesthesiol 13:17
46. Monge Garcia MI, Guijo Gonzalez P, Gracia Romero M et al (2015) Effects of fluid administration on arterial load in septic shock patients. Intensive Care Med 41:1247–1255
47. Aya HD, Ster IC, Fletcher N et al (2016) Pharmacodynamic analysis of a fluid challenge. Crit Care Med 44:880–891
48. van Genderen ME, Engels N, van der Valk RJ et al (2015) Early peripheral perfusion-guided fluid therapy in patients with septic shock. Am J Respir Crit Care Med 191:477–480
49. Georger JF, Hamzaoui O, Chaari A et al (2010) Restoring arterial pressure with norepinephrine improves muscle tissue oxygenation assessed by near-infrared spectroscopy in severely hypotensive septic patients. Intensive Care Med 36:1882–1889

Use of 'Tidal Volume Challenge' to Improve the Reliability of Pulse Pressure Variation

S. N. Myatra, X. Monnet, and J.-L. Teboul

Introduction

Fluid loading is usually the first step in the resuscitation of patients with acute circulatory failure. Fluid responsiveness is defined as the ability of the left ventricle to increase its stroke volume in response to fluid administration [1]. Fluids are administered with the aim of increasing cardiac output and oxygen delivery. Thus giving fluid is not beneficial if cardiac output does not increase. According to the Frank-Starling principle, increasing preload increases the left ventricular (LV) stroke volume if the ventricle is functioning on the steep portion of the Frank-Starling curve. Once the left ventricle is functioning on the flat portion of the curve, further fluid loading has little effect on the stroke volume. In a normal heart, both ventricles generally operate on the steep portion of the Frank-Starling curve and the patient is fluid responsive, unless large fluid volumes have already been administered (Fig. 1). In this case, the ventricles may operate on the flat part of the curve (Fig. 1). A failing heart operates on the flat portion of the curve, except for very low preload values and thus the same increase in cardiac preload induced by volume expansion may result in a negligible increase in stroke volume (Fig. 1).

Studies have shown that only about 50% of unstable critically ill patients will actually respond positively to a fluid challenge [1]. Uncorrected hypovolemia may result in inappropriate administration of vasopressor infusions, which may in turn affect tissue oxygenation, leading to organ dysfunction and death [2, 3]. On the other hand, excessive fluid loading is associated with increased complications, mortality and duration of intensive care unit (ICU) stay [4, 5]. Thus, it is important to

S. N. Myatra
Department of Anesthesiology, Critical Care and Pain, Tata Memorial Hospital
Mumbai, India

X. Monnet · J.-L. Teboul (✉)
Service de Réanimation Médicale, AP-HP, Hôpitaux Universitaires Paris-Sud, Hôpital de Bicêtre
78 rue du Général Leclerc, 94270 Le Kremlin-Bicêtre, France
e-mail: jean-louis.teboul@aphp.fr

J.-L. Vincent (ed.), *Annual Update in Intensive Care and Emergency Medicine 2017*,
DOI 10.1007/978-3-319-51908-1_7

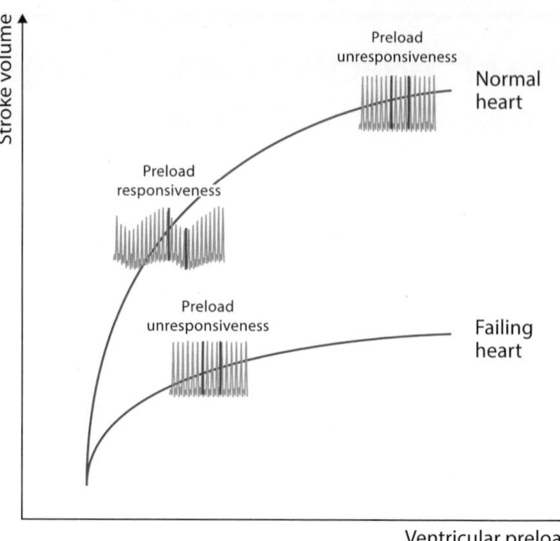

Fig. 1 Frank-Starling curves in a normal and failing heart. The same increase in cardiac preload induced by volume expansion may result in a significant increase (*normal heart*) or a negligible increase (*failing heart*) in stroke volume, depending upon the shape of the curve

identify fluid responders to know who can benefit from fluid administration and to avoid fluid overload in those who are not fluid responsive. However, identifying which patients will respond to volume expansion presents a daily challenge in ICUs today.

Dynamic changes in arterial waveform-derived variables during mechanical ventilation, such as systolic pressure variation (SPV), pulse pressure variation (PPV) and stroke volume variation (SVV), have proven to be superior to traditionally used static indices, such as central venous pressure (CVP) and pulmonary artery occlusion pressure (PAOP), to predict fluid responsiveness [1, 6–8]. Of these indices, PPV and SVV are commonly used in clinical practice, with PPV being more reliable and having a higher level of evidence [7, 9, 10].

Heart-lung Interactions During Mechanical Ventilation: Physiological Principles Underlying PPV and SVV

The PPV is calculated as the difference between the maximal and the minimal pulse pressure value over one ventilator cycle divided by their average value [6]. It can be automatically calculated by newer hemodynamic monitors. The SVV is derived from the arterial pressure waveform analysis and is automatically calculated by calibrated and uncalibrated pulse contour analysis cardiac output monitors. The principle mechanisms underlying how these parameters work are based on heart-lung interactions during mechanical ventilation [11].

Intermittent positive-pressure ventilation produces cyclic changes in the loading conditions of both the ventricles. The intrathoracic and transpulmonary pressures increase during inspiration leading to variable changes in the loading conditions of both the ventricles. Increase in intrathoracic pressures during mechanical insufflation decreases venous return and in turn decreases the right ventricular (RV) preload, whereas an increase in transpulmonary pressure increases RV afterload resulting in decreased RV stroke volume, which will be at its lowest at the end of inspiration [11–16]. At the same time, an increase in the intrathoracic and transpulmonary pressures results in decreased LV afterload and a transient increase in LV preload due to squeezing out of alveolar blood, leading to increased LV stroke volume, which will be at its maximum at the end of inspiration [11]. The reduction in RV stroke volume during inspiration leads to decreased LV filling after a lag period of two to three heart beats due to the pulmonary transit time [17]. This leads to decreased LV stroke volume, which will be its lowest during expiration.

Thus, intermittent positive-pressure ventilation produces cyclic changes in LV stroke volume, which is maximum during inspiration and lowest during expiration. The magnitude of change in LV stroke volume, or of its surrogates, such as pulse pressure, will be magnified when the patient is preload-dependent. Therefore, a high PPV value should be associated with preload responsiveness and a low PPV value with preload unresponsiveness (Fig. 1). A threshold value greater than 12–13% has been reported to be highly predictive of volume responsiveness [7, 9, 10].

Comparison of Dynamic Changes of Arterial Waveform-derived Variables During Mechanical Ventilation (SPV, PPV and SVV)

Since the earliest studies about PPV and SVV [6, 17], both indices have been consistently shown to be reliable predictors of fluid responsiveness. The first systematic review by Marik et al. [7] comparing PPV, SPV and SVV for prediction of fluid responsiveness in mechanically ventilated patients showed that the areas under the receiver operating characteristic curves (AUC) were 0.94, 0.84, and 0.86, respectively. The AUC for PPV was significantly greater than that for either the SPV or the SVV ($p<0.001$). Another meta-analysis [9] comparing SVV and PPV as diagnostic indicators of fluid responsiveness in mechanically ventilated critically ill patients showed AUC values of 0.84 for SVV and 0.88 for PPV. A recent meta-analysis [10] that included only ICU patients ventilated with tidal volumes > 8 ml/kg, showed that PPV predicted fluid responsiveness accurately with an AUC of 0.94. A comparison of the predictive value of variables used to determine fluid responsiveness in these three systematic reviews [7, 9, 10] is given in Table 1. Among PPV, SVV and SPV, PPV has been most extensively studied and is more reliable.

Table 1 Comparison of predictive value of variables used to determine fluid responsiveness in mechanically ventilated patients in three systematic reviews

Systematic review/meta-analysis	Publication year	Types of studies	Patient type	Variable	AUC (95% confidence interval)
Marik et al. [7]	2009	29 studies 685 patients variable tidal volume	ICU and OR patients	**PPV**	**0.94 (0.93–0.95)**
				SPV	0.86 (0.82–0.90)
				SVV	0.84 (0.78–0.88)
				LVEDA	0.64 (0.53–0.74)
				GEDV	0.56 (0.37–0.67)
				CVP	0.55 (0.48–0.62)
Hong et al. [9]	2014	19 studies 850 patients variable tidal volume	Only ICU patients	**PPV**	**0.88 (0.84–0.92)**
				SVV	0.84 (0.79–0.89)
Yang and Du [10]	2014	22 studies 807 patients tidal volume > 8 ml/kg	Only ICU patients	**PPV**	**0.94 (0.91–0.95)**

AUC: area under the curve; *ICU*: intensive care unit; *OR*: operating room; *PPV*: pulse pressure variation; *SPV*: systolic pressure variation; *SVV*: stroke volume variation; *LVEDA*: left ventricular end-diastolic area; *GEDV*: global end-diastolic volume; *CVP*: central venous pressure

Limitations with the Use of PPV to Predict Fluid Responsiveness

The PPV works on heart-lung interactions and has several limitations for use in predicting fluid responsiveness, which are enumerated in Table 2. Recent studies [18–20] have questioned the applicability of PPV and SVV in the ICU. Tests like passive leg raising (PLR) [21–23] and end-expiratory occlusion [24–26] can reliably predict fluid responsiveness and have been proposed as alternatives to be performed in these situations. PLR can help overcome most of the limitations of PPV. However, it requires continuous cardiac output monitoring and cannot be used in patients with neurotrauma or those requiring immobilization [27, 28]. The end-expiratory occlusion test is not suitable for patients who are not intubated, whereas PLR can be reliably used in these patients. A mini-fluid challenge [29] may also be used as an alternative to PPV, but requires a very precise technique for monitoring cardiac output. Using respiratory variations in the diameters of the superior [31] and inferior [30] vena cavae diameter obtained from transesophageal or transthoracic echocardiography to predict fluid responsiveness has share the same limitations as PPV, except that they can be used in patients with cardiac arrhythmias. Although alternative tests have been proposed, few attempts have been made to improve the reliability of PPV itself in situations where it is currently not recommended for use [32].

Table 2 Limitations with the use of pulse pressure variation (PPV) to predict fluid responsiveness

	Limitations	Mechanisms for failure	Type of error
1	Spontaneous breathing activity	Irregular variations in intrathoracic pressure and thus the variation in stroke volume cannot correlate with preload dependency	False positive (may occasionally be false negative depending on the type of breathing)
2	Cardiac arrhythmias	The variation in stroke volume is related more to the irregularity in diastole than to the heart-lung interactions	False positive
3	Mechanical ventilation using low tidal volume (< 8 ml/kg)	The small variations in intrathoracic pressure due to the low tidal volume are insufficient to produce significant changes in the intrathoracic pressure	False negative
4	Low lung compliance	The transmission of changes in alveolar pressure to the intrathoracic structures is attenuated	False negative
5	Open thorax	No change in intrathoracic pressure during the respiratory cycle	False negative
6	Increased intra-abdominal pressure	Threshold values of PPV will be elevated	False positive
7	Low HR/RR ratio < 3.6 (severe bradycardia or high frequency ventilation)	If the RR is very high, the number of cardiac cycles per respiratory cycle may be too low to allow variation in stroke volume	False negative

HR: heart rate; *RR*: respiratory rate

Using a 'Tidal Volume Challenge' to Overcome the Limitations Associated with PPV During Low Tidal Volume Ventilation

Several studies have shown that PPV does not reliably predict fluid responsiveness during low tidal volume ventilation [25, 33–37]. De Backer et al. [33] showed that PPV was a reliable predictor of fluid responsiveness, provided that the tidal volume was at least 8 ml/kg predicted body weight (PBW). During low tidal volume ventilation, PPV may indicate a non-responsive status even in responders as the tidal volume might be insufficient to produce a significant change in the intrathoracic pressure [38, 39]. However, Freitas et al. [40] showed that PPV was a reliable marker of fluid responsiveness in septic patients with acute respiratory distress syndrome (ARDS) during low tidal volume ventilation using a lower cut-off value of 6.5%.

Among the limitations with use of PPV during controlled mechanical ventilation in the ICU, the use of low tidal volume is the most common. Today the indications for use of low tidal volume in ICU are expanding [41, 42]. Two multicenter studies [18, 19] showed that the number of ICU patients in whom PPV was suitable for use was very low, with as many as 72–87% of the patients on controlled mechanical ventilation being unsuitable for use of this parameter, because of use of low tidal volume ventilation. Two recent studies [43, 44] that used the 'gray zone' approach to investigate the clinical value of PPV, included several patients ventilated with low tidal volume. Biais et al. [44], in a subgroup analysis, showed that the gray zone was larger in patients ventilated with a low tidal volume than in patients with a tidal volume of at least 8 ml/kg PBW. These studies may mislead one to conclude that PPV has limited clinical value [32].

The 'tidal volume challenge' is a novel test proposed to improve the reliability of PPV during low tidal volume ventilation [45]. The test involves transiently increasing tidal volume from 6 ml/kg PBW to 8 ml/kg PBW for one minute and observing the change in PPV (ΔPPV_{6-8}) from baseline (PPV_6) to that at 8 ml/kg PBW (PPV_8). In a recent study testing the tidal volume challenge [45], 30 sets of measurements were recorded in 20 patients with acute circulatory failure receiving low tidal volume ventilation using volume assist-control ventilation and without spontaneous breathing activity. Fluid responsiveness was defined as an increase in thermodilution cardiac output > 15% after giving a fluid bolus after reducing tidal volume back to 6 m/kg PBW. As expected, the PPV_6 could not predict fluid responsiveness, with an AUC of 0.69. Importantly, there was a significant increase in PPV (ΔPPV_{6-8}), following the tidal volume challenge only in fluid responders. The ΔPPV_{6-8} discriminated responders from non-responders with an AUC of 0.99 (sensitivity 94% and specificity 100%) with a cut off value of 3.5% [45]. The tidal volume challenge thus improved the reliability of PPV in predicting fluid responsiveness in patients receiving low tidal volume ventilation. Similar results were also seen using SVV (ΔSVV_{6-8}) obtained from a pulse contour analysis cardiac output device with an AUC of 0.97 (sensitivity 88% and specificity 100%) with a cut off value of 2.5% [45]. The change in PPV after giving a fluid bolus (ΔPPV_{fb}) also accurately confirmed fluid responsiveness with an AUC of 0.98 (sensitivity 94% and specificity 100%) with a cut off value of 1.5%.

How to Perform and Interpret the Tidal Volume Challenge

This test is performed to assess fluid responsiveness in patents in shock, ventilated using low tidal volume without spontaneous breathing activity. The PPV is noted from the bedside monitor at baseline (tidal volume 6 ml/kg PBW). The tidal volume is then transiently increased from 6 ml/kg PBW to 8 ml/kg PBW for one minute. The PPV is recorded at 8 ml/kg PBW and the tidal volume is reduced back to 6 ml/kg PBW. The ΔPPV_{6-8} after performing the tidal volume challenge is recorded. A ΔPPV_{6-8} greater than 3.5% predicts fluid responsiveness with high accuracy.

PPV is unreliable in patients with low lung compliance, especially in patients with ARDS [38]. In these patients, airway pressure transmission is reduced, such that the cyclic changes in intrathoracic pressure may be attenuated even with marked changes in alveolar pressure [46]. Monnet et al. [25] showed that the predictive value of PPV was related to compliance of the respiratory system and if compliance was $< 30\,ml/cmH_2O$, PPV was less accurate in predicting fluid responsiveness. In our study, although the median compliance of the respiratory system was $< 30\,ml/cmH_2O$ (25 [23–33]) during low tidal volume ventilation, it increased to $> 30\,ml/cmH_2O$ (32 [24–40]) after the tidal volume challenge. Thus, the tidal volume challenge may help identify responders even when compliance of the respiratory system is low in patients receiving low tidal volume ventilation with recruitable lungs. This needs to be confirmed in an adequately powered study. Whether this approach will also work in patients who do not increase compliance of the respiratory system after giving a tidal volume challenge needs to be tested. Whether PPV will be reliable during spontaneous breathing attempts after giving a tidal volume challenge or in other situations where use of PPV is limited also needs to be tested.

Advantages of Using the Tidal Volume Challenge

Use of a tidal volume challenge increases the reliability of PPV to predict fluid responsiveness during low tidal volume ventilation, which is now common practice in the ICU. It is a simple test that can be performed easily at the bedside. Importantly, observing the changes in PPV (obtained from a simple bedside hemodynamic monitor) during this test does not require a cardiac output monitor, making this test applicable even in resource-limited settings. The ΔPPV_{fb} accurately confirms fluid responsiveness. Thus, a combination of ΔPPV_{6-8} with ΔPPV_{fb} can help predict and thereafter confirm fluid responsiveness when continuous cardiac output monitoring is unavailable.

Limitations of the Tidal Volume Challenge

The tidal volume challenge may not be able to overcome the other limitations associated with the use of PPV, such as spontaneous breathing, cardiac arrhythmias, open chest, and raised intra-abdominal pressure and needs to be evaluated in these settings. Alternative techniques, such as PLR or end-expiratory occlusion, when applicable, may be considered in these situations.

Conclusion

The PPV is a dynamic parameter that can be easily recorded from a bedside monitor and reliably predicts preload responsiveness. In addition, it does not require continuous cardiac output monitoring or any other tools or maneuvers to be performed. One of the major limitations with its use in patients receiving controlled mechanical ventilation is that it is unreliable during low tidal volume ventilation, which is now widely practiced in ICU patients. Discarding this useful parameter would, however, be like throwing the baby out with the bathwater. This major limitation can be easily overcome by using the 'tidal volume challenge' a simple bedside test, following which PPV can reliably predict fluid responsiveness. Whether this test may also have the potential to overcome other limitations associated with the use of PPV needs to be further studied. Alternative methods to assess preload responsiveness may be required to overcome the other limitations with the use of PPV.

References

1. Michard F, Teboul JL (2002) Predicting fluid responsiveness in ICU patients: a critical analysis of the evidence. Chest 121:2000–2008
2. Murakawa K, Kobayashi A (1998) Effects of vasopressors on renal tissue gas tensions during hemorrhagic shock in dogs. Crit Care Med 16:789–792
3. Pinsky MR, Brophy P, Padilla J, Paganini E, Pannu N (2008) Fluid and volume monitoring. Int J Artif Organs 31:111–126
4. Wiedemann HP, Wheeler AP, Bernard GR et al (2006) Comparison of two fluid-management strategies in acute lung injury. N Engl J Med 354:2564–2575
5. Acheampong A, Vincent JL (2015) A positive fluid balance is an independent prognostic factor in patients with sepsis. Crit Care 19:251
6. Michard F, Boussat S, Chemla D et al (2000) Relation between respiratory changes in arterial pulse pressure and fluid responsiveness in septic patients with acute circulatory failure. Am J Respir Crit Care Med 162:134–138
7. Marik PE, Cavallazzi R, Vasu T, Hirani A (2009) Dynamic changes in arterial waveform derived variables and fluid responsiveness in mechanically ventilated patients. A systematic review of the literature. Crit Care Med 37:2642–2647
8. Perel A, Pizov R, Cotev S (2014) Respiratory variations in the arterial pressure during mechanical ventilation reflect volume status and fluid responsiveness. Intensive Care Med 40:798–807
9. Hong JQ, He HF, Chen ZY et al (2014) Comparison of stroke volume variation with pulse pressure variation as a diagnostic indicator of fluid responsiveness in mechanically ventilated critically ill patients. Saudi Med J 35:261–268
10. Yang X, Du B (2014) Does pulse pressure variation predicts fluid responsiveness in critically ill patients: a critical review and meta-analysis. Crit Care 18:650
11. Michard F, Teboul JL (2000) Using heart lung interactions to assess fluid responsiveness during mechanical ventilation. Crit Care 4:282–289
12. Morgan BC, Martin WE, Hornbein TF, Crawford EW, Guntheroth WG (1966) Hemodynamic effects of intermittent positive pressure ventilation. Anesthesiology 27:584–590
13. Jardin F, Delorme G, Hardy A, Auvert B, Beauchet A, Bourdarias JP (1990) Reevaluation of hemodynamic consequences of positive pressure ventilation: emphasis on cyclic right ventricular afterloading by mechanical lung inflation. Anesthesiology 72:966–970
14. Permutt S, Wise RA, Brower RG (1989) How changes in pleural and alveolar pressure cause changes in afterload and preload. In: Scharf SM, Cassidy SS (eds) Heart-Lung Interactions in Health and Disease. Marcel Dekker, New York, pp 243–250
15. Jardin F, Farcot JC, Gueret P, Prost JF, Ozier Y, Bourdarias JP (1983) Cyclic changes in arterial pulse during respiratory support. Circulation 68:266–274
16. Scharf SM, Brown R, Saunders N, Green LH (1980) Hemodynamic effects of positive-pressure inflation. J Appl Physiol 49:124–131
17. Berkenstadt H, Margalit N, Hadani M et al (2001) Stroke volume variation as a predictor of fluid responsiveness in patients undergoing brain surgery. Anesth Analg 92:984–989
18. Mahjoub Y, Lejeune V, Muller L et al (2014) Evaluation of pulse pressure variation validity criteria in critically ill patients: a prospective observational multicentre point prevalence study. Br J Anaesth 112:681–685
19. Fischer MO, Mahjoub Y, Boisselier C et al (2015) Arterial pulse pressure variation suitability in critical care: A French national survey. Anaesth Crit Care Pain Med 34:23–28

20. Benes J, Zatloukal J, Kletecka J, Simanova A, Haidingerova L, Pradl R (2013) Respiratory induced dynamic variations of stroke volume and its surrogates as predictors of fluid responsiveness: applicability in the early stages of specific critical states. J Clin Monit Comput 28:225–231
21. Monnet X, Marik P, Teboul JL (2016) Passive leg raising for predicting fluid responsiveness: a systematic review and meta-analysis. Intensive Care Med 42:1935–1947
22. Monnet X, Teboul JL (2008) Passive leg raising. Intensive Care Med 34:659–663
23. Monnet X, Teboul JL (2015) Passive leg raising: five rules, not a drop of fluid! Crit Care 19:18
24. Monnet X, Osman D, Ridel C, Lamia B, Richard C, Teboul JL (2009) Predicting volume responsiveness by using the end-expiratory occlusion in mechanically ventilated intensive care unit patients. Crit Care Med 37:951–956
25. Monnet X, Bleibtreu A, Ferré A et al (2012) Passive leg-raising and end-expiratory occlusion tests perform better than pulse pressure variation in patients with low respiratory system compliance. Crit Care Med 40:152–157
26. Silva S, Jozwiak M, Teboul JL, Persichini R, Richard C, Monnet X (2013) End-expiratory occlusion test predicts preload responsiveness independently of positive end-expiratory pressure during acute respiratory distress syndrome. Crit Care Med 41:1692–1701
27. Guerin L, Monnet X, Teboul JL (2013) Monitoring volume and fluid responsiveness: From static to dynamic indicators. Best Pract Res Clin Anaesthesiol 27:177–185
28. De Backer D, Pinsky MR (2007) Can one predict fluid responsiveness in spontaneously breathing patients? Intensive Care Med 33:1111–1113
29. Muller L, Toumi M, Bousquet PJ et al (2011) An increase in aortic blood flow after an infusion of 100 ml colloid over 1 minute can predict fluid responsiveness: the mini-fluid challenge study. Anesthesiology 115:541–547
30. Feissel M, Michard F, Faller JP, Teboul JL (2004) The respiratory variation in inferior vena cava diameter as a guide to fluid therapy. Intensive Care Med 30:1834–1837
31. Vieillard-Baron A, Chergui K, Rabiller A et al (2004) Superior vena caval collapsibility as a gauge of volume status in ventilated septic patients. Intensive Care Med 30:1734–1739
32. Michard F, Chemla D, Teboul JL (2015) Applicability of pulse pressure variation: how many shades of grey? Crit Care 19:144
33. De Backer D, Heenen S, Piagnerelli M, Koch M, Vincent J (2005) Pulse pressure variations to predict fluid responsiveness: influence of tidal volume. Intensive Care Med 31:517–523
34. Vallée F, Richard JC, Mari A et al (2009) Pulse pressure variations adjusted by alveolar driving pressure to assess fluid responsiveness. Intensive Care Med 35:1004–1010
35. Lakhal K, Ehrmann S, Benzekri-Lefèvre D et al (2011) Respiratory pulse pressure variation fails to predict fluid responsiveness in acute respiratory distress syndrome. Crit Care 15:R85
36. Lansdorp B, Lemson J, vanPutten MJ, de Keijzer A, van der Hoeven JG, Pickkers P (2012) Dynamic indices do not predict volume responsiveness in routine clinical practice. Br J Anaesth 108:395–401
37. Reuter DA, Bayerlein J, Goepfert MS et al (2003) Influence of tidal volume on left ventricular stroke volume variation measured by pulse contour analysis in mechanically ventilated patients. Intensive Care Med 29:476–480
38. Teboul JL, Monnet X (2013) Pulse pressure variation and ARDS. Minerva Anestesiol 79:398–407
39. Pinsky MR (2004) Using ventilation-induced aortic pressure and flow variation to diagnose preload responsiveness. Intensive Care Med 30:1008–1010
40. Freitas FG, Bafi AT, Nascente AP et al (2013) Predictive value of pulse pressure variation for fluid responsiveness in septic patients using lung-protective ventilation strategies. Br J Anaesth 110:402–408
41. Serpa Neto A, Cardoso SO, Manetta JA et al (2012) Association between use of lung-protective ventilation with lower tidal volumes and clinical outcomes among patients without acute respiratory distress syndrome: a meta-analysis. JAMA 308:1651–1659

42. Futier E, Pereira B, Jaber S (2013) Intraoperative low-tidal-volume ventilation. N Engl J Med 369:1862–1863
43. Cannesson M, Le Manach Y, Hofer C et al (2011) Assessing the diagnostic accuracy of pulse pressure variations for the prediction of fluid responsiveness: a "gray zone" approach. Anesthesiology 115:231–241
44. Biais M, Ehrmann S, Mari A et al (2014) Clinical relevance of pulse pressure variations for predicting fluid responsiveness in mechanically ventilated intensive care unit patients: the grey zone approach. Crit Care 18:587
45. Myatra SN, Prabu NR, Divatia JV, Monnet X, Kulkarni AP, Teboul JL (2016) The changes in pulse pressure variation or stroke volume variation after a "tidal volume challenge" reliably predict fluid responsiveness during low tidal volume ventilation. Crit Care Med. doi:10.1097/CCM0000000000002183
46. Teboul JL, Pinsky MR, Mercat A et al (2000) Estimating cardiac filling pressure in mechanically ventilated patients with hyperinflation. Crit Care Med 28:3631–3636

Distribution of Crystalloids and Colloids During Fluid Resuscitation: All Fluids Can be Good and Bad?

I. László, N. Öveges, and Z. Molnár

Introduction

Early fluid resuscitation remains the cornerstone of the treatment of severe hypovolemia, bleeding and septic shock. Although during these circumstances fluid administration is a life-saving intervention, it can also exert a number of adverse and potentially life-threatening effects; hence fluid therapy by-and-large is regarded a "double-edged sword" [1]. Unfortunately, for the three fundamental questions of: 'when', 'what' and 'how much', there are no universally accepted answers. Nevertheless, not giving enough volume may result in inadequate cardiac output and oxygen delivery (DO_2) and hence severe oxygen debt; while fluid overload can cause edema formation both in vital organs and in the periphery, hence impairing tissue perfusion. Despite broad acceptance of the importance of using appropriate parameters to guide treatment during resuscitation, current practice seems rather uncoordinated worldwide as was recently demonstrated in the FENICE trial [2]. In addition to using appropriate hemodynamic parameters to guide fluid resuscitation, the type of the infusion fluid should also be chosen carefully.

Fundamentally, crystalloids *or* colloids are suitable for fluid resuscitation. Theoretically, colloids have better volume expansion effects, therefore they restore the circulating blood volume and hence DO_2 faster than crystalloids do. The natural colloid, albumin, is very expansive compared to crystalloids, but the cheaper synthetic colloids have several potential adverse effects. Ever since colloids appeared on the scene the 'crystalloid-colloid debate' started, which seems like a never-ending story. At present, the gigantic pendulum that swings our opinion between 'good' and 'bad' based on current evidence, points more to the latter where synthetic colloids are concerned.

I. László · N. Öveges · Z. Molnár (✉)
Department of Anesthesiology and Intensive Care, University of Szeged
6 Semmelweis St., 6725 Szeged, Hungary
e-mail: zsoltmolna@gmail.com

J.-L. Vincent (ed.), *Annual Update in Intensive Care and Emergency Medicine 2017*,
DOI 10.1007/978-3-319-51908-1_8

According to Starling's '3-compartment model', crystalloids, with their sodium content similar to that of the serum, are distributed in the extracellular space, while colloids should remain intravascular because of their large molecular weight. Therefore, theoretically one unit of blood loss can be replaced by 3–4 units of crystalloid and one unit of colloid solution [3]. This theory has a long history and has been widely accepted worldwide since the 1960s [4]. However, several clinical trials including thousands of critically ill patients seemed to disapprove this principle as there were no large differences in the volumes of crystalloids versus colloids needed to stabilize these patients.

Understanding physiology, especially the role of the recently discovered multiple functions of the endothelial glycocalyx layer, may cast a different light on these controversies. The purpose of this chapter is to highlight several issues, which should be taken into account when we are interpreting the results of recent clinical trials on crystalloid and colloid fluid resuscitation.

Starling's Hypothesis Revisited in the Context of the Glycocalyx

Fundamentally, there are three infusion solutions that can be administered intravenously: water, in the form of 5% dextrose; crystalloids, containing sodium ions in similar concentration to that of the plasma; and colloids, which are macromolecules of either albumin or synthetic colloid molecules, such as hydroxyethyl starches (HES), dextrans or gelatin solutions.

According to the classic Starling view, the main determinants of fluid transport between the three main fluid compartments of the intracellular, interstitial and intravascular spaces are determined mainly by the two semipermeable membranes: the endothelium and the cell membrane (Fig. 1). Water and glucose molecules can pass freely from the vasculature to the cells, hence they are distributed in the total body water. Sodium containing crystalloids can pass the endothelium but not the cell membrane, hence these are distributed in the extracellular space, proportionally to the volume of the interstitial and intravascular compartments to the total extracellular fluid volume (Fig. 2). Colloids, because of their large molecular weight should remain intravascularly (Fig. 3).

The filtration rate per unit area across the capillary wall is mainly determined by hydrostatic and colloid osmotic pressures as indicated by the classic Starling's equation:

$$J_v = K_f((P_c - P_i) - \sigma(\pi_i - \pi_c))$$

where J_v is the fluid movement; $(P_c - P_i) - \sigma(\pi_i - \pi_c)$ is the driving force; P_c is the capillary hydrostatic pressure; P_i is the interstitial hydrostatic pressure; π_i is the interstitial oncotic pressure; π_c is the capillary oncotic pressure; K_f is the filtration coefficient; and σ is the reflection coefficient.

However, there is some evidence that in most tissues lymphatic flow would be insufficient to handle the extravasation of the amount of fluid as predicted by Starling, a phenomenon also termed the "low lymph flow paradox" [5, 6]. It has

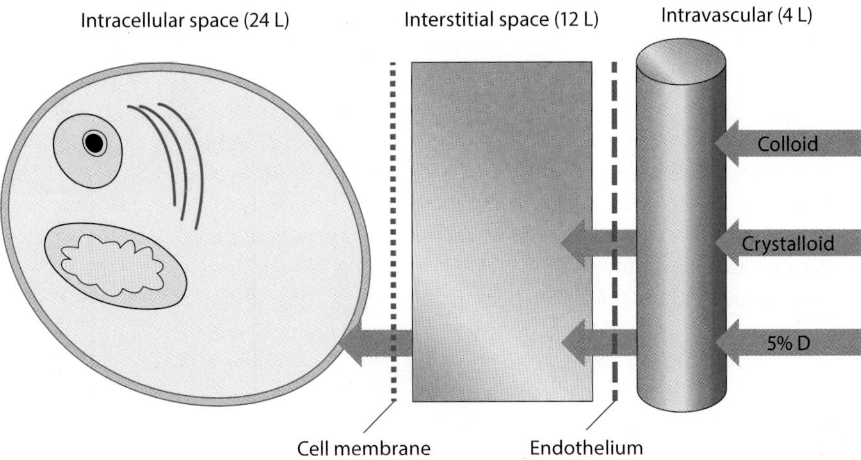

Fig. 1 Fluid distribution in the three main fluid compartments. In a normal (70 kg) adult, the total body water is about 60% of the total body weight, approximately 40 L, divided into intracellular (~24 L), interstitial (~12 L) and intravascular (~4 L) spaces separated by the endothelium and the cell membrane. According to Starling's classic '3 compartmental model' fluid distribution is mainly determined by these semipermeable membranes. Therefore, colloids stay in the intravascular compartment, crystalloids are distributed in the extracellular space, and water, in the form of 5% dextrose (5%D), is distributed in total body water

Fig. 2 Crystalloid distribution between the 3 compartments in normal subjects. Crystalloid solutions can pass the endothelium freely, but not the cell membrane because of their sodium ion content, hence they cannot enter the intracellular (IC) compartment. Therefore, they are distributed in the intravascular (IV) and the interstitial (IS) compartments. The rate of distribution between these two compartments is determined by how each relates in volume to the total extracellular fluid volume (12 + 4 = 16 L in our example in Fig. 1). Accordingly, for every unit of infused crystalloid, one fourth will remain intravascularly and three fourths interstitially

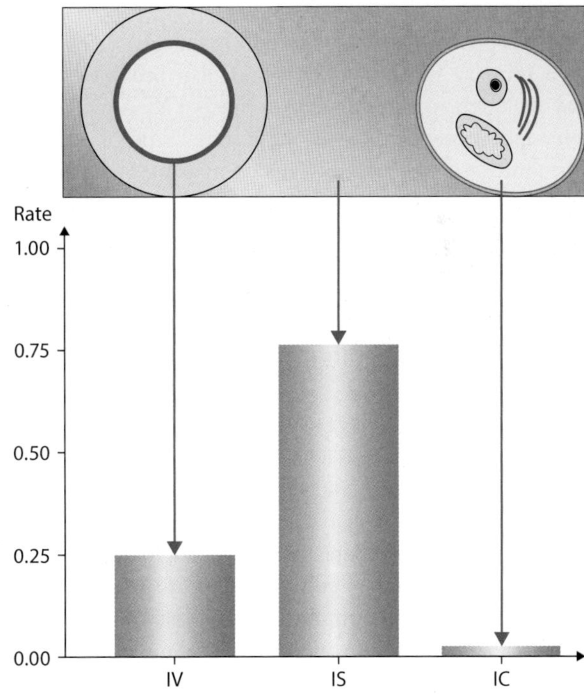

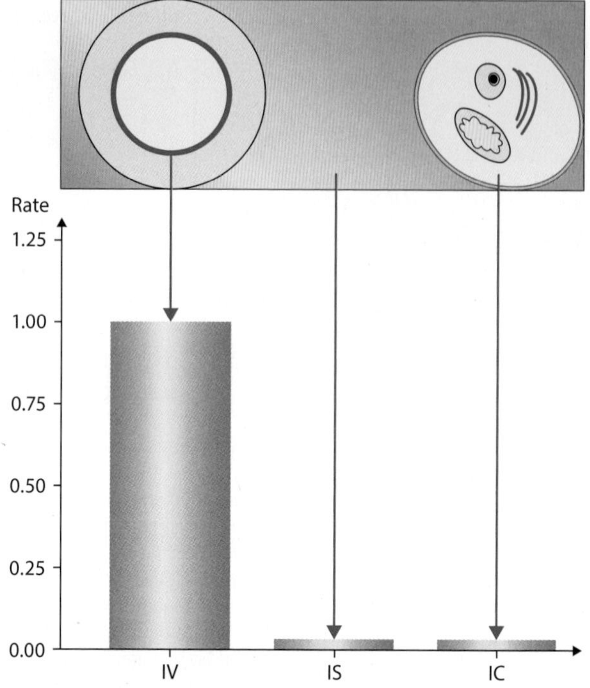

Fig. 3 Colloid distribution in normal subjects. Theoretically, due to their molecular weight, colloids should remain in the intravascular space. *IV*: intravascular; *IS*: interstitial; *IC*: intracellular spaces

been proposed that it is the endothelial glycocalyx layer that plays a pivotal role as a primary molecular filter and also provides an oncotic gradient, which was not included in Starling's hypothesis [7]. A web of membrane-bound glycoproteins and proteoglycans on the luminal side of endothelium has been identified to form the glycocalyx layer. This compartment consists of many highly sulfated glycosaminoglycan chains providing a negative charge for the endothelium. Due to these electrostatic properties, the subglycocalyx space produces a colloid oncotic pressure that may be an important determinant of vascular permeability and thus fluid balance [8]. The structure and function of the endothelial glycocalyx varies substantially among different organ systems, and it is also affected by several inflammatory conditions [9].

In a recent experiment on isolated guinea pig heart, Jacob et al. observed a very interesting phenomenon [10]. They perfused the coronaries with colloid free buffer, isotonic saline, albumin and HES solution, and measured extravascular transudate and edema formation. The experiment was then repeated when the glycocalyx was stripped from the vessel wall by treating it with heparinase. With intact glycocalyx, the net transudate, measured as hydraulic conductivity, was found to be 9.14 µl/min/g tissue for colloid free perfusion, which was dramatically reduced to 1.04 µl/min/g when albumin was added in physiological concentration to the perfusate. It was also attenuated by HES supplementation but to a significantly lesser degree, to 2.67 µl/min/g. The observation that adding colloids to the perfusate reduced extravasation, seemingly confirms Starling's hypothesis, but interestingly, this effect did not correlate with the colloid osmotic pressure: albumin, which is a much smaller molecule than HES, had significantly better effects in preventing transudate formation. This phenomenon is termed the "colloid osmotic pressure paradox", and cannot be fully explained by Starling's hypothesis and equation. One of the possible explanations is that the charges exposed by molecules forming the glycocalyx are mainly negative, whereas albumin carries molecules such as arginine and lysine with positive charges. There is some experimental evidence that these arginine groups are responsible for the effects of albumin on vascular permeability. By contrast, HES molecules are uniformly negatively charged, which may explain the significant difference in hydraulic conductivity observed by Jacob and coworkers [10].

These authors also suggested modifying the Starling equation to:

$$J_v/A = L_p((P_c - P_t) - (\pi_e - \pi_g))$$

where J_v / A is the filtration rate per unit area; L_p the hydraulic conductivity of the vessel wall; $P_c - P_t$ the difference in hydrostatic pressure between the capillary lumen (c) and tissue (t); π_e the colloid osmotic pressure in the endothelial surface layer; and π_g the colloid osmotic pressures directly below the endothelial surface layer in the glycocalyx.

Nevertheless, under normal circumstances, when the glycocalyx is intact, the Starling concept is still valid and fluid transport is determined by the 'Starling forces' (Fig. 4a), and the volume-replacement ratio should be several times higher for colloids compared to crystalloids. Indeed, several experimental studies mainly in bleeding-resuscitation animal models reported the volume-replacement ratios

Table 1 Experimental studies

Trial	Modell	Type of Fluids	VRR	Comments
Kocsi (n = 13) [12]	Controlled bleeding on pigs	Voluven (6% HES)	1:1	The 1:1 blood loss:colloid VRR maintained baseline GEDV throughout the experiment
Simon (n = 25) [11]	Controlled animal study in septic shock in pigs	– RL – HES 700/6:1 – HES 130 – HES 700/2.5:1	1:11.12 1:3.08 1:2.97 1:3.78	In comparison to RL, all HES solutions were more effective at maintaining plasma volume
Ponschab (n = 24) [13]	Bleeding-resuscitation pig model	Balanced crystalloid, in 1:1 or 1:3 replacement ratio	1:1.08 1:2.85	High volume (1:3) caused more pronounced cooling and impaired coagulation
Fodor (n = 25) [14]	Bleeding-resuscitation in rats	– Blood – HES 6% – NaCl 0.9%	1:1	No difference between colloids and crystalloids on pulmonary function. However, detailed invasive hemodynamic assessment was not performed

VRR: volume-replacement ratio; *GEDV*: global end diastolic volume; *HES*: hydroxyethyl starch; *RL*: Ringer's lactate for colloids as predicted by Starling's hypothesis [11–14]. These are summarized briefly in Table 1. The explanation could be that, in animal models, because of the relatively short experimental time, and because most models investigated hypovolemia, bleeding and resuscitation, the glycocalyx has no time for degradation. Nevertheless, these studies had different aims than to test Starling's hypothesis, and this should be performed in the future.

The glycocalyx has a pivotal role not just in regulating endothelial permeability but in several others functions: it modulates shear force induced nitric oxide

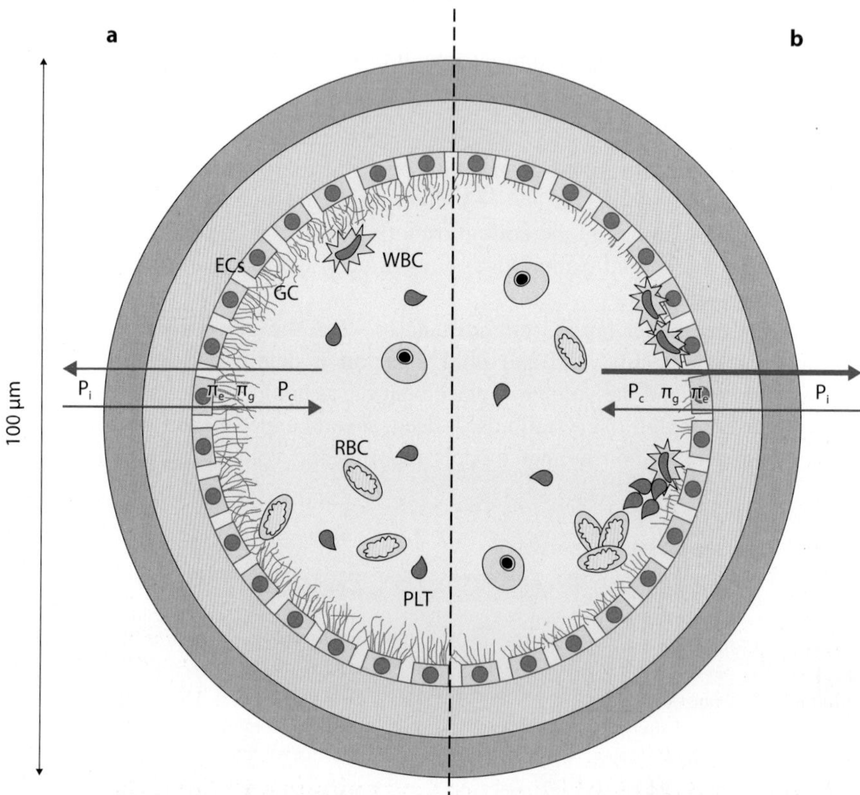

Fig. 4 Schematic transection of a capillary. **a** In normal subjects, the glycocalyx (GC) is intact and Starling's concept is more-or-less valid so that fluid transport is mainly determined by the Starling equation (see text). **b** In several critical illness conditions, both the glycocalyx and the endothelium become damaged. During these conditions, the regulating functions of the endothelium and glycocalyx are partially or totally lost. These will affect fluid transport across the vessel walls with excessive fluid and protein extravasation, will cause leukocyte adherence and platelet adhesion, further impairing capillary blood flow, and the complex function of the endothelium and the microcirculation. *ECs*: endothelial cells; *RBC*: red blood cells; *PLT*: platelets; *WBC*: white blood cells; *Pi*: interstitial hydrostatic pressure; π_e: colloid osmotic pressures in the endothelial surface layer; π_g: colloid osmotic pressures directly below the endothelial surface layer in the glycocalyx

(NO)-synthesis and dismutation of oxygen free radicals in the endothelial cells and controls coagulation and inflammation by preventing platelet adhesion and leukocyte adherence to the vessel walls [15]. It is, therefore, not surprising that whenever the glycocalyx layer is damaged, important pathophysiological changes take place, which can have serious effects on the function of the affected organ, or organs.

The Glycocalyx in the Critically Ill

There is mounting evidence that the glycocalyx becomes impaired or destroyed in several critical illness conditions, including inflammation (both infectious and non-infectious), trauma, sepsis, ischemia-reperfusion injuries, but also persistent hypo-, and hypervolemia [16]. During these conditions, the regulating functions of the endothelium and glycocalyx are lost, which can have serious effects on permeability and hence fluid transport across the vessel walls with excessive fluid and protein extravasation (Fig. 4b), but other functions like leukocyte adherence and platelet adhesion are also affected. There is experimental evidence that during these conditions, the interstitial space becomes overwhelmed with colloid molecules [10]. Although albumin seemed to be somewhat more able to interact with these conditions than HES, nevertheless it could not prevent colloid extravasation, which was also enforced by increasing hydrostatic pressures. These experimental findings are in agreement with the results of our clinical study, in which patients with septic shock and acute respiratory distress syndrome (ARDS) were administered either HES (molecular weight of 250 kDa) or gelatin (30 kDa) to treat hypovolemia. We used detailed hemodynamic monitoring and observed no difference in the volume-replacing effects of these colloids, and no change in the extravascular fluid volume, despite the huge difference in their molecular weight and colloid osmotic pressure [17]. This was possibly due to the very severe and long-standing (several days) condition of these patients, when it is highly likely that the glycocalyx was already severely damaged, hence 'size' (i. e., molecular weight) no longer mattered.

These observations are important when we try to interpret the results of recent large clinical trials comparing crystalloids and colloids in the critically ill.

Volume-replacement Effects of Crystalloids and Colloids in the Critically Ill

Although most recent large clinical trials had end-points of 28-day mortality or organ dysfunction, it is worthwhile analyzing the results from a different perspective. One of the landmark trials was the SAFE study, published in 2004, in which investigators compared the safety of albumin to normal saline in ICU patients (n = 6,997). The results showed no significant differences between the groups in hemodynamic resuscitation endpoints, such as mean arterial pressure (MAP) or heart rate, although the use of albumin was associated with a significant but clinically small increase in central venous pressure (CVP). The study showed no significant difference between albumin and normal saline regarding 28-day mortality rate or development of new organ failure [18]. The SAFE study was followed by the VISEP [19], CHEST [20] and 6S [21] trials, all reaching a more or less similar conclusion. Results showed a strong association between acute kidney injury, increased use of renal replacement therapy (RRT) and the use of HES solution, which was also accompanied with unfavorable patient outcome [19–21]. By contrast, in the CRISTAL trial, which was designed to test mortality related to colloid and crystalloid based fluid replacement in ICU patients, investigators detected a difference in death rate after 90 days, favoring the use of colloids. Furthermore, patients spent significantly fewer days on mechanical ventilation and needed shorter durations of vasopressor therapy in the colloid group than in the crystalloid group [22].

There are several common features in these studies. First of all, the ratio of the administered volume of crystalloid and colloids was completely different to what would have been expected according to the Starling principle (Table 2). In general, 30–50% more crystalloid seemed to have the same volume-expanding effect as colloids. Based on these results, a common view was formed that HES does not have higher potency for volume expansion than crystalloids, but carries a greater risk of renal dysfunction and mortality [18–25].

However, it is important to note that none of these trials used detailed hemodynamic monitoring, which is the second common feature of these studies. The administration of intravenous fluids was mainly based on clinicians' subjective decision [18, 19, 21, 22, 25], or on parameters such as heart rate [20], blood pressure [19, 21, 23], CVP [19, 21, 23], urine output [18–21, 23], lactate levels [20] or central venous oxygen saturation [19, 21, 23]. Cardiac output and stroke volume were not measured in most of the trials, which is essential to prove volume responsiveness, and none of the applied indices listed above are good monitoring tools of fluid therapy [1, 26]. Therefore, it is possible that a considerable number of these patients was treated inappropriately. Although it is not the task of the current review, it is important to note that the methods used as indications for fluid administration, also reflect our everyday practice, as was nicely confirmed in a recent observational study [2]. In this large international survey, it was revealed that fluid therapy is mainly guided by inadequate indices during our daily clinical routine. Therefore, one cannot exclude that in these trials a considerable proportion of patients were not hypovolemic at all. Indeed, in the CHEST trial the mean values of the target parameters were as follows: heart rate of 89/min, MAP 74 mmHg, CVP 9 mmHg and serum lactate 2 mmol/l. [20] None of these values suggests hypovolemia, or at least it is highly unlikely that any of us would commence fluid resuscitation based on these values. There is some evidence that in healthy male subjects colloid solutions provided a four times greater increase in blood volume compared to saline, and extravasation was significantly higher after saline infusion [27]. Therefore, if we consider that a considerable proportion of these patients were critically ill, hence their glycocalyx was impaired, and although they were not hypovolemic they still received colloids, this may have led to excessive extravasation. Furthermore, if fluid was administered to normovolemic patients, this could have caused increased hydrostatic pressures in the microcirculation leading to excessive HES extravasation

Table 2 Human randomized controlled trials

Trial	Population	Types of fluid	Cr/Co	Invasive hemo-dynamic monitoring
Finfer (n = 6,933) [18]	ICU patients	Albumin, saline	1.32	No
Brunk-horst (n = 537) [19]	ICU patients with severe sepsis	HES, RL	1.32	No
Myburgh (n = 7,000) [20]	ICU patients	HES 130/0.4, saline	1.20	No
Guidet (n = 174) [23]	Patients with severe sepsis	HES 130/0.4, saline	1.23	No
Perner (n = 798) [21]	ICU patients with severe sepsis	HES 130/0.42, Ringer's acetate	1.00	No
Annane (n = 2,857) [22]	ICU patients with hypovolemic shock	Colloids (gelatins, dextrans, HES, 4 or 20% albumin), crystalloids (isotonic or hypertonic saline, Ringer's lactate)	1.5	No
Yates (n = 202) [24]	High-risk surgical patients	HES 130/0.4, Hartman's solution	1.69	No
Caironi (n = 1,810) [25]	Severe sepsis, septic shock	20% albumin, crystalloid	1.02	No
Lobo (n = 10) [27]	Healthy male subjects	Gelofusin or HES 6%, saline	1.00	No

Cr/Co: ratio of crystalloid/colloid; *HES*: hydroxyethyl starch; *ICU*: intensive care unit

and deposit of colloid molecules in the tissues, further amplifying its adverse/toxic effects.

Clinical Implications

These observations can have an important impact on our daily clinical practice. These results suggest that, in addition to global and regional hemodynamic parameters, the role of the glycocalyx should be taken into account during the management of fluid resuscitation. Measuring several degradation markers (Table 3) in the blood [28–33] and even visualizing the microvasculature (Table 4) has now become pos-

Table 3 Glycocalyx degradation markers

Trial	Model	Methods	Conclusions, comments
Johansson (n = 75) (n = 80) [28, 29]	Prospective observational study in trauma patients	syndecan-1 (ng/ml); ELISA	Trauma is associated with endothelial damage, glycocalyx degradation
Ostrowski (n = 29) [30]	Experimental human endotoxemia (n = 9) and septic patients (n = 20)	syndecan-1 (ng/ml); ELISA	Endotoxemia did not but sepsis did cause endothelial damage, indicated by biomarkers that correlated with disease severity
Steppan (n = 150) [31]	Septic patients (n = 104), major abdominal surgery (n = 28), healthy volunteers (n = 18)	syndecan-1 (ng/ml); ELISA HS (μg/ml); ELISA	Significant flaking of the endothelial glycocalyx occurred in patients with sepsis, and to a lesser extent in surgical patients
Yagmur (n = 225) [32]	Critically ill patients (n = 164) and healthy controls (n = 61)	HA (μg/L); automated latex agglutination assay	Authors suggest that HA might have implications in the pathogenesis of critical illness and sepsis
Schmidt (n = 17) [33]	Mechanically ventilated ICU patients	CS (μg/ml) HS (μg/ml) Mass spectrometry	Circulating glycosaminoglycans may provide insight into respiratory pathophysiology

CS: chondroitin sulfate; *ELISA*: enzyme-linked immunosorbent assay; *HA*: hyaluronic acid; *HS*: heparan sulfate; *ICU*: intensive care unit

Table 4 Techniques to visualize the endothelial glycocalyx

Trial	Model	Method	Conclusions
Donati (n = 66) [34]	Septic patients (n = 32) Non-septic ICU patients (n = 18)	Sublingual sidestream dark field (SDF)	Correlation between PBR and number of rolling leukocytes postcapillary, confirming that glycocalyx shedding enhances leukocyte-endothelium interaction
Reitsma (n = 22) [15]	Endothelial glycocalyx structure in the intact carotid artery on C57B16/J mouse	Electron microscopy	The EG can be adequately imaged and quantified using two-photon laser scanning microscopy in intact, viable mounted carotid arteries
Gao [35]	Male Wistar rats, weighing 200–300 g	Brightfield images	The removal of heparan sulfate may cause collapse of the glycocalyx
Yen [36]	Ex vivo experiment on rat and mouse aortas	High resolution confocal microscopy	The surface glycocalyx layer is continuously and evenly distributed on the aorta wall but not on the microvessel wall

EG: endothelial glycocalyx; *EM*: electron microscopy; *PBR*: perfused boundary region; *RL*: rolling leukocyte sible [15, 34–36], and may become part of bedside routine in the not too distant future. Theoretically, for example in an acutely bleeding patient in the emergency room or in the operating room, the glycocalyx may be intact, which could be proven by novel investigations, and fluid resuscitation with colloids may be more beneficial and more effective compared to crystalloids. By contrast, during circumstances when the glycocalyx is impaired, colloids should be avoided. However, rather than just assuming the condition of the glycocalyx, its routine measurement could have an important impact on our daily practice and even on patient outcome.

Conclusion

Transport of fluids across the vessel wall was first described by Ernest Starling. Although his hypothesis is predominantly still valid, especially under physiological circumstances, the "low lymph flow paradox" and the "colloid osmotic pressure paradox" cannot be explained by simply applying the Starling equation. The discovery of the glycocalyx and its multiple roles in maintaining an intact and appropriately functioning endothelial surface layer has shone new light on vascular physiology. Therefore, in the future a paradigm shift will become necessary in order to appropriately assess and better guide fluid therapy. Without a detailed evaluation of the global effects of hypovolemia and fluid resuscitation, and assessment of the function of the microcirculation and the function of the glycocalyx, one cannot give adequate answers to the questions of 'when, what and for how long' should we administer fluids to our patients. We have to accept that, despite the significant results of large trials that are valid for the majority of the investigated population, at the bedside we should take an appropriate physiological parameter-based individualized approach. Thus, it turns out that all fluids can be good *and* bad depending on the specific circumstances.

References

1. Benes J, Kirov M, Kuzkov V et al (2015) Fluid therapy: double-edged sword during critical care? Biomed Res Int 2015:729075
2. Cecconi M, Hofer C, Teboul JL et al (2015) Fluid challenges in intensive care: the FENICE study: A global inception cohort study. Intensive Care Med 41:1529–1537
3. Woodcock TE, Woodcock TM (2012) Revised Starling equation and the glycocalyx model of transvascular fluid exchange: An improved paradigm for prescribing intravenous fluid therapy. Br J Anaesth 108:384–394
4. Moore FD, Dagher FJ, Boyden CM et al (1966) Hemorrhage in normal man. I. distribution and dispersal of saline infusions following acute blood loss: clinical kinetics of blood volume support. Ann Surg 163:485–504
5. Adamson RH, Lenz JF, Zhang X et al (2004) Oncotic pressures opposing filtration across non-fenestrated rat microvessels. J Physiol 557:889–907
6. Levick JR (2004) Revision of the Starling principle: new views of tissue fluid balance. J Physiol 557:704
7. Michel C (1997) Starling: the formulation of his hypothesis of microvascular fluid exchange and its significance after 100 years. Exp Physiol 82:1–30

8. Levick JR, Michel CC (2010) Microvascular fluid exchange and the revised Starling principle. Cardiovasc Res 87:198–210
9. Ince C (2014) The rationale for microcirculatory guided fluid therapy. Curr Opin Crit Care 20:301–308
10. Jacob M, Bruegger D, Rehm M et al (2007) The endothelial glycocalyx affords compatibility of Starling's principle and high cardiac interstitial albumin levels. Cardiovasc Res 73:575–586
11. Simon TP, Schuerholz T, Haugvik SP, Forberger C, Burmeister MA, Marx G (2013) High molecular weight hydroxyethyl starch solutions are not more effective than a low molecular weight hydroxyethyl starch solution in a porcine model of septic shock. Minerva Anestesiol 79:44–52
12. Kocsi S, Demeter G, Fogas J et al (2012) Central venous oxygen saturation is a good indicator of altered oxygen balance in isovolemic anemia. Acta Anaesthesiol Scand 56:291–297
13. Ponschab M, Schöchl H, Keibl C, Fischer H, Redl HSC (2015) Preferential effects of low volume versus high volume replacement with crystalloid fluid in a hemorrhagic shock model in pigs. BMC Anesthesiol 15:133
14. Fodor GH, Babik B, Czövek D et al (2016) Fluid replacement and respiratory function. Eur J Anaesthesiol 33:34–41
15. Reitsma S, Oude Egbrink MGA, Vink H et al (2011) Endothelial glycocalyx structure in the intact carotid artery: A two-photon laser scanning microscopy study. J Vasc Res 48:297–306
16. Tánczos K, Molnár Z (2013) Do no harm: use starches? Minerva Anestesiol 79:1101–1102
17. Molnár Z, Mikor A, Leiner T, Szakmány T (2004) Fluid resuscitation with colloids of different molecular weight in septic shock. Intensive Care Med 30:1356–1360
18. Finfer S, Bellomo R, Boyce N et al (2004) A comparison of albumin and saline for fluid resuscitation in the intensive care unit. N Engl J Med 350:2247–2256
19. Brunkhorst FM, Engel C, Bloos F et al (2008) Intensive insulin therapy and pentastarch resuscitation in severe sepsis. N Engl J Med 358:125–139
20. Myburgh JA, Finfer S, Bellomo R et al (2012) Hydroxyethyl starch or saline for fluid resuscitation in intensive care. N Engl J Med 367:1901–1911
21. Perner A, Haase N, Guttormsen AB et al (2012) Hydroxyethyl starch 130/0.42 versus Ringer's acetate in severe sepsis. N Engl J Med 367:124–134
22. Annane D, Siami S, Jaber S et al (2013) Effects of fluid resuscitation with colloids vs crystalloids on mortality in critically ill patients presenting with hypovolemic shock: the CRISTAL randomized trial. JAMA 310:1809–1817
23. Guidet B, Martinet O, Boulain T et al (2012) Assessment of hemodynamic efficacy and safety fluid replacement in patients with severe sepsis : The CRYSTMAS study. Crit Care 16:R94
24. Yates DRA, Davies SJ, Milner HE, Wilson RJT (2014) Crystalloid or colloid for goal-directed fluid therapy in colorectal surgery. Br J Anaesth 112:281–289
25. Caironi P, Tognoni G, Masson S et al (2014) Albumin replacement in patients with severe sepsis or septic shock. N Engl J Med 370:1412–1421
26. Benes J, Chytra I, Altmann P et al (2010) Intraoperative fluid optimization using stroke volume variation in high risk surgical patients: results of prospective randomized study. Crit Care 14:R118
27. Lobo DN, Stanga Z, Aloysius MM et al (2010) Effect of volume loading with 1 liter intravenous infusions of 0.9% saline, 4% succinylated gelatine (Gelofusine) and 6% hydroxyethyl starch (Voluven) on blood volume and endocrine responses: a randomized, three-way crossover study in healthy volunteers. Crit Care Med 38:464–470
28. Johansson PI, Sørensen AM, Perner AWK et al (2011) Elderly trauma patients have high circulating noradrenaline levels but attenuated release of adrenaline, platelets, and leukocytes in response to increasing injury severity. Ann Surg 254:194
29. Johansson PI, Stensballe J, Rasmussen LS, Ostrowski SR (2011) A high admission syndecan-1 level, a marker of endothelial glycocalyx degradation, is associated with inflammation, protein c depletion, fibrinolysis, and increased mortality in trauma patients. Ann Surg 254:194–200

30. Ostrowski SR, Berg RMG, Windeløv NA et al (2013) Coagulopathy, catecholamines, and biomarkers of endothelial damage in experimental human endotoxemia and in patients with severe sepsis: A prospective study. J Crit Care 28:586–596
31. Steppan J, Hofer S, Funke B et al (2011) Sepsis and major abdominal surgery lead to flaking of the endothelial glycocalix. J Surg Res 165:136–141
32. Yagmur E, Koch A, Haumann M et al (2012) Hyaluronan serum concentrations are elevated in critically ill patients and associated with disease severity. Clin Biochem 45:82–87
33. Schmidt EP, Li G, Li L et al (2014) The circulating glycosaminoglycan signature of respiratory. J Biol Chem 289:8194–8202
34. Donati A, Damiani E, Domizi R et al (2013) Alteration of the sublingual microvascular glycocalyx in critically ill patients. Microvasc Res 90:86–89
35. Gao L, Lipowsky HH (2010) Composition of the endothelial glycocalyx and its relation to its thickness and diffusion of small solutes. Microvasc Res 80:394–401
36. Yen WY, Cai B, Zeng M et al (2012) Quantification of the endothelial surface glycocalyx on rat and mouse blood vessels. Microvasc Res 83:337–346

Part IV
Renal Issues

New Diagnostic Approaches in Acute Kidney Injury

M. Meersch and A. Zarbock

Introduction

Acute kidney injury (AKI) is a serious and well-recognized complication in critically ill patients with a large impact on morbidity and mortality. Early detection allows for timely intervention and may improve patient outcome. During the last few years, renal biomarkers have been developed and evaluated for early detection of AKI. Analysis of the biomarkers kidney injury molecule-1 (KIM-1), liver-type fatty acid binding protein (L-FABP), interleukin-18 (IL-18), neutrophil gelatinase-associated lipocalin (NGAL), tissue inhibitor of metalloproteinase-2 (TIMP-2) and insulin-like growth factor-binding protein (IGFBP7) has brought new insights into the molecular mechanisms of this complex and heterogeneous disease. Biomarker-based AKI models have the potential to expand options for the diagnosis of AKI and to optimize AKI management in critically ill patients.

Acute Kidney Injury

AKI is characterized by an acute and rapid loss of renal function within hours or days often in the context of other acute conditions of critical illness. A deterioration of kidney function results in an accumulation of waste products, electrolyte and fluid disturbances and impairment of the immune system, all impacting on patient outcome. The incidence of AKI in critically ill patients reaches up to 50%, depending on the underlying baseline characteristics and the cause of critical illness. One to five percent of all AKI patients require renal replacement therapy (RRT) [1, 2]. AKI is independently associated with the development of chronic kidney disease

M. Meersch · A. Zarbock (✉)
Department of Anesthesiology, Intensive Care and Pain Medicine, University of Münster
Albert-Schweitzer-Campus 1, Gebäude A1, 48149 Münster, Germany
e-mail: zarbock@uni-muenster.de

J.-L. Vincent (ed.), *Annual Update in Intensive Care and Emergency Medicine 2017*,
DOI 10.1007/978-3-319-51908-1_9

Table 1 Risk factors for the development of AKI

Preoperative factors	Perioperative factors	Other factors

– Female sex
– ACE therapy
– Congestive heart failure
– LVEF < 35%
– IABP
– Preoperative sCr > 2.1 mg/dl
– IDDM
– Emergency surgery
– Valve surgery
– Combination CABG + valve
– Other cardiac surgery
	– Hemodynamic instability
	– Aortic cross clamping
	– Hypertension
	– Infection
	– Sepsis
	– MODS
		– Antibiotics
		  – Amphotericin
		  – Aminoglycosides
		  – Vancomycin
		– Nephrotoxic agents
		– Transfusion
		– Hyperchloremic fluids

ACE: angiotensin converting enzyme; *LVEF*: left ventricular ejection fraction; *IABP*: intra-aortic balloon pump; *sCr*: serum creatinine; *IDDM*: insulin dependent diabetes mellitus; *CABG*: coronary artery bypass graft; *MODS*: multiorgan dysfunction syndrome

(CKD), with an approximately 8-fold increased risk, and a higher mortality (up to 60%) [3].

The development of AKI is not attributable to a single etiologic factor but arises as the result of multiple preconditions. The prognosis depends on comorbid factors (e. g., chronic obstructive pulmonary disease [COPD], diabetes mellitus, CKD), the respective clinical setting (e. g., sepsis, cardiothoracic surgery), concomitant medication (e. g., angiotensin converting enzyme blockers), use of nephrotoxic drugs (aminoglycosides, contrast agents) and severity of AKI (need for dialysis). Over the last two decades several risk predicting models have been evaluated, which are all closely related to the development of AKI (Table 1).

Diagnosis

In the past, insufficient knowledge about AKI and the lack of a consensus definition resulted in underdiagnosis of AKI. In 2004, the Acute Dialysis Quality Initiative (ADQI) proposed a first consensus definition based on serum-creatinine and urinary output: the RIFLE classification (Risk, Injury, Failure, Loss and End-stage renal disease) [4]. The subsequent recognition that even small increases in serum creatinine levels are associated with worse outcome [5] resulted, in 2007, in the evolution of the RIFLE criteria towards the Acute Kidney Injury Network (AKIN) criteria [6]. In 2012, the Kidney Disease: Improving Global Outcomes (KDIGO) workgroup reconciled the RIFLE and AKIN criteria and developed the KDIGO criteria. According to the KDIGO guidelines, AKI is diagnosed when at least one of the following conditions is met: serum-creatinine elevation of ≥ 0.3 mg/dl within 48 h or a 1.5-fold increase in serum creatinine compared to baseline within 7 days, or urinary output < 0.5 ml/kg/h ≥ 6 h ([7]; Table 2). A recent trial including 32,000 critically ill patients confirmed the importance of both criteria [8]. The results showed that the risk

Table 2 KDIGO criteria for the diagnosis of AKI [7]

Stage	Serum creatinine	Urine output
1	Increase of ≥ 0.3 mg/dl within 48 h *or* Increase of 1.5–1.9-times baseline within 7 days	< 0.5 ml/kg/h for ≥ 6 h
2	Increase of 2.0–2.9-times baseline within 7 days	< 0.5 ml/kg/h for ≥ 12 h
3	Increase of 3-times baseline within 7 days *or* Increase to ≥ 4.0 mg/dl with an acute increase of 0.5 mg/dl *or* Initiation of renal replacement therapy *or* Decrease of eGFR to < 35 ml/min/1.73 m^2 in patients < 18 years of age	< 0.3 ml/kg/h for ≥ 24 h *or* anuria for ≥ 12 h

for RRT and death was highest in patients meeting both KDIGO criteria, especially if these persisted for a period of more than 3 days.

However, the classical biomarkers, serum creatinine and urinary output, have important limitations that should not be disregarded. Serum creatinine is a metabolic product of creatine, which serves as an energy reservoir and is excreted through the kidneys. Its concentration is influenced by multiple factors including age, muscle mass and meat intake. The level of serum creatinine does not accurately reflect kidney function as an increase does not occur until 50% of the glomerular filtration rate (GFR) has been lost. It is also worth mentioning that in critically ill patients, serum creatinine production is reduced as compared to in healthy individuals.

What applies to serum creatinine also applies to urinary output, a clinically important but nevertheless non-specific marker of kidney function. Urinary output often persists until renal function ceases completely, and its interpretation is often confused by clinical conditions, such as hypovolemia, extended surgery, trauma or the use of diuretics. To put it concisely, the fact that the classical biomarkers change late during the course of AKI development considerably restricts their suitability as a diagnostic tool. The emergence of new renal biomarkers tackles exactly this problem and makes a vital contribution to the early and timely diagnosis of AKI [9].

Renal Biomarkers

Over the last few years, significant progress has been made in the field of novel biomarkers to prevent or detect AKI early (Fig. 1). The ADQI has assigned the highest research priority to the evaluation of new biomarkers [10]. Abundant trials investigating different biomarkers have been performed, with most of them defining AKI using serum creatinine definitions [11]. Several promising biomarkers have been identified, which make it possible to diagnose AKI up to 48 h earlier than would have been possible on the basis of a significant change in serum creatinine. Predicting AKI early would offer the opportunity to strictly implement hemodynamic optimization models in an effort to prevent a manifest functional loss of the

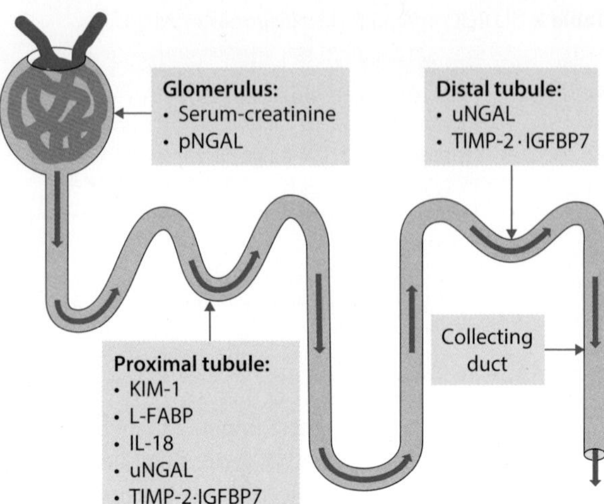

Fig. 1 Localization of new biomarkers. The classic biomarker, serum creatinine, and plasma neutrophil gelatinase-associated lipocalin (p-NGAL) are detectable in the blood. All other mentioned biomarkers are detected in the urine. *KIM*: kidney injury molecule; *L-FABP*: liver-type fatty acid binding protein; *IL-18*: interleukin-18; *TIMP-2*: tissue inhibitor of metalloproteinase-2; *IGFBP7*: insulin-like growth factor-binding protein; *uNGAL*: urinary NGAL

kidneys. Furthermore, there is evidence that some biomarkers may predict the need for RRT, which can help to make the decision when to initiate RRT.

Kidney Injury Molecule-1

KIM-1 is a transmembrane protein that is almost undetectable in healthy kidneys. Its expression is upregulated in dedifferentiated epithelial cells of the proximal tubule after ischemic and nephrotoxic injuries. The extracellular segment is detached by matrix-metalloproteinases (MMP) and eliminated through the urine [12]. Forty-eight hours after the primary injury, elevated KIM-1 levels can be detected in the urine.

After cardiothoracic surgery, significant KIM-1 increases could be demonstrated in patients with postoperative AKI and in patients with already established AKI. The predictive value for the development of AKI and the severity of the injury in septic patients was lower for KIM-1 than for other biomarkers. In addition, no bedside test is available for KIM-1.

Thus, KIM-1 might not be an adequate marker for the prediction of AKI in clinical routine.

Liver-type Fatty Acid Binding Protein

L-FABP is a 14 kilo-Dalton (kDa) protein expressed in the proximal tubular epithelial cells. Elevated expression and excretion was first detected in pediatric patients with AKI after cardiopulmonary bypass (CPB). High sensitivity and specificity have been demonstrated for L-FABP, particularly in patients with already established AKI. Furthermore, patients with higher L-FABP values had a worse outcome (need for RRT and mortality) [13]. This finding has also been demonstrated in patients with septic shock and AKI [14]. However, the excretion of L-FABP was elevated in patients with AKI as well as in patients with CKD resulting in a difficult clinical differentiation. In addition, L-FABP needs to be measured in the laboratory due to the lack of bedside tests. Therefore, it has not yet been implemented in clinical practice.

Interleukin-18

IL-18 is a proinflammatory cytokine of the IL-1 super family. It is produced in the proximal tubular epithelial cells, activated through the enzyme caspase-1 and secreted into the urine after ischemic insults [15].

Significant IL-18 elevation is detectable 24 h before an increase of serum creatinine in patients with AKI [16]. Patients developing AKI showed higher IL-18 values compared to patients with CKD or nephrotoxic syndrome [17]. However, the excretion of IL-18 varies considerably depending on the clinical setting. Septic patients in particular showed high IL-18 values, independent of the presence of AKI [18]. Although IL-18 is specific for AKI caused by ischemia, the clinical benefit of this biomarker remains unclear.

Neutrophil Gelatinase-associated Lipocalin

NGAL is a 25 kDa protein of the lipocalin family linked to neutrophil gelatinase in specific leukocyte granules. It is also expressed in different epithelial cells of the respiratory and intestinal tissue. The molecule is filtered to the primary urine and reabsorbed via megalin-receptors of the tubular epithelial cells. It is almost undetectable in the urine of patients with normal kidney function. Ischemic and nephrotoxic insults lead to an increase in NGAL-mRNA expression. A reduced GFR results in a diminished NGAL clearance and consequently in an accumulation of NGAL in the urine and plasma [19]. Depending on the extent of the injury, higher NGAL elevations can be detected in the urine than in the plasma. Several studies, which have been performed in different clinical scenarios (critical illness [20], trauma [21], cardiothoracic surgery [22], radiocontrast exposure [23]) have shown that NGAL is rapidly upregulated in the kidneys very early after AKI (2–3 h). Moreover, there is growing evidence that urine NGAL is directly associated with the need for RRT.

NGAL has been designated the troponin of the kidneys, but unlike myocardial infarction, AKI etiology is not limited to ischemia [24]. NGAL is a highly sensitive marker but its specificity still remains vague. In septic patients with AKI, NGAL values were higher than in septic patients without AKI. However, several studies showed that NGAL was also elevated in patients with systemic inflammatory response syndrome (SIRS), sepsis and septic shock independent of the presence of AKI [25, 26]. This might be explained by the fact that systemic inflammation leads to a reduced resorption capacity of the tubular epithelial cells and consequently to higher NGAL values. Moreover, older patients with comorbidities, such as hypertension or diabetes mellitus, and patients with CKD show different NGAL values than younger patients without these conditions [27, 28].

Despite the many unanswered questions, current findings imply that NGAL is a valuable biomarker for the early prediction of AKI and for the clinical decision to initiate RRT. Recently, de Geus et al. proposed an NGAL-score to detect acute tubular damage early in cardiac surgery patients [29]. It is conceivable to apply such an approach to critically ill patients in the ICU.

Tissue Inhibitor of Metalloproteinases-2 and Insulin-like Growth Factor Binding Protein 7

TIMP-2 and IGFBP7 are both markers of G1 cell cycle arrest. After ischemic and inflammatory insults, renal tubular epithelial cells enter the G1 cell cycle arrest to avoid cell division with damaged deoxyribonucleic acid (DNA). These cells sustain the modus until the DNA is completely repaired. TIMP-2 and IGFBP7 are both expressed in the early phase of AKI, signaling damage of tubular epithelial cells.

Both markers have been evaluated in a validation trial analyzing different biomarkers for the early detection of AKI in critically ill patients [30]. The combination of TIMP-2 and IGFBP7 showed best predictive performance for the prediction of moderate and severe AKI. TIMP-2·IGFBP7 > 0.3 demonstrated high sensitivity and specificity for the development of AKI. This was confirmed in further studies performed in other clinical settings (cardiac [31] and abdominal surgery [32]). Moreover, there is growing evidence that TIMP-2 and IGFBP7 might also predict the need for RRT [31, 33], but further confirmatory analyses are needed to substantiate these findings. A bedside test to measure TIMP-2·IGFBP7 is commercially available, with results ready within 20 min.

Biomarkers in Daily Clinical Practice

Although existing data strongly support the use of new biomarkers in routine clinical practice, many clinicians still express skepticism. Biomarkers enable an accurate diagnosis to be made at a very early stage and offer new insights into the severity and prognosis of AKI. Therefore, the 10th ADQI Consensus Conference proposed to utilize both function (classic) and damage (new) biomarkers to define and characterize AKI (Fig. 2) and integrate them into preventive and therapeutic strategies (Fig. 3; [9]).

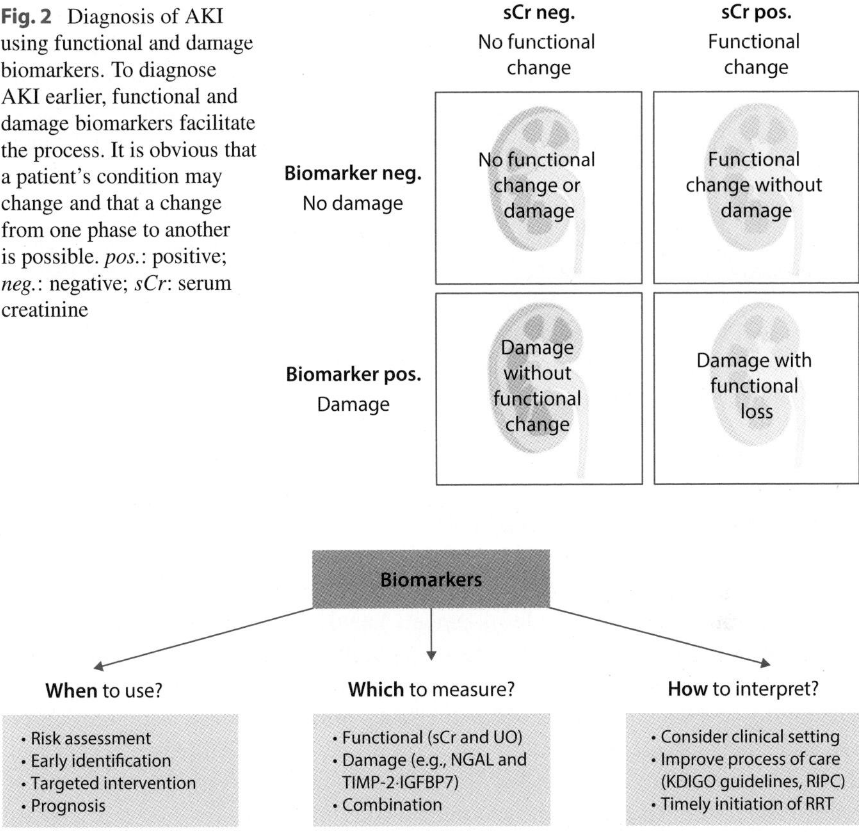

Fig. 2 Diagnosis of AKI using functional and damage biomarkers. To diagnose AKI earlier, functional and damage biomarkers facilitate the process. It is obvious that a patient's condition may change and that a change from one phase to another is possible. *pos.*: positive; *neg.*: negative; *sCr*: serum creatinine

Fig. 3 Decision guide for the utilization of biomarkers [9]. *sCr*: serum-creatinine; *UO*: urinary output; *NGAL*: neutrophil gelatinase associated lipocalin; *TIMP-2*: tissue inhibitor of metalloproteinase-2; *IGFBP*: insulin-like growth factor binding protein; *RIPC*: remote ischemic preconditioning; *RRT*: renal replacement therapy

Strategies for the Prevention of AKI

Over the last few years, reasonable efforts have been made to identify interventions, drugs and strategies for the prevention of AKI, unfortunately with little success. The bundle of preventive strategies proposed by the KDIGO guidelines includes the discontinuation and avoidance of nephrotoxic agents, the assurance of volume status and perfusion pressure, the consideration of functional hemodynamic monitoring, close monitoring of the functional markers, serum creatinine and urinary output, and avoidance of hyperglycemia [7]. The true clinical benefit of these recommendations is as yet scientifically not established. Aside from, and in addition to the KDIGO bundle, existing data suggest that remote ischemic preconditioning might be effective in the prevention of AKI in high-risk patients.

Nevertheless, the fundamental aspect for the prevention of AKI is to identify patients at risk by using new biomarkers. New biomarkers help to identify patients at risk for AKI before the occurrence of functional loss. Their implementation would allow for earlier and more timely execution of the bundle of preventive measures proposed by the KDIGO guidelines, which would be a great step forward. Vijayan et al. [34] proposed the bedside measurement of TIMP-2·IGFBP7 in patients with at least one risk factor for AKI, especially after cardiac and major high-risk surgery and in patients with sepsis, to detect acute tubular damage early.

Currently, a large randomized controlled trial is underway addressing exactly this particular issue (German Clinical Trials Register: DRKS00006139). Hopefully, this trial will provide more definitive answers as to whether and to what extent adherence to the KDIGO guidelines is truly effective, and whether it is sufficient to implement these strategies only in patients with elevated biomarker levels and a high risk for AKI.

Strategies for the Initiation of RRT

The lack of a broad consensus definition results in wide practice variation for starting RRT in the course of AKI development. The decision is influenced by several factors, including serum creatinine, urinary output, patient condition, and is more than anything a question of the preferences of the intensivist in charge of the patient. The timing of RRT initiation has been the focus of many studies. Data from observational studies suggest a trend toward early initiation of RRT [35–37]. However, the conclusions were based on heterogeneous studies with varying definitions of 'early' and 'late'. Recently, two randomized controlled trials have been performed analyzing the effect of early initiation of RRT on patient outcome (the Artificial Kidney Initiation in Kidney Injury [AKIKI] and Early vs Late Initiation of Renal Replacement Therapy in Critically Ill Patients With Acute Kidney Injury [ELAIN] trials) [38, 39]. These trials came to different conclusions. Gaudry et al. (AKIKI trial) showed no survival benefit at day 60, whereas Zarbock et al. (ELAIN trial) demonstrated a significantly reduced 90-day mortality with the early initiation of RRT. The difference might be caused by the stage of AKI severity at which RRT was initiated. In the AKIKI trial, patients were enrolled once they achieved KDIGO stage 3, an advanced stage in the chain of AKI development. In the ELAIN trial, patients were enrolled at KDIGO stage 2. Furthermore, to avoid the inclusion of patients likely recovering spontaneously from AKI, a biomarker-based model was used and patients were included if NGAL levels exceeded 150 ng/ml. As mentioned above, the elevation of NGAL is strongly associated with the need for RRT. Selecting patients for RRT using a combination of function and damage biomarkers, effectively reduced the 90-day all-cause mortality in patients at KDIGO stage 2 who were treated early with RRT.

This interesting approach serves as an example of how to incorporate biomarker measurements into clinical algorithms. Ideally, future studies should address two questions: which patients do not need RRT treatment because they will likely recover spontaneously from AKI, and which patients with severe renal injury will benefit from early treatment with RRT.

Conclusion

AKI is a common and severe complication in critically ill patients with a high impact on patient outcome. Great efforts have been devoted to identify new biomarkers and to integrate them in new strategies for the early diagnosis and optimization of preventive and therapeutic strategies. The two biomarkers NGAL and TIMP-2·IGFBP7 can be measured at the bedside within a few minutes. They have demonstrated promising results for both the early detection and prognostication of the development of AKI. Consequently, in patients at risk for AKI renoprotective treatment strategies (maintenance of hemodynamic stability, optimization of intravascular volume status, avoidance of nephrotoxic agents) should strictly be implemented to avoid a loss of kidney function. In high risk critically ill patients with already established AKI and elevated biomarker levels an early initiation of RRT should be considered.

References

1. Hoste EA, Kellum JA (2006) Acute kidney injury: epidemiology and diagnostic criteria. Curr Opin Crit Care 12:531–537
2. Hoste EA, Bagshaw SM, Bellomo R et al (2015) Epidemiology of acute kidney injury in critically ill patients: the multinational AKI-EPI study. Intensive Care Med 41:1411–1423
3. Coca SG, Singanamala S, Parikh CR (2012) Chronic kidney disease after acute kidney injury: a systematic review and meta-analysis. Kidney Int 81:442–448
4. Bellomo R, Ronco C, Kellum JA, Mehta RL, Palevsky P (2004) Acute Dialysis Quality Initiative w. Acute renal failure – definition, outcome measures, animal models, fluid therapy and information technology needs: the Second International Consensus Conference of the Acute Dialysis Quality Initiative (ADQI) Group. Crit Care 8:R204–212
5. Lassnigg A, Schmidlin D, Mouhieddine M et al (2004) Minimal changes of serum creatinine predict prognosis in patients after cardiothoracic surgery: a prospective cohort study. J Am Soc Nephrol 15:1597–1605
6. Mehta RL, Kellum JA, Shah SV et al (2007) Acute Kidney Injury Network: report of an initiative to improve outcomes in acute kidney injury. Crit Care 11:R31
7. KDIGO Workgroup (2012) KDIGO clinical practice guideline for acute kidney injury. Kidney Int Suppl 2:1–138
8. Kellum JA, Sileanu FE, Murugan R, Lucko N, Shaw AD, Clermont G (2015) Classifying AKI by urine output versus serum creatinine level. J Am Soc Nephrol 26:2231–2238
9. Murray PT, Mehta RL, Shaw A et al (2014) Potential use of biomarkers in acute kidney injury: report and summary of recommendations from the 10th Acute Dialysis Quality Initiative consensus conference. Kidney Int 85:513–521
10. McCullough PA, Shaw AD, Haase M et al (2013) Diagnosis of acute kidney injury using functional and injury biomarkers: workgroup statements from the tenth Acute Dialysis Quality Initiative Consensus Conference. Contrib Nephrol 182:13–29
11. Coca SG, Yalavarthy R, Concato J, Parikh CR (2008) Biomarkers for the diagnosis and risk stratification of acute kidney injury: a systematic review. Kidney Int 73:1008–1016

12. Bailly V, Zhang Z, Meier W, Cate R, Sanicola M, Bonventre JV (2002) Shedding of kidney injury molecule-1, a putative adhesion protein involved in renal regeneration. J Biol Chem 277:39739–39748
13. Ferguson MA, Vaidya VS, Waikar SS et al (2010) Urinary liver-type fatty acid-binding protein predicts adverse outcomes in acute kidney injury. Kidney Int 77:708–714
14. Doi K, Noiri E, Maeda-Mamiya R et al (2010) Urinary L-type fatty acid-binding protein as a new biomarker of sepsis complicated with acute kidney injury. Crit Care Med 38:2037–2042
15. Liu Y, Guo W, Zhang J et al (2013) Urinary interleukin 18 for detection of acute kidney injury: a meta-analysis. Am J Kidney Dis 62:1058–1067
16. Parikh CR, Abraham E, Ancukiewicz M, Edelstein CL (2005) Urine IL-18 is an early diagnostic marker for acute kidney injury and predicts mortality in the intensive care unit. J Am Soc Nephrol 16:3046–3052
17. Parikh CR, Jani A, Melnikov VY, Faubel S, Edelstein CL (2004) Urinary interleukin-18 is a marker of human acute tubular necrosis. Am J Kidney Dis 43:405–414
18. Siew ED, Ikizler TA, Gebretsadik T et al (2010) Elevated urinary IL-18 levels at the time of ICU admission predict adverse clinical outcomes. Clin J Am Soc Nephrol 5:1497–1505
19. Haase-Fielitz A, Haase M, Devarajan P (2014) Neutrophil gelatinase-associated lipocalin as a biomarker of acute kidney injury: a critical evaluation of current status. Ann Clin Biochem 51:335–351
20. Cruz DN, de Cal M, Garzotto F et al (2010) Plasma neutrophil gelatinase-associated lipocalin is an early biomarker for acute kidney injury in an adult ICU population. Intensive Care Med 36:444–451
21. Makris K, Markou N, Evodia E et al (2009) Urinary neutrophil gelatinase-associated lipocalin (NGAL) as an early marker of acute kidney injury in critically ill multiple trauma patients. Clin Chem Lab Med 47:79–82
22. Mishra J, Ma Q, Prada A et al (2003) Identification of neutrophil gelatinase-associated lipocalin as a novel early urinary biomarker for ischemic renal injury. J Am Soc Nephrol 14:2534–2543
23. Hirsch R, Dent C, Pfriem H et al (2007) NGAL is an early predictive biomarker of contrast-induced nephropathy in children. Pediatr Nephrol 22:2089–2095
24. Devarajan P (2010) Review: neutrophil gelatinase-associated lipocalin: a troponin-like biomarker for human acute kidney injury. Nephrology 15:419–428
25. Vanmassenhove J, Glorieux G, Lameire N et al (2015) Influence of severity of illness on neutrophil gelatinase-associated lipocalin performance as a marker of acute kidney injury: a prospective cohort study of patients with sepsis. BMC Nephrol 16:18
26. Otto GP, Hurtado-Oliveros J, Chung HY et al (2015) Plasma neutrophil gelatinase-associated lipocalin is primarily related to inflammation during sepsis: a translational approach. PLoS One 10:e0124429
27. Malyszko J, Bachorzewska-Gajewska H, Malyszko JS, Pawlak K, Dobrzycki S (2008) Serum neutrophil gelatinase-associated lipocalin as a marker of renal function in hypertensive and normotensive patients with coronary artery disease. Nephrology 13:153–156
28. Haase M, Bellomo R, Devarajan P, Schlattmann P, Haase-Fielitz A (2009) Accuracy of neutrophil gelatinase-associated lipocalin (NGAL) in diagnosis and prognosis in acute kidney injury: a systematic review and meta-analysis. Am J Kidney Dis 54:1012–1024
29. de Geus HR, Ronco C, Haase M, Jacob L, Lewington A, Vincent JL (2016) The cardiac surgery-associated neutrophil gelatinase-associated lipocalin (CSA-NGAL) score: A potential tool to monitor acute tubular damage. J Thorac Cardiovasc Surg 151:1476–1481
30. Kashani K, Al-Khafaji A, Ardiles T et al (2013) Discovery and validation of cell cycle arrest biomarkers in human acute kidney injury. Crit Care 17:R25
31. Meersch M, Schmidt C, Van Aken H et al (2014) Urinary TIMP-2 and IGFBP7 as early biomarkers of acute kidney injury and renal recovery following cardiac surgery. PLoS One 9:e93460

32. Gocze I, Koch M, Renner P et al (2015) Urinary biomarkers TIMP-2 and IGFBP7 early predict acute kidney injury after major surgery. PLoS One 10:e0120863
33. Koyner JL, Davison DL, Brasha-Mitchell E et al (2015) Furosemide Stress Test and Biomarkers for the Prediction of AKI Severity. J Am Soc Nephrol 26:2023–2031
34. Vijayan A, Faubel S, Askenazi DJ et al (2016) Clinical use of the urine biomarker [TIMP-2] x [IGFBP7] for Acute kidney injury risk assessment. Am J Kidney Dis 68:19–28
35. Gibney N, Hoste E, Burdmann EA et al (2008) Timing of initiation and discontinuation of renal replacement therapy in AKI: unanswered key questions. Clin J Am Soc Nephrol 3:876–880
36. Palevsky PM (2008) Indications and timing of renal replacement therapy in acute kidney injury. Crit Care Med 36(4 Suppl):S224–S228
37. Seabra VF, Balk EM, Liangos O, Sosa MA, Cendoroglo M, Jaber BL (2008) Timing of renal replacement therapy initiation in acute renal failure: a meta-analysis. A J Kidney Dis 52:272–284
38. Gaudry S, Hajage D, Schortgen F et al (2016) Initiation strategies for renal-replacement therapy in the intensive care unit. N Engl J Med 375:122–133
39. Zarbock A, Kellum JA, Schmidt C et al (2016) Effect of early vs delayed initiation of renal replacement therapy on mortality in critically ill patients with acute kidney injury: The ELAIN randomized clinical trial. JAMA 315:2190–2199

When Should Renal Replacement Therapy Start?

J. Izawa, A. Zarbock, and J. A. Kellum

Introduction

The use of renal replacement therapy (RRT) must be tailored as two recent randomized controlled trials (RCTs) demonstrated [1, 2]. In a study where the vast majority of patients received RRT, early initiation resulted in improved survival [1], whereas, in a study where only a fraction of patients ever required RRT, a 'wait and see' approach appeared to be preferred [2]; however, even in this situation, those requiring late therapy generally do worse.

For patients with 'less severe' acute kidney injury (AKI), who are not judged as requiring RRT, outcomes are generally better. However, less severe AKI may still be in the causal pathway for morbidity and mortality in critically ill patients [3]. Effects of renal dysfunction on immune function, fluid balance, and drug clearance may result in a myriad of complications, prolonging hospitalization and increasing risk of death. Evolution in disease management from severe to 'less severe' is familiar to us all. The emergence of non-ST segment myocardial infarction and 'precancerous syndromes' are both examples of evolving pathonomenclature as the epidemiology and pathobiology of diseases like coronary artery disease and cancer advance. We

J. Izawa
Intensive Care Unit, Department of Anesthesiology, Jikei University School of Medicine
105-8471 Minato-ku, Tokyo, Japan
Department of Preventive Services, Kyoto University School of Public Health
606-8501 Sakyo-ku, Kyoto, Japan

A. Zarbock
Department of Anesthesiology, Intensive Care Medicine and Pain Medicine, University Hospital Münster
48149 Münster, Germany

J. A. Kellum (✉)
Center for Critical Care Nephrology, University of Pittsburgh Medical Center
604 Scaife Hall, 3550 Terrace Street, Pittsburgh, PA 15261, USA
e-mail: kellumja@upmc.edu

J.-L. Vincent (ed.), *Annual Update in Intensive Care and Emergency Medicine 2017*,
DOI 10.1007/978-3-319-51908-1_10

should expect the same as we move from acute renal failure to AKI and ultimately to acute kidney disease [4].

Benefits and Harms of Early-timing RRT

The potential benefits and harms of RRT are shown in Box 1. Early initiation of RRT might therefore lead to certain benefits but also cause certain harms. Although there are few RCTs about the effects of fluid removal, fluid overload is definitely harmful for the prognosis of critically ill patients with and without AKI [5–13]. Ultrafiltration by early RRT could achieve adequate fluid removal even when diuretic therapy and fluid restriction do not succeed. In addition, fluid removal itself might encourage renal recovery because studies have indicated that the increase in central venous pressure (CVP) would play an important role in the progression of renal injury [14–16]. Conversely, complications associated with RRT (hemodynamic instability, infection) might adversely affect renal recovery.

Box 1. Potential benefits and harms associated with renal replacement therapy

Benefits

- Fluid removal
- Removal of uremic toxins
- Stabilizing electrolyte levels and acid-base balance
- Elimination of other toxins (e. g., cytokines)

Harms

- Hemodynamic instability, especially in intermittent hemodialysis
- Excess removal of electrolytes such as potassium or phosphate
- Removal of drugs
- Complications of catheter insertion, catheter-related infections
- Cost

How Should We Define the Timing of RRT?

In early clinical research in this area, 'late', also called 'delayed', initiation of RRT, was often defined as at the time of "life-threatening indications," also called "absolute indications" or "classic indications." Life-threatening indications were suggested in the Kidney Disease: Improving Global Outcomes (KDIGO) practice guidelines as follows: hyperkalemia, acidemia, pulmonary edema, and uremic complications [17]. However, there are no clear, standardized thresholds that absolutely indicate RRT initiation [18]. Furthermore, most guidelines have emphasized the importance of avoiding these complications rather than trying to reverse them once they have occurred.

A lot of critically ill patients with AKI have a progressive decline in kidney function and they do not develop these 'absolute indications'. Unfortunately, the definition of 'early' strategy is much more uncertain than that of late initiation. Some studies chose biochemistry levels, such as blood urea nitrogen (BUN) and serum creatinine, as early initiation criteria and other studies defined time from AKI or from advanced stage AKI, for example using the Risk, Injury, Failure, Loss and End-stage kidney disease (RIFLE) [19] or the Acute Kidney Injury Network (AKIN) [20] criteria [18]. In a recent systematic review about the timing of RRT, Wierstra and colleagues conducted meta-analyses including recent RCTs [18]. In their systematic review, a meta-analysis of nine high-quality studies defined by the authors (seven RCTs and two observational studies) showed that early initiation was not significantly different from later initiation in terms of survival (random effects OR 0.665, 95% CI 0.384–1.153, $p=0.146$). However, high statistical heterogeneity ($I^2=72.5\%$) was observed making any definitive conclusions difficult. In addition, we should consider that clinical heterogeneity was also high because there were various definitions of the timing of RRT in the included studies. Therefore, it is difficult to evaluate meta-analyses even if new RCTs are included, unless or until standardization of clinical protocols is achieved.

The AKIKI Trial

The Artificial Kidney Initiation in Kidney Injury (AKIKI) trial was conducted in 31 ICUs in France from September 2013 through January 2016 [2]. In the study, 620 patients with severe AKI (KDIGO stage 3) and with mechanical ventilation, vasopressors (epinephrine or norepinephrine), or both were randomly allocated to "early strategy" or "delayed strategy" of RRT, and 619 patients were analyzed. The main exclusion criteria were life-threatening indications for dialysis on enrollment as follows: severe hyperkalemia, metabolic acidosis, pulmonary edema, or BUN > 112 mg/dl. In the early-group, RRT was immediately started after randomization. In the late-group, if the abnormalities aforementioned in the exclusion criteria or oliguria > 72 hours developed, RRT was initiated. If the spontaneous urine output was ≥ 500 ml per 24 h, discontinuation of RRT was considered in the two groups. Discontinuation was highly recommended if the spontaneous urine output was ≥ 1,000 ml per 24 h without using diuretics, or if the urine output was ≥ 2,000 ml per 24 h with diuretics.

No difference between the two groups was observed in terms of 60-day overall survival, the primary outcome: death at day-60 was 48.5% (150/311) in the early-group and 49.7% (153/308) in the late-group. Importantly, 49% (151/311) of patients in the late-group never received RRT. Analyzing only those patients who received RRT, mortality at 60 days was 48.5% in the early and 61.8% in the delayed group. Those patients never receiving RRT had the lowest mortality (37.1%), but were less ill at baseline compared to the other groups as shown by sequential organ failure assessment (SOFA) scores ($p < 0.0001$). In addition, in the early-group, there were more catheter-related blood stream infections (10% [31/311] vs. 5% [16/308], $p = 0.03$) and cases of hypophosphatemia (22% [69/311] vs. 15% [46/308], $p = 0.03$). Patients in the late-group achieved adequate diuresis without the need for RRT earlier than in the early-group ($p < 0.001$).

The ELAIN Trial

Another important recent RCT, the Early vs Late Initiation of Renal Replacement Therapy in Critically Ill Patients With Acute Kidney Injury (ELAIN) trial, was conducted at a single center in Germany between August 2013 and July 2015, and the result were published at almost the same time as the AKIKI trial results [1]. The inclusion criteria were patients aged 18–90 years with KDIGO stage 2 and plasma neutrophil gelatinase-associated lipocalin (NGAL) > 150 ng/ml, in addition to at least one of the following conditions: severe sepsis, high doses of catecholamines, fluid overload, or non-renal SOFA score > 2.

RRT was initiated within 8 h after randomization and diagnosis of KDIGO stage 2 for patients in the early-group. For patients in the late-group, RRT was started within 12 h after developing KDIGO stage 3 or any of the following absolute indications: BUN > 100 mg/dl, severe hyperkalemia (K > 6 mEq/l), severe hypermagnesemia (Mg > 8 mEq/l), urine output < 200 ml per 12 h, and organ edema resistant to loop diuretics. Renal recovery was defined by spontaneous urine output > 400 ml per 24 h or urine output 2,100 ml per 24 h with diuretics, and recovered creatinine clearance (> 20 ml/min). RRT was discontinued if the renal recovery occurred.

In the ELAIN trial, 231 patients were randomly allocated and eligible in the intention-to-treat analyses. The method was continuous venovenous hemofiltration with citrate as the anticoagulation among all patients who received RRT, and 90.8% (108/119) of the patients even in the late-group eventually received RRT. The 90-day mortality rate as the primary outcome was significantly lower in the early-group compared to the late-group (39.3% [44/112] vs. 54.7% [65/119], $p = 0.03$). More patients in the early-group recovered renal function by day 90 than in the late-group (53.6% [60/112] vs. 38.7% [46/119], $p = 0.02$). The duration of RRT in the early-group was shorter than in the late-group (9 days vs. 25 days, $p = 0.04$). Levels of selected plasma proinflammatory mediators, such as interleukin (IL)-6 and IL-8, were reduced in the early-group. Although the clinical significance of changes in IL-6 and IL-8 are uncertain, these molecules have been found to be associated with survival and recovery of renal function [21] and are not influenced by intensity of RRT (within the range tested in recent dosing trials) [22].

Limitations of AKIKI and ELAIN

Given the results of these two trials, should we adopt a 'wait and see' approach for all patients with severe AKI according to the results of AKIKI [2] or should we initiate RRT early as per ELAIN [1]? Before we decide, we should consider some points before generalizing the results to patients in our real world. First, the initial mode of RRT in the AKIKI study was intermittent RRT (IRRT) for over 50% of the patients who received RRT in both groups. Moreover, continuous RRT (CRRT) was used as the sole method in only about 30% of the patients. Given that 85% of patients enrolled in AKIKI were receiving vasopressors (i. e., hemodynamically unstable), we would expect the vast majority of patients to be treated using CRRT – as per KDIGO and other guidelines [17]. Thus, it is possible that potential benefits of early initiation of RRT were negated by potential harms (Box 1). Second, in a *post-hoc* analysis of the trial, the mortality at day 60 was lowest among patients randomized to the 'late' group who never received RRT (37.1% [56/151]), and highest among patients who received late RRT (61.8% [97/157]). Mortality for patients in the early group was in-between (48.5% [150/311]). Therefore, the early-group included patients who would never have received RRT had they been randomized to the late-group (Fig. 1). On the other hand, RRT initiation might have been too delayed for patients who ultimately received RRT in the late-group. In other words, there is both a risk of unnecessary treatment using a strategy of early initiation, and a risk of harmful delay when using a strategy of 'wait and see'.

Obviously, the ELAIN trial has some limitations as well. First, most patients were postoperative cardiac surgery patients so generalizability might be limited. A second threat to generalizability is the single center study design. An interesting aspect of ELAIN was that investigators used a biomarker (plasma NGAL) to exclude low-risk patients. This enrichment approach has been advocated in the conduct of clinical trials in AKI [23]. However, this marker is relatively novel and few nephrologists or intensivists around the world have access to it.

Comparison of the Two Studies

Both studies, AKIKI and ELAIN, were RCTs, making the potential for bias from unobservable and unmeasured confounders small. However, we should consider the phenomenon of 'interaction' or 'effect modification' even in randomized trials. Patient severity could modify the effect of timing of RRT on clinical outcomes. When we compare the two trials, it seems that each trial included patients with rather different severity and time course. Fig. 1 is a conceptual model for understanding the patient selection in each trial. In the figure, the early-group of the ELAIN trial included many typical patients (shown in white) and several very sick patients (striped), but obviously excluded patients with emergent indications (dark gray). The late-group included some patients who spontaneously recovered renal function (light gray) and also some patients who developed emergent indications between the time that they were enrolled and the time they met 'late RRT' criteria. In the AKIKI

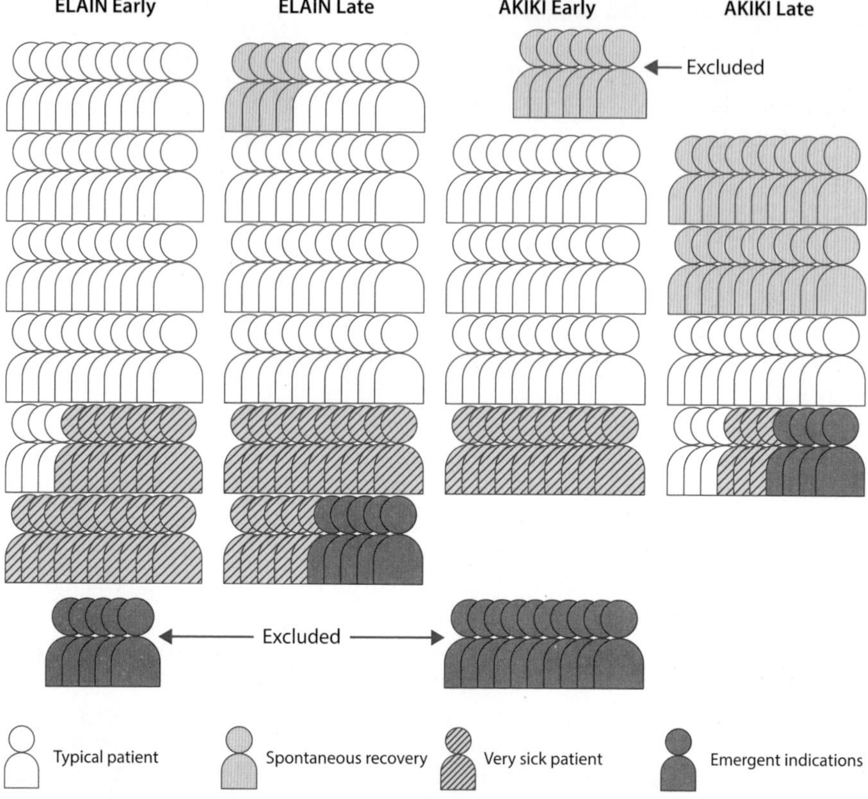

Fig. 1 Conceptual model for recent trial results on timing of renal replacement therapy (RRT). When you compare the two trials you can see that they looked at rather different patients. Starting on the far left, the early arm of the ELAIN trial [1] included many typical patients (shown in *white*) and several very sick patients (*striped*) but obviously excluded patients with emergent indications (*dark gray*). The late arm includes some patients who spontaneously recovered renal function (*light gray*) and also some patients who developed emergent indications. The AKIKI 'early' arm would have excluded those early recovery patients and also those with emergent indications prior to enrollment. The remaining patients are less sick and may have spontaneous recovery before reaching criteria for 'late' initiation

early-group, we would have excluded those early recovery patients and also those with emergent indications prior to enrollment. Indeed, as the supplement to the paper shows, more patients were excluded because of emergent indications (n = 663) than were ultimately randomized (n = 620). Not surprisingly, the remaining patients were less sick and may have had spontaneous recovery before reaching the criteria for late initiation (life-threatening indications).

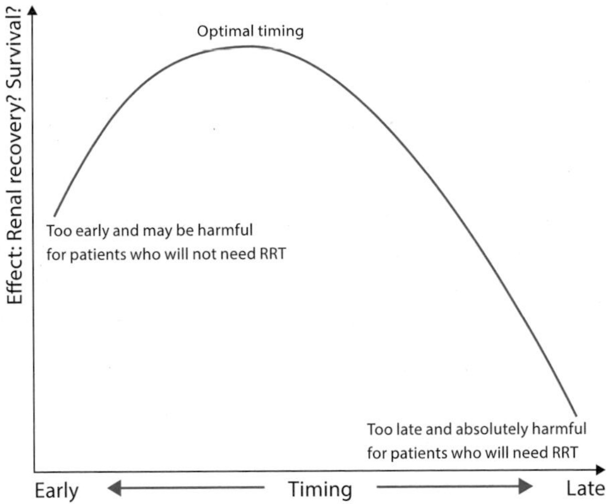

Fig. 2 Optimal timing of initiation of renal replacement therapy. This graph suggests that the relationship between the timing of renal replacement therapy (RRT) and its effects may not be linear. The horizontal axis indicates timing of RRT. In this graph, 'timing' includes various meanings: not just 'time' from certain AKI stages but also the 'severity' of the patients. The vertical axis indicates the potential effects of RRT: for example, renal recovery and improving survival. Timing may be too early and not necessary for less severe patients who might spontaneously recover. On the other hand, timing might be too late for more severely ill patients who will develop an emergent need for RRT

Future RCTs

As of September 2016, two larger RCTs are progressing (STARRT-AKI: NCT02568722 [24] and IDEAL-ICU: NCT01682590 [25]). Unless the problems of inclusion criteria and effect modification are solved, however, any new RCTs or new meta-analyses will continue to be limited in their ability to draw firm conclusions that will alter clinical practice. Given the results of the two RCTs, AKIKI and ELAIN, we can conclude the following: we should not start RRT early for patients who will not need RRT, and we should not delay RRT for patients who will need it (Fig. 2). Determining who will or will not ultimately need RRT therefore becomes a critical issue. Tools that can predict whether AKI patients will need RRT within a few days or biomarkers that do this would be quite helpful. Using such tools, we would be able to include patients who will need RRT more precisely and provide more precision RRT – as well as conduct more informative trials.

Optimal Timing of RRT: From a 'Time-centered' to a 'Patient-centered' Approach

For staging AKI, the standardized criteria by KDIGO will be useful for future AKI research [17]. The "AKI checklist" as recently proposed will also be helpful to diagnose AKI [26]. However, even global criteria have limitations for predicting whether patients will need RRT. For example, with the KDIGO criteria, a patient with AKI and a serum creatinine of 4.0 mg/dl will be classified as 'Stage 3' whether they have a baseline creatinine of 3.7 or 1.0 mg/dl. Obviously, these patients will not have the same AKI severity even if they have similar 'renal impairment'. They may also have very different recovery potential.

It is time to move from a 'time-centered' to a 'patient-centered' approach. Biomarkers, such as NGAL, may play a role but their clinical utility for this indication has not yet been established. Risk prediction models, such as the Cleveland Clinic Foundation Score [27] or the Renal Angina Index [28], may be useful in certain populations but they have not been widely validated. Dynamic parameters such as the furosemide stress test may also be efficient to predict the future-need for RRT [29]. Koyner and colleagues found that 2-hour urine output after intravenous administration of furosemide (1.0–1.5 mg/kg) significantly predicted RRT and the predictability was significantly better than any other novel biomarkers, including plasma NGAL [30]. However, although their findings deserve attention, the results still require external validation. Ultimately, the best prediction model might be some combination of ICU parameters (e. g., cumulative and recent fluid balances, recent urine output, severity of illness), along with biomarkers and/or furosemide stress test.

Conclusion

Despite the results of the recent RCTs, AKIKI and ELAIN, we cannot yet provide a definitive answer about the timing of RRT initiation. Furthermore, we may not be any more certain once the results of currently ongoing RCTs become available because of the challenges this kind of research involves. For the present, if the population in each clinical practice has a low proportion of RRT ($\leq 50\%$) then a 'wait and see' approach may be best, but if the population is more likely to receive RRT ($> 70\%$) then it probably makes sense to start early. Tools for the precise prediction of RRT, whether biomarkers, clinical scores or both, are definitely needed.

References

1. Zarbock A, Kellum JA, Schmidt C et al (2016) Effect of early vs delayed initiation of renal replacement therapy on mortality in critically ill patients with acute kidney injury: The ELAIN randomized clinical trial. JAMA 315:2190–2199
2. Gaudry S, Hajage D, Schortgen F et al (2016) Initiation strategies for renal-replacement therapy in the intensive care unit. N Engl J Med 375:122–133

3. Kellum JA, Murugan R (2016) Effects of non-severe acute kidney injury on clinical outcomes in critically ill patients. Crit Care 20:159
4. Kellum JA, Ronco C, Bellomo R (2016) Acute kidney disease and the community. Lancet 387:1974–1976
5. Boyd JH, Forbes J, Nakada TA, Walley KR, Russell JA (2011) Fluid resuscitation in septic shock: a positive fluid balance and elevated central venous pressure are associated with increased mortality. Crit Care Med 39:259–265
6. Bellomo R, Cass A, Cole L et al (2012) An observational study fluid balance and patient outcomes in the Randomized Evaluation of Normal vs. Augmented Level of Replacement Therapy trial. Crit Care Med 40:1753–1760
7. Rahbari NN, Zimmermann JB, Schmidt T, Koch M, Weigand MA, Weitz J (2009) Meta-analysis of standard, restrictive and supplemental fluid administration in colorectal surgery. Br J Surg 96:331–341
8. Wiedemann HP, Wheeler AP, Bernard GR et al (2006) Comparison of two fluid-management strategies in acute lung injury. N Engl J Med 354:2564–2575
9. Heung M, Wolfgram DF, Kommareddi M, Hu Y, Song PX, Ojo AO (2012) Fluid overload at initiation of renal replacement therapy is associated with lack of renal recovery in patients with acute kidney injury. Nephrol Dial Transplant 27:956–961
10. Vaara ST, Korhonen AM, Kaukonen KM et al (2012) Fluid overload is associated with an increased risk for 90-day mortality in critically ill patients with renal replacement therapy: data from the prospective FINNAKI study. Crit Care 16:R197
11. Teixeira C, Garzotto F, Piccinni P et al (2013) Fluid balance and urine volume are independent predictors of mortality in acute kidney injury. Crit Care 17:R14
12. Bouchard J, Soroko SB, Chertow GM et al (2009) Fluid accumulation, survival and recovery of kidney function in critically ill patients with acute kidney injury. Kidney Int 76:422–427
13. Wang N, Jiang L, Zhu B, Wen Y, Xi XM (2015) Fluid balance and mortality in critically ill patients with acute kidney injury: a multicenter prospective epidemiological study. Crit Care 19:371
14. Chen KP, Cavender S, Lee J et al (2016) Peripheral edema, central venous pressure, and risk of AKI in critical illness. Clin J Am Soc Nephrol 11:602–608
15. Damman K, van Deursen VM, Navis G, Voors AA, van Veldhuisen DJ, Hillege HL (2009) Increased central venous pressure is associated with impaired renal function and mortality in a broad spectrum of patients with cardiovascular disease. J Am Coll Cardiol 53:582–588
16. Mullens W, Abrahams Z, Francis GS et al (2009) Importance of venous congestion for worsening of renal function in advanced decompensated heart failure. J Am Coll Cardiol 53:589–596
17. Kidney Disease: Improving Global Outcomes (2012) KDIGO Clinical Practice Guideline for Acute Kidney Injury. Kidney Int Suppl 2:1–141
18. Wierstra BT, Kadri S, Alomar S, Burbano X, Barrisford GW, Kao RL (2016) The impact of "early" versus "late" initiation of renal replacement therapy in critical care patients with acute kidney injury: a systematic review and evidence synthesis. Crit Care 20:122
19. Bellomo R, Ronco C, Kellum JA, Mehta RL, Palevsky P (2004) Acute renal failure – definition, outcome measures, animal models, fluid therapy and information technology needs: the Second International Consensus Conference of the Acute Dialysis Quality Initiative (ADQI) Group. Crit Care 8:R204–212
20. Mehta RL, Kellum JA, Shah SV et al (2007) Acute Kidney Injury Network: report of an initiative to improve outcomes in acute kidney injury. Crit Care 11:R31
21. Murugan R, Wen X, Shah N et al (2014) Plasma inflammatory and apoptosis markers are associated with dialysis dependence and death among critically ill patients receiving renal replacement therapy. Nephrol Dial Transplant 29:1854–1864
22. Murugan R, Wen X, Keener C et al (2015) Associations between intensity of RRT, inflammatory mediators, and outcomes. Clin J Am Soc Nephrol 10:926–933

23. Kellum JA, Devarajan P (2014) What can we expect from biomarkers for acute kidney injury? Biomark Med 8:1239–1245
24. Wald R, Adhikari NK, Smith OM et al (2015) Comparison of standard and accelerated initiation of renal replacement therapy in acute kidney injury. Kidney Int 88:897–904
25. Barbar SD, Binquet C, Monchi M, Bruyere R, Quenot JP (2014) Impact on mortality of the timing of renal replacement therapy in patients with severe acute kidney injury in septic shock: the IDEAL-ICU study (initiation of dialysis early versus delayed in the intensive care unit): study protocol for a randomized controlled trial. Trials 15:270
26. Kellum JA, Bellomo R, Ronco C (2016) Does this patient have acute kidney injury? An AKI checklist. Intensive Care Med 42:96–99
27. Thakar CV, Arrigain S, Worley S, Yared JP, Paganini EP (2005) A clinical score to predict acute renal failure after cardiac surgery. J Am Soc Nephrol 16:162–168
28. Chawla LS, Goldstein SL, Kellum JA, Ronco C (2015) Renal angina: concept and development of pretest probability assessment in acute kidney injury. Crit Care 19:93
29. Chawla LS, Davison DL, Brasha-Mitchell E et al (2013) Development and standardization of a furosemide stress test to predict the severity of acute kidney injury. Crit Care 17:R207
30. Koyner JL, Davison DL, Brasha-Mitchell E et al (2015) Furosemide stress test and biomarkers for the prediction of AKI severity. J Am Soc Nephrol 26:2023–2031

An Overview of Complications Associated with Continuous Renal Replacement Therapy in Critically Ill Patients

S. De Rosa, F. Ferrari, and C. Ronco

Introduction

Acute kidney injury (AKI) is a frequent event in the intensive care unit (ICU) with a prevalence of approximately 40–57%. Approximately 13% of AKI patients receive extracorporeal treatment, associated with prolonged hospitalization and a high risk of death [1–5]. Renal replacement therapy (RRT) in critically ill patients is conducted as either intermittent hemodialysis or continuous renal replacement therapy (CRRT).

There is still ongoing debate concerning the optimal time to start RRT or which modality to use in the course of critical illness complicated by AKI. A recent systematic review showed that 'early' initiation of RRT in critical illness complicated by AKI did not improve patient survival or confer reductions in ICU or hospital lengths of stay [6]. Concerning the choice of modality, it should be made individually and on the basis of specific clinical situations. CRRT enables excess fluid to be removed more gradually and provides more efficient removal of small and large metabolites, Intermittent RRT is more practical, flexible, and cost-effective minimizing anticoagulation and thus bleeding risks and enabling more efficient removal of small solutes, such as potassium [7]. A recent prospective study compared mortality and short- and long-term renal recovery in patients treated with CRRT or intermittent hemodialysis. Results showed that CRRT did not appear to improve

S. De Rosa (✉) · F. Ferrari
International Renal Research Institute Vicenza (IRRIV)
Vicenza, Italy
Department of Anaesthesia and Intensive Care, San Bortolo Hospital
Viale Rodolfi 37, 36100 Vicenza, Italy
e-mail: derosa.silvia@ymail.com

C. Ronco
International Renal Research Institute Vicenza (IRRIV)
Vicenza, Italy
Department of Nephrology, Dialysis and Transplantation, San Bortolo Hospital
Vicenza, Italy

J.-L. Vincent (ed.), *Annual Update in Intensive Care and Emergency Medicine 2017*,
DOI 10.1007/978-3-319-51908-1_11

Table 1 Technical-clinical complications of renal replacement therapy

Technical	Clinical
Vascular access	Bioincompatibility and immune activation
Decreased filter lifespan and dialysis dose	Hypothermia
Air embolism	Hemodynamic instability
Imbalance of fluids and electrolyte	Hematological complications
	Electrolyte and acid-base disturbances
	Nutritional losses
	Errors in fluid management
	Drug removal

30-day or 6-month patient outcomes. CRRT seems beneficial for patients with fluid overload, but may be deleterious in the absence of hemodynamic failure [8]. CRRT also has complications. Because of the complexity of these patients, it is often difficult to distinguish between complications related to the extracorporeal treatment (technical complications) and those occurring as the result of the underlying disease process (clinical complications) (Table 1). In addition, the continuing evolution of technology, new indications for treatment and the need for a team expert in extracorporeal therapy have led gradually to parallel changes in the frequency and relative degree of the various complications, so it is more appropriate to define them together as technical-clinical complications. In the past, the dialytrauma concept was developed to enable early identification of harmful adverse events related to CRRT and to propose strategies to minimize them [9]. The present chapter details the existing evidence on technical-clinical complications related to CRRT to provide practical knowledge for those managing CRRT in the ICU.

Vascular Access

An adequately functioning temporary vascular access is an essential component for effective CRRT in AKI, but it is important to preserve the patient's vascular network in case of evolution to end-stage renal disease [10]. Central venous catheters (CVC) used in the ICU to perform extracorporeal treatment are high flow, temporary, not tunneled and dual.

Venous access sites include the subclavian, internal jugular and femoral veins. The Kidney Disease: Improving Global Outcomes (KDIGO) guidelines suggest the use of ultrasound for the placement of high flow CVCs in the right internal jugular vein to perform extracorporeal treatment. A femoral catheter is preferred to a catheter in the left internal jugular vein to reduce catheter failure, and the subclavian vein should be considered as a last option. In addition, it is suggested that a chest x-ray be performed after placement and before using a catheter in the subclavian vein or jugular vein [11].

Complications may be related to dysfunction (acute malfunction) or infection of the catheter [12, 13]. Catheter dysfunction, due to blood recirculation through the double lumen, causes hemoconcentration. Short femoral catheters (9–13 cm) have a higher recirculation rate than longer femoral catheters (18–25 cm) [14].

Any distortion or kinking of the catheter can result in the generation of different flows and pressures; this causes a reduction in laminar flow associated with deposition of fibrin, an increase in negative pressure in the artery and in positive pressure in the vein but also a decrease in both the length of the catheter and the filter lifespan with a decrease in dialysis dose [15].

The risk of nosocomial infections increases with increasing duration of extracorporeal treatment: patients may develop catheter colonization or catheter-related systemic infection. Colonization and infection risk may be influenced by the insertion site, the duration of use, and the CRRT modality. Recent evidence suggests that double lumen jugular and femoral CVCs used for RRT (including intermittent dialysis) in the ICU do not differ significantly with respect to these risks [16]. However, the results may not be so relevant to patients receiving RRT in whom a second double lumen CVC is positioned or replaced on the guide wire inserted in an existing catheter. A recent study by Chua et al. showed that in the initial and prolonged use of CRRT, double lumen femoral CVCs, compared with non-femoral, were safe and viable options, supported by low colonization and infectious profiles compared to non-femoral sites [5]. The replacement of femoral catheters to maintain venous access for CRRT is associated with an acceptable risk of colonization and infection [5]. Although guide-wire exchange compared to venepuncture insertion did not contribute to dialysis catheter colonization or infection, it was associated with a more than twofold increase in catheter dysfunction [17]. However, repeated use and prolonged femoral CVCs may be less appropriate in obese patients because of the high risk of colonization [5]. These important findings may help guide the choice of vascular access for RRT in critically ill patients.

Reduced Filter Life

Circuit clotting increases nursing workload, cost of therapy and blood loss [18]. It is not rare for a filter to have reduced efficiency with a consequent reduction in the effective dialysis time and dose. In addition, the prescribed dialysis dose may also be reduced, not only because of malfunctioning of the device, but also because of treatment interruptions for diagnostic procedures or because of the presence of non-expert personnel [15, 19]. The effectiveness of the filter decreases with the passage of time: clearance of solutes is also impaired as the sieving coefficients decrease with increasing time. Accordingly, ultrafiltration is reduced due to the formation of a protein layer from the deposition of proteins (i. e., clogging), which enhances the blockage of hollow fibers [18].

Air Embolism

After priming, air may remain in the extracorporeal circuit or may enter because of losses present in parts of the extracorporeal circuit (pre-pump, pump). Microbubbles originating in the extracorporeal lines of dialysis machines may be endogenous in cases of decompression sickness or mechanical heart valves [20]. Microbubbles obstruct blood flow in the capillaries, thus causing tissue ischemia, followed by an inflammatory response and complement activation, obstruction of the microcirculation and tissue damage [20].

All devices can detect the presence of air bubbles inside the circuit with consequent interruption of flow and emission of an audible alarm. The air detectors protect patients from massive air embolism, but are not designated to prevent infusion of microbubbles.

Fluid Balance

The reliability and safety of CRRT machines have improved, but there still remains the potential for fluid balance errors during treatment [21]. The new generations of CRRT machines are more reliable but may still cause some problems, such as the 'water balance error' alarm that can appear on several occasions without requiring discontinuation of treatment. Recent software versions force the operator to discontinue therapy after a given number of repeated alarms. However, most CRRT machines do not stop the treatment and allow the user to override the alarm repeatedly, which represents a potential risk to the patient. An accurate fluid management system may be particularly useful in the pediatric population: often clinicians adapt approved adult CRRT devices for use in children because of lack of safer alternatives [22]. Unfortunately, this may result in inaccurate fluid balance. Moreover, the extracorporeal blood volume used in current adult CRRT devices, which exceeds 15% of the total blood volume in many children, represents a health hazard to the smaller patients due to risks associated with clotting, hypotension, hypothermia and transfusion complications [22]. The need for adequate practical training, and clear protocols and procedures for RRT cannot be underestimated.

Hemodynamics

Hemodynamic instability and tissue hypoperfusion are major features of the critically ill patient. The following factors can influence hemodynamic stability: patient blood volume, which is directly influenced by the speed of ultra-filtration; aggressive removal of fluids, which results in a depression of the intravascular volume but also, in the presence of compromised myocardial function, may lead to a reduction in systemic perfusion [23]. Invasive blood pressure monitoring, evaluation of central venous pressure (CVP), urine output and systemic perfusion are useful to help maintain stable hemodynamics and optimize volume status [15]. A prospective observational study evaluated the impact of the "Slow blood flow safety protocol" on the start of CRRT and dependence on vasopressors in critically ill patients with AKI. A total of 205 circuits were studied in 52 patients. The slow blood flow safety protocol consisted of the following steps: 1) the blood pump set at speeds equal to 50 ml/min until the circuit is completely filled with blood; 2) increased blood pump speed of 20–50 ml/min every 5–10 min until 200 ml/min is reached. During the first 4 h of treatment following initiation of CRRT, there were no significant changes in mean arterial pressure (MAP), heart rate, CVP, or vasopressor dose compared to baseline. Only 16 circuits initiated in 13 patients were associated with a MAP > 20%. The implementation of a slow blood flow protocol might therefore be useful to limit episodes of hemodynamic compromise [24].

Biocompatibility

Bioincompatibility involves a complex series of humoral and cellular reactions (coagulation, the complement cascade, leukocytes and platelets) triggered by exposure of blood to foreign material. Use of biomaterials with direct blood contact results in activation of the blood coagulation system and in an inflammatory reaction. These responses are the result of the natural response of the host defense mechanism against foreign surfaces. Inadequate control by natural inhibitors results in pathological processes, including microthrombi generation or thrombosis, bleeding complications, hemodynamic instability, fever, edema, and organ damage. These adverse events become manifest during prolonged and intensive foreign material contact with vascular implants and extracorporeal blood circulation [25]. These reactions are very complex and not completely understood. Contact between the active material and blood cytokines and proteases causes an increase in protein and energy expenditure. To reduce bioincompatibility reactions, the membrane pore size has been increased and biomaterials improved (e. g., microfluidics and membraneless systems, living membranes, etc.) [26]. These changes optimize the removal of low molecular weight proteins and the direct removal of inflammatory mediators. The literature reports rare anaphylactoid reactions to dialysis membranes from activation of bradykinin, especially in patients previously treated with angiotensin converting enzyme inhibitors [27].

Hypothermia

Heat loss, heat conservation, and heat generation interact to maintain a narrow optimum range for cell functions [28]; in 5–50% of cases, RRT may expose the blood of the patient to an ambient temperature for a prolonged period of time [15]. The associated heat loss involves loss of energy, with increased oxygen demands, vasoconstriction, and inhibition of leukocyte function and coagulation. For this reason, it is recommended that body temperature is monitored and, if possible, external heating used. New devices are equipped with external heaters but these may not be sufficient. Intravenous infusion of heated liquid is not mandatory and does not prevent hypothermia during CRRT [14, 29].

Bleeding

Hemorrhagic complications have been reported in up to 30% of critically ill patients with AKI undergoing RRT with systemic anticoagulation [30]. Bleeding is a hematological complication that can occur during an extracorporeal treatment, and may be the result of clotting of the circuit and of the hemofilter, ineffective or excessive anticoagulant therapy, and inadvertent disconnection of the CRRT system. In addition, critically ill patients can also develop a procoagulant state due to sepsis, hyperviscosity syndrome or antiphospholipid antibody syndrome [18].

Furthermore, despite obvious progress regarding biocompatibility, all current membranes induce more or less activation of coagulation. Although studies have assessed associations between circuit coagulation, platelet counts and platelet transfusion, the interpretation of studies evaluating the duration of the extracorporeal circulation is hindered by the complexity of interactions with the various causal factors mentioned previously. Critically ill patients may not all require some form of anticoagulation, but if it is necessary, systemic anticoagulation should be performed using unfractionated heparin that has a short biological half-life and can be monitored using routine laboratory tests. Unfortunately, unfractionated heparin has a complex effect on platelets causing direct activation or immune-mediated thrombocytopenia [31].

Regional heparinization is another alternative that could be performed, using an infusion of protamine on the return line of the extracorporeal circuit, but it is not very successful. Low molecular weight heparins, widely used as antithrombotic therapy, have a more predictable pharmacokinetic and anticoagulant response, with an increased half-life that is more dependent on renal function, and a decreased likelihood of heparin-induced thrombocytopenia [32]. An alternative to heparin is citrate, which inhibits coagulation by chelating ionized calcium, and inducing profound hypocalcemia in the filter, thus maintaining circuit patency and reducing the risk of bleeding. The anticoagulant effect of citrate is regional in that it is partially removed by the CRRT and in part metabolized. It can be recommended for CRRT if and when metabolic monitoring is adequate and protocols are followed [30, 33].

Several non-randomized trials and two smaller randomized trials have shown a reduction in bleeding and need for transfusions in patients receiving regional citrate anticoagulation. A recent meta-analysis showed that the efficacy of citrate and heparin anticoagulation during CRRT was similar. Citrate anticoagulation decreased the risk of bleeding with no significant increase in the incidence of metabolic alkalosis [34]. The KDIGO guidelines recommend anticoagulation with citrate in critically ill patients in whom it is not contraindicated [11]. Citrate inhibits cellular activation induced by bioincompatibility and attenuates the inflammatory response. Potential complications related to citrate include hypocalcemia, metabolic alkalosis, hypernatremia and intoxication. Despite these concerns, there

Table 2 Measures to preserve circuit life

Reduction of flow stasis	Optimization of extracorporeal treatment
Vascular access	CVVHDF (less hemoconcentration)
Nursing training	Filtration fraction (less than 25%) or hematocrit post-filter
	Pre-dilution versus post-dilution
	Clogging
	Kind of membrane
	Filter size

CVVHDF: continuous veno-venous hemodiafiltration

is increasing evidence of the safety of citrate in patients with severe liver failure/liver transplant or severe septic shock with liver hypoperfusion [30]. Although anticoagulation is important to preserve circuit life, it is also important to adopt measures that ensure circuit life (Table 2).

Electrolyte Imbalance

AKI is associated with electrolyte and acid-base disturbances such as hyperkalemia, metabolic acidosis, hypocalcemia and hyperphosphatemia. The initiation of dialysis in AKI can efficiently treat these complications but can also trigger significant electrolyte and acid-base disorders, such as hypokalemia, hypophosphatemia and metabolic alkalosis, which may require changes in fluid delivery and composition [35]. Electrolyte complications of CRRT can be classified into two categories [36]:

1) Complications caused by the removal of electrolytes during dialysis or hemofiltration with inadequate substitution;
2) Complications caused by the use of trisodium citrate as an anticoagulant.

Patients with liver failure, in particular, have a reduced ability to metabolize citrate, leading to hypercitratemia and resulting in hypocalcemia and metabolic acidosis. Citrate has unique properties as an anticoagulant by forming a complex with calcium, an important substance in the coagulation cascade, which is then removed by the filter. The difference between chelation with citrate and post-filter calcium infusion is responsible for calcium imbalance [30].

Nutritional Losses

Nutritional losses should be considered in critically ill patients with AKI receiving CRRT. These losses can be caused by several factors including hypercatabolic state, loss of nutrients through the dialysis membrane, and secondary to lean protein catabolism particularly due to insulin resistance, the release of inflammatory mediators and metabolic acidosis [15].

In patients receiving RRT, the dose of protein should be between 1 and 1.5 g/kg/day. Energy provision should be between 20 and 25 kcal/kg/day. Nutritional support during CRRT should be based on extracorporeal losses of glucose, amino acids, and micronutrients. Amino acid loss through the filter accounts for 10–20% of administered protein. Larger proteins, such as albumin, are lost during extracorporeal treatment; high ultrafiltration rate and the use of new membranes with increased permeability can cause a significant negative nitrogen balance [37].

Critically ill patients are often hyperglycemic due to insulin resistance and increased hepatic gluconeogenesis. Dialysate solutions, in order to avoid significant diffusive losses, contain dextrose in 100–180 mg/dl concentrations equivalent to about 40–80 g/day which generally cause an increase in the patient's blood glucose. By contrast, glucose-free solutions are usually responsible for hypoglycemia and inadequate nutritional intake. The use of such solutions induces gluconeogenesis, primarily using amino acids as substrates, and their use is not recommended [15]. Water-soluble vitamins and trace elements are easily filtered out and may be lost during CRRT. Antioxidant mediators, including zinc, selenium, copper, manganese, chromium and vitamin E, are all freely lost through the dialysis membrane. Losses of thiamine may amount to 1.5 times the recommended intake, whereas the clinical significance of vitamin C losses remains unclear. Vitamin A supplementation is not recommended because of the risk of toxic accumulation. Amounts of active vitamin D are reduced in CRRT and preventive replacement will limit systemic breakdown [36].

Drug Removal

Drug removal during RRT remains largely unexplored. The impact of CRRT on drug removal is variable depending on the CRRT modality, the ultrafiltrate and dialysate flow rates, the filter and the patient's residual renal function [38]. The degree of removal of drugs is directly proportional to the surface of the device and dependent on the mode of replacement fluid (pre-dilution or post-dilution) and on ultrafiltration and/or speed of flow of dialysate applied [38]. If available, serum drug concentrations should be monitored along with patient clinical status.

RRT drug removal is clinically relevant for most hydrophilic antimicrobial agents (e. g., β-lactams, aminoglycosides, glycopeptides), whereas it is less relevant for lipophilic compounds (e. g., fluoroquinolones, oxazolidinones), which generally are not cleared by the kidney [39]. The impact of CRRT on drug removal is complicated and pharmacist dosing adjustment for these patients may be advantageous.

Conclusion

Adverse effects of CRRT are related to bioincompatibility, bleeding, metabolic disequilibrium, loss of heat but also human error. The dialytrauma concept should be emphasized and used to elaborate programs of early identification of adverse events and to propose new strategies in order to avoid complications. Continuous training of doctors and nurses for better understanding of how to prevent CRRT complications and avoid human error is recommended.

References

1. Hoste EA, Bagshaw SM, Bellomo R et al (2015) Epidemiology of acute kidney injury in critically ill patients: the multinational AKI-EPI study. Intensive Care Med 41:1411–1423
2. Nisula S, Kaukonen KM, Vaara ST et al (2013) Incidence, risk factors and 90-day mortality of patients with acute kidney injury in Finnish intensive care units: the FINNAKI study. Intensive Care Med 39:420–428
3. Kellum JA, Angus DC (2002) Patients are dying of acute renal failure. Crit Care Med 30:2156–2157
4. De Corte W, Dhondt A, Vanholder R et al (2016) Long-term outcome in ICU patients with acute kidney injury treated with renal replacement therapy: a prospective cohort study. Crit Care 20:256
5. Chua HR, Schneider AG, Sherry NL et al (2014) Initial and extended use of femoral versus nonfemoral double-lumen vascular catheters and catheter-related infection during continuous renal replacement therapy. Am J Kidney Dis 64:909–917
6. Wierstra BT, Kadri S, Alomar S et al (2016) The impact of "early" versus "late" initiation of renal replacement therapy in critical care patients with acute kidney injury: a systematic review and evidence synthesis. Crit Care 20:122
7. Vanholder R, Van Biesen W, Hoste E et al (2011) Pro/con debate: continuous versus intermittent dialysis for acute kidney injury: a never-ending story yet approaching the finish? Crit Care 15:204
8. Truche AS, Darmon M, Bailly S et al (2016) Continuous renal replacement therapy versus intermittent hemodialysis in intensive care patients: impact on mortality and renal recovery. Intensive Care Med 42:1408–1417
9. Maynar Moliner J, Honore PM, Sanchez-Izquierdo Riera JA et al (2012) Handling continuous renal replacement therapy-related adverse effects in intensive care unit patients: the dialytrauma concept. Blood Purif 34:177–185
10. Canaud B, Desmeules S, Klouche K et al (2004) Vascular access for dialysis in the intensive care unit. Best Pract Res Clin Anaesthesiol 18:159–174
11. Khwaja A (2012) KDIGO clinical practice guidelines for acute kidney injury. Nephron Clin Pract 120:c179–c184
12. Canaud B, Leray-Moragues H, Leblanc M et al (1998) Temporary vascular access for extracorporeal renal replacement therapies in acute renal failure patients. Kidney Int Suppl 66:142–150
13. Schetz M (2007) Vascular access for HD and CRRT. Contrib Nephrol 156:275–286
14. Little MA, Conlon PJ, Walshe JJ (2000) Access recirculation in temporary hemodialysis catheters as measured by the saline dilution technique. Am J Kidney Dis 36:1135–1139
15. Finkel KW, Podoll AS (2009) Complications of continuous renal replacement therapy. Sem Dial 22:155–159
16. Marik PE, Flemmer M, Harrison W (2012) The risk of catheter-related bloodstream infection with femoral venous catheters as compared to subclavian and internal jugular venous catheters: a systematic review of the literature and meta-analysis. Crit Care Med 40:2479–2485
17. Coupez E, Timsit JF, Ruckly S et al (2016) Guidewire exchange vs new site placement for temporary dialysis catheter insertion in ICU patients: is there a greater risk of colonization or dysfunction? Crit Care 20:230

18. Joannidis M, Oudemans-van Straaten HM (2007) Clinical review: Patency of the circuit in continuous renal replacement therapy. Crit Care 11:218
19. Page M, Rimmele T, Prothet J et al (2014) Impact of a program designed to improve continuous renal replacement therapy stability. Ann Fr Anesth Reanim 33:626–630
20. Barak M, Katz Y (2005) Microbubbles: pathophysiology and clinical implications. Chest 128:2918–2932
21. Cruz D, Bobek I, Lentini P et al (2009) Machines for continuous renal replacement therapy. Sem Dial 22:123–132
22. Santhanakrishnan A, Nestle TT, Moore BL et al (2013) Development of an accurate fluid management system for a pediatric continuous renal replacement therapy device. ASAIO J 59:294–301
23. Fieghen HE, Friedrich JO, Burns KE et al (2010) The hemodynamic tolerability and feasibility of sustained low efficiency dialysis in the management of critically ill patients with acute kidney injury. BMC Nephrol 11:32
24. Kim IB, Fealy N, Baldwin I et al (2011) Circuit start during continuous renal replacement therapy in vasopressor-dependent patients: the impact of a slow blood flow protocol. Blood Purif 32:1–6
25. van Oeveren W (2013) Obstacles in haemocompatibility testing. Scientifica (Cairo) 2013:392584
26. Oudemans-van Straaten HM (2007) Primum non nocere, safety of continuous renal replacement therapy. Curr Opin Crit Care 13:635–637
27. Brunet P, Jaber K, Berland Y et al (1992) Anaphylactoid reactions during hemodialysis and hemofiltration: role of associating AN69 membrane and angiotensin I-converting enzyme inhibitors. Am J Kidney Dis 19:444–447
28. Jones S (2004) Heat loss and continuous renal replacement therapy. AACN Clin Issues 15:223–230
29. Rickard CM, Couchman BA, Hughes M, al at (2004) Preventing hypothermia during continuous veno-venous haemodiafiltration: a randomized controlled trial. J Adv Nurs 47:393–400
30. Morabito S, Pistolesi V, Tritapepe L et al (2014) Regional citrate anticoagulation for RRTs in critically ill patients with AKI. Clin J Am Soc Nephrol 9:2173–2188
31. Hirsh J, Warkentin TE, Shaughnessy SG et al (2001) Heparin and low-molecular-weight heparin: mechanisms of action, pharmacokinetics, dosing, monitoring, efficacy, and safety. Chest 119:64S–94S
32. Schetz M (2001) Anticoagulation for continuous renal replacement therapy. Curr Opin Anaesthesiol 14:143–149
33. Zhang Z, Hongying N (2012) Efficacy and safety of regional citrate anticoagulation in critically ill patients undergoing continuous renal replacement therapy. Intensive Care Med 38:20–28
34. Wu MY, Hsu YH, Bai CH et al (2012) Regional citrate versus heparin anticoagulation for continuous renal replacement therapy: a meta-analysis of randomized controlled trials. Am J Kidney Dis 59:810–818
35. Claure-Del Granado R, Bouchard J (2012) Acid-base and electrolyte abnormalities during renal support for acute kidney injury: recognition and management. Blood Purif 34:186–193
36. Fall P, Szerlip HM (2010) Continuous renal replacement therapy: cause and treatment of electrolyte complications. Sem Dial 23:581–585
37. Oudemans-van-Straaten H, Chua HR, Joannes-Boyau O, Bellomo R (2015) Metabolic aspects of CRRT. In: Oudemans-van Straaten HM, Forni LG, Groeneveld ABJ, Bagshaw SM, Joannidis M (eds) Acute Nephrology for the Critical Care Physician Part IV. Springer International, Heidelberg, pp 203–216
38. Thompson AJ (2008) Drug dosing during continuous renal replacement therapies. J Pediatr Pharmacol Ther 13:99–113
39. Pea F, Viale P, Pavan F et al (2007) Pharmacokinetic considerations for antimicrobial therapy in patients receiving renal replacement therapy. Clin Pharmacokinet 46:997–1038

Measuring Quality in the Care of Patients with Acute Kidney Injury

M. H. Rosner

Introduction

All clinicians are interested in providing the highest quality care to our patients. In recent years, there has been an increased focus on developing metrics to define quality and benchmark performance of individual clinicians and institutions against one another. In some cases, these metrics have not been scientifically defined and may be of questionable value to the patient and not directly linked to an outcome of significance (such as mortality). Thus, a rigorous process of evaluating quality measures must exist to ensure that these measures are of value and can be measured appropriately. Furthermore, the reporting of these quality measures must be linked to continued process improvement. As a centering point to focus efforts in the quality domain, the Institute of Medicine has defined a quality measure as "the degree to which health care services for individuals and populations increase the likelihood of desired health outcomes and are consistent with current professional knowledge" [1]. In the area of acute kidney injury (AKI), little has been written in terms of appropriate quality measures, yet this condition is associated with significant short and long-term consequences and available data suggest that current care is sub-optimal [2].

AKI, depending upon the patient population studied, has an incidence in hospitalized patients that ranges from 3–20% [3–6]. For those patients admitted to the intensive care unit (ICU), the incidence of AKI ranges from 16–67% [7–9]. Furthermore, the available evidence suggests that the incidence of AKI is growing [10]. Of paramount importance is that the development of AKI is associated with significant increases in morbidity and mortality, even with small decreases in kidney function [3, 6, 10–14]. Despite this clinical importance, there are very few effective interventions either to prevent AKI in at-risk populations or to treat established AKI, other

M. H. Rosner (✉)
Division of Nephrology, University of Virginia Health System
Charlottesville, VA 22908, Virginia, USA
e-mail: mhr9r@virginia.edu

J.-L. Vincent (ed.), *Annual Update in Intensive Care and Emergency Medicine 2017*,
DOI 10.1007/978-3-319-51908-1_12

than dialysis [15]. Thus, it would seem that if we could develop measures to better define what quality of care was for patients with AKI, and if we could implement these care measures, we might see better outcomes independent of having effective therapeutics for this condition.

Quality Measure Domains

In order to better define quality of care, the Institute of Medicine has defined quality measure domains that are used to assess the performance of individual clinicians, clinical delivery teams, delivery organizations, or health insurance plans in the provision of care to their patients or enrollees [16]. These measure domains should be supported by evidence demonstrating that the measure indicates better or worse care. Unfortunately, for many measures, data supporting whether they, in fact, measure quality is lacking or may be debated. However, consensus among experts may exist that supports moving forward with these measures while evidence is gathered, with full recognition that the measure may change with time and experience.

The five domains include [16]:

- *Process*: A process of care is a health care-related activity performed for, on behalf of, or by a patient. Process measures are supported by evidence that the clinical process – that is the focus of the measure – has led to improved outcomes. An example may be: the percentage of patients with chronic stable coronary artery disease who were prescribed lipid-lowering therapy.
- *Access*: Access to care is the attainment of timely and appropriate health care by patients or enrollees of a health care organization or clinician. An example may be: the percentage of members 12 months to 19 years of age who had a visit with a primary care practitioner in the past year.
- *Outcome measures*: An outcome of care is a health state of a patient resulting from health care. These measures are supported by evidence that the measure had been used to detect the impact of a clinical intervention.
- *Structure*: Structure of care is a feature of a health care organization or clinician related to the capacity to provide high quality health care. This could include such measures as whether a health care system uses computerized physician order entry.
- *Patient Experience*: Experience of care is a patient's report of observations of and participation in health care, or assessment of any resulting change in their health. Such a measure may include how often or how well a physician communicated with a patient.

Applying these domains to the care processes in AKI is challenging and for the purposes of this chapter, the focus will largely be restricted to process of care elements that may be linked to outcome measures.

The Current State of AKI Care

Data that describe the current state of care for the patient with AKI are lacking although it is likely that significant variability in care processes and outcomes are present. There is a lack of consensus about what constitutes high quality processes that are essential for detection, management and prevention of AKI. For example, the Kidney Disease Improving Global Outcomes (KDIGO) 2012 Clinical Practice Guidelines for AKI set forth recommendations for care processes in this domain [17]. This was followed by numerous commentaries that differed with some of the recommendations [18, 19]. The UK National Institute for Health and Care Excellence (NICE) also issued their own set of guidelines in 2013 for the prevention, detection and management of AKI [20]. While there is significant overlap with many of these guidelines, there is no clear consensus on valid process of care indicators that are critical to assess the quality of care so that it can be measured, monitored and targeted for improvement.

The imperative to improve care was highlighted by the UK National Confidential Enquiry into Patient Outcome and Death (NCEPOD) study on AKI in 2009 [21, 22]. This report highlighted the process of care of patients who died in hospital with a primary diagnosis of AKI. It took a critical look at areas where the care of patients might have been improved and identified remediable factors in the clinical and the organizational care of these patients. In this study, only 50% of AKI care was considered at a level of "good" and there was poor assessment of risk factors for AKI, delay in AKI recognition, and failure to diagnose complications of AKI. The authors believed that 20% of patients had AKI that was predictable and avoidable. A more recent study highlighted that up to 30% of AKI cases are preventable and related to sub-optimal care [2]. These include mistakes such as failure to use fluid volume resuscitation/prophylaxis to prevent contrast-induced nephropathy, inappropriate medication use and dosage errors in patients at high-risk for AKI and inappropriate treatment of volume depletion. Clearly, there are opportunities to do better and directly defining care processes and outcome measures is one step along this pathway to improved care.

A common criticism of much of the work in the development of process and outcome measures in that there is little objective data to support inclusion of certain measures. However, given that we know that care can be improved, we have to start somewhere and that place can be helped by expert and consensus opinion that develops measures for inclusion in care pathways that can be subsequently studied and refined. Ideally, protocols to assess their influence on outcomes need to be developed and tested. Furthermore, protocols are needed to decrease variability of practice in order to determine what works and what does not work in improving outcomes. The community of AKI experts can lead the charge in developing these protocols. There are also some excellent examples of regional development of protocols, such as that developed by the UK National Health System with its AKI care bundle [23]. The development of these protocols and outcome measures can be supplemented by rigorous evidence-grading and also through Delphi methods that allow experts to grade and assess the validity of various options. The latter method was successfully used by the Canadian Society of Nephrology to develop care measures in surgically-associated AKI [24].

The Mission of AKI Care

In order to best define what process measures may be useful for AKI care, it is important to note what the care goals for AKI should be. These may include the following: (1) preventable causes of AKI should be eliminated; (2) early stages of AKI should not progress to later stages; (3) AKI care should be multidisciplinary; (4) AKI care should be based on evidence-based protocols and studied for best practice; (5) patients should recover from AKI; and (6) those patients not recovering should have aggressive follow-up care to monitor kidney function. With these goals in mind, potential process of care measures could be outlined and developed as in Fig. 1 and can be defined in four main areas: prevention of AKI, early diagnosis of AKI, management of AKI, and follow-up care for AKI.

What follows are some possible care measures that can be brought forward as items that could be defined and studied and most importantly bundled together to improve outcomes.

Prevention of AKI

Given that there are no effective therapies for the treatment of established AKI, preventative measures are critical to improve outcomes. These might include the following:

1. Obtain a serum creatinine and urinalysis before any potentially nephrotoxic insult (surgery, contrast administration, chemotherapy, etc.).
2. Use a risk stratification tool to 'flag' high-risk patients in the medical record. An example of such a risk assessment instrument is that developed by Inohara

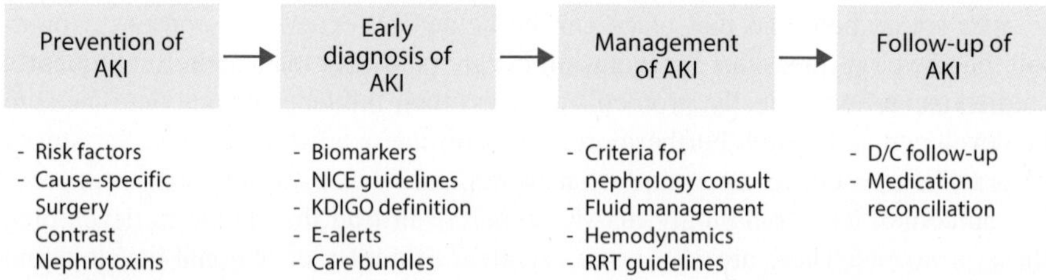

Fig. 1 Potential process of care measures. *RRT*: renal replacement therapy; *D/C*: discharge; *AKI*: acute kidney injury

and colleagues for contrast-induced AKI associated with percutaneous coronary interventions [25].

3. Use isotonic (balanced) crystalloids to expand intravascular volume prior to nephrotoxin exposure, such as contrast administration. Clinicians should also monitor a patient's volume status and avoid volume depletion after any nephrotoxic insult.
4. Monitor serum creatinine, fluid balance and urine output daily after nephrotoxic insult (surgery, contrast, chemotherapy, etc.).

Certain circumstances may require specific preventative strategies. For example, the use of nephrotoxic medications may require the following care processes to be instituted:

- Administer aminoglycoside drugs using a daily dosage and monitor levels with limited length of exposure.
- Discontinue non-steroidal anti-inflammatory drugs (NSAIDs) prior to nephrotoxic exposure.
- Monitor serum creatinine after exposure to nephrotoxic medications and stop potential agents with any changes in serum creatinine.
- Avoid multiple nephrotoxic drugs.
- Monitor levels of nephrotoxins if methods available.

For those patients undergoing surgical procedures where there is a substantial risk of AKI, the following care process measures could be developed and even placed into a bundle in an effort to systematize care and measure effectiveness.

- Obtain a serum creatinine (estimated glomerular filtration rate [eGFR] measurement) prior to surgery.
- Use a risk scoring system to assess AKI risk.
- Withhold NSAIDs and diuretics before surgery.
- Withhold RAAS blockers before surgery (evidence is controversial [26]).
- Provide intravenous crystalloids to restore effective circulating volume and blood pressure in patients with signs of effective volume depletion.
- Use vasopressors/inotropes in patients with vasomotor shock unresponsive to intravenous fluids.
- Consider targeting higher mean blood pressure for patients with history of hypertension.
- Avoid excessive positive fluid balance.
- Use a methodology to measure fluid responsiveness and monitor effectiveness of intravenous fluid therapy to measure their effectiveness in preventing AKI.

Many of these process measures, clinicians will view as 'obvious' and part of routine care. However, only by measuring how often these measures are really instituted in the care of patients will we know if they are effective in preventing AKI and provide feedback to clinicians regarding their care.

Early Diagnosis of AKI

While there are few data to state that early recognition and diagnosis of AKI improves outcomes, common sense would dictate that those patients in whom AKI is diagnosed would have greater attention to kidney-specific issues and may benefit from strategies to limit injury. Some potential quality process measures that could be included for an AKI care bundle would include:

- For those patients potentially at risk for AKI, measure serum creatinine, kidney function daily or, rarely, more frequently.
- Stage AKI severity using KDIGO methodology.
- Measure urine output, fluid balance at least daily.
- Monitor for electrolyte disorders (such as hyperkalemia) and acid-base disorders at least daily.

For those patients meeting criteria for AKI, early management issues should be instituted at once.

Early Management of AKI

The focus here is on limiting kidney damage, avoiding complications and improving outcomes. Thus, certain measure should be considered as care processes that should be routinely implemented and compliance with these processes should be monitored:

- Avoid nephrotoxin exposure after diagnosis of AKI.
- Use diuretics only when clearly indicated for volume overload.
- Perform careful review of medication exposures and drugs (ideally with electronic medical record [EMR] with computerized physician order entry [CPOE] and decision support).
- Maximize hemodynamics to ensure adequate renal perfusion pressure:
  - Provide intravenous crystalloids to restore effective circulating volume and blood pressure in patients with signs of effective volume depletion.
  - Use vasopressors/inotropes in patients with vasomotor shock unresponsive to intravenous fluids.
  - Consider targeting higher mean blood pressure for patients with history of hypertension.
  - Avoid excessive positive fluid balance.
  - Use a methodology to measure fluid responsiveness and monitor effectiveness of intravenous fluid therapy.
- Nephrology consultation should be obtained for patients with AKI especially if the etiology is not clear or worsening despite early interventions.

Management of later stages of AKI, especially when renal replacement therapy (RRT) is required is not covered in this manuscript but even this management should be broken down into key component parts that can be developed into care pathways where compliance and quality can be measured. For example, in the placement and use of temporary dialysis catheters, one could envision clear process steps that all hospitals would utilize to ensure safe placement as well as avoidance of catheter-related infections. Furthermore, in all patients receiving dialysis for AKI, the delivered dose should be measured and a minimum dose should be delivered [27]. Finally, all medications should be dosed and timed appropriately based upon dialysis modality. Ideally, this is accomplished in conjunction with an experienced pharmacist and an EMR with CPOE and decision support capabilities. Whenever possible, drug levels should be monitored for patients receiving dialysis.

Follow-up Care for Patients with AKI

Recent data have made it clear that patients who suffer an episode of AKI may not have complete recovery of kidney function and may subsequently develop progressive chronic kidney disease (CKD) [28]. Given the mortality and morbidity associated with CKD, it is imperative that patients with AKI have appropriate follow-up care and the following care measures could be considered as requirements for a high-quality program:

- For patients discharged from the hospital on dialysis, the patient should be monitored for signs of renal recovery and dialysis therapy should be frequently assessed to determine if it can be stopped.
- All survivors after an episode of AKI should have follow-up with a nephrologist to assess:
  - return of kidney function,
  - risk for progressive CKD with management of risk factors,
  - risk for mortality and morbidity with management of risk factors for these outcomes.

It would be anticipated that such post-AKI care processes would lead to improved outcomes for the patient.

Do Such Quality Interventions Improve Outcomes for AKI?

Unfortunately, data are lacking as to whether implementation of care pathways or even individual care processes can improve outcomes. A recent study that reported on a multicenter quality improvement intervention to lower the incidence of contrast-induced AKI provides some evidence that such multi-pronged efforts can be successful [29]. Through implementation of a standardized care pathway and protocol for AKI prevention (including such items as eliminating ventriculography, ensuring proper pre-procedure hydration and staging multiple procedures that required contrast), the centers were able to demonstrate that such an intervention lowered the rates of contrast-induced AKI by 21%. Importantly, the authors commented on what drove successful change in their model. They cited: multidisciplinary teams, having strong physician champions, standardized order sets to limit variability and providing quality improvement training.

Holding Ourselves Accountable for Outcomes

Protocols and standards for the care of patients with AKI can be developed. Through expert panels and consensus, we can develop these care pathways, study what is effective and improve outcomes. We can compare outcomes between centers and we can take advantage of EMRs and data mining to define outcomes and link them to care processes. What we cannot do is be complacent about the current state of care and accept current outcomes for patients with AKI.

Conclusion

AKI is a serious, morbid outcome and can be prevented in a substantial number of cases. For those patients with established AKI, it can be treated with a focus on best practices to optimize outcomes and clinicians can tailor care based upon protocols and a multidisciplinary care team. We need to seriously study what care processes work and develop best practices that can be shared and widely adopted.

What should not happen are uncoordinated efforts to improve care that will only lead to numerous protocols that are not well studied. Furthermore, we should not allow continued extreme variation in care leading to questions on what works and what does not work. We can clearly do better to foster excellent outcomes.

References

1. The Six Domains of Health Care Quality (2016) http://www.ahrq.gov/professionals/quality-patient-safety/talkingquality/create/sixdomains.html. Accessed November 6, 2016
2. Yamout H, Levin ML, Rosa RM et al (2015) Physician prevention of acute kidney injury. Am J Med 128:1001–1006
3. Ali T, Khan I, Simpson W et al (2007) Incidence and outcomes in acute kidney injury: a comprehensive population-based study. J Am Soc Nephrol 18:1292–1298
4. Lafrance JP, Miller DR (2010) Acute kidney injury associates with increased long-term mortality. J Am Soc Nephrol 21:345–352
5. Waikar SS, Liu KD, Chertow GM (2008) Diagnosis, epidemiology and outcomes of acute kidney injury. Clin J Am Soc Nephrol 3:844–861
6. Wonnacott A, Meran S, Amphlett B et al (2014) Epidemiology and outcomes in community-acquired versus hospital-acquired AKI. Clin J Am Soc Nephrol 9:1007–1014
7. Susantitaphong P, Cruz DN, Cerda J et al (2013) World incidence of AKI: a meta-analysis. Clin J Am Soc Nephrol 8:1482–1493
8. Bagshaw SM, George C, Dinu I, Bellomo R (2008) A multicenter evaluation of the RIFLE criteria for early acute kidney injury in critically ill patients. Nephrol Dial Transplant 23:1203–1210

9. Ostermann M, Chang RW (2007) Acute kidney injury in the intensive care unit according to RIFLE. Crit Care Med 35:1837–1843
10. Piccini P, Cruz DN, Grammaticopolo S et al (2011) Prospective multicenter study on epidemiology of acute kidney injury in the ICU: a critical care nephrology Italian collaborative effort (NEFROINT). Minerva Anestesiol 77:1072–1083
11. Rewa O, Bagshaw SM (2014) Acute kidney injury – epidemiology, outcomes and economics. Nature Nephrol Rev 10:193–207
12. Nisula S, Kaukonen KM, Vaara ST et al (2013) Incidence, risk factors and 90 day mortality of patients with acute kidney injury in Finnish intensive care units: the FINNAKI study. Intensive Care Med 39:420–428
13. Thakar CV, Christianson A, Freyberg R et al (2009) Incidence and outcomes of acute kidney injury in intensive care units: a Veterans Administration study. Crit Care Med 37:2552–2558
14. Hoste EA, Clermont G, Kersten A et al (2006) RIFLE criteria for acute kidney injury are associated with hospital mortality in critically ill patients: a cohort analysis. Crit Care 10:R73
15. Hsu CY, Chertow GM, McCulloch CE et al (2009) Nonrecovery of kidney function and death after acute on chronic renal failure. Clin J Am Soc Nephrol 4:891–898
16. Crossing the Quality Chasm: A New Health System for the 21st Century (2016) http://www.nationalacademies.org/hmd/Reports/2001/Crossing-the-Quality-Chasm-A-New-Health-System-for-the-21st-Century.aspx. Accessed November 6, 2016
17. KDIGO Clinical Practice Guideline for Acute Kidney Injury (2016) http://www.kdigo.org/clinical_practice_guidelines/pdf/KDIGO%20AKI%20Guideline.pdf. Accessed November 6, 2016
18. James M, Bouchard J, Ho K et al (2013) Canadian Society of Nephrology commentary on the 2012 KDIGO clinical practice guideline for acute kidney injury. Am J Kidney Dis 61:673–685
19. Palevsky PM, Liu KD, Brophy PD et al (2013) KDOQI US commentary on the 2012 KDIGO clinical practice guideline for acute kidney injury. Am J Kidney Dis 61:649–672
20. Acute kidney injury: prevention, detection and management (2016) Clinical guideline [CG169]. https://www.nice.org.uk/guidance/cg169. Accessed November 6, 2016
21. Acute Kidney Injury: Adding Insult to Injury (2016) http://www.ncepod.org.uk/2009aki.html. Accessed November 6, 2016
22. MacLeod A (2009) NCEPOD report on acute kidney injury – must do better. Lancet 374:1405–1406
23. Selby NM, Kolhe NV (2016) Care bundles for acute kidney injury: Do they work? Nephron 134:195–199
24. James MT, Pannu M, Barry R et al (2015) A modified Delphi process to identify process of care indicators for the identification, prevention and management of acute kidney injury after major surgery. Can J Kidney Health Dis 2:11
25. Inohara T, Kohsaka S, Abe T et al (2015) Development and validation of a pre-percutaneous coronary intervention risk model of contrast-induced acute kidney injury with an integer scoring system. Am J Cardiol 115:1636–1642
26. Zacharias M, Mugawar M, Herbison GP et al (2013) Interventions for protecting renal function in the perioperative period. Cochrane Database Syst Rev CD003590
27. Claure-Del Granado R, Mehta RL (2011) Assessing and delivering dialysis dose in acute kidney injury. Semin Dial 24:157–163
28. Chawla LS, Eggers PW, Star RA, Kimmel PL (2014) Acute kidney injury and chronic kidney disease as interconnected syndromes. N Engl J Med 371:58–66
29. Brown JR, Solomon RJ, Sarnak MJ et al (2014) Reducing contrast-induced acute kidney injury using a regional multicenter quality improvement intervention. Circ Cardiovasc Qual Outcomes 7:693–700

Characteristics and Outcomes of Chronic Dialysis Patients Admitted to the Intensive Care Unit

M. Chan, M. Varrier, and M. Ostermann

Introduction

The incidence and prevalence of end-stage renal disease (ESRD) is rising worldwide, mainly due to increasing rates of diabetes, cardiovascular disease, an aging population and general advances in the care of patients with chronic kidney disease (CKD) [1, 2]. Patients with ESRD now constitute approximately 0.2% of the adult population [1]. When compared to patients with normal renal function, ESRD patients experience higher rates of hospitalization, cardiovascular events and all cause mortality [3, 4]. It is estimated that 2% of chronic dialysis patients require admission to the intensive care unit (ICU) every year [5]. Dara et al. followed 476 ESRD patients for 7 years and reported that 20% required ICU admission during this period [6].

In this chapter, we will summarize the epidemiology of chronic dialysis patients in the ICU and highlight pertinent studies in the literature.

Admission Rates to the ICU

Chronic dialysis patients have significantly higher critical care admission rates than the general population. In an analysis of the Intensive Care National Audit & Research Centre (ICNARC) Case Mix Programme Database including 276,731 ad-

M. Chan
Centre for Nephrology, Royal Free Hospital
London, NW3 2QG, UK

M. Varrier
Department of Critical Care Medicine, Guy's & St Thomas' Hospital
London, SE1 7EH, UK

M. Ostermann (✉)
Department of Critical Care Medicine, King's College London, Guy's & St Thomas' Hospital
London, SE1 7EH, UK
e-mail: Marlies.Ostermann@gstt.nhs.uk

J.-L. Vincent (ed.), *Annual Update in Intensive Care and Emergency Medicine 2017*,
DOI 10.1007/978-3-319-51908-1_13

missions in England, Wales and Northern Ireland during the period 1995–2004, Hutchison et al. showed that 1.3% of admissions were chronic dialysis patients [4]. This was estimated to be equivalent to six ICU admissions or 32 ICU bed days per 100 dialysis patient-years. Compared to the annual ICU admission rate of the general population (2 per 1,000), this represents a 30-fold difference in critical care requirements.

An analysis of 41,972 admissions in the UK and Germany concluded that approximately 1.9% were individuals with ESRD [7]. Smaller studies from mostly single centers have reported higher admission rates of 3.4 to 8.6% confirming that ICU admission for critical illness is more common in ESRD patients than in the general population [8–10].

Characteristics of Critically Ill Dialysis Patients Admitted to the ICU

Reasons for Admission to the ICU

Sepsis and cardiovascular emergencies constitute the most common reasons for admission to the ICU [1, 2, 11, 12]. Patients with ESRD are particularly susceptible to infections due to uremia-related immune deficiency, defective phagocytic function, immunosuppressive medications and comorbidities including liver disease and diabetes mellitus. Sepsis accounts for up to 46% of all admissions [4, 6, 8, 9, 14–18]. A small study from Brazil reported that the lung was the most frequent source of sepsis, followed by soft tissue, catheter-related/blood-stream and abdominal sources [17].

Cardiovascular disease is very common in dialysis patients. In an analysis of 34,965 ICU admissions, Strijack et al. showed that ESRD patients admitted to the ICU had higher rates of diabetes mellitus (52.3% versus 22.4%), coronary artery disease (15.7% versus 14.3%), peripheral vascular disease (29.7% versus 12.7%) and strokes (10.3% versus 7.2%) compared to patients without ESRD [8]. Each of these conditions can lead to ICU admission as well as complicate ICU care. Studies have estimated that the proportion of ESRD patients admitted to the ICU with a cardiovascular emergency (including pulmonary edema) ranges from 5.1–31% [4, 6, 8, 9, 14–17]. ICU admission after cardiopulmonary resuscitation (CPR) is also more common in ESRD patients (13.6% versus 7.3%, $p<0.001$) [4]. The reasons for this observation are multifactorial but excessive inter-dialytic weight gain and fluid and electrolyte shifts during and between dialysis sessions play an important role. Other predisposing factors are left ventricular hypertrophy, ischemic heart disease, autonomic dysfunction, hypertension, diabetes, and being male [19].

Gastrointestinal bleeding is the third most common reason for chronic dialysis patients to require critical care, with studies estimating rates of 2.7–20% [6, 9, 16, 17].

It is difficult to ascertain precisely how often ESRD patients require critical care intervention for complications directly related to end-stage renal failure. It is increasingly recognized that hemodialysis patients on a traditional thrice weekly schedule are at increased risk of admission and mortality after the 2-day weekend gap. The commonest reason for these admissions is fluid overload [20]. Data on how many such patients require critical care admission is lacking. Hyperkalemia accounted for 4.3% and 3% of ESRD patients admitted to single ICUs in France and Australia, respectively [9, 14]. Clearly, these statistics depend not only on severity of illness but also on patients' wishes, ICU admission policy, ICU capacity and access to a renal unit.

Severity of Illness on Admission to the ICU

Several studies have used prognostication models such as the Acute Physiology and Chronic Health Evaluation (APACHE) II score to quantify the severity of illness of dialysis patients admitted to the ICU (Table 1). Hutchison et al. reported that both the APACHE II score (24.7 versus 16.6, $p < 0.001$) and the Simplified Acute Physiology Score (SAPS; 17.2 versus 12.6, $p < 0.001$) were significantly higher in dialysis patients than in patients without ESRD [4]. Similar conclusions were made in a Canadian historical cohort study in which patients with ESRD had a higher APACHE II score than those without ESRD (24 versus 15, $p < 0.0001$) [8]. The difference persisted even after removal of the renal component of the score (20 versus 14, $p < 0.0001$).

Outcomes

ICU Mortality

Critically ill patients with ESRD have higher ICU and hospital mortality rates than critically ill patients without ESRD [1, 4, 11, 12]. Analysis of the UK ICNARC database showed an ICU mortality rate of 26.3% in patients with ESRD compared to 20.8% in those without ESRD ($p < 0.001$) [4]. Risk factors for ICU mortality in chronic dialysis patients include increasing age, number of non-renal organ system failures, cardiac arrest, an abnormal serum phosphorus level (high or low), higher severity of illness, duration of mechanical ventilation and non-surgical status [1, 9, 10, 14]. This implies that the increased mortality risk relates to underlying comorbidities and severity of the acute illness rather than the presence of ESRD *per se* [1].

Length of Stay

The reported average length of stay of chronic dialysis patients in the ICU ranges from 1.9 to 9 days which is comparable to that of the general population [4, 8–10, 14, 17, 21–23]. Clearly, some of the discrepancies may be due to differences in

Table 1 Comparison of studies assessing outcomes of chronic dialysis patients admitted to the intensive care unit (ICU)

Study	Country	Study period	Number of ESRD patients	Mean age (years)	Mean severity of illness score on admission to ICU	ICU mortality (%)	Hospital mortality (%)	30-day mortality (%)
Bagshaw et al. [24]	Canada	1999–2002	92	66	APACHE II 29.7	16	34	–
Chapman et al. [21]	UK	1999–2004	199	59	APACHE II 27.6	44	56	–
Clermont et al. [10]	USA	2000–2001	57	58	APACHE III 64	11	14	–
Dara et al. [6]	USA	1997–2002	93	66	APACHE III 64	9	16	22
Hutchison et al. [4]	UK	1995–2004	3,420	57	APACHE II 24.7	26	45	–
Juneja et al. [16]	India	2007–2009	73	54	APACHE II 27.1	27	–	41
Manhes et al. [9]	France	1996–1999	92	63	SAPS II 49.4	28	38	–
O'Brien et al. [22]	UK	1995–2008	8,991	59	APACHE II 24.6	24	42	–
Ostermann et al. [7]	UK/Germany	1989–1999	797	55	SOFA 8	21	35	–
Rocha et al. [17]	Brazil	2004–2007	54	66	SAPS II 43.9	20	24	–
Senthuran et al. [14]	Australia	2001–2006	70	57	APACHE II 26.1	17	29	–
Sood et al. [18]	Canada	2000–2006	578	61	Renal-adjusted APACHE II 19	13	–	–
Strijack et al. [8]	Canada	2000–2006	619	62	APACHE II 24	–	16	–
Uchino et al. [5]	Australia	2002	38	45	APACHE II 22	22	38	–
Walcher et al. [23]	USA	2002–2010	28	58	–	36	39	39

APACHE: Acute Physiology Assessment and Chronic Health Evaluation; *ESRD*: end stage renal disease; *SOFA*: sequential organ failure assessment; *SAPS*: Simplified Acute Physiology Score discharge policies, levels of staffing on the receiving ward and availability of a bed in a renal unit.

ICU Readmission Rate

ESRD patients have an increased risk of ICU readmission during the same hospital stay following discharge from the ICU [4, 8, 14]. Strijack et al. reported twice the frequency of readmissions to the ICU within three days in ESRD patients compared to those without ESRD [8]. In addition to increased health care costs, readmissions to ICU are also associated with poor outcomes.

Prognosis After ICU Discharge

Hospital mortality rates have been found to be significantly higher in chronic dialysis patients compared to the non-ESRD population after ICU discharge (45.3 versus 31.2%, $p < 0.001$) [4]. Chapman et al. reported that the majority of deaths occurred within the first month of ICU admission [21]. Hemodialysis patients who survived to one month or hospital discharge, had long-term survival rates equivalent to ESRD patients who had not been admitted to the ICU. Bagshaw et al. reported that chronic dialysis patients had a similar 1-year mortality rate to those without ESRD after adjustment for age, severity of illness and admission type [24]. The main prognostic factors following ICU admission are older age, admission after emergency surgery, chronic health problems, need for CPR in the 24 hours preceding admission to the ICU, stay in hospital for at least 7 days prior to ICU admission and the number of failed non-renal organ systems [4, 6, 10, 17]. Mechanical ventilation and need for inotropic support are also significantly associated with mortality at 30 days [16].

Bell et al. investigated the effect of ICU admission on long-term prognosis in 245 ESRD patients admitted with a critical illness [15]. In multivariate analysis, ICU admission was not significantly associated with long-term mortality. Similarly, Senthuran et al. concluded that the long-term survival of dialysis patients who survived to hospital discharge following ICU admission was similar to that of the general dialysis population [14].

Comparison Between Acute Kidney Injury and ESRD Patients

Acute kidney injury (AKI) is common in critically ill patients and a frequent reason for admission to the ICU [25]. It is associated with an increased risk of mortality, especially if renal replacement therapy (RRT) is required. Clermont et al. were among the first to examine ICU mortality in patients with AKI, ESRD and those with normal renal function [10]. In spite of similar illness severity scores, ICU mortality rates were five times higher in AKI patients who required RRT than in those on chronic dialysis and ten times higher when compared to those with normal renal function (57% versus 11% vs. 5%, respectively). Similarly, Rocha et al. showed that ICU and hospital mortality rates were twice as high in AKI patients requiring RRT compared to ESRD patients when matched for age, severity of illness and number of organ dysfunctions (42% versus 20% and 50% versus 24%, respectively) [17].

A large retrospective database analysis found similar results when comparing outcomes of 1847 critically ill patients with AKI on RRT to 797 ESRD patients admitted to the ICU [7]. ESRD patients had approximately half the ICU and hospital mortality rates of AKI patients on RRT (20.8% versus 54.1%, $p < 0.0001$ and 34.5% versus 61.6%, $p < 0.0001$, respectively). As expected, increasing ICU mortality was seen with an increasing number of organ failures in both cohorts; however, among patients with AKI requiring RRT, the proportion of patients with more than two non-renal organ failures was significantly higher compared to the ESRD cohort (75.4% versus 25.6%, respectively). Length of stay in both ICU and hospital also tends to be significantly higher in patients with severe AKI compared to ESRD [7, 17, 23]. These data suggest that the prognosis of ESRD and AKI patients is related to severity of illness and comorbidities rather than lack of renal function *per se*. There may also be a contribution from the systemic effects of AKI on other organs (i. e., organ cross-talk) that do not occur in ESRD [26].

Severity of Illness Scores in ESRD

ICU illness severity and organ dysfunction scoring systems, including APACHE II and III [27, 28], SAPS II [29] and Sequential Organ Failure Assessment (SOFA) [30] scores, are primarily used within the critical care setting. Whilst these scoring systems have been validated in a wide variety of different subspecialties, their application to ESRD patients remains limited and controversial. Hutchison and co-workers evaluated the role of the APACHE II score to predict mortality in chronic dialysis patients admitted to the ICU [4]. They reported an area under the receiver operating characteristics curve (AUC) of 0.721 for the ESRD cohort, compared to 0.805 in the non-ESRD group. The APACHE III score has been found to overestimate 30-day mortality in ESRD patients [6, 10].

Data on the validity of the SOFA score in patients with ESRD are also conflicting. Juneja et al. reported an AUC of 0.92 [16] whereas Dara et al. [6] noted that the SOFA score was less accurate than the APACHE III score with an AUC of 0.66. These studies confirm that there is a clear need for more specific tools to assess severity of illness and predict the outcome of dialysis patients referred for ICU admission.

Conclusion

Critically ill patients with ESRD are frequently admitted to the ICU. Although they display worse outcomes than those with normal renal function, their prognosis is better than that of patients with AKI. Mortality is related primarily to the severity of the underlying illness and comorbid diseases rather than to lack of renal function *per se*. Having survived an episode of critical illness, data suggest that their longer-term prognosis is acceptable but little is known about quality of life and performance status after discharge from the ICU. Prognostic scoring systems used in critical care appear to overestimate mortality in the chronic dialysis population and should be used with caution. Current evidence suggests that the presence of ESRD should not prejudice against prompt referral or admission to ICU.

References

1. Hotchkiss JR, Palevsky PM (2012) Care of the critically ill patient with advanced chronic kidney disease or end-stage renal disease. Curr Opin Crit Care 18:599–606
2. Collins AJ, Foley RN, Herzog C et al (2011) US Renal Data System 2010 Annual Data Report. Am J Kidney Dis 57(Suppl 1):A8,e1–526
3. Go AS, Chertow GM, Fan D, McCulloch CE, Hsu CY (2004) Chronic kidney disease and the risks of death, cardiovascular events, and hospitalization. N Engl J Med 351:1296–1305
4. Hutchison CA, Crowe AV, Stevens PE, Harrison DA, Lipkin GW (2007) Case mix, outcome and activity for patients admitted to intensive care units requiring chronic renal dialysis: a secondary analysis of the ICNARC Case Mix Programme Database. Crit Care 11:R50
5. Uchino S, Morimatsu H, Bellomo R, Silvester W, Cole L (2003) End-stage renal failure patients requiring renal replacement therapy in the intensive care unit: incidence, clinical features, and outcome. Blood Purif 21:170–175
6. Dara SI, Afessa B, Bajwa AA, Albright RC (2004) Outcome of patients with end-stage renal disease admitted to the intensive care unit. Mayo Clin Proc 79:1385–1390
7. Ostermann ME, Chang R (2008) Renal failure in the intensive care unit: acute kidney injury compared to end-stage renal failure. Crit Care 12:432
8. Strijack B, Mojica J, Sood M et al (2009) Outcomes of chronic dialysis patients admitted to the intensive care unit. J Am Soc Nephrol 20:2441–2447
9. Manhes G, Heng AE, Aublet-Cuvelier B, Gazuy N, Deteix P, Souweine B (2005) Clinical features and outcome of chronic dialysis patients admitted to an intensive care unit. Nephrol Dial Transplant 20:1127–1133
10. Clermont G, Acker CG, Angus DC, Sirio CA, Pinsky MR, Johnson JP (2002) Renal failure in the ICU: comparison of the impact of acute renal failure and end-stage renal disease on ICU outcomes. Kidney Int 62:986–996
11. Chan M, Ostermann M (2013) Outcomes of chronic haemodialysis patients in the Intensive Care Unit. Crit Care Res Pract 2013:715807
12. Arulkumaran N, Annear NM, Singer M (2013) Patients with end-stage renal disease admitted to the intensive care unit: systematic review. Br J Anaesth 110:13–20
13. Sarnak MJ, Jaber BL (2000) Mortality caused by sepsis in patients with endstage renal disease compared with the general population. Kidney Int 58:1758–1764
14. Senthuran S, Bandeshe H, Ranganathan D, Boots R (2008) Outcomes for dialysis patients with end-stage renal failure admitted to an intensive care unit or high dependency unit. Med J Aust 188:292–295
15. Bell M, Granath F, Schon S, Lofberg E, Ekbom A, Martling CR (2008) Endstage renal disease patients on renal replacement therapy in the intensive care unit: short- and long-term outcome. Crit Care Med 36:2773–2778
16. Juneja D, Prabhu MV, Gopal PB, Mohan S, Sridhar G, Nayak KS (2010) Outcome of patients with end stage renal disease admitted to an intensive care unit in India. Ren Fail 32:69–73

17. Rocha E, Soares M, Valente C et al (2009) Outcomes of critically ill patients with acute kidney injury and end-stage renal disease requiring renal replacement therapy: a case-control study. Nephrol Dial Transplant 24:1925–1930
18. Sood MM, Miller L, Komenda P et al (2011) Long-term outcomes of end-stage renal disease patients admitted to the ICU. Nephrol Dial Transplant 26:2965–2970
19. Herzog CA (2003) Cardiac arrest in dialysis patients: approaches to alter an abysmal outcome. Kidney Int Suppl May:S197–S200
20. Fotheringham J, Fogarty D, El Nahas M et al (2015) The mortality and hospitalization rates associated with the long interdialytic gap in thrice-weekly hemodialysis patients. Kidney Int 88:569–575
21. Chapman RJ, Templeton M, Ashworth S, Broomhead R, McLean A, Brett SJ (2009) Long-term survival of chronic dialysis patients following survival from an episode of multiple-organ failure. Crit Care 13:R65
22. O'Brien AJ, Welch CA, Singer M, Harrison DA (2012) Prevalence and outcome of cirrhosis patients admitted to UK intensive care: a comparison against dialysis-dependent chronic renal failure patients. Intensive Care Med 38:991–1000
23. Walcher A, Faubel S, Keniston A, Dennen P (2011) In critically ill patients requiring CRRT, AKI is associated with increased respiratory failure and death versus ESRD. Ren Fail 33:935–942
24. Bagshaw SM, Mortis G, Doig CJ, Godinez-Luna T, Fick GH, Laupland KB (2006) One-year mortality in critically ill patients by severity of kidney dysfunction: a population-based assessment. Am J Kidney Dis 48:402–409
25. Hoste EA, Bagshaw SM, Bellomo R et al (2015) Epidemiology of acute kidney injury in critically ill patients: the multinational AKI-EPI study. Intensive Care Med 41:1411–1423
26. Doi K, Rabb H (2016) Impact of acute kidney injury on distant organ function: recent findings and potential therapeutic targets. Kidney Int 89:555–564
27. Knaus WA, Draper EA, Wagner DP, Zimmerman JE (1985) APACHE II: a severity of disease classification system. Crit Care Med 13:818–829
28. Knaus WA, Wagner DP, Draper EA et al (1991) The APACHE III prognostic system. Risk prediction of hospital mortality for critically ill hospitalized adults. Chest 100:1619–1636
29. Le Gall J, Lemeshow S, Saulnier F (1993) A new simplified acute physiology score (SAPS II) based on a European/North American multicenter study. JAMA 270:2957–2963
30. Vincent JL, de Mendonça A, Cantraine F et al (1998) Use of the SOFA score to assess the incidence of organ dysfunction/failure in intensive care units: results of a multicenter, prospective study. Working group on "sepsis-related problems" of the European Society of Intensive Care Medicine. Crit Care Med 26:1793–1800

Part V
Metabolic Support

Energy Expenditure During Extracorporeal Circulation

E. De Waele, P. M. Honore, and H. D. Spapen

Introduction

Nutritional therapy has become as important as other life-saving interventions (e. g., antibiotics, fluids, mechanical ventilation and renal replacement therapy [RRT]) in the treatment of the critically ill patient [1]. Knowledge of 'critical care nutrition' is evolving fast and 'nutrition pharmacology' has become a distinct specialty and research field [2]. Adequate nutrition is thought to improve outcomes whilst inappropriate feeding may expose the patient to unwarranted or deleterious effects [3]. Energy and protein supply in the critically ill depend on clearly formulated and decisive feeding guidelines. Within a nutritional care plan, optimal energy-protein targeting is imperative [4] and correct assessment of the patient's energy expenditure is required for setting caloric goals. Substrate and energy metabolism are sex-specific and weight-dependent [5, 6]. Adipose tissue barely contributes to resting energy expenditure (REE) [6]. As such, adjusted REE decreases with increased body mass index (BMI): 25 kcal/kg in normal weight, 20.4 kcal/kg in obese, and 16 kcal/kg in morbidly obese patients.

Leading experts in the field of clinical nutrition concur that indirect calorimetry is currently the best method for estimating energy expenditure [7]. From a practical viewpoint, only spontaneously breathing patients or patients who are mechanically ventilated with no other gas exchange site than the native lungs [8] qualify for indirect calorimetry. This theoretically excludes an increasing number of critically ill patients who receive some form of extracorporeal treatment. We briefly review the basic mechanisms of metabolism and metabolic rate and discuss recent evidence on the evaluation of energy expenditure during extracorporeal therapy.

E. De Waele (✉) · P. M. Honore · H. D. Spapen
ICU Department, Universitair Ziekenhuis Brussel, Vrije Universiteit Brussel
101 Laarbeeklaan, 1090 Brussels, Belgium
e-mail: elisabeth.dewaele@uzbrussel.be

J.-L. Vincent (ed.), *Annual Update in Intensive Care and Emergency Medicine 2017*,
DOI 10.1007/978-3-319-51908-1_14

Energy Expenditure

Body Energy Production

Body metabolism is the aggregation of anabolic processes responsible for synthesis and catabolic pathways that degrade molecules to release energy [9]. The global concept of energy production is based on the fact that nutrient molecules contain energy, which is converted through chemical reactions into a readily available form. Adenosine triphosphate (ATP) is the molecule that participates in most energy exchanges to support cellular activities. Glucose is, by cellular respiration, the main source of intracellular ATP. Glycolysis, the citrate acid cycle, and the electron transport chain provide ATP. Glycolysis uses two ATP molecules to form pyruvic acid, adenosine diphosphate (ADP) and four ATP molecules. This process is oxygen-independent and a prelude to the Krebs cycle. In this aerobic pathway, pyruvic acid is decarboxylated to form acetyl Co-enzyme A (acetylCoA) with carbon dioxide (CO_2) as a waste product. The Krebs cycle runs in the mitochondrial matrix as a series of oxidation/reduction reactions that generate energy from acetate derived from carbohydrates, fats and proteins:

$$C_6H_{12}O_6 + 6\,O_2 + 36 \text{ or } 38 \text{ ADP} + 36 \text{ or } 38\ P \rightarrow 6\,CO_2 + 6\,H_2O + 36 \text{ or } 38 \text{ ATP}.$$

This includes the electron transport chain where energy released as electrons is passed from one carrier to the next and is used to synthetize ATP from ADP and phosphate. Oxygen is consumed and water and CO_2 are released.

Energy Expenditure in Critically Ill Patients

Although scientific publications still refer to an 'ebb and flow' phase of shock, no strict correlation exists between measured metabolic rate and acute illness [10]. Energy expenditure can be influenced by medication (e. g., barbiturates) [11] and may vary considerably in patients undergoing therapeutic hypothermia for severe acute cerebral injury or after successful resuscitation from cardiac arrest. A 1 °C drop in temperature causes a 6% reduction in basal metabolism [12]. In contrast, REE increases with rising body temperature [13]. During mechanical ventilation, REE did not significantly differ in medical versus surgical or trauma patients. Indirect calorimetry measurements are not influenced by the ventilation mode (i. e., volume or pressure-controlled ventilation) [14]. Infection may not alter the metabolic rate measured by indirect calorimetry [15]. However, differences between calculated and indirect calorimetry-measured REE were positively correlated with C-reactive protein (CRP) levels in septic patients, suggesting that REE in critically ill patients corresponds with the degree of inflammation [16]. There are large individual variations in energy expenditure in critically ill patients.

Assessment of Energy Expenditure in Critically Ill Patients

Direct calorimetry provides direct measurement of body heat production. However, this technique is restricted to specialized research centers and logistically not feasible in a clinical, let alone critical care, setting [17]. Indirect calorimetry is increasingly recognized as the gold standard to objectify energy expenditure in clinical practice. In mechanically ventilated patients, metabolic rate can be measured by analysis of in- and exhaled gases. Determination of oxygen consumption (VO_2) and carbon dioxide production (VCO_2) enables the respiratory quotient (RQ) and REE to be established [8]. The modified Weir equation (energy expenditure $= [VO_2 \times 3.941] + [VCO_2 \times 1.11]$) is used for metabolic rate measurement.

However, most hospitals do not have access to indirect calorimetry mainly because of doubts regarding investment of time, complexity and cost. Instead, clinicians continue to rely on a wide array of predictive equations and formulas to estimate target energy uptake for nutritional support.

When metabolic rate is used as a nutritional target, caloric estimations are typically based on body weight (e. g., 25 kcal/kg body weight/day according to the European Society for Clinical Nutrition and Metabolism [ESPEN] guidelines) [18]. In general, formulas can be divided into two categories. The first approach is formulas using 'static' variables that predict REE in healthy humans (e. g., height, weight, sex and age). REE in critically ill subjects is then 'adjusted' by adding stress factors related to disease severity [19]. The second approach uses a combination of variables based in part on REE estimation in health but also incorporating disease-dependent 'dynamic' parameters (e. g., body temperature, minute ventilation and heart rate) [20]. Interestingly, a remarkably poor correlation is observed between REE values calculated by formulas and those measured by indirect calorimetry: the correlation coefficient varies between 0.24 and 0.51 [21]. None of the formula-based calculated energy requirements reached a clinically acceptable spread in limits of agreement. Accordingly, the weight-based REE estimation adopted in the Early Parenteral Nutrition Completing Enteral Nutrition in Adult Critically Ill Patients (EPaNIC) study showed very low correlation with measured REE [22]. In elderly, obese or underweight critically ill patients, correlation tended to be even worse. This underpins a more prominent role of indirect calorimetry in the intensive care unit (ICU).

Energy Expenditure and Assessment During Extracorporeal Treatment

Extracorporeal Membrane Oxygenation

ICU physicians increasingly use extracorporeal membrane oxygenation (ECMO) when faced with respiratory, cardiac, or cardiopulmonary failure refractory to classic treatment modalities. This approach is not without success because the Extracorporeal Life Support Organization (ELSO) recently reported an overall 54% survival rate in 70,000 adult patients undergoing extracorporeal life support (ECLS) [23]. ECMO provides pump-driven lung or heart-lung bypass support. Gas exchange occurs both in the native and artificial lung. The need for an individualized nutritional therapy protocol to prevent over- and underfeeding in this frail ICU subpopulation is evident. The widespread belief that ECMO patients are hypercatabolic is probably based on data obtained using a closed-circuit indirect calorimetry technique in ECMO-treated neonates, which revealed highly variable metabolic rates within and among neonates over time [24]. Measurement of VO_2 and VCO_2 enabled assessment of pulmonary function and predicted weaning from ECMO in this particular population. The concept that ECLS induces a metabolic 'rest state' (because 80% of cardiopulmonary work is provided 'mechanically') has been refuted by isotope tracer techniques [25]. Energy expenditure obtained during (88.6 ± 7.7 kcal/kg/d) and after (84.3 ± 9.2 kcal/kg/d) initiating ECMO indicated a hypermetabolic state. Recent work in pediatric cardiac failure reported a small increase in energy expenditure during consecutive ECMO support. Respiratory mass spectrometry enabled information to be gathered on energy expenditure and RQ [26] and permitted inadequate feeding to be avoided. Isotope dilution methods enabled comparison of the energy expenditure of ECLS-dependent neonates with that of hemodynamically stable, non-ventilated, postsurgical controls [27]; the mean energy expenditure was 53 ± 5.1 kcal/kg/d in controls and 55 ± 20 kcal/kg/d in ECLS patients ($p = 0.83$). Thus, no increased energy expenditure was objectified in the 'stressed' ECMO-dependent neonates. The observation that surplus caloric intake in ECMO-treated neonates did not affect protein catabolism whilst increasing CO_2 production rate is cumbersome [28].

A key question regarding nutrition in ECMO is whether predictive equations are still useful in this condition. A study on the adequacy of feeding in ECMO patients reported that only 55% of nutritional targets were covered [29]. However, caloric goals were set by the Schofield equation corrected for stress. The level of agreement between this calculated value and real energy expenditure is unknown. The ELSO guidelines remain vague in guiding treatment by merely stating 'to guarantee full caloric and protein nutritional support' but without specifying how this should be accomplished.

Indirect calorimetry has never been studied in an adult ECMO setting, mainly because of the technical challenge imposed by the presence of two simultaneously active gas exchange locations: the native and the artificial lung. To overcome these issues, we developed an innovative technical set-up coupled to a novel mathematical approach [30]. Respiratory gas exchange analysis was performed separately at the ventilator and the artificial lung in a patient with severe respiratory failure treated by ECMO (Fig. 1). Applying the Weir formula on the combined data produced a "composite" REE of 1,703 kcal/day. Introducing the manual-derived VO_2 and VCO_2 membrane oxygenator characteristics into the Weir formula retrieved a REE of 1,729 kcal/day.

The effect of ECMO on oxidative metabolism and protein synthesis has been studied in animals [31]. ECMO caused metabolic disturbances that contributed to total body wasting and protein loss. ECMO also decreased pulse pressure and

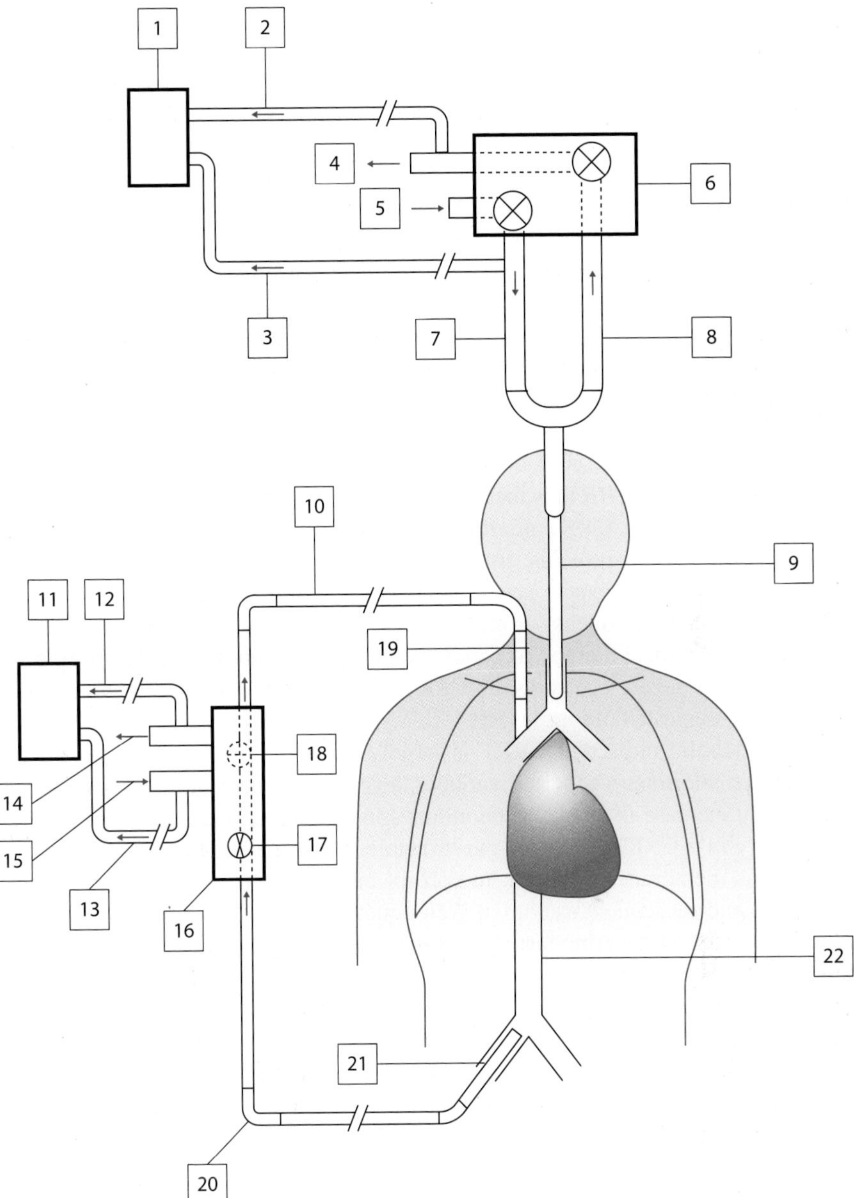

Fig. 1 Schematic representation of patient, indirect calorimeter, and extracorporeal membrane oxygenation (ECMO) system. *1* indirect calorimeter in position 1; *2* outflow sampler; *3* inflow sampler; *4* outflow of mechanical ventilator; *5* oxygen/air; *6* mechanical ventilator (including internal circuit); *7* inspiratory tubing; *8* expiratory tubing; *9* endotracheal tube; *10* venous return tubing ECMO; *11* indirect calorimeter in position 2; *12* outflow sampler; *13* inflow sampler; *14* outflow of oxygenator; *15* inflow of oxygenator; *16* ECMO; *17* pump; *18* oxygenator; *19* return cannula; *20* ECMO tubing; *21* venous drainage cannula; *22* inferior vena cava. Modified from [30] with permission

lowered myocardial VO_2 by approximately 40% indicating decreased overall mitochondrial oxidative metabolism. The influence of ECMO on metabolic rate in clinical conditions has not been determined. This is not surprising because large metabolic variations are already present in a 'general' critically ill population.

Continuous Renal Replacement Therapy

Acute kidney injury (AKI) is diagnosed in 10 to 30% of patients hospitalized in European ICUs. Although prevention, general management, and RRT have all substantially improved in recent years, mortality associated with AKI remains high [32]. AKI induces metabolic and physiological disturbances that are superimposed on those produced by the initial disease. In addition, AKI therapy *per se*, in particular when not carefully monitored for quality and safety, may be harmful or cause unwarranted side-effects (e. g., the so-called 'dialytrauma' concept) [33].

Continuous RRT (CRRT) is increasingly used to treat AKI in hemodynamically unstable patients [34]. CRRT produces a significant loss of glucose, amino acids, low-molecular-weight proteins, trace elements and water-soluble vitamins. Non-selective molecular transport across CRRT membranes also enhances clearance of certain blood components at elimination rates varying with operational characteristics. Nutritional therapy of patients on CRRT remains markedly unexplored. Information on dietary needs during CRRT is scarce and only basic recommendations can be suggested (Table 1) [35].

The metabolic impact of CRRT is largely unknown. Early investigations using indirect calorimetry reported variable degrees of hyper- and hypo-catabolism and a daily increase in energy expenditure [36]. However, the validity of indirect calorimetry in a CRRT setting is questionable. In particular, CO_2 removal across the dialysis membrane is thought to corrupt interpretation of gas exchange measurements and subsequent use of the Weir equation. Currently, indirect calorimetry is not advocated by the American Association for Respiratory Care (AARC) guidelines.

In a recent study, indirect calorimetry was performed at admission, immediately before and 6 h after starting CRRT in a septic patient [37]. A significant downregulation of REE/body weight was observed, which was positively correlated with the variation of extracellular water decrease and CRRT duration. Measured REE values were higher than calculated ones suggesting a 'cooling' effect of CRRT on the sepsis-induced hypermetabolic state. The RQ shifted to 0.85, reflecting mixed-substrate but no lipid use as the main energy source. Thus, CRRT seems to downregulate hypermetabolism in sepsis but no conclusions can be drawn on the impact of the technique itself.

Further research should focus on specific issues, such as CRRT dosing, flow rate and type of substitution fluid. The impact of citrate as regional anticoagulant during CRRT must also be determined. Indeed, as a crucial component of the Krebs cycle, excess administration of citrate may alter mitochondrial function because cit-

Table 1 Summary recommendations for nutrient doses in CRRT. From [35] with permission

Energy	Indirect calorimetry 25–35 kcal/kg body weight/day	60–70% carbohydrates 30–40% lipids
Protein	1.5–1.8 g/kg body weight/day	
Electrolytes		
K	Serum level > 4 mEq/l	i. v. supplements K-rich replacement fluid K-rich substitution fluid
P		i. v. supplements substitution fluid enteral supplements
Mg		i. v. bolus 2–4 g/day
Glucose		Strict glycemic control
Amino acids	+0.2–2.5 g/kg body weight/day glutamine (alanyl-glutamine dipeptide) 0.3–0.6 g/kg body weight/day	
Lipids		Close triglyceride monitoring
Vitamins		
Water-soluble	Vitamin B_1: 100 mg/day Vitamin B_2: 2 mg/day Vitamin B_3: 20 mg/day Vitamin B_5: 10 mg/day Vitamin B_6: 100 mg/day	Vitamin B_7 (biotin): 200 mg/day Vitamin B_9 (folic acid): 1 mg/day Vitamin B_{12}: 4 µg/day Vitamin C: 250 mg/day
Fat-soluble	Vitamin E: 10 IU/day Vitamin K: 4 mg/week	Vitamin A: reduce supplementation
Trace elements	Selenium: +100 µg/day Zinc: 50 mg/day Copper: 5 mg/day	Triple dose of i. v. trace elements-containing solutions
Body temperature	> 37 °C	

i. v.: intravenous

rate censors ATP production and controls anabolic and catabolic pathways through feedback reactions [38].

Conclusion

ECMO and CRRT are increasingly used in our ICUs. The metabolic impact of these treatment modalities remains largely unknown. Nevertheless, nutritional therapy must be implemented even in the absence of 'evidence-based' guidance. Indirect calorimetry cannot be advocated for routine measurement of REE during extracorporeal treatment. However, primary experience with a distinct indirect calorimetry setup in an ECMO patient is promising. In the meantime, REE assumptions are an acceptable alternative. More research time should be spent to better understand physiologic changes, to solve technical challenges, and to avoid pitfalls that currently hamper or preclude adequate assessment of energy expenditure in critically ill patients on CRRT.

References

1. Iapichino G, Radrizzani D, Giacomini M, Pezzi A, Zaniboni M, Mistraletti G (2006) Metabolic treatment of critically ill patients: energy expenditure and energy supply. Minerva Anestesiol 72:559–565
2. Wischmeyer PE, Heyland DK (2010) The future of critical care nutrition therapy. Crit Care Clin 26:433–441
3. Ridley E, Gantner D, Pellegrino V (2015) Nutrition therapy in critically ill patients – a review of current evidence for clinicians. Clin Nutr 34:565–571
4. Singer P, Hiesmayr M, Biolo G et al (2014) Pragmatic approach to nutrition in the ICU: expert opinion regarding which calorie protein target. Clin Nutr 33:246–251
5. Drolz A, Wewalka M, Horvatits T et al (2014) Gender-specific differences in energy metabolism during the initial phase of critical illness. Eur J Clin Nutr 68:707–711
6. Zauner A, Schneeweiss B, Kneidinger N, Lindner G, Zauner C (2006) Weight-adjusted resting energy expenditure is not constant in critically ill patients. Intensive Care Med 32:428–434
7. Preiser JC, van Zanten AR, Berger MM et al (2015) Metabolic and nutritional support of critically ill patients: consensus and controversies. Crit Care 19:35
8. American Association for Respiratory Care (1994) AARC clinical practice guideline. Metabolic measurement using indirect calorimetry during mechanical ventilation. Respir Care 39:1170–1175
9. Tortora GJ, Grabowski SR (1993) Principles of Anatomy and Physiology, 7th edn. vol. 862. Harper Collins College, New York, p 822
10. Vandervelden S, Malbrain ML (2015) Initial resuscitation from severe sepsis: one size does not fit all. Anaesthesiol Intensive Ther 47:s44–s55
11. Ashcraft CM, Frankenfield DC (2013) Energy expenditure during barbiturate coma. Nutr Clin Pract 28:603–668
12. Saur J, Leweling H, Trinkmann F, Weissmann J, Borggrefe M, Kaden JJ (2008) Modification of the Harris-Benedict equation to predict the energy requirements of critically ill patients during mild therapeutic hypothermia. In Vivo (Brooklyn) 22:143–146
13. Oshima T, Furukawa Y, Kobayashi M, Sato Y, Nihei A, Oda S (2015) Fulfilling caloric demands according to indirect calorimetry may be beneficial for post cardiac arrest patients under therapeutic hypothermia. Resuscitation 88:81–85
14. Clapis FC, Auxiliadora-Martins M, Japur CC, Martins-Filho OA, Evora PR, Basile-Filho A (2010) Mechanical ventilation mode (volume × pressure) does not change the variables obtained by indirect calorimetry in critically ill patients. J Crit Care 25:659.e9–659.16
15. Raurich JM, Ibáñez J, Marsé P, Riera M, Homar X (2007) Resting energy expenditure during mechanical ventilation and its relationship with the type of lesion. JPEN J Parenter Enteral Nutr 31:58–62
16. Hickmann CE, Roeseler J, Castanares-Zapatero D, Herrera EI, Mongodin A, Laterre PF (2014) Energy expenditure in the critically ill performing early physical therapy. Intensive Care Med 40:548–555
17. Oshima T, Berger MM, De Waele E (2016) Indirect calorimetry in nutritional therapy. A position paper by the ICALIC study group. Clin Nutr June 22, Epub ahead of print
18. Singer P, Berger MM, Van den Berghe G et al (2009) ESPEN. ESPEN Guidelines on Parenteral Nutrition: intensive care. Clin Nutr 28:387–400
19. Harris JA, Benedict JA (1919) Biometric studies of basal metabolism in man. Carnegie Institute of Washington, Washington (Publication no 270)

20. Walker RN, Heuberger RA (2009) Predictive equations for energy needs for the critically ill. Respir Care 54:509–521
21. De Waele E, Opsomer T, Honore PM et al (2015) Measured versus calculated resting energy expenditure in critically ill adult patients. Do mathematics match the gold standard? Minerva Anestesiol 81:272–282
22. Casaer MP, Mesotten D, Hermans G et al (2011) Early versus late parenteral nutrition in critically ill adults. N Engl J Med 365:506–517
23. ELSO Guidelines for Cardiopulmonary Extracorporeal Life Support Extracorporeal Life Support Organization, Version 1.3 November 2013. Available at: http://www.elso.org/resources/Guidelines.aspx. Accessed 10 November 2016
24. Cilley RE, Wesley JR, Zwischenberger JB, Bartlett RH (1988) Gas exchange measurements in neonates treated with extracorporeal membrane oxygenation. J Pediatr Surg 23:306–311
25. Keshen TH, Miller RG, Jahoor F, Jaksic T (1997) Stable isotopic quantitation of protein metabolism and energy expenditure in neonates on- and post-extracorporeal life support. J Pediatr Surg 32:958–962
26. Li X, Yu X, Cheypesh A, Li J (2015) Non-invasive measurements of energy expenditure and respiratory quotient by respiratory mass spectrometry in children on extracorporeal membrane oxygenation – a pilot study. Artif Organs 39:815–819
27. Jaksic T, Shew SB, Keshen TH, Dzakovic A, Jahoor F (2001) Do critically ill surgical neonates have increased energy expenditure? J Pediatr Surg 36:63–67
28. Shew SB, Keshen TH, Jahoor F, Jaksic T (1999) The determinants of protein catabolism in neonates on extracorporeal membrane oxygenation. J Pediatr Surg 34:1086–1090
29. Lukas G, Davies AR, Hilton AK, Pellegrino VA, Scheinkestel CD, Ridley E (2010) Nutritional support in adult patients receiving extracorporeal membrane oxygenation. Crit Care Resusc 12:230–234
30. De Waele E, van Zwam K, Mattens S et al (2015) Measuring resting energy expenditure during extracorporeal membrane oxygenation: preliminary clinical experience with a proposed theoretical model. Acta Anaesthesiol Scand 59:1296–1302
31. Priddy CM, Kajimoto M, Ledee DR et al (2013) Myocardial oxidative metabolism and protein synthesis during mechanical circulatory support by extracorporeal membrane oxygenation. Am J Physiol Heart Circ Physiol 304:H406–H414
32. Bozfakioğlu S (2001) Nutrition in patients with acute renal failure. Nephrol Dial Transplant 16(Suppl 6):21–22
33. Maynar Moliner J, Honore PM, Sánchez-Izquierdo Riera JA, Herrera Gutiérrez M, Spapen HD (2012) Handling continuous renal replacement therapy-related adverse effects in intensive care unit patients: the dialytrauma concept. Blood Purif 34:177–185
34. Schneider AG, Bellomo R (2013) Acute kidney injury: new studies. Intensive Care Med 39:569–571
35. Honoré PM, De Waele E, Jacobs R et al (2013) Nutritional and metabolic alterations during continuous renal replacement therapy. Blood Purif 35:279–284
36. Scheinkestel CD, Kar L, Marshall K (2003) Prospective randomized trial to assess caloric and protein needs of critically Ill, anuric, ventilated patients requiring continuous renal replacement therapy. Nutrition 19:909–916
37. Wu C, Wang X, Yu W et al (2016) Short-term consequences of continuous renal replacement therapy on body composition and metabolic status in sepsis. Asia Pac J Clin Nutr 25:300–307
38. Icard P, Poulain L, Lincet H (2012) Understanding the central role of citrate in the metabolism of cancer cells. Biochim Biophys Acta 1825:111–116

Vitamin D, Hospital-Acquired Infections and Mortality in Critically Ill Patients: Emerging Evidence

G. De Pascale, M. Antonelli, and S. A. Quraishi

Introduction

Hospital-acquired infections (HAIs) represent a major cause of morbidity and mortality worldwide. With a reported incidence of 22 new episodes per 100,000 admissions, this equates to approximately 2 million new cases of HAI each year, and is the cause of nearly 100,000 deaths annually in the United States alone [1]. Catheter-associated urinary tract infections (CAUTIs) are the most common cause of HAIs, followed by surgical site infections (SSIs), hospital-acquired pneumonia (HAP), and hospital-acquired bloodstream infections (HABSIs). Additional healthcare expenditure due to HAIs in the United States is estimated at between $28 and $45 billion annually, and is mainly driven by an increase in hospital length of stay (LOS).

Current HAI reduction strategies principally include behavioral interventions (e. g., removal of unnecessary devices), increased staff education (directed towards medical and nursing providers), reduction of microbial transmission through infection control measures (e. g., use of bundle kits for placement of central venous catheters), improvements to hand hygiene, and the adoption of antibiotic stewardship programs. And although hospitalized patients are known to exhibit varying degrees of immune dysfunction, few modifiable risk factors have been identified to improve this state [2]. Recently, however, sub-optimal vitamin D status has been

G. De Pascale · M. Antonelli (✉)
Department of Intensive Care and Anesthesiology, Catholic University of the Sacred Heart, Agostino Gemelli Hospital
Largo A. Gemelli 8, 00168 Rome, Italy
e-mail: Massimo.Antonelli@unicatt.it

S. A. Quraishi
Department of Anesthesia, Critical Care and Pain Medicine, Massachusetts General Hospital
Boston, MA, USA
Department of Anaesthesia, Harvard Medical School
Boston, MA, USA

J.-L. Vincent (ed.), *Annual Update in Intensive Care and Emergency Medicine 2017*,
DOI 10.1007/978-3-319-51908-1_15

Table 1 Main investigations on vitamin D, hospital-acquired infections and mortality in the critically ill patient setting

First author	Year	Design of the study	Sample size	Results
Vitamin D and sepsis in hospitalized patients				
Ginde [9]	2011	Prospective cohort study	81 septic patients admitted from the ED	25(OH)D < 30 ng/ml (n = 64) was associated with severity of sepsis (p = 0.005)
Braun [19]	2011	Retrospective cohort study	2,399 hospital admitted patients (1,160 subgroup who had blood cultures taken)	25(OH)D < 15 ng/ml was associated with HABSI (p = 0.03) occurrence and mortality (p < 0.001)
Cecchi [13]	2011	Prospective cohort study	170 ICU patients (92 with severe sepsis/septic shock)	Lower 25(OH)D levels in septic patients. No association with mortality in multivariable analysis
Flynn [17]	2012	Prospective cohort study	66 ICU patients	Hypovitaminosis D (74%) was associated with a trend to higher infection/sepsis rate (p = 0.09)
Nair [10]	2013	Prospective cohort study	100 ICU patients (26 with sepsis)	25(OH)D admission levels correlated with higher SAPS II, APACHE II scores (p < 0.001; p = 0.02) and fewer hospital-free days (OR 3.15; 95% CI 1.18–8.43)
Lange [14]	2013	Retrospective cohort study	5,628 hospital admitted patients	25(OH)D ≤ 15 ng/ml associated with increased odds of sepsis (OR, 1.29; 95% CI 1.06–1.57; p = 0.01)
Nguyen [15]	2013	Prospective cohort study	91 septic hospital admitted patients	Low 1,25(OH)$_2$D levels associated with increased 30-day mortality (p < 0.01)
Quraishi [20]	2013	Retrospective cohort study	2,135 hospitalized patients	25(OH)D < 10 ng/ml associated with significantly increased odds of HABSI occurrence
Moromizato [16]	2014	Retrospective cohort study	3,386 ICU patients	Preadmission 25(OH)D level an independent predictor of sepsis development in ICU (p = 0.009)
Amrein [18]	2014	Retrospective cohort study	655 ICU patients	Death prevalent in septic patients with vitamin D deficiency

Table 1 (Continued)

First author	Year	Design of the study	Sample size	Results
Vitamin D and SSI and CDI				
Quraishi [26]	2013	Retrospective cohort study	770 gastric bypass surgery patients	Patients with 25(OH)D < 30 ng/ml at higher risk of HAI [OR 3.05 (95% CI 1.34–6.94)] and SSI [OR 4.14 (95% CI 1.16–14.83)]
Zittermann [27]	2016	Prospective cohort study	3,340 cardiac surgical patients	1,25(OH)$_2$D levels independent risk factors for post-surgical infections (OR 2.57, 95% CI 1.47–4.49)
Quraishi [28]	2014	Retrospective cohort study	5,047 patients admitted to the hospital	25(OH)D levels < 10 ng/ml and 10–19.9 ng/ml increased CDI risk (OR 4.96; 95% CI 1.84–13.38 and OR 3.36; 95% CI 1.28–8.85)
Wang [30]	2014	Prospective cohort study	62 hospitalized patients with CDI	Normal 25(OH)D levels predicted CDI resolution ($p=0.028$)
Van der Wilden [32]	2015	Prospective cohort study	100 hospitalized patients with CDI	25(OH)D$_3$ levels significantly correlated with disease severity (OR 0.92; CI 0.87–0.98; $p=0.008$); 1 ng/ml increase in 25(OH)D$_3$ decreased by 8% the risk of severe CDI
Vitamin D and in-hospital mortality				
McKinney [41]	2011	Retrospective cohort study	136 ICU patients	Risk of death significantly higher in ICU patients with vitamin D deficiency (RR 1.81)
Venkatram [42]	2011	Retrospective cohort study	437 ICU patients	Hospital mortality higher in patients with 25(OH)D deficiency ($p=0.01$)
Arnson [45]	2012	Prospective cohort study	130 ICU patients	Shorter survival curves in patients with 25(OH)D < 20 ng/ml ($p<0.05$)
Remmelts [36]	2012	Prospective cohort study	272 hospitalized patients	25(OH)D < 20 ng/ml independent predictor of 30-day mortality (AUC 0.69; 95% CI 0.71–0.94)
Braun [43]	2012	Retrospective cohort study	1,325 ICU patients	25(OH)D < 15 ng/ml associated with increased mortality ($p=0.01$)
Higgins [46]	2012	Prospective cohort study	196 ICU patients	Higher levels of 25(OH)D were associated with a shorter time-to-alive ICU discharge (HR 2.11; 95% CI, 1.27–3.51)

Table 1 (Continued)

First author	Year	Design of the study	Sample size	Results
Matthews [47]	2012	Prospective cohort study	258 ICU patients	Severe/moderate deficiency status (<26 ng/ml) was associated with significantly increased ICU costs ($p=0.027/p=0.047$)
Aygencel [44]	2013	Prospective cohort study	201 ICU patients	25(OH)D <20 ng/ml was associated with increased mortality rate (43% vs 26%; $p=0.027$)
Lange [14]	2013	Retrospective cohort study	26,603 hospitalized patients	25(OH)D <15 ng/ml and 25(OH)D 15–30 ng/ml were associated with increased all cause 30-day mortality ($p<0.001$; $p=0.003$)
Amrein [40]	2013	Retrospective cohort study	24,094 hospitalized patients	25(OH)D levels <20 and ≥ 60 ng/ml before hospitalization associated with increased odds of 90-day mortality (U shaped relationship)
Quraishi [4]	2014	Prospective cohort study	100 ICU patients	Significant association of 25(OH)D with readmission (OR per 1 ng/ml, 0.84; 95% CI, 0.74–0.95) and mortality (OR per 1 ng/ml, 0.84; 95% CI 0.73–0.97)
Amrein [51]	2014	Randomized controlled trial	492 ICU patients	Lower mortality associated with vitamin D supplementation in patients with severe vitamin D deficiency ($p=0.04$)
De Pascale [48]	2016	Retrospective cohort study	107 ICU septic patients	Extremely low 25(OH)D level independent predictor of sepsis-related mortality ($p=0.01$)

25(OH)D: 25-hydroxyvitamin D; *ED*: emergency department; *HABSI*: hospital-acquire bloodstream infection; *ICU*: intensive care unit; *SAPS II*: Simplified Acute Physiology Score II; *APACHE II*: Acute Physiology and Chronic Health Evaluation II; *SSI*: skin and soft tissue infection; *CDI*: *Clostridium difficile* infection; *OR*: odds ratio; *CI*: confidence interval investigated as a potential risk factor for HAIs and other undesirable clinical outcomes [3].

Indeed, growing evidence suggests that low vitamin D status, as characterized by serum 25-hydroxyvitamin D [25(OH)D] levels < 20 ng/m, increases the risk of cardiovascular disease, cancer, and pulmonary ailments in community dwelling individuals. There is now also increasing evidence of a strong relationship between hypovitaminosis D and increased morbidity as well as higher mortality in hospitalized patients (Table 1). This may be due to the central role that vitamin D plays in regulating innate and adaptive immune responses [4]. As such, the objective of this chapter is to provide a comprehensive account of the emerging evidence regarding the relationship of vitamin D status with HAIs and mortality in the critical care setting.

Vitamin D as an Immune Regulator

Vitamin D production and function is dependent on a complex regulatory system. It is derived from endogenous or exogenous prehormones, requiring extensive tissue modification, which includes an active intermediate molecule [25(OH)D], and is potentially influenced by numerous modulators, such as parathyroid hormone (PTH), calcium, phosphorus, and fibroblast growth factor-23. Calcitriol or 1,25-dihydroxyvitamin D [1,25$(OH)_2$D] is the most biologically active metabolite of the vitamin D pathway. However, plasma levels of 1,25$(OH)_2$D are not only 500–1,000 times lower than those of 25(OH)D, but its half-life is also significantly shorter than the monohydroxylated form. As such, and under normal circumstances, 25(OH)D levels are used to represent total body vitamin D status. Both 25(OH)D and 1,25$(OH)_2$D are largely protein-bound to vitamin D binding protein (DBP) and, much less so (~ 10%), to albumin, while less than 1% of each molecule is found unbound in the circulation. Since the binding affinity of vitamin D metabolites to albumin is significantly lower than it is to DBP, it is postulated that during times of acute need, only the unbound and albumin-bound 25(OH)D and/or 1,25$(OH)_2$D is biologically active, and therefore referred to as the bioavailable fraction of vitamin D [3]. Epithelial, mucosal and innate immune cells, such as leukocytes, monocytes and macrophages, all of which represent the first barrier against infections, express the vitamin D receptor (VDR) and produce 1-α-hydroxylase, which facilitates conversion of 25(OH)D to 1,25$(OH)_2$D for paracrine and autocrine use within the target cells. Stimulation of the VDR through production of 1,25$(OH)_2$D can attenuate the proliferation and differentiation of both T and B lymphocytes, which likely improves outcome in autoimmune diseases. Furthermore, vitamin D metabolites activate Toll-like receptors (TLRs) in order to stimulate innate immunity and upregulate the production of potent antimicrobial peptides, such as cathelicidin and β-defensin 2 [3]. LL-37, the only know human cathelicidin, expresses a wide-range of antimicrobial activity against pathogens, including Gram-positive and Gram-negative bacteria, fungi, mycobacteria and viruses. LL-37 is not only expressed systemically by cells of the immune system, but is also produced by epithelial cells at barrier sites including skin, respiratory tract, and gastrointestinal mucosa. Recent evidence suggests that LL-37 production is optimized with 25(OH)D levels of ~ 30–35 ng/ml.

Bloodstream Infections

Bloodstream infections (BSIs) represent a major concern among all causes of HAIs. It is estimated that the incidence of BSIs is 0.6 cases per 100 admissions across all units, and 9.7 per 100 admissions in the intensive care unit (ICU), with attributable LOS and hospital costs of approximately 10 days and €5,000 (US ~ $5,500), respectively [1]. To-date, most preventive strategies are focused on the control of environmental factors, such as hand hygiene, skin decontamination, antiseptic-impregnated catheters, and non-pharmacological bundles. And, although immune dysfunction is recognized as a key element for susceptibility to infection, few modifiable immunomodulatory factors have been identified to reduce HABSIs.

Low serum 25(OH)D levels may be an important risk factor for HABSI development. A prospective study looking at vitamin D status in 49 critically ill patients and 21 healthy controls found that 25(OH)D and LL-37 concentrations were significantly lower in ICU patients than in controls, with a positive correlation between the two [5]. Moreover, a retrospective cohort analysis of acute care patients hospitalized in non-federal US hospitals with a diagnosis of sepsis during a 24 year period found that the incidence of sepsis and mortality rate increased by 16.5 and 40% respectively during the winter. Indeed, low vitamin D status, due to reduced exposure to ultraviolet B radiation, which is necessary for endogenous 25(OH)D production, has been proposed as a possible underlying cause of such observations [6]. Similarly, in a prospective review of 106 French ICU patients, spring admission, low albumin levels, and high Simplified Acute Physiology Score (SAPS II) were independent predictors of low 25(OH)D levels [7]. Furthermore, preclinical data support the relationship between sepsis incidence or severity and vitamin D status. In a mouse study, DBP levels were shown to correlate with disease severity and the administration of vitamin D3 improved survival rates by 40% [8].

Prospective studies have also investigated the relationship between vitamin D status and sepsis. A pilot study assessed 25(OH)D levels in 81 patients admitted to an emergency department with suspected infection. Subjects with 25(OH)D levels < 75 nmol/l (23.5 ng/ml) were more likely to develop severe sepsis within 24 h of presentation compared to subjects with normal values [9]. These findings are further supported by another study, which found that the degree of hypovitaminosis D in critically ill patients was associated with higher SAPS II, Acute Physiology and Chronic Health Evaluation (APACHE) II scores, and fewer hospital-free days [10]. Conversely, a recent randomized controlled trial (RCT), which included 67 critically ill septic patients found that a single intravenous administration of 2 μg of calcitriol did not improve mortality rates or blood cathelicidin levels after 48 h but it did increase plasma $1,25(OH)_2D$ and anti-microbial protein mRNA levels [11]. Nevertheless, a case-control study that included 240 patients with severe sepsis found no significant differences in outcomes between patients with normal or low vitamin D levels. However, this investigation only evaluated samples taken the morning after admission, and the mean serum level for the top quartile was 58.3 nmol/l (23.3 ng/ml), therefore still below an optimal value [12]. Interestingly, an Italian study found that the median 25(OH)D levels at admission for 172 ICU patients were lower in the severe sepsis and septic shock group than in trauma patients (10.1 ng/ml vs. 18.4 ng/ml): the univariate analysis revealed that, after adjusting for age, sex and SAPS II score, low vitamin D status was associated with a higher mortality rate [13].

Retrospective studies have also found a strong correlation between sepsis and vitamin D levels. An analysis of 5,628 patients reported that pre-hospital 25(OH)D levels ≤ 15 ng/ml were associated with a 1.3-fold increased risk of developing a community-acquired BSI requiring hospitalization compared to patients with levels > 15 ng/ml [14]. Similarly, all 91 outpatients admitted to the emergency department of a large US hospital with sepsis met vitamin D deficiency or insufficiency criteria, and, in this population, low 1,25(OH)$_2$D levels were associated with increased 30-day mortality and PTH insensitivity [15]. A two-center study analyzed 3,386 critically ill patients admitted to ICUs and verified that deficient vitamin D levels three days prior and seven days after ICU admission were strong independent predictors of sepsis [16]; similar results have been observed in surgical ICU patients with vitamin D levels < 20 ng/ml [17]. Conversely, a recent cohort study of 655 critically ill patients did not find any association between 25(OH)D levels and LOS, but all 20 patients who died of sepsis had vitamin D levels less than 30 ng/ml [18].

Even though a growing body of evidence supports a strong relationship between low vitamin D status and sepsis, few data are available regarding nosocomial bacteremia. The results of an observational study that analyzed 2,399 patients admitted to two university hospitals in Boston showed that, for the 1,160 subjects who had blood cultures, hypovitaminosis D was significantly associated with a higher risk of BSI development (OR 1.64; CI 1.05–2.55; $p = 0.03$) [19].

Furthermore, in a retrospective analysis of 2,135 patients, the odds of developing a HABSI in the 323 patients with 25(OH)D levels < 10 ng/ml was 2.3-fold higher than in patients with levels ≥ 30 ng/ml despite adjusting for age, sex, race, Deyo-Charlson Comorbidity index and admission cause [20]. And finally, a recent meta-analysis of 14 observational reports found that 25(OH)D < 20 ng/ml was significantly associated with an increased risk of sepsis in critically ill patients (RR 1.46, 95% CI 1.27 to 1.68) [21].

Although definitive data from large RCTs are lacking, the available observational evidence and preliminary RCTs suggest a potential beneficial effect of vitamin D on sepsis outcomes in ICU patients.

Surgical Site Infections

SSIs are a leading cause of morbidity and mortality during the 30 days following surgery. It is estimated that up to 40% of all patients and around 15% of hospitalized patients may develop an SSI following an invasive procedure. Surgical stress, pain, and exposure to general anesthesia are only a few example of the myriad of factors that can affect immune regulation in the perioperative period. And immunocompetence as well as barrier site (skin or anastomosis) integrity are known risk factors for developing SSIs. Therefore, due to its immunomodulatory effects, vitamin D may be involved in the mechanisms that are involved in attenuating post-operative immunoparalysis and that may promote wound protection as well as repair.

Suboptimal vitamin D status before surgery may be a highly prevalent issue of concern. An analysis of patients undergoing bariatric surgery during a five year period found that 84% of 127 patients had low 25(OH)D baseline levels and that this deficiency was significantly correlated with preoperative body mass index and PTH levels [22]. Similar results were documented in a review of 379 obese individuals undergoing bariatric surgery between 2002 and 2004, which identified low vitamin D status in 68% of patients [23]. On the other hand, in a retrospective review of 723 patients undergoing orthopedic surgery, preoperative 25(OH)D < 32 ng/ml was present in almost half of all patients, while levels < 20 ng/ml were observed in 40% of individuals in this cohort [24].

There is a growing body of literature that has investigated the association of vitamin D status with post-surgical health. A prospective analysis in Germany of 190 patients who came into an orthopedic clinic for either total hip, knee, or shoulder prosthesis due to aseptic loosening of the joint or periprosthetic infection, demonstrated that 64, 52, and 86% of patients, respectively, had 25(OH)D levels < 20 ng/ml. Moreover, the mean 25(OH)D level of the 43 patients with joint infections was significantly lower than that of patients with aseptic loosening [25]. Recent evidence also suggests that surgical stress may be associated with a significant reduction in circulating 25(OH)D levels when compared with preoperative values. Moreover, the derangement in perioperative 25(OH)D levels may be sustained for up to 3 months after surgery.

A retrospective analysis of the association between preoperative 25(OH)D levels and HAIs following Roux-en-Y gastric bypass surgery was performed at a major Boston teaching hospital [26]. During the five-year study period, 770 patients underwent surgery and had their 25(OH)D levels checked within 30 days before surgery. Forty-one cases of HAI were diagnosed, with 20 cases identified as SSIs and the other 21 were either urinary tract infections (UTIs), pneumonia, or bacteremia. Using a propensity score matching approach, subjects with baseline 25(OH)D levels < 30 ng/ml demonstrated a 3-fold and 4-fold increased risk of HAIs and SSI development, respectively, compared to patients with levels ≥ 30 ng/ml (OR 3.05; CI, 1.34–6.94). The validity of these findings has recently been bolstered in a cohort of 3,340 consecutive patients undergoing cardiac surgery. In their analysis, the study investigators found that low 1,25$(OH)_2$D levels were independently associated with an increased risk of post operative-infection [27]. So, although limited, emerging data support the potential beneficial effect of optimizing vitamin D status in the perioperative setting.

Clostridium Difficile Infections

C. difficile is the major cause of nosocomial diarrhea in North America. During the last decade, the incidence of hospital-acquired *C. difficile* infection (HACDI) has increased dramatically, with more than 300,000 new cases and almost 15,000 deaths being reported annually [1].

Vitamin D is thought to be involved in innate gastrointestinal immune defenses by promoting the maturation of T cell populations, and protection of macrophages from the deleterious effects of *C. difficile* toxins. Furthermore, VDR activation within the gastrointestinal tract is thought to upregulate macrophage and epithelial LL-37 as well as β-defensin expression, which attenuates interleukin (IL)-1β release.

A recent retrospective cohort study investigating CDIs in 568 adults admitted to two Boston teaching hospitals found that only 13% of patients had 25(OH)D $\geq$ 30 ng/ml [28]. After adjusting for age, sex, race, patient type, and the Deyo-Charlson Comorbidity index, 25(OH)D levels < 10 ng/ml were strongly associated with HACDI occurrence, with the odds of infection being 3-fold higher than those of patients with levels $\geq$ 30 ng/ml. Another recent analysis looked at the association between CDI and vitamin D status in 3,188 patients who had inflammatory bowel disease and at least one 25(OH)D test on record at two US teaching hospitals. The 35 patients in this cohort who developed CDI had a mean 25(OH)D level of 20.4, which was significantly lower than in non-CDI patients [29].

Prospective studies on this topic have recently been conducted as well. An analysis of data from 62 hospitalized patients with *C. difficile*-associated diarrhea found that 25(OH)D levels > 21 ng/ml were significantly associated with higher *C. difficile* disease resolution; indeed, in these patients, low vitamin D status was associated with a higher risk of recurrence and an almost 6-fold increased risk of death compared to patients with more optimal 25(OH)D levels [30]. Vitamin D status may also be a predictor of CDI severity. A recent study enrolled 100 patients with confirmed CDI while admitted to a large teaching hospital in Boston between 2011 and 2013. Multivariable regression analysis demonstrated that 25(OH)D_3 levels were significantly associated with disease severity and each 1 ng/ml increase in 25(OH)D_3 was observed to decrease the risk of severe CDI by 8% (OR 0.92; CI 0.87–0.98). However, no association was observed between total 25(OH)D or 25(OH)D_2 levels, supporting the hypothesis that vitamin D_3 is the biological driver of vitamin D-related immune function [32]. Similarly, a longer course of CDI-associated diarrhea has been observed in patients with low vitamin D status compared to a matched group with more optimal 25(OH)D levels [31]. And finally, in a recent meta-analysis of 8 observational studies, including both community and nosocomial CDIs, patients with lower vitamin D status were shown to have significantly higher odds of developing severe CDI compared with those with more optimal 25(OH)D levels [33]. Although, at present, there are no RCTs that have investigated the effect of vitamin D supplementation in patients with CDI, within the given limits of observational cohort studies there is a strong signal that vitamin D optimization in patients affected by or at high risk for CDIs may be clinically relevant.

Other Nosocomial Infections

CAUTIs are the most common HAIs worldwide, accounting for almost 50% of all nosocomial infectious complications. Nearly 25% of patients with bacteriuria develop CAUTI, followed, in 4% of cases, by bacteremia. These episodes are responsible for an estimated health care-related cost of between $676 and $2,836 per patient. Preliminary investigations have shown a relationship between vitamin D status and UTIs. In a study of 92 patients diagnosed with a UTI, a significant relationship between VDR gene polymorphism and infection was observed, and a significant increase in LL-37 expression after a three-month period of vitamin D supplementation was observed in bladder biopsies of patients infected with *Escherichia coli* [34]. Additionally, a significant association between hypovitaminosis D and recurrent UTIs was observed in premenopausal women. Although previous studies demonstrated an upregulation of LL-37 with chronic UTI [34], increased β-defensin 2 expression may be more profound in the acute setting. To date, no RCTs have investigated whether vitamin D supplementation may reduce the incidence, severity, or duration of CAUTI.

HAP represents a leading cause of morbidity and mortality in ICU patients. In the critically ill, nosocomial pneumonias, including ventilator-associated pneumonia (VAP), are responsible for increased ICU LOS, patient-related resource utilization and mortality. Vitamin D significantly contributes to innate immune function in respiratory mucosa and many recent studies have identified hypovitaminosis D as a determining risk factor for pulmonary infections. A retrospective analysis of 16,975 individuals with documented 25(OH)D levels from the third National Health and Nutrition Examination Survey (NHANES) revealed that patients with levels <30 ng/ml had a 56% higher chance of developing community-acquired pneumonia (CAP) [35]. Similarly, a prospective cohort study including 272 hospitalized patients with CAP observed that, after controlling for commonly used biomarkers and prognostic scores, vitamin D deficiency was independently associated with 30-day mortality [36]. Interestingly, although there are no published investigations about the potential role of vitamin D as a risk indicator and prognostic marker of HAP, vitamin D levels <50 nm/l have been frequently observed in hospitalized critically ill patients with acute respiratory distress syndrome (ARDS) [37].

New data relating vitamin D deficiency and other infection types are also emerging. A large retrospective population study observed that, after adjusting for potential confounding variables, vitamin D status was associated with the risk of methicillin-resistant *Staphylococcus aureus* (MRSA) nasal carriage. Similarly, in a prospective observation involving 201 critically ill patients, hypovitaminosis D and invasive mechanical ventilation were the two independent risk factors for *Acinetobacter baumannii* infections [38]. A French study analyzed the vitamin D levels of 88 patients with cirrhosis who attended a liver clinic, finding a 56.8% rate of severe 25(OH)D deficiency, defined as < 10 ng/ml. These subjects were more likely to be hospitalized due to a severe infection than those with a normal vitamin D status [39].

Mortality and Critical Care Outcomes

It is well know that vitamin D deficiency is associated with all-cause mortality in the general population, mainly due to its relationship with chronic conditions including cardiovascular disease and cancer. Recent evidence supports its role as a major determinant of poor outcome in hospitalized patients, especially in the ICU setting. A retrospective cohort study of 24,915 hospitalized adult patients with mean and median pre-hospital serum 25(OH)D levels of 27.9 and 26 ng/ml, respectively, found that 13% of the enrolled patients were ICU admitted [40]. In a cohort study of patients with pre-hospital admission 25(OH)D levels, those with levels ≤ 15 ng/ml had a 1.45 greater odds of 30-day in-hospital mortality compared to those with levels > 15 ng/ml, after adjusting for major potential influencing covariates [14]. Furthermore, in a retrospective study of 136 veterans, ICU survivors had a significantly lower rate of suboptimal vitamin D status compared to non-survivors, and also had a shorter ICU LOS [41]. Another cohort study of 523 critically ill patients admitted to a medical ICU demonstrated a significant relationship between low vitamin D status and mortality [42], as did another large observational study from Boston, which included 1,325 study patients. In the latter study, low pre-hospital 25(OH)D levels were an independent risk factor for 30-day mortality (OR 1.85; CI 1.25–2.98) [43].

Prospective data from a Turkish cohort demonstrated that among 139 adults admitted to a medical ICU, the median serum 25(OH)D level was 14.9 ng/ml; 69% of these patients had 25(OH)D levels < 20 ng/ml [44] and had more comorbidities, needed more invasive procedures and had a higher incidence of septic shock. However, no difference in mortality was observed. However, in patients with 25(OH)D levels < 20 ng/ml, a higher mortality rate and a shorter survival course (15.3 days vs. 24.2 days) was observed compared to those with 25(OH)D ≥ 20 ng/ml in a cohort of 130 critically ill patients admitted to a mixed ICU [45]. Similarly, in another analysis of 196 patients admitted to a medical/surgical ICU, low 25(OH)D levels were associated with greater ICU LOS and a trend towards increased risk of ICU-acquired infections [46]. Additionally, among 100 critically ill patients enrolled in a multicenter prospective Australian study, the observed rate of 25(OH)D < 30 and < 20 ng/ml was 54% and 24%, respectively, confirming a significant relationship between hypovitaminosis and both worse disease severity and fewer hospital-free days [10]. Although there are fewer data on just critically ill surgical patients, a prospective study which assessed the vitamin D status of 258 patients admitted to a surgical ICU reported a severe/moderate vitamin D deficiency status in 91.8% of cases. Low vitamin D status in these patients was associated with higher mortality (11.9 vs. 0%) and greater health care costs ($51,413 ± $75,123 vs. $20,414 ± $25,714), compared to patients with more optimal 25(OH)D levels [47]. More recently, another prospective cohort study of 100 patients in two surgical ICUs of a single institution demonstrated that 25(OH)D levels upon admission were inversely associated with LOS, 90-day readmission, and 90-day mortality rate [4].

Finally a recent observational study analyzed the vitamin D profile of 107 critically ill patients with severe sepsis and septic shock. At ICU admission, vitamin D deficiency (≤ 20 ng/ml) was observed in 93.5% of the patients and 57 showed levels < 7 ng/ml. Severe vitamin D deficiency was associated with lower microbiological eradication and significantly higher sepsis-related mortality [48].

Future Directions

Although emerging data suggest a relationship between low vitamin D status and an increased risk of infection, little is known about optimal 25(OH)D levels for immune function during acute stress and critical illness. 25(OH)D levels around 35 ng/ml are thought to optimize vitamin D-dependent cathelicidin expression, while patients with levels ≥ 60 ng/ml have been shown to be at higher risk of 90-day mortality compared to patients with levels between 30–50 ng/ml [40]. Usually, adults need a daily supplementation of 1,500–2,000 IU of vitamin D to maintain blood levels above 30 ng/ml and oral intakes up to 5,000 IU a day have been observed to be absolutely safe [40].

Recent data have demonstrated that critically ill patients undergoing very high supplementation regimens (> 200,000 UI in a single oral dose) had their vitamin D deficiency rapidly corrected without increasing risk of hypocalcemia or hypercalciuria [49, 50], but a large randomized clinical trial enrolling 492 vitamin D deficient ICU patients found that oral vitamin D (540,000 IU bolus followed by 90,000 IU monthly doses) increased 25(OH)D levels without improving ICU and hospital LOS and mortality rates. However, such supplementation did improve 6-month mortality rates in severely deficient patients with serum 25(OH)D levels ≤ 12 ng/ml [51].

Single intramuscular or intravenous vitamin D administration has also been observed to effectively correct hypovitaminosis in critically ill patients [11]. Hence, although a strong relationship seems to link vitamin D and immune system function, there is limited and conflicting evidence supporting its use as adjunctive therapy in high-risk patients for severe systemic infections, such as hospitalized critically ill subjects. Investigations in this research field have to carefully consider multiple possible biases (such as baseline vitamin D status, dosages administered, and plasmatic levels obtained), which can influence the appropriateness of final observations.

Conclusion

Preclinical research and observational studies highlight the key role of vitamin D for optimal function of the human immune system. The incidence and prognosis of HAIs may benefit from hypovitaminosis D correction, especially in the critically ill setting where low 25(OH)D levels appear to significantly influence outcome. However, evidence supporting vitamin D supplementation as a tool to improve morbidity and mortality is still lacking. Further studies aimed at defining target populations where functional vitamin D insufficiency is detrimental and to provide new insights regarding optimal administration regimens are needed in order to definitively determine the antimicrobial properties of this intriguing molecule.

Acknowledgements

This work was partially supported US National Institutes of Health grant number L30 TR001257.

References

1. Klevens RM, Edwards JR, Richards CL Jr et al (2007) Estimating health care-associated infections and deaths in U.S. hospitals, 2002. Public Health Rep 122:160–166
2. De Pascale G, Cutuli SL, Pennisi MA, Antonelli M (2013) The role of mannose-binding lectin in severe sepsis and septic shock. Mediators Inflamm 2013:625083
3. Quraishi SA, Camargo CA Jr (2012) Vitamin D in acute stress and critical illness. Curr Opin Clin Nutr Metab Care 15:625–634
4. Quraishi SA, Bittner EA, Blum L, McCarthy C, Bhan I, Camargo CA Jr (2014) Prospective study of vitamin D status at initiation of care in critically ill surgical patients and risk of 90-day mortality. Crit Care Med 42:1365–1371
5. Jeng L, Yamshchikov AV, Judd SE et al (2009) Alterations in vitamin D status and antimicrobial peptide levels in patients in the intensive care unit with sepsis. J Transl Med 7:28
6. Danai PA, Sinha S, Moss M, Haber MJ, Martin GS (2007) Seasonal variation in the epidemiology of sepsis. Crit Care Med 35:410–415
7. Lucidarme O, Messai E, Mazzoni T, Arcade M, du Cheyron D (2010) Incidence and risk factors of vitamin D deficiency in critically ill patients: results from a prospective observational study. Intensive Care Med 36:1609–1611
8. Horiuchi H, Nagata I, Komoriya K (1991) Protective effect of vitamin D3 analogues on endotoxin shock in mice. Agents Actions 33:343–348
9. Ginde AA, Camargo CA Jr, Shapiro NI (2011) Vitamin D insufficiency and sepsis severity in emergency department patients with suspected infection. Acad Emerg Med 18:551–554
10. Nair P, Lee P, Reynolds C et al (2013) Significant perturbation of vitamin D-parathyroid-calcium axis and adverse clinical outcomes in critically ill patients. Intensive Care Med 39:267–274
11. Leaf DE, Raed A, Donnino MW, Ginde AA, Waikar SS (2014) Randomized controlled trial of calcitriol in severe sepsis. Am J Respir Crit Care Med 190:533–541
12. Barnett N, Zhao Z, Koyama T et al (2014) Vitamin D deficiency and risk of acute lung injury in severe sepsis and severe trauma: a case-control study. Ann Intensive Care 4:5

13. Cecchi A, Bonizzoli M, Douar S et al (2011) Vitamin D deficiency in septic patients at ICU admission is not a mortality predictor. Minerva Anestesiol 77:1184–1189
14. Lange N, Litonjua AA, Gibbons FK, Giovannucci E, Christopher KB (2013) Pre-hospital vitamin D concentration, mortality, and bloodstream infection in a hospitalized patient population. Am J Med 126:e19–27
15. Nguyen HB, Eshete B, Lau KH, Sai A, Villarin M, Baylink D (2013) Serum 1,25-dihydroxyvitamin D: an outcome prognosticator in human sepsis. PLoS One 8:e64348
16. Moromizato T, Litonjua AA, Braun AB, Gibbons FK, Giovannucci E, Christopher KB (2014) Association of low serum 25-hydroxyvitamin d levels and sepsis in the critically ill. Crit Care Med 42:97–107
17. Flynn L, Zimmerman LH, McNorton K et al (2012) Effects of vitamin D deficiency in critically ill surgical patients. Am J Surg 203:379–382
18. Amrein K, Zajic P, Schnedl C et al (2014) Vitamin D status and its association with season, hospital and sepsis mortality in critical illness. Crit Care 18:R47
19. Braun A, Chang D, Mahadevappa K et al (2011) Association of low serum 25-hydroxyvitamin D levels and mortality in the critically ill. Crit Care Med 39:671–677
20. Quraishi SA, Litonjua AA, Moromizato T et al (2013) Association between prehospital vitamin D status and hospital-acquired bloodstream infections. Am J Clin Nutr 98:952–959
21. de Haan K, Groeneveld AB, de Geus HR, Egal M, Struijs A (2014) Vitamin D deficiency as a risk factor for infection, sepsis and mortality in the critically ill: systematic review and meta-analysis. Crit Care 18:660
22. Fish E, Beverstein G, Olson D, Reinhardt S, Garren M, Gould J (2010) Vitamin D status of morbidly obese bariatric surgery patients. J Surg Res 164:198–202
23. Flancbaum L, Belsley S, Drake V, Colarusso T, Tayler E (2006) Preoperative nutritional status of patients undergoing Roux-en-Y gastric bypass for morbid obesity. J Gastrointest Surg 10:1033–1037
24. Bogunovic L, Kim AD, Beamer BS, Nguyen J, Lane JM (2010) Hypovitaminosis D in patients scheduled to undergo orthopaedic surgery: a single-center analysis. J Bone Joint Surg Am 92(13):2300–2304
25. Maier GS, Horas K, Seeger JB, Roth KE, Kurth AA, Maus U (2015) Vitamin D insufficiency in the elderly orthopaedic patient: an epidemic phenomenon. Int Orthop 39:787–792
26. Quraishi SA, Bittner EA, Blum L, Hutter MM, Camargo CA Jr (2014) Association between preoperative 25-hydroxyvitamin D level and hospital-acquired infections following Roux-en-Y gastric bypass surgery. JAMA Surg 149:112–118
27. Zittermann A, Kuhn J, Ernst JB et al (2016) Circulating 25-hydroxyvitamin D and 1,25-dihydroxyvitamin D concentrations and postoperative infections in cardiac surgical patients: The CALCITOP-Study. PLoS One 11:e0158532
28. Quraishi SA, Litonjua AA, Moromizato T et al (2015) Association between prehospital vitamin D status and hospital-acquired Clostridium difficile infections. JPEN Parenter Enteral Nutr 39:47–55
29. Ananthakrishnan AN, Cagan A, Gainer VS et al (2014) Higher plasma vitamin D is associated with reduced risk of Clostridium difficile infection in patients with inflammatory bowel diseases. Aliment Pharmacol Ther 39:1136–1142
30. Wang WJ, Gray S, Sison C et al (2014) Low vitamin D level is an independent predictor of poor outcomes in Clostridium difficile-associated diarrhea. Therap Adv Gastroenterol 7:14–19
31. Wilden GM van der, Fagenholz P et al (2015) Vitamin D status and severity of Clostridium difficile infections: a prospective cohort study in hospitalized adults. JPEN J Parenter Enteral Nutr 39:465–470
32. Wong KK, Lee R, Watkins RR, Haller N (2016) Prolonged Clostridium difficile infection may be associated with vitamin D deficiency. J Parenter Enteral Nutr 40:682–687
33. Furuya-Kanamori L, Wangdi K, Yakob L et al (2015) 25-hydroxyvitamin D concentrations and Clostridium difficile infection: A meta-analysis. JPEN J Parenter Enteral Nutr Dec 23, Epub ahead of print

34. Hertting O, Holm Å, Lüthje P et al (2010) Vitamin D induction of the human antimicrobial peptide cathelicidin in the urinary bladder. PLoS One 14:e15580
35. Quraishi SA, Bittner EA, Christopher KB, Camargo CA Jr (2013) Vitamin D status and community-acquired pneumonia: results from the third National Health and Nutrition Examination Survey. PLoS One 8:e81120
36. Remmelts HH, van de Garde EM et al (2012) Addition of vitamin D status to prognostic scores improves the prediction of outcome in community-acquired pneumonia. Clin Infect Dis 55:1488–1494
37. Dancer RC, Parekh D, Lax S et al (2015) Vitamin D deficiency contributes directly to the acute respiratory distress syndrome (ARDS). Thorax 70:617–624
38. Türkoğlu M, Aygencel G, Dizbay M et al (2013) Is vitamin D deficiency associated with development of Acinetobacter baumannii infections in critically ill patients? J Crit Care 28:735–740
39. Anty R, Tonohouan M, Ferrari-Panaia P et al (2014) Low levels of 25-hydroxy vitamin D are independently associated with the risk of bacterial infection in cirrhotic patients. Clin Transl Gastroenterol 5:e56
40. Amrein K, Quraishi SA, Litonjua AA et al (2014) Evidence for a U-shaped relationship between pre-hospital vitamin D status and mortality: a cohort study. J Clin Endocrinol Metab 99:1461–1469
41. McKinney JD, Bailey BA, Garrett LH, Peiris P, Manning T, Peiris AN (2011) Relationship between vitamin D status and ICU outcomes in veterans. J Am Med Dir Assoc 12:208–211
42. Venkatram S, Chilimuri S, Adrish M, Salako A, Patel M, Diaz-Fuentes G (2011) Vitamin D deficiency is associated with mortality in the medical intensive care unit. Crit Care 15:R292
43. Braun AB, Litonjua AA, Gibbons FK, Litonjua AA, Giovannucci E, Christopher KB (2012) Low serum 25-hydroxyvitamin D at critical care initiation is associated with increased mortality. Crit Care Med 40:179
44. Aygencel G, Turkoglu M, Tuncel AF, Candır BA, Bildacı YD, Pasaoglu H (2013) Is vitamin d insufficiency associated with mortality of critically ill patients? Crit Care Res Pract 2013:856747
45. Arnson Y, Gringauz I, Itzhaky D, Amital H (2012) Vitamin D deficiency is associated with poor outcomes and increased mortality in severely ill patients. QJM 105:633–639
46. Higgins DM, Wischmeyer PE, Queensland KM, Sillau SH, Sufit AJ, Heyland DK (2012) Relationship of vitamin D deficiency to clinical outcomes in critically ill patients. JPEN J Parenter Enteral Nutr 36:713–720
47. Matthews LR, Ahmed Y, Wilson KL, Griggs DD, Danner OK (2012) Worsening severity of vitamin D deficiency is associated with increased LOS, surgical intensive care unit cost, and mortality rate in surgical intensive care unit patients. Am J Surg 204:37–43
48. De Pascale G, Vallecoccia MS, Schiattarella A et al (2016) Clinical and microbiological outcome in septic patients with extremely low 25-hydroxyvitamin D levels at initiation of critical care. Clin Microbiol Infect 22:456
49. Quraishi SA, De Pascale G, Needleman JS et al (2015) Effect of cholecalciferol supplementation on vitamin D Status and cathelicidin levels in sepsis: a randomized, placebo-controlled trial. Crit Care Med 43:1928–1937
50. Amrein K, Sourij H, Wagner G et al (2011) Short-term effects of high-dose oral vitamin D3 in critically ill vitamin D deficient patients: a randomized, double-blind, placebo-controlled pilot study. Crit Care 15:R104
51. Amrein K, Schnedl C, Holl A et al (2014) Effect of high-dose vitamin D3 on hospital length of stay in critically ill patients with vitamin D deficiency: the VITdAL-ICU randomized clinical trial. JAMA 312:1520–1530

Part VI

Cardiac Conditions

Anemia and Blood Transfusion in the Critically Ill Patient with Cardiovascular Disease

A. B. Docherty and T. S. Walsh

Introduction

Anemia and Cardiovascular Disease

Approximately seven million people in the United Kingdom, and 30% of patients admitted to the ICU have co-existing cardiovascular disease (CVD) [1–3] and this proportion may rise as the average age of both the general population and patients admitted to the ICU increase. Patients with CVD will have impaired compensatory mechanisms to enable maximum oxygen delivery to the tissues in the event of anemia (Fig. 1). Anemia causes an increase in cardiac output, which stresses the heart to increase heart rate and stroke volume. In acute illness, global oxygen demand is increased, further stressing the heart. This is exacerbated by the frequent presence of tachycardia and hypotension, which reduce blood flow to the coronary arteries, and by catecholamines that increase myocardial work. Significant left ventricular coronary flow occurs only during diastole and the subendocardial region is particularly at risk of ischemia because of the high pressure in the left ventricle [4]. At rest, the myocardium extracts approximately 75% of the oxygen delivered by coronary blood flow [5], and there is therefore little reserve when myocardial oxygen consumption is increased in critical illness. Atheroma-related flow limitation further compromises myocardial oxygen delivery.

A. B. Docherty (✉) · T. S. Walsh
Dept of Anaesthesia, Critical Care, Pain Medicine, and Intensive Care Medicine, University of Edinburgh
Edinburgh, UK
Centre for Inflammation Research, University of Edinburgh
Edinburgh, UK
e-mail: annemarie.docherty@ed.ac.uk

J.-L. Vincent (ed.), *Annual Update in Intensive Care and Emergency Medicine 2017*,
DOI 10.1007/978-3-319-51908-1_16

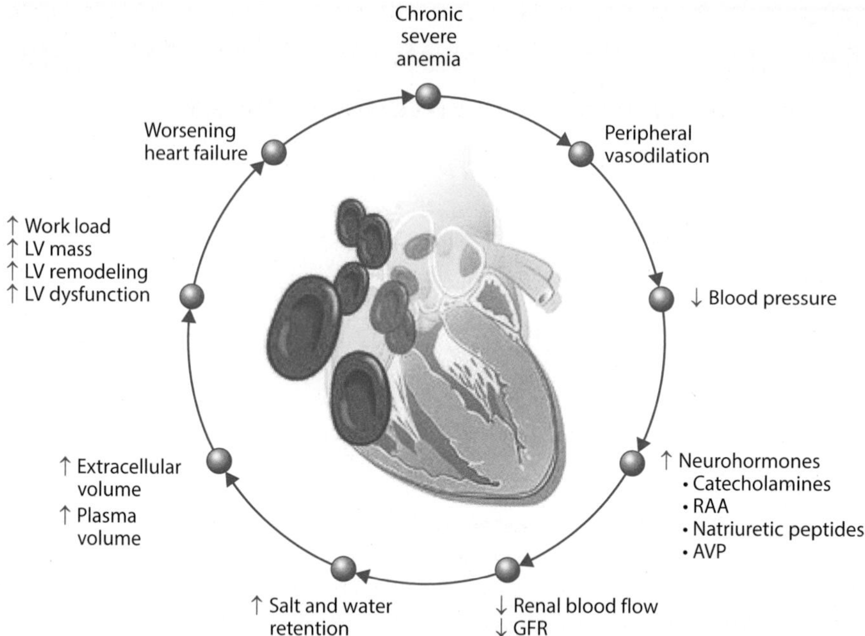

Fig. 1 The impact of chronic severe anemia on myocardial function. *LV*: left ventricular; *AVP*: arginine vasopressin; *RAA*: renin-angiotensin-aldosterone; *GFR*: glomerular filtration rate. Reproduced from [50] with permission

Anemia and Outcomes in Patients with Cardiovascular Disease

Anemia is associated with worse outcomes in patients with CVD, both in terms of severity of illness, and mortality. Anemia is a significant risk factor in ischemic heart disease (IHD), correlating with advanced IHD, chronic heart failure, rhythm disturbance and higher mortality rate in comparison to non-anemic patients [6]. Anemia is also an independent predictor of major adverse cardiovascular events in patients across the spectrum of acute coronary syndrome (ACS) [7]. Anemia in heart failure is associated with impaired functional capacity and cardiac function, renal dysfunction, increased rate of hospitalizations and poor prognosis [8]. However, these studies are all observational, and the direction of causality is difficult to ascertain – anemia may cause the worse outcomes, or it may be a reflection of the severity of the underlying chronic disease. It therefore follows that correction with red blood cells (RBCs) may not improve patient prognosis.

Evidence from Transfusion Trials

All major RBC transfusion trials have compared restrictive with liberal transfusion strategies based on higher versus lower hemoglobin thresholds for transfusion

[9–13]. Trials based in the ICU have shown that a more restrictive transfusion threshold of 7.0 g/dl is as safe as a more liberal threshold for the general ICU population [9, 11, 14]. A recent systematic review did not find any association with mortality, overall morbidity or myocardial infarction when comparing restrictive transfusion strategies with liberal transfusion strategies; however, the overall quality of evidence was low [15]. A Cochrane review indicated that restrictive transfusion strategies were not associated with an increased rate of adverse events (mortality, cardiac events, stroke, pneumonia and thromboembolism) compared with liberal transfusion strategies. Restrictive transfusion strategies were associated with a reduction in hospital mortality but not in 30-day mortality [16]. A review published in 2014 using restrictive hemoglobin transfusion triggers of 7 g/dl showed reductions in in-hospital mortality, total mortality, rebleeding, ACS, pulmonary edema, and bacterial infections compared with liberal transfusion [17].

However, these trials were based in general ICU cohorts, and there is the risk of practice misalignment, whereby inclusion of heterogeneous populations in trials can mask potentially divergent effects in subpopulations [18]. Both of the major transfusion trials in ICUs had underpowered pre-defined subgroups that suggested that a more liberal transfusion threshold may be beneficial in patients with CVD [9, 11]. Evidence is also limited by the under-representation of patients with CVD in trials. Observational studies suggest the prevalence of CVD in ICU patients is around 30% [1, 3]; however patients with CVD accounted for only 20% of patients recruited to the Transfusion Requirements in Critical Care (TRICC) trial compared with 29% of patients excluded [9], and only 14% of patients recruited to the Transfusion Requirements in Septic Shock (TRISS) trial [11]. A trial undertaken in patients presenting with acute gastrointestinal bleeding trial excluded all patients with significant CVD [12].

Evidence in Patients with Co-existing Cardiovascular Disease

There have been few trials aimed specifically at transfusion thresholds in critically ill patients with co-existing CVD. Two recent systematic reviews in cardiac surgery [19] and in perioperative transfusion practice (including cardiac surgery) [20] reported higher mortality with a restrictive transfusion threshold. Our systematic review [21] found only 11 blood transfusion threshold randomized controlled trials (RCTs) that included patients with co-existing CVD, either as the whole population [10, 22–24], as a pre-defined subgroup [9, 11, 25] or as a high proportion of patients [14, 26–28]. We found no evidence of a difference in 30-day mortality between restrictive and liberal transfusion thresholds. However, we found an increased risk of new ACS in patients with co-existing CVD who were randomized to a restrictive blood transfusion threshold (Figs. 2 and 3). The restrictive transfusion threshold for most of the included trials was 8 g/dl compared with a liberal transfusion threshold of 10 g/dl. These trials do not, therefore, provide high quality evidence that the widely recommended 'default' transfusion trigger of 7 g/dl is as safe as higher thresholds for preventing ACS in patients with CVD. There was

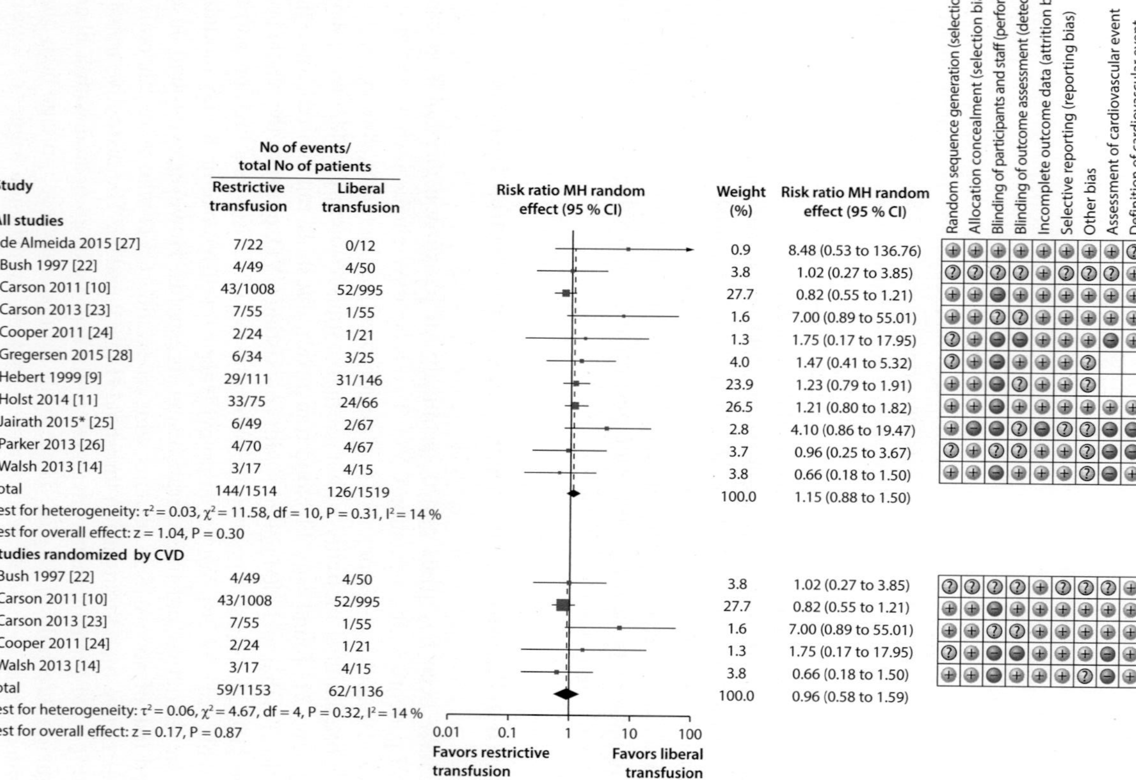

Fig. 2 Systematic review: Blood transfusion thresholds in patients with cardiovascular disease (CVD). Forest plot showing risk ratios for 30-day mortality, and risk of bias assessment for each study. *Additional risk of bias assessed as to completeness of patients recruited into clusters (this was graded as low risk). Modified from [21] with permission

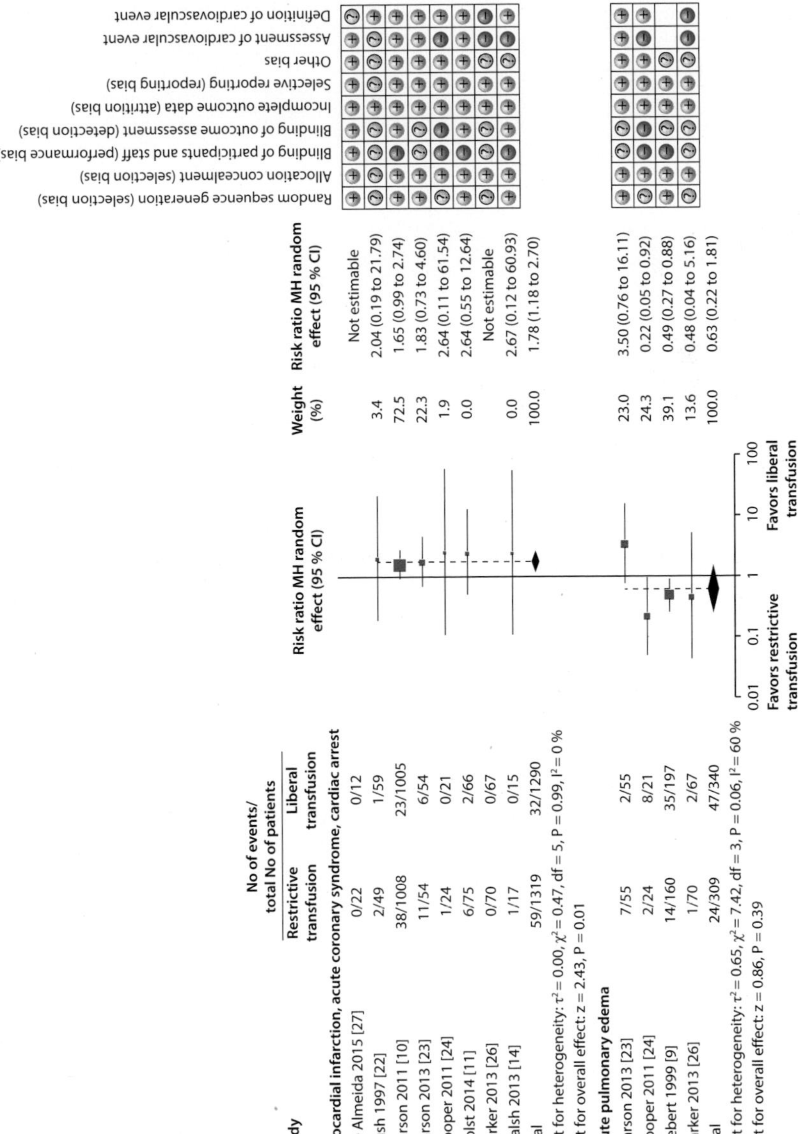

Fig. 3 Systematic review: Blood transfusion thresholds in patients with cardiovascular disease (CVD). Forest plot showing risk ratios for adverse cardiovascular events and risk of bias assessment for each study. Modified from [21] with permission

Table 1 Table of guidelines for red blood cell transfusion in patients with cardiovascular disease

Organization	Year	Recommendation for general	Recommendation for CVD
British Committee for Standards in Haematology [38]	2013	7.0 g/dl, target 7.0–9.0 g/dl	Stable angina should have a Hb maintained >7.0 g/dl
NICE: National Institute for Health and Clinical Excellence [52]	2015	7.0 g/dl, target 7.0–9.0 g/dl	ACS: transfusion threshold of 8.0 g/dl, target of 8.0–10.0 g/dl Chronic: further research
Association of Anaesthetists of Great Britain and Ireland [53]	2016	7.0 g/dl	Uncertainty remains for patients with ischemic heart disease, higher thresholds (8.0 g/dl) may be appropriate
American Association of Blood Banks (AABB) [51]	2016	7.0 g/dl	Patients with symptoms or a Hb level of 8.0 g/dl or less

ACS: acute coronary syndrome; *CVD*: cardiovascular disease; *Hb*: hemoglobin

no difference in the incidence of pulmonary edema between restrictive and liberal thresholds; however pulmonary edema can result from both transfusion-related circulatory overload and ACS, and these were not reported separately in the different trials.

Current guidelines reflect the paucity of evidence in patients with co-existing cardiovascular disease (Table 1).

Clinician Variability in Decision Making

Audits of blood transfusion practice in the UK have consistently shown that around 20% of blood product usage is outside guideline recommendations [29]. This variation in practice was evident in an analysis of the ABLE trial (Age of transfused blood in critically ill adults), which found that the presence of co-existing CVD modified transfusion thresholds [30].

Future Trial Design

A pragmatic RCT of restrictive versus liberal blood transfusion thresholds in patients with CVD with mortality as a primary outcome is likely to encounter the same difficulties as previous trials. In order to find a 5% reduction in mortality (32 to 27%, 90% power), a two-arm trial would require nearly 2,000 patients. Within this population will be patients with differing severity of cardiovascular disease, and differing severity of acute illness, and there is again the risk of practice misalignment. Using the 'PICO' model, we address some of the difficulties a future trial might encounter and offer some potential solutions.

Population

Critically ill patients with co-existing CVD are not all the same. There is a spectrum of severity of both CVD and critical illness, and it follows that the balance of risks and benefits of transfusion may change along this spectrum.

One approach could be to limit the trial population to the highest risk group, such as those with high severity of illness scores at presentation to the ICU (e. g., APACHE II score > 19), or those with known coronary artery disease. This would mean that we are focusing on the group in which we are most likely to see a difference in outcome between restrictive and liberal thresholds. In addition to this, these patients have high hospital and longer-term mortality, which may make trial numbers more manageable. If no difference is found, then we could say with confidence that patients with CVD do not benefit from higher transfusion thresholds. However, if there is a benefit in this high-risk group (and from previous trials, we have seen no benefit in patients without CVD), we would be unable to recommend practice for the low-risk CVD group – patients who are either less critically ill or have milder co-existing CVD. A subsequent trial would potentially need to be undertaken in this group.

It is physiologically appealing to design a trial that individualizes transfusion based on patient risk of mortality or ACS. Those patients at high risk would be transfused at a higher threshold than those at lower risk. Significant work would need to be carried out modelling risk in this population to inform the trial design, and observational studies are ongoing [31]. An adaptive trial design, allowing the risk algorithm to be informed by previous participants in the trial would reduce the risk to patients of being randomized to a harmful threshold and would be more cost-effective.

Intervention

RBC transfusion is current standard practice for correcting anemia in critically ill patients, and it would be logical to continue this in a future trial. Iron therapy plus or minus erythropoietin would be another potential intervention. There is a functional iron deficiency in critical illness and a theoretical increased risk of bacterial infection with the use of iron, and although there is an ongoing trial into intravenous iron in critical illness [32], use of iron or erythropoietin is not standard during the acute phase of critical illness. Previous large trials of erythropoietin have not shown efficacy for significantly reducing RBC transfusions and/or increasing hemoglobin by clinically relevant amounts [33]. A limitation of both iron and erythropoietin is their slow impact on erythropoiesis and hemoglobin level in the context of acute illness. It seems likely that RBC transfusion will remain the therapy of choice for acutely increasing hemoglobin concentration in critical illness.

Comparator

Previous transfusion trials have all compared liberal with restrictive transfusion hemoglobin thresholds. There are limitations in using hemoglobin, given that the concentration is significantly affected by fluid resuscitation, however this is a pragmatic approach which is reproducible and routinely measured. In a population in which patients are not sedated and ventilated, an alternative could be to transfuse based on symptomatology, or potentially anaerobic threshold, but this is unlikely to be feasible in the ICU.

Thresholds have varied between trials (restrictive 7.0–9.7 g/dl, liberal 9.0–11.3 g/dl [21]), with overlap between restrictive thresholds in some trials and liberal in others. The larger the difference in thresholds, the more likely a difference will be shown, and a trial of 7 g/dl (current practice excepting ACS) vs 90 g/l would need fewer patients than 7.5–8.0 g/dl vs 9.0 g/dl. Clinicians need equipoise, and if clinicians are unwilling to randomize patients with CVD to a low threshold of 7.0 g/dl then a higher threshold must be agreed on, otherwise high-risk patients may be excluded from the trial.

Outcomes

Mortality

The majority of blood transfusion threshold trials have used 30-day mortality as their primary outcome. There are many causes of mortality in critically ill patients and it is difficult to argue that mortality during the first few days of critical illness is anything other than a result of the severity of presenting illness. A 10–20% difference in hemoglobin concentration seems to lack biological plausibility to alter this substantially. Longer-term mortality may be a more appropriate endpoint either in isolation or combination with measures of quality of life.

Acute Coronary Syndrome

ACS is an appropriate outcome for blood transfusion trials, particularly in patients with co-existing CVD. However, diagnosis of ACS in critically ill patients is not straightforward. Standard diagnosis comprises patient symptoms and signs, evidence of ischemia on the electrocardiogram (EKG), and a rise and fall pattern of cardiac biomarker (usually troponin I or troponin T) [34]. Standard symptoms are often masked by sedation, delirium or analgesia. EKGs are not performed routinely and there is significant interobserver variability [35]. Troponin release is prevalent in the critically ill [1, 36] and there are multiple causes. Potential cardiac mechanisms include increased thrombogenicity leading to coronary plaque rupture and

Table 2 Acute coronary syndrome (ACS) in patients with co-existing cardiovascular disease in critical care blood transfusion threshold trials. Diagnosis made by Investigator (I) or Clinician (C)

Author, year	Population	Blinded y/n	Diagnosis of ACS	Incidence of new ACS
de Almeida, 2015 [27]	Major abdominal cancer surgery	Y (I)	Clinical symptoms suggesting myocardial ischemia with ≥ 1 of the following: increase/decrease in cTnI (≥ 1 value > 99th centile upper reference limit); EKG changes: new Q waves, ST elevation, new LBBB; Image-based evidence of new loss of viable myocardium	R: 0/22 L: 0/12
Hebert, 1999 [9]	General ICU	? (I)	Unclear	*
Holst, 2014 [11]	Septic shock	Y (I)	Symptoms, EKG signs, or elevated biomarker levels resulting in an intervention	R: 6/75 L: 2/66
Walsh, 2013 [14]	Older, mechanically ventilated	N (C)	Troponin rise, new EKG change	R: 1/17 L: 0/15

*All complications, including shock, myocardial infarction, unstable angina and cardiac arrest, with the exception of acute pulmonary edema (9 vs. 18%; $p<0.01$), were comparable in both groups ($p>0.05$). *LBBB*: left bundle branch block; *R*: restrictive; *L*: liberal; *Tn*: troponin; *EKG*: electrocardiogram

thrombosis (type I myocardial infarction) or underlying critical coronary artery disease leading to an oxygen supply/demand imbalance (type II myocardial infarction) [34]. However, elevated troponin is also recognized in sepsis, end-stage renal disease, acute exacerbations of chronic obstructive pulmonary disease (COPD) and acute intracerebral pathology [37]. This finding may be as a result of underlying cardiac disease, but there is also evidence of troponin release as a result of direct toxicity from cytokines, stretch-mediated troponin release, or ongoing subclinical myocardial injury due to uremia and impaired excretion [37]. Our systematic review found that cardiovascular events were diagnosed by unblinded clinicians in a third of trials, and that the criteria for the diagnosis of myocardial infarction were inconsistent (Table 2), and this resulted in a low GRADE quality of evidence [21]. The diagnosis of ACS in high-risk patients who are unable to communicate their symptoms, have non-specific EKG changes, and multiple causes for troponin elevation is challenging and often arbitrary. Before we are able to use ACS as an objective endpoint, we need to be able to diagnose its presence or absence with accuracy and precision.

Duration of Mechanical Ventilation

Weaning consists of liberation from mechanical ventilation and extubation. Patients with CVD may develop myocardial ischemia associated with the increased sym-

Table 3 Duration of mechanical ventilation, length of stay in ICU/hospital (LOS) in patients with co-existing cardiovascular disease in critical care blood transfusion threshold trials

Author, year	Population	ICU LOS	Hospital LOS
Hebert, 1999 [9]	General ICU	R: 9.3 (9.7) L: 10.4 (10.3)	R: 28.8 (19.5) L: 30.6 (18.8)
Walsh, 2013 [14]	Older, mechanically ventilated	R: 36.5 (26.7) L: 53.3 (40.1)	R: 25.6 (18.1) L: 36.3 (28.3)

R: restrictive; *L*: liberal

pathetic activation associated with difficulty weaning from the ventilator. Studies have suggested an association between anemia and failure to wean, and between RBC transfusion and reduction in the work of breathing [38]; however this is not a consistent finding. Transfusion in anemic patients with CVD prior to weaning could potentially reduce the incidence of ACS, as well as being both clinically effective and cost-effective. No published ICU trials have commented on duration of mechanical ventilation specifically for patients with CVD. Data regarding ICU and hospital length of stay are also scarce (Table 3).

Health-related Quality of Life (HRQOL)

There are few data regarding the prevalence and time course of anemia after intensive care. One study showed that 77% of patients were still anemic at hospital discharge and that nearly half the patients who were in the ICU for seven or more days had hemoglobin concentrations <10.0 g/dl [39]. In a study looking at patients mechanically ventilated >24 h and discharged from ICU with hemoglobin concentrations <10.0 g/dl, half the patients were still anemic at six months [40]. The anemia was predominantly normochromic and normocytic, consistent with ongoing inflammation, inappropriate erythropoietin response and poor marrow RBC production, although the contribution of iron deficiency is difficult to ascertain in these states. These patients had a reduced mean SF-36 score at both 3 and 6 months compared to the normal population. Studies looking at HRQOL for anemia and other chronic disease such as malignancy [41] and end-stage renal disease [42] consistently show an association between hemoglobin concentrations and HRQOL. Fatigue is a prevalent symptom among survivors, and many of the physical features of the post-ICU syndrome are typical of anemia [43]. However, the causal association between anemia and fatigue, and reduced HRQOL, in this patient group are not well studied. Equally, there are no high quality studies exploring whether interventions to treat and correct anemia, whether with RBC transfusion or non-transfusion interventions such as iron or erythropoietin, can modify these important outcomes.

Cost-effectiveness

The cost of a unit of blood is around £120 in the UK, but this does not take into account the complications avoided and complications arising from transfusion. Evaluation of the cost-effectiveness of RBC transfusion is essential. The combination of very high hospital costs for critically ill survivors [44] and low HRQOL during the months following survivorship means that the loss of quality-adjusted life years (QALYs) is substantial following critical illness. The rationale for blood transfusion is to decrease both deaths and complications, such as new ACS, which might impact further on quality of life, thus improving HRQOL and cost-effectiveness. Few completed ICU studies have included health economic evaluations. Cost-effectiveness analysis of the Transfusion Indication Threshold Reduction (TITRe) II blood transfusion threshold in cardiac surgery trial found no clear difference between restrictive and liberal arms up to three months after surgery [45]. Hemoglobin concentration remained different at hospital discharge in the Restrictive and Liberal Transfusion Strategies in Intensive Care (RELIEVE) trial [14], suggesting that longer term exposure to anemia and its effect on HRQOL is potentially important for survivors. It seems logical for future transfusion trials during critical illness to include an economic evaluation in addition to measuring clinical outcomes, especially in exploring the hypothesis that treating anemia might improve quality of life among survivors.

Future Areas for Research

Imaging

The mechanism of troponin release in critically ill patients with cardiovascular disease is not yet fully understood and the relative contribution of ischemic versus inflammatory injury is unknown. This has potentially important therapeutic implications. At present, imaging is mainly limited to bedside transthoracic echocardiography (TTE) due to concerns regarding transferring unstable patients to isolated locations such as the computed tomography (CT) scanner or for angiography. Standard TTE is technically more difficult in these patients, and has only moderate diagnostic accuracy.

Strain Echocardiography

Strain TTE, is a relatively novel imaging technique and describes the lengthening, shortening or thickening, also known as regional deformation, of the myocardium [46]. It uses the unique 'speckle' pattern visible in the myocardium on routine echo images. It follows the movement of blocks of speckle pattern over time frames and is able to capture longitudinal, circumferential and radial strain (rate of deformation). This algorithm results in objective analyses of myocardial function, and is more sensitive than standard TTE evaluation of left ventricular function. It has been successfully used to demonstrate left ventricular dysfunction in septic patients in critical care [47], and stress cardiomyopathy in patients with subarachnoid hemorrhage [48].

Cardiac Magnetic Resonance

Cardiac magnetic resonance is another non-invasive imaging technique that allows for accurate visualization of tissue changes in patients with acute myocardial disease. In the context of troponin elevation in critical illness, it is of particular value in distinguishing myocardial infarction from other myocardial abnormalities such as myocarditis, due to the ability to distinguish between subendocardial and other patterns of fibrosis. Cardiac magnetic resonance is able to detect the increased tissue edema in acute myocardial infarction that lasts up to five weeks and the scar from myocardial necrosis [49]. This means that patients would be able to be scanned in the recovery period for troponin elevations that occurred in acute critical illness.

Blood Transfusion in Recovery from Critical Illness

Given the long trajectory of anemia in critical care survivors, another important area to study is the impact of blood transfusion in patients once they have recovered from their critical illness. It would be possible to look at both physiological parameters and patient HRQOL before and after RBC transfusion. Continuous pulmonary exercise testing (C-PEX) can give an objective assessment of anaerobic threshold, as well as monitor for ischemia by EKG monitoring. Important patient outcomes, such as fatigue and breathlessness, can be explored with qualitative patient interviews or more structured questionnaires.

Conclusion

There is biological plausibility that patients with CVD may benefit from higher transfusion thresholds than patients without CVD. Evidence from a systematic review and meta-analysis in this population suggest that there is no difference in 30-day mortality, but there is an increased risk of ACS in patients with CVD who were randomized to a restrictive transfusion threshold compared with a more liberal threshold. We suggest that a more liberal transfusion threshold (> 80 g/l) in this population should be used until a high-quality trial including endpoints for longer term mortality, ACS, quality of life and cost effectiveness has been performed.

References

1. Ostermann M, Lo J, Toolan M et al (2014) A prospective study of the impact of serial troponin measurements on the diagnosis of myocardial infarction and hospital and six-month mortality in patients admitted to ICU with non-cardiac diagnoses. Crit Care 18:R62
2. British Heart Foundation (2015) Cardiovascular Disease Statistics 2015. https://www.bhf.org.uk/publications/statistics/cvd-stats-2015. Accessed September 2016
3. Walsh TS, McClelland DB, Lee RJ et al (2005) Prevalence of ischaemic heart disease at admission to intensive care and its influence on red cell transfusion thresholds: multicentre Scottish Study. Br J Anaesth 94:445–452
4. Walsh TS, McClelland DB (2003) When should we transfuse critically ill and perioperative patients with known coronary artery disease? Br J Anaesth 90:719–722
5. Tune JD, Gorman MW, Feigl EO (2004) Matching coronary blood flow to myocardial oxygen consumption. J Appl Physiol 97:404–415

6. Zeidman A, Fradin Z, Blecher A, Oster HS, Avrahami Y, Mittelman M (2004) Anemia as a risk factor for ischemic heart disease. Isr Med Assoc J 6:16–18
7. Sabatine MS, Morrow DA, Giugliano RP et al (2005) Association of hemoglobin levels with clinical outcomes in acute coronary syndromes. Circulation 111:2042–2049
8. Ezekowitz JA, McAlister FA, Armstrong PW (2003) Anemia is common in heart failure and is associated with poor outcomes: insights from a cohort of 12 065 patients with new-onset heart failure. Circulation 107:223–225
9. Hebert PC, Wells G, Blajchman MA et al (1999) A multicenter, randomized, controlled clinical trial of transfusion requirements in critical care. Transfusion Requirements in Critical Care Investigators, Canadian Critical Care Trials Group. N Engl J Med 340:409–417
10. Carson JL, Terrin ML, Noveck H et al (2011) Liberal or restrictive transfusion in high-risk patients after hip surgery. N Engl J Med 365:2453–2462
11. Holst LB, Haase N, Wetterslev J et al (2014) Lower versus higher hemoglobin threshold for transfusion in septic shock. N Engl J Med 371:1381–1391
12. Villanueva C, Colomo A, Bosch A et al (2013) Transfusion strategies for acute upper gastrointestinal bleeding. N Engl J Med 368:11–21
13. Murphy GJ, Pike K, Rogers CA et al (2015) Liberal or restrictive transfusion after cardiac surgery. N Engl J Med 372:997–1008
14. Walsh TS, Boyd JA, Watson D et al (2013) Restrictive versus liberal transfusion strategies for older mechanically ventilated critically ill patients: a randomized pilot trial. Crit Care Med 41:2354–2363
15. Holst LB, Petersen MW, Haase N, Perner A, Wetterslev J (2015) Restrictive versus liberal transfusion strategy for red blood cell transfusion: systematic review of randomised trials with meta-analysis and trial sequential analysis. BMJ 350:h1354
16. Carson JL, Carless PA, Hebert PC (2012) Transfusion thresholds and other strategies for guiding allogeneic red blood cell transfusion. Cochrane Database Syst Rev CD002042
17. Salpeter SR, Buckley JS, Chatterjee S (2014) Impact of more restrictive blood transfusion strategies on clinical outcomes: a meta-analysis and systematic review. Am J Med 127(e123):124–131
18. Deans KJ, Minneci PC, Suffredini AF et al (2007) Randomization in clinical trials of titrated therapies: unintended consequences of using fixed treatment protocols. Crit Care Med 35:1509–1516
19. Patel NN, Avlonitis VS, Jones HE et al (2015) Indications for red blood cell transfusion in cardiac surgery: a systematic review and meta-analysis. Lancet Haematol 2:e543–e553
20. Fominskiy E, Putzu A, Monaco F et al (2015) Liberal transfusion strategy improves survival in perioperative but not in critically ill patients. A meta-analysis of randomised trials. Br J Anaesth 115:511–519
21. Docherty AB, O'Donnell R, Brunskill S et al (2016) Effect of restrictive versus liberal transfusion strategies on outcomes in patients with cardiovascular disease in a non-cardiac surgery setting: systematic review and meta-analysis. BMJ 352:i1351
22. Bush RL, Pevec WC, Holcroft JW (1997) A prospective, randomized trial limiting perioperative red blood cell transfusions in vascular patients. Am J Surg 174:143–148
23. Carson JL, Brooks MM, Abbott JD et al (2013) Liberal versus restrictive transfusion thresholds for patients with symptomatic coronary artery disease. Am Heart J 165:964–971 (e961)
24. Cooper HA, Rao SV, Greenberg MD et al (2011) Conservative versus liberal red cell transfusion in acute myocardial infarction (the CRIT Randomized Pilot Study). Am J Cardiol 108:1108–1111
25. Jairath V, Kahan BC, Gray A et al (2015) Restrictive versus liberal blood transfusion for acute upper gastrointestinal bleeding (TRIGGER): a pragmatic, open-label, cluster randomised feasibility trial. Lancet 386:137–144
26. Parker MJ (2013) Randomised trial of blood transfusion versus a restrictive transfusion policy after hip fracture surgery. Injury 44:1916–1918

27. de Almeida JP, Vincent JL, Galas FR et al (2015) Transfusion requirements in surgical oncology patients: a prospective, randomized controlled trial. Anesthesiology 122:29–38
28. Gregersen M, Damsgaard EM, Borris LC (2015) Blood transfusion and risk of infection in frail elderly after hip fracture surgery: the TRIFE randomized controlled trial. Eur J Orthop Surg Traumatol 25:1031–1038
29. National Comparative Audit of Blood Transfusion (2011) Audit of Blood in Adult Medical Patients-Part 1. http://hospital.blood.co.uk/media/26862/nca-medical_use_audit_part_1_report.pdf. Accessed September 2016
30. Wilton K, Fowler RA, Walsh T, Lacroix J, Callum J (2014) Variation of red blood cell transfusion thresholds for critically ill patients. Crit Care 18:106
31. Docherty AB, Stanworth SJ, Lone NI, Walsh TS (2016) TROPICCAL: TROPonin I in cardiovascular patients in CriticAL care. https://www.ukctg.nihr.ac.uk. Accessed September 2016
32. Litton E, Baker S, Erber W et al (2014) The IRONMAN trial: a protocol for a multicentre randomised placebo-controlled trial of intravenous iron in intensive care unit patients with anaemia. Crit Care Resusc 16:285–290
33. Corwin HL, Gettinger A, Pearl RG et al (2002) Efficacy of recombinant human erythropoietin in critically ill patients: a randomized controlled trial. JAMA 288:2827–2835
34. Thygesen K, Alpert JS, Jaffe AS et al (2012) Third universal definition of myocardial infarction. Eur Heart J 33:2551–2567
35. Mehta S, Granton J, Lapinsky SE et al (2011) Agreement in electrocardiogram interpretation in patients with septic shock. Crit Care Med 39:2080–2086
36. Lim W, Qushmaq I, Cook DJ et al (2005) Elevated troponin and myocardial infarction in the intensive care unit: a prospective study. Crit Care 9:R636–644
37. Agewall S, Giannitsis E, Jernberg T, Katus H (2011) Troponin elevation in coronary vs. noncoronary disease. Eur Heart J 32:404–411
38. Retter A, Wyncoll D, Pearse R et al (2013) Guidelines on the management of anaemia and red cell transfusion in adult critically ill patients. Br J Haematol 160:445–464
39. Walsh TS, Saleh EE, Lee RJ, McClelland DB (2006) The prevalence and characteristics of anaemia at discharge home after intensive care. Intensive Care Med 32:1206–1213
40. Bateman AP, McArdle F, Walsh TS (2009) Time course of anemia during six months follow up following intensive care discharge and factors associated with impaired recovery of erythropoiesis. Crit Care Med 37:1906–1912
41. Sabbatini P (2000) The relationship between anemia and quality of life in cancer patients. Oncologist 5(Suppl 2):19–23
42. Finkelstein FO, Story K, Firanek C et al (2009) Health-related quality of life and hemoglobin levels in chronic kidney disease patients. Clin J Am Soc Nephrol 4:33–38
43. Walsh TS, Salisbury LG, Merriweather JL et al (2015) Increased hospital-based physical rehabilitation and information provision after intensive care unit discharge: The RECOVER randomized clinical trial. JAMA Intern Med 175:901–910
44. Lone NI, Gillies MA, Haddow C et al (2016) Five-year mortality and hospital costs associated with surviving intensive care. Am J Respir Crit Care Med 194:198–208
45. Stokes EA, Wordsworth S, Bargo D et al (2016) Are lower levels of red blood cell transfusion more cost-effective than liberal levels after cardiac surgery? Findings from the TITRe2 randomised controlled trial. BMJ Open 6:e011311
46. Gorcsan J 3rd, Tanaka H (2011) Echocardiographic assessment of myocardial strain. J Am Coll Cardiol 58:1401–1413
47. De Geer L, Engvall J, Oscarsson A (2015) Strain echocardiography in septic shock – a comparison with systolic and diastolic function parameters, cardiac biomarkers and outcome. Crit Care 19:122
48. Cinotti R, Piriou N, Launey Y et al (2016) Speckle tracking analysis allows sensitive detection of stress cardiomyopathy in severe aneurysmal subarachnoid hemorrhage patients. Intensive Care Med 42:173–182

49. Friedrich MG (2008) Tissue characterization of acute myocardial infarction and myocarditis by cardiac magnetic resonance. JACC Cardiovasc Imaging 1:652–662
50. Anand IS (2008) Anemia and chronic heart failure implications and treatment options. J Am Coll Cardiol 52:501–511
51. Carson JL, Guyatt G, Heddle NM et al (2016) Clinical Practice Guidelines From the AABB: Red Blood Cell Transfusion Thresholds and Storage. JAMA 316:2025–2035
52. National Institute for Health and Clinical Excellence (2015) Transfusion. http://www.nice.org.uk/guidance/ng24/evidence/full-guidance-2177160733. Accessed November 2016
53. Klein AA, Arnold P, Bingham RM et al (2016) AAGBI Guidelines: the use of blood components and their alternatives 2016. Anaesthesia 71:829–842

Right Ventriculo-Arterial Coupling in the Critically Ill

F. Guarracino, P. Bertini, and M. R. Pinsky

Introduction

Hemodynamic instability is one of the most common and important clinical issues the intensivist has to face in the treatment of the critically ill. Standard hemodynamic evaluation of such unstable patients is often based on hemodynamic monitoring that reports mean arterial pressure (MAP), central venous pressure (CVP), heart rate (HR), cardiac index (CI), and occasionally venous oxygen saturation and serum lactate values. However, these global cardiovascular measures do not define the very relevant relationship between ventricular pump function and arterial pressure and flow. This relationship, referred to as ventriculo-arterial coupling is a primary determinant of cardiovascular function. For example, left ventricular (LV) stroke volume is a function of LV end-diastolic volume, intrinsic LV contractility, often quantified as end-systolic elastance and arterial pressure. Similarly, arterial pressure is a function of LV stroke volume, heart rate and arterial tone, often quantified as arterial elastance. Thus, LV stoke volume is both limited by and defines arterial pressure. This interaction is referred to as ventriculo-arterial coupling. Ventriculo-arterial coupling represents the efficiency of the heart and vascular system to create the necessary flow under pressure (e. g., workload). These factors can be visualized by displaying the LV pressure-loop relationship during a single cardiac cycle relative to the resultant arterial pressure (Fig. 1). Maximal LV myocardial energetic efficiency, defined as the amount of external work performed for myocardial oxygen consumption, occurs when arterial elastance is approximately half LV elastance [1]. Although the physiological foundations of ventriculo-arterial coupling as a ma-

F. Guarracino (✉) · P. Bertini
Department of Anesthesia and Critical Care Medicine, Cardiothoracic and Vascular Anesthesia and Intensive Care, Azienda Ospedaliero Universitaria Pisana
56126 Pisa, Italy
e-mail: fabiodoc64@hotmail.com

M. R. Pinsky
Department of Critical Care Medicine, University of Pittsburgh
Pittsburgh, PA, USA

J.-L. Vincent (ed.), *Annual Update in Intensive Care and Emergency Medicine 2017*,
DOI 10.1007/978-3-319-51908-1_17

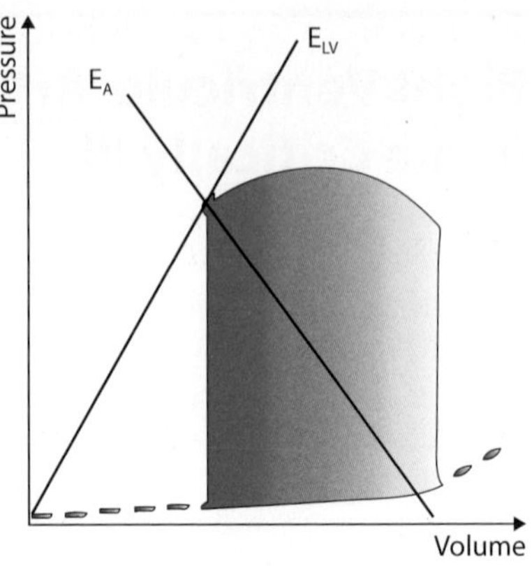

Fig. 1 Left ventricular pressure volume loop. Arterial elastance (E_A) and ventricular elastance (E_{LV}) are displayed

jor determinant of cardiovascular health are well described [2], until recently, its bedside measurement was not possible. Previously, clinical studies required complex and highly invasive measures of LV pressure-volume loops only possible in well-equipped cardiac catheterization laboratories. Importantly, with the advent of echocardiographic imaging of the heart such ventriculo-arterial coupling analyses are possible non-invasively at the bedside [3, 4]. Using this non-invasive approach we recently showed that critically ill patients in septic shock have a profoundly uncoupled LV ventriculo-arterial pressure relation, which may explain some of the impaired LV function seen in sepsis [5]. However, although left ventriculo-arterial coupling estimates are readily available, estimates of left ventriculo-arterial coupling or their use in bedside clinical decision making are not routinely performed.

The major advantage of using measures of left ventriculo-arterial coupling as part of hemodynamic monitoring of the critically ill is that it separates arterial pressure from ventricular function, such that both can be assessed separately as a functional unit. Such analyses should also improve pathophysiological interpretation of the hemodynamic alterations occurring in the critically ill patient and, subsequently, enable a more focused and potentially more efficient treatment based on the specific pathophysiological guidance. For example, if a patient in septic shock has primarily decreased arterial tone, quantified as arterial elastance, then a vasopressor should be the primary pharmacologic intervention; however, if both arterial elastance and LV contractility are reduced, for the same MAP, then both an inotrope and vasopressor may need to be started simultaneously. Although increased acceptance of this approach has focused on LV pathophysiology, the right heart has always been considered to have little influence on the hemodynamic derangement. However, as was recently shown, right ventricular (RV) dysfunction is a common and often primary cause of cardiovascular insufficiency in the critically ill [6].

Right ventriculo-arterial coupling has been used to assess RV function in patients with pulmonary hypertension. Indeed, impaired coupling is the best predictor of death or the need for lung transplantation in patients with pulmonary hypertension, independent of pulmonary arterial pressure measures [7]. We describe below efforts to expand RV ventriculo-arterial coupling analyses into bedside analysis for clinical decision making. Though not yet ready for bedside monitoring, awareness of this evolving and clinically-relevant analysis needs to occur as we move forward.

The Right Ventricle

RV function, which has been historically underestimated as relevant to cardiovascular homeostasis, has recently drawn the attention of intensivists because of the growing awareness of its role in several acute and chronic states. For example, RV dysfunction is universally present to some degree in all critically ill patients with acute respiratory failure requiring positive-pressure ventilation. Similarly, many septic shock and post-cardiac surgery patients display RV dysfunction. To what degree ventriculo-arterial coupling plays a role in each of these disease states is unknown, but will define patient response to specific therapies. In general, taking into consideration RV contractility, defined as end-systolic elastance, and pulmonary arterial elastance, we can classify right heart impairment as due to increase in pulmonary artery elastance, a reduction in RV elastance or both. Excess differences in these two elastances reflect uncoupling causing inefficient ventricular loading that itself causes heart failure, independent of pulmonary arterial pressure or baseline RV elastance.

Measuring Right Ventricular Arterial Coupling

Unlike left ventriculo-arterial coupling, which is relatively easy to measure using only echocardiographic data and simple measures of systolic arterial pressure, measuring RV function is relatively difficult. Several methods are available to indirectly assess RV performance, including RV ejection fraction (RVEF), estimated by thermodilution [8], pulmonary artery occlusion pressure (PAOP) estimated by a pulmonary artery catheter (PAC) or echocardiography, tricuspid annual plane systolic excursion (TAPSE) or the measurement of RV diameters using ultrasound, and tissue Doppler imaging of RV wall stress and strain. Regrettably, none of these techniques accurately assess RV systolic function or estimate RV functional reserve [9–12].

Additionally, to measure right ventriculo-arterial coupling, other measures are required. As in the past with the left ventricle, measures of right ventriculo-arterial coupling require measurements of specific aspects of the RV pressure–volume loop during one cardiac cycle. From these data one can then extrapolate the RV end systolic pressure–volume relationship. The most accurate methods are based on cardiac magnetic resonance imaging (MRI), which measure RV end-diastolic and end-systolic volumes, plus a PAC that measures the end-systolic arterial pressure [13]. Unfortunately, these methods, though accurate, are not applicable in a critical care setting. RV volumes can be measured by conductance catheters placed in the right ventricle and when added to the PAC-derived measures of RV pressure, can also define right ventriculo-arterial coupling [14]. In the literature, we were able to find only one brief report on the use of the PAC alone to measure right heart pressures and volumes every 20 s using thermodilution [15]. Alternatively, one can estimate RV maximal systolic arterial pressure during a hypothetical RV isovolumic contraction by extrapolation of the right ventricular pressure profile [7].

Right ventriculo-arterial mismatch can occur as a result of RV failure (decrease in RV elastance), pulmonary arterial hypertension (increase in pulmonary artery elastance) or both. Regardless of the cause of right ventriculo-arterial uncoupling, there will be a reduction in the energetic efficiency between the right heart and the pulmonary circuit, ultimately leading to right heart failure and potentially the need for inotropic support, use of selective pulmonary vasodilators or mechanical assistance. Furthermore, right ventriculo-arterial uncoupling can be a problem alone, due to primary LV dysfunction, or part of global cardiovascular collapse (e. g., adrenal insufficiency).

Causes of Decreased Right Ventricular Elastance

Primary Left Heart Failure

The majority of right heart failure patients have left heart dysfunction. The left heart has thicker walls dispersing wall stress and markedly decreases in diameter during systole making it ideally suited to handle the higher intra-luminal LV pressures need to sustain a high systemic MAP [16]. In contrast, the right heart has thinner walls and decreases in diameter less during systole, such that it cannot handle similar intra-luminal pressures. Importantly, under normal conditions, RV pressures are very low (~ 10–15 mmHg). However, its capacity to handle sudden increases in pulmonary artery pressure is limited and if coupled with increased volume may rapidly spiral into acute *cor pulmonale* and cardiac standstill, a common terminal event in patients with massive pulmonary emboli. Pathologies involving the left heart, especially if they occur suddenly, often result in a passive increase in the pulmonary artery pressure, leading, subsequently, to right ventriculo-arterial uncoupling.

Primary Right Heart Failure

Primary right heart failure can occur if the supply of oxygenated blood to the right heart is stopped due to a right-sided acute coronary syndrome (ACS). RV infarction is often difficult to diagnose, especially in the perioperative period. Routine electrocardiographic (EKG) analysis is often insufficient to identify an ST-T mismatch as it is poorly displayed for the right heart. Only if associated LV inferior wall ischemia or infarction is present is RV infarction readily diagnosed by EKG. Although easily identified as impaired contractility by echocardiography, right heart echocardiography is usually not considered the first line of diagnosis in this setting. Owing to the low RV intra-luminal systolic pressures, RV myocardial blood flow primarily occurs in systole, unlike LV myocardial perfusion, which only occurs in diastole [17]. Thus, systolic hypotension or any condition in which systemic systolic arterial pressure is less than pulmonary systolic arterial pressure will result in RV myocardial ischemia.

The Cardiac Surgical Patient

Patients undergoing heart surgery are usually very complex and in need of a higher number of therapies including mechanical ventilation, inotropic support, and, on occasion, mechanical circulatory support devices [18]. Since the right ventricle has an anterior position in the mediastinum, if cold cardioplegia does not fully cover the RV free wall, it is at risk for postoperative selective RV stunning which presents as transitory right heart impairment. Nonetheless, a right heart issue can persist, and this has to be known by the intensivist to reduce the causes of further hemodynamic derangement, such as aggressive ventilation in the immediate postoperative period or fluid overload or, in the case of initiating countermeasures (prostaglandins, nitric oxide, pharmaceutical or mechanical support), to restore right ventriculo-arterial coupling.

Causes of Increases in Pulmonary Arterial Elastance

Pulmonary Artery Embolism

A pulmonary arterial embolism is a relatively frequent complication in critically ill patients in general and in the postoperative period in particular. It can lead to pulmonary artery hypertension and right ventriculo-arterial uncoupling. Early recognition of this condition is crucial, although, in severe cases, it is usually relatively easy to diagnose by cardiac ultrasonography. RV bulging, septal flattening and paradoxical septal motion are universally seen in hemodynamically significant pulmonary emboli [19]. Intra-luminal thrombi may also be visible in both the right heart and main pulmonary artery. In mild or moderate conditions, however, diagnosis can be carried out using advanced imaging techniques, such as a high-resolution computed tomography (CT) scan or perfusion pulmonary scintigraphy. However, a right ventriculo-arterial evaluation at the bedside may provide clues about the condition along with a clinical examination and routine analysis [20].

Pulmonary Hypertension

Although many critically ill patients with pulmonary hypertension are usually known ahead of time, it is not uncommon to identify pulmonary hypertension (defined as a systolic pulmonary artery pressure >35 mmHg) during the routine management of the critically ill. Importantly, if a patient has high pulmonary arterial pressure consistent with increased pulmonary arterial elastance and their CVP is < 8 mmHg, then they are in a compensated state and probably are not uncoupled [21]. Nevertheless, right ventriculo-arterial decoupling due to increased pulmonary arterial elastance is the primary predictor of death in patients with pulmonary hypertension [22].

The Ventilated Patient

Mechanical ventilatory support of acute and chronic respiratory failure is often lifesaving and is routinely used during surgery requiring general anesthesia. However, mechanical ventilation, by increasing intrathoracic pressure and altering lung volumes also profoundly alters RV preload and pulmonary arterial elastance. Hyperinflation, due to excess tidal volumes, inadequate expiratory time or high levels of end-expiratory airway pressure may all increase pulmonary arterial elastance [23]. This topic is too large to be covered further here but needs to be considered in every ventilated patient who presents with hemodynamic insufficiency. Most often, when a patient needs mechanical ventilation, intensivists are prone to think of it as a pure lung issue, and right heart problems can be underestimated. Yet, it is an equally important part of the story; frequently, RV problems can be exacerbated or even caused by the respiratory support.

Conclusion

Although evaluation of the right heart has not become mainstream and integrated into traditional hemodynamic monitoring owing to the difficulties present in its measurement, RV assessment is instrumental in defining the effect of cardiovascular treatment of the critically ill patient. The assessment of right ventriculo-arterial coupling may play a key role in understanding the pathophysiology of several patterns of hemodynamic derangement from severe sepsis to acute respiratory distress syndrome (ARDS), and should become a commonly available hemodynamic tool in the near future.

References

1. Burkhoff D, Sagawa K (1986) Ventricular efficiency predicted by an analytical model. Am J Physiol 250:R1021–1027
2. Starling MR (1993) Left ventricular-arterial coupling relations in the normal human heart. Am Heart J 125:1659–1666
3. Chen CH, Fetics B, Nevo E et al (2001) Noninvasive single-beat determination of left ventricular end-systolic elastance in humans. J Am Coll Cardiol 38:2028–2034
4. Chirinos JA (2013) Ventricular-arterial coupling: Invasive and non-invasive assessment. Artery Res. doi:10.1016/j.artres.2012.12.002

5. Guarracino F, Ferro B, Morelli A, Bertini P, Baldassarri B, Pinsky MR (2014) Ventriculoarterial decoupling in human septic shock. Crit Care 18:R80
6. Pinsky MR (2016) The right ventricle: interaction with the pulmonary circulation. Crit Care 20:266
7. Brimioulle S, Wauthy P, Ewalenko P et al (2003) Single-beat estimation of right ventricular end-systolic pressure-volume relationship. Am J Physiol Heart Circ Physiol 284:H1625–1630
8. Jardin F, Gueret P, Dubourg O, Farcot JC, Margairaz A, Bourdarias JP (1985) Right ventricular volumes by thermodilution in the adult respiratory distress syndrome. A comparative study using two-dimensional echocardiography as a reference method. Chest 88:34–39
9. Ostenfeld E, Flachskampf FA (2015) Assessment of right ventricular volumes and ejection fraction by echocardiography: from geometric approximations to realistic shapes. Echo Res Pract 2:R1–R11
10. Champion HC, Michelakis ED, Hassoun PM (2009) Comprehensive invasive and noninvasive approach to the right ventricle-pulmonary circulation unit: state of the art and clinical and research implications. Circulation 120:992–1007
11. Bellofiore A, Chesler NC (2013) Methods for measuring right ventricular function and hemodynamic coupling with the pulmonary vasculature. Ann Biomed Eng 41:1384–1398
12. Milan A, Magnino C, Veglio F (2010) Echocardiographic indexes for the non-invasive evaluation of pulmonary hemodynamics. J Am Soc Echocardiogr 23:225–239
13. Kuehne T, Yilmaz S, Steendijk P et al (2004) Magnetic resonance imaging analysis of right ventricular pressure-volume loops: in vivo validation and clinical application in patients with pulmonary hypertension. Circulation 110:2010–2016
14. Solda PL, Pantaleo P, Perlini S et al (1992) Continuous monitoring of right ventricular volume changes using a conductance catheter in the rabbit. J Appl Physiol 73:1770–1775
15. Mehmood MB, Biederman RW, McCarthy MC, Tchorz KM (2015) Right ventricular-vascular coupling in acute hemodynamic stress: a simple method of estimation and relationship with right ventricular ejection fraction and afterload. Circulation 132(Suppl 3):A13214 (abst)
16. Ponikowski P, Voors AA, Anker SD et al (2016) 2016 ESC Guidelines for the diagnosis and treatment of acute and chronic heart failure: The Task Force for the diagnosis and treatment of acute and chronic heart failure of the European Society of Cardiology (ESC). Developed with the special contribution of the Heart Failure Association (HFA) of the ESC. Eur J Heart Fail 18:891–975
17. Brooks H, Kirk ES, Vokonas PS, Urschel CW, Sonnenblick EH (1971) Performance of the right ventricle under stress: relation to right coronary flow. J Clin Invest 50:2176–2183
18. Kormos RL, Teuteberg JJ, Pagani FD et al (2010) Right ventricular failure in patients with the HeartMate II continuous-flow left ventricular assist device: incidence, risk factors, and effect on outcomes. J Thorac Cardiovasc Surg 139:1316–1324
19. Jardin F, Dubourg O, Gueret P, Delorme G, Bourdarias JP (1987) Quantitative two-dimensional echocardiography in massive pulmonary embolism: emphasis on ventricular interdependence and leftward septal displacement. J Am Coll Cardiol 10:1201–1206
20. Vieillard-Baron A, Page B, Augarde R et al (2001) Acute cor pulmonale in massive pulmonary embolism: incidence, echocardiographic pattern, clinical implications and recovery rate. Intensive Care Med 27:1481–1486
21. Simon MA, Pinsky MR (2011) Right ventricular dysfunction and failure in chronic pressure overload. Cardiol Res Pract 2011:568095
22. Vanderpool RR, Pinsky MR, Naeije R et al (2015) RV-pulmonary arterial coupling predicts outcome in patients referred for pulmonary hypertension. Heart 101:37–43
23. Vieillard-Baron A, Prin S, Chergui K, Dubourg O, Jardin F (2002) Echo-Doppler demonstration of acute cor pulmonale at the bedside in the medical intensive care unit. Am J Respir Crit Care Med 166:1310–1319

Part VII
Cardiopulmonary Resuscitation

Antiarrhythmic Drugs for Out-of-Hospital Cardiac Arrest with Refractory Ventricular Fibrillation

T. Tagami, H. Yasunaga, and H. Yokota

Introduction

Out-of-hospital cardiac arrest (OHCA) affects approximately 300,000 people in the United States, 280,000 people in Europe and 110,000 people in Japan each year [1–3]. Among all the presentations of cardiac arrest (asystole, pulseless electrical activity [PEA], ventricular fibrillation [VF], and pulseless ventricular tachycardia [pVT]), VF and pVT are considered the most treatment responsive, but the rate of survival to hospital discharge after OHCA remains markedly low [1–3]. To overcome this time-sensitive and severe condition that has a low survival rate, the "chain of survival" concept was first introduced by Newman [4] in the 1980s as follows: (1) early access to emergency medical care; (2) early cardiopulmonary resuscitation (CPR); (3) early defibrillation; and (4) early advanced cardiac life support. Even after three decades of accumulation of evidence, the 2015 International Liaison Committee on Resuscitation (ILCOR) guidelines still recommend immediate defibrillation with CPR as the treatment of choice for VF/pVT in OHCA patients and that antiarrhythmic drugs can be used as advanced life support during cardiac arrest

T. Tagami (✉)
Department of Emergency and Critical Care Medicine, Nippon Medical School, Tama Nagayama Hospital
2068512 Tama-shi, Tokyo, Japan
Department of Clinical Epidemiology and Health Economics, School of Public Health, Graduate School of Medicine, The University of Tokyo
1138555 Bunkyo-ku, Tokyo, Japan
e-mail: t-tagami@nms.ac.jp

H. Yasunaga
Department of Clinical Epidemiology and Health Economics, School of Public Health, Graduate School of Medicine, The University of Tokyo
1138555 Bunkyo-ku, Tokyo, Japan

H. Yokota
Department of Emergency and Critical Care Medicine, Nippon Medical School
1138603 Bunkyo-ku, Tokyo, Japan

J.-L. Vincent (ed.), *Annual Update in Intensive Care and Emergency Medicine 2017*,
DOI 10.1007/978-3-319-51908-1_18

Table 1 Classification and recommendations for the three antiarrhythmic drugs

	Amiodarone	Lidocaine	Nifekalant
Vaughan Williams classification	Class III	Class Ib	Class III
2015 ILCOR treatment recommendation [5]	Suggest use of amiodarone in adult patients with refractory VF/pVT to improve rates of ROSC.	Suggest use of lidocaine as an alternative to amiodarone in adult patients with refractory VF/pVT.	Suggest use of nifekalant as an alternative to amiodarone in adult patients with refractory VF/pVT.
Level of recommendation	Weak recommendation, moderate-quality evidence	Weak recommendation, very-low-quality evidence	Weak recommendation, very-low-quality evidence

ILCOR: International Liaison Committee on Resuscitation; *VF*: ventricular fibrillation; *pVT*: pulseless ventricular tachycardia

in patients with refractory ventricular dysrhythmias [5, 6]. Refractory VF/pVT is generally defined as failure to terminate VF/pVT with one to three stacked shocks [5].

Antiarrhythmic drugs that may be used include amiodarone, lidocaine, and nifekalant ([5, 6]; Table 1). The ILCOR guidelines recommend the use of amiodarone as first-choice treatment for adult patients with refractory VF/pVT to improve the rate of return of spontaneous circulation (ROSC) [5, 6]. Lidocaine and nifekalant are recommended as alternatives to amiodarone in the treatment of refractory VF/pVT in adult patients. However, as mentioned in the knowledge gap section of the latest resuscitation guidelines [5], existing evidence is not enough to suggest that amiodarone is superior to lidocaine and/or nifekalant in terms of the critical outcome of survival to discharge. In a trial involving OHCA patients with VF/pVT, Dorian et al. [7] reported that the rate of survival to admission was significantly higher in the amiodarone group than in the lidocaine group but found no significant difference in the rate of survival to discharge between the two groups. More recently, Kudenchuk et al. [8] reported survival data for patients with OHCA due to initial VF/pVT in the prehospital setting and found that survival rates with amiodarone or lidocaine administration were not significantly higher than with placebo.

Thus, the provision of amiodarone, lidocaine, or nifekalant to OHCA patients with refractory VF/pVT is still controversial in clinical practice. In this chapter, we review the recent evidence from randomized trials and observational studies for the efficacy of antiarrhythmic drugs for OHCA patients with refractory VF/pVT.

Characteristics and Evidence of the Efficacy of Antiarrhythmic Drugs

Lidocaine was traditionally used as the drug of choice for the treatment of OHCA in patients with persistent VF/pVT until the early 2000s [9]. Lidocaine is classified as a class Ib agent in the Vaughan-Williams classification. Although lidocaine is low-cost and simple to administer, evidence is not enough to suggest its superiority to other antiarrhythmic drugs or placebo in terms of rate of survival to hospital discharge of OHCA patients with persistent VF/pVT. One retrospective study suggested that lidocaine may improve the success rate of resuscitation [10], contrary to the negative results reported in other studies [11, 12]. After the reports of two landmark studies on amiodarone [7, 13], resuscitation guidelines were revised with preference for amiodarone over lidocaine in the treatment of cardiac arrest patients with persistent VF/pVT [5, 6, 9].

Amiodarone and nifekalant are both classified as class III antiarrhythmic agents (potassium channel blockers) in the Vaughan-Williams classification [14, 15]. However, these two class III antiarrhythmic drugs have different pharmacological characteristics. Amiodarone has several effects on ion channels, receptors, and sympathetic activity, in addition to blocking the rapid components of delayed rectifier potassium currents, such as sodium and calcium channel-blocking effects, and α- and β-receptor blocking actions. In other words, amiodarone has negative inotropic and vasodilatory effects, which may negatively affect hemodynamic status after ROSC in OHCA patients. On the other hand, nifekalant is a pure potassium channel blocker that specifically blocks the rapid component of delayed rectifier potassium currents without blocking sodium or calcium channels [16]. Laboratory studies suggest that nifekalant has no negative inotropic effects and no effect on cardiac conduction and hemodynamic status, whereas amiodarone has these effects via its β-blocking action [17, 18]. Although some animal model studies suggested that amiodarone did not contribute to the decrease in defibrillation threshold, nifekalant was found to decrease the defibrillation threshold of ventricular fibrillation [19–21]. Therefore, nifekalant may have advantages over amiodarone for the treatment of refractory VF/pVT via defibrillation and post-resuscitation hemodynamic management from a pharmacological point of view. However, data from clinical studies have provided limited robust results [22, 23].

Only a few studies have compared the efficacy of amiodarone with that of nifekalant for the treatment of refractory VF/pVT [22–25]. Amino et al. [22] reported no significant differences in the success rate of defibrillation and rate of survival to discharge between nifekalant and amiodarone in OHCA patients with refractory VF/pVT. However, they reported that the interval between antiarrhythmic drug administration and defibrillation success in the amiodarone group was significantly longer than that in the nifekalant group [22]. This finding was also reported in a retrospective study by Harayama et al. [23], who found that nifekalant achieved faster ROSC after refractory VF/pVT than did amiodarone. More recently, Amino et al. [25] evaluated the results of a large multicenter prospective study (SOS-KANTO 2012 [26]). These investigators retrospectively investigated nifekalant potency and differential effects of two initial amiodarone doses (150 or 300 mg) as compared with lidocaine doses in the Japanese population. The odds ratios (ORs) for survival to admission were significantly higher in the 150-mg nifekalant or amiodarone group than in the lidocaine group. The authors also reported that 24-hour survival was significantly higher in the nifekalant, 150-mg amiodarone, or 300-mg amiodarone groups than in the lidocaine group. Amino et al. [27] published another *post hoc* analysis from the SOS-KANTO 2012 study. They evaluated the effect of administration of antiarrhythmic drugs (defined as any one among or a combination of lidocaine, nifekalant, and amiodarone) during CPR on 1-month outcome by using propensity score analyses. Logistic regression with propensity scoring demonstrated an OR of 1.92 for 1-month survival in the antiarrhythmic drug group ($p = 0.01$) and 1.44 for favorable neurological outcome at 1 month ($p = 0.26$).

The ROC-ALPS Study

Recently, Resuscitation Outcomes Consortium (ROC) investigators published the results of the Amiodarone, Lidocaine or Placebo Study (ALPS), a randomized double-blind trial [8]. Amiodarone, lidocaine, or placebo was administered by paramedics in the prehospital setting for OHCA patients with refractory VF/pVT in 10 North American sites. The investigators evaluated 3,026 patients, of whom 974 were assigned to the amiodarone group, 993 to the lidocaine group, and 1,059 to the placebo group. Of these patients, 24.4%, 23.7%, and 21.0%, respectively, survived to hospital discharge (primary outcome). The difference in survival rate was 3.2 percentage points for amiodarone compared with placebo (95% confidence interval [CI] −0.4 to 7.0; $p = 0.08$), 2.6 percentage points for lidocaine compared with placebo (95% CI −1.0 to 6.3; $p = 0.16$), and 0.7 percentage points for amiodarone compared with lidocaine (95% CI −3.2 to 4.7; $p = 0.70$).

The survival rates with favorable neurological status (secondary outcome) were similar in the amiodarone group (182 patients [18.8%]), lidocaine group (172 [17.5%]), and placebo group (175 [16.6%]). The risk difference for the secondary outcome was 2.2 percentage points for amiodarone compared with placebo (95% CI −1.1 to 5.6; $p = 0.19$), 0.9 percentage points for lidocaine compared with placebo (95% CI −2.4 to 4.2; $p = 0.59$), and 1.3 percentage points for amiodarone compared with lidocaine (95% CI −2.1 to 4.8; $p = 0.44$).

Kudenchuk et al. [8] concluded the ROC-ALPS study as follows: neither amiodarone nor lidocaine resulted in a survival rate or favorable neurological outcome that was significantly better than that achieved with placebo among patients with OHCA due to initial shock-refractory VF/pVT. However, the study also provided insightful data to the field of resuscitation. The authors reported that among 1,934 patients with bystander-witnessed arrest, the survival rate was higher with amiodarone (27.7%) or lidocaine administration (27.8%) than with placebo (22.7%). This absolute risk difference was significant for amiodarone compared with placebo (5.0 percentage points; 95% CI 0.3–9.7; $p = 0.04$) and for lidocaine compared with placebo (5.2 percentage points; 95% CI 0.5–9.9, p = 0.03). The survival rate was also higher among amiodarone recipients than among placebo recipients with emergency medical services (EMS)-witnessed arrest, with a risk difference of 21.9 percentage points (95% CI 5.8–38.0; p = 0.01). Considering that OHCA with refractory VF/pVT is a time-sensitive condition with a low survival rate, determining whether OHCA was witnessed or not is a reasonable method of performing subanalyses. The authors also reported that among 839 patients with unwitnessed OHCA, survival did not differ significantly between trial groups. These data may indicate that both amiodarone and lidocaine therapies may be effective for shock-refractory bystander-witnessed OHCA but may be useless in unwitnessed OHCA.

Analyses of Data from a Japanese Nationwide Database: Comparisons Between Amiodarone and Nifekalant and Between Amiodarone and Lidocaine

Nifekalant was developed and approved for clinical use in Japan in 1999. Thus, nifekalant and lidocaine were the traditionally used drugs of choice for VF/pVT until the Japanese Ministry of Health, Labour and Welfare approved the use of intravenous amiodarone in June 2007. Thus, Japan is the only country in which amiodarone, nifekalant, and lidocaine are all approved for clinical use. We therefore decided to analyze the effectiveness of antiarrhythmic drugs by using real-world clinical data from cardiogenic OHCA patients with refractory VF/pVT on hospital arrival across the country.

We retrospectively evaluated data from the Japanese Diagnosis Procedure Combination (DPC) database, which is a nationwide in-hospital patient administrative database [28–30]. The DPC database includes administrative claims and discharge abstract data for all patients (including OHCA patients who die in the emergency room) discharged from more than 1,000 participating hospitals, covering all 82 academic hospitals and more than 90% of all tertiary-care emergency hospitals in Japan. The database includes the following information for each patient, recorded using a uniform data submission form: age, sex, medical procedures (e. g., defibrillation, therapeutic hypothermia, and percutaneous coronary angiogram/intervention), daily records of all drugs administered and devices used (e. g., amiodarone, nifekalant, lidocaine, extracorporeal membrane oxygenation [ECMO], and intra-aortic balloon pumping [IABP]), length of hospital stay, and discharge status (home, transfer to another hospital, death in the emergency room, or death after admission) [28–30].

We compared the rates of survival to discharge among cardiogenic OHCA patients with persistent VF/pVT on hospital arrival following treatment with either amiodarone or nifekalant [28], and amiodarone or lidocaine [29].

In the study that compared amiodarone and nifekalant [28], we identified 2,961 patients with cardiogenic OHCA who had VF/pVT on hospital arrival between July 2007 and March 2013. Patients were categorized into amiodarone (n = 2,353) and nifekalant groups (n = 608), from which 525 propensity score-matched pairs were generated. We found a significant difference in admission rate between the nifekalant and amiodarone groups in the propensity score-matched groups (75.6 vs. 69.3%; difference 6.3%; 95% CI 0.9–11.7). An analysis that used the in-hospital administration rate of nifekalant/amiodarone as an instrumental variable found that receiving nifekalant was associated with an improved admission rate (22.2%; 95% CI 11.9–32.4). However, we found no significant difference in in-hospital mortality between the nifekalant and amiodarone groups (81.5 vs. 82.1%; difference −0.6%; 95% CI −5.2 to 4.1). Instrumental variable analysis showed that receiving nifekalant was not associated with reduced in-hospital mortality (6.2%, 95% CI −2.4 to 14.8). We concluded that although nifekalant may potentially improve hospital admission rates compared with amiodarone for these patients, no significant association with in-hospital mortality was found between nifekalant and amiodarone for cardiogenic OHCA patients with VF/pVT on hospital arrival.

In the study that compared amiodarone and lidocaine [29], we identified 3,951 patients from 795 hospitals who experienced cardiogenic OHCA and had refractory ventricular fibrillation on hospital arrival. The patients were categorized into amiodarone (n = 1,743) and lidocaine (n = 2,208) groups, from which 801 propensity score-matched pairs were generated. No significant difference in the rate of survival to hospital discharge was found between the amiodarone and lidocaine groups (15.2 vs. 17.1%; difference −1.9%; 95% CI −5.5 to 1.7) in the propensity score-matched analyses. Thus, we concluded that the amiodarone and lidocaine groups had no significant difference in the rate of survival to hospital discharge.

As compared with those reported in the ROC-ALPS study, the survival rates of our two nationwide observational studies were lower (approximately 17–18% in our studies [28, 29] vs. 24% in the ROC-ALPS study [8]). These differences may be attributed to the differences in the EMS of the countries in which the studies were conducted. The ROC-ALPS study [8] was conducted in North America, whereas we analyzed Japanese data. In the ROC-ALPS study [8], patients were randomized at the scene by the responding paramedics. This is in contrast to our study, in which antiarrhythmic drugs were provided after hospital arrival because paramedics are not allowed to administer any antiarrhythmic drugs in prehospital settings in Japan. Thus, the times from cardiac arrest to first administration of the antiarrhythmic drug were much longer in our studies [28, 29] than in the ROC-ALPS study [8].

Recent Systematic Review and Meta-analyses

Huang et al. [31] reviewed 10 randomized controlled trials and 7 observational trials in 2013. They found that amiodarone (relative risk [RR] 0.82; 95% CI 0.54–1.24), lidocaine (RR 2.26; 95% CI 0.93–5.52) and nifekalant therapies did not improve survival to hospital discharge compared with placebo, but amiodarone, lidocaine, and nifekalant therapies were beneficial to initial resuscitation, as assessed based on the rate of ROSC and survival to hospital admission, with amiodarone being superior to lidocaine (RR 1.28; 95% CI 0.57–2.86) and nifekalant (RR 0.50; 95% CI 0.19–1.31).

Amino et al. reported a systematic review of the use of intravenous amiodarone and nifekalant in 2014 [32]. They reviewed 9 articles, including those written in the Japanese language. They found that amiodarone and nifekalant therapies were equally effective in preventing electrical storm (67 vs. 67%). The defibrillation effect on CPR was also equal in the two groups (60 vs. 54%). More cases of hypotension and bradycardia were recorded as adverse effects in the amiodarone group (9.5 and 5.3%) than in the nifekalant group [32].

After publication of the results of the ROC-ALPS study, two systematic reviews with meta-analyses were published in 2016 [33, 34]. Laina et al. [34] reported that amiodarone therapy significantly improved survival to hospital admission (OR 1.402; 95% CI 1.068–1.840; $Z=2.43$; $p=0.015$), but neither survival to hospital discharge (RR 0.850; 95% CI 0.631–1.144; $Z=1.07$; $p=0.284$) nor neurological outcome (OR 1.114; 95% CI 0.923–1.345; $Z=1.12$; $p=0.475$) were significantly improved by amiodarone therapy compared with placebo or nifekalant therapy. Sanfilippo et al. [33] reported another review regarding this issue. They reported that amiodarone was as beneficial as lidocaine for survival to hospital admission (primary analysis OR 1.02; 95% CI 0.86–1.23; $p=0.40$) and discharge (primary analysis OR 1.06; 95% CI 0.87–1.30; $p=0.56$; secondary analysis OR 1.04; 95% CI 0.86–1.27; $p=0.67$). Compared with placebo, survival to hospital admission was higher with both amiodarone (primary analysis OR 1.32; 95% CI 1.12–1.54; $p<0.0001$; secondary analysis OR 1.25; 95% CI 1.07–1.45; $p<0.005$) and lidocaine (secondary analysis only OR 1.34; 95% CI 1.14–1.58; $p=0.0005$) therapies. With regard to hospital discharge, no significant differences were observed between placebo and amiodarone (primary outcome OR 1.19; 95% CI 0.98–1.44; $p=0.08$; secondary outcome OR 1.11; 95% CI 0.92–1.33; $p=0.28$) or lidocaine (secondary outcome only OR 1.19; 95% CI 0.97–1.45; $p=0.10$) therapy.

These recent four systematic reviews with meta-analyses suggested that amiodarone, lidocaine and nifekalant therapies equally improved survival to hospital admission as compared with placebo. However, none of these antiarrhythmic drugs improved long-term outcomes.

Is Earlier Provision of Antiarrhythmic Drugs Better?

After publication of the results of the ROC-ALPS study, several corresponding editorials and comments were published in response [35–38]. As pointed out by several comments, the key finding of the ROC-ALPS study was that both amiodarone and lidocaine therapies may be effective for shock-refractory VF/pVT in bystander-witnessed arrest but might be useless in the later phase of resuscitation [35, 37]. The first dose of the trial drugs was given a mean (±SD) of 19.3 ± 7.4 min after the initial call to EMS and after a median of three shocks in the overall population of the ROC-ALPS study [8]. Kudenchuk et al. speculated that such delays may attenuate the effectiveness of antiarrhythmic interventions as patients progress to the metabolic phase of OHCA when cellular injury and physiological derangements may be irreversible despite restored circulation [39]. The potential benefit of treatment could have been underestimated among patients with unwitnessed OHCA. Patients with witnessed OHCA who received earlier initiation of resuscitation and a shorter interval to antiarrhythmic drug administration (12 min) had significantly higher rates of survival to hospital discharge by about 5%.

Conclusion

Recent guidelines on resuscitation recommend immediate defibrillation with CPR as the treatment of choice for OHCA patients with VF/pVT and that antiarrhythmic drugs (including amiodarone, lidocaine and nifekalant) can be used as advanced life support during cardiac arrest in patients with refractory ventricular dysrhythmias. Recent systematic reviews and meta-analyses suggest that amiodarone, lidocaine, and nifekalant therapies equally improve survival to hospital admission compared with placebo. However, none of these antiarrhythmic drugs improved long-term outcomes. The landmark study, ROC-ALPS, concluded that compared with placebo, neither amiodarone nor lidocaine therapy resulted in a significantly higher rate of survival or more favorable neurological outcome among patients with OHCA due to refractory VF/pVT. However, the authors also reported that among patients with bystander-witnessed cardiac arrest, the survival rate was higher with amiodarone or lidocaine than with placebo. Although further studies are required to confirm this speculation, earlier administration of antiarrhythmic drugs may result in better outcomes.

References

1. Atwood C, Eisenberg MS, Herlitz J, Rea TD (2005) Incidence of EMS-treated out-of-hospital cardiac arrest in Europe. Resuscitation 67:75–80
2. Kitamura T, Iwami T, Kawamura T et al (2012) Nationwide improvements in survival from out-of-hospital cardiac arrest in Japan. Circulation 126:2834–2843
3. Nichol G, Thomas E, Callaway CW et al (2008) Regional variation in out-of-hospital cardiac arrest incidence and outcome. JAMA 300:1423–1431
4. Newman M (1989) The chain of survival concept takes hold. JEMS 14:11–13
5. Callaway CW, Soar J, Aibiki M et al (2015) Part 4: Advanced Life Support: 2015 International Consensus on Cardiopulmonary Resuscitation and Emergency Cardiovascular Care Science With Treatment Recommendations. Circulation 132:84–S145
6. Soar J, Nolan JP, Bottiger BW et al (2015) European Resuscitation Council Guidelines for Resuscitation 2015: Section 3. Adult advanced life support. Resuscitation 95:100–147
7. Dorian P, Cass D, Schwartz B, Cooper R, Gelaznikas R, Barr A (2002) Amiodarone as compared with lidocaine for shock-resistant ventricular fibrillation. N Engl J Med 346:884–890
8. Kudenchuk PJ, Brown SP, Daya M et al (2016) Amiodarone, lidocaine, or placebo in out-of-hospital cardiac arrest. N Engl J Med 374:1711–1722
9. The American Heart Association in collaboration with the International Liaison Committee on Resuscitation (2000) Guidelines 2000 for Cardiopulmonary Resuscitation and Emergency Cardiovascular Care. Part 6: advanced cardiovascular life support: section 5: pharmacology I: agents for arrhythmias. Circulation 102:I112–128

10. Herlitz J, Ekstrom L, Wennerblom B et al (1997) Lidocaine in out-of-hospital ventricular fibrillation. Does it improve survival? Resuscitation 33:199–205
11. Harrison EE (1981) Lidocaine in prehospital countershock refractory ventricular fibrillation. Ann Emerg Med 10:420–423
12. Weaver WD, Fahrenbruch CE, Johnson DD, Hallstrom AP, Cobb LA, Copass MK (1990) Effect of epinephrine and lidocaine therapy on outcome after cardiac arrest due to ventricular fibrillation. Circulation 82:2027–2034
13. Kudenchuk PJ, Cobb LA, Copass MK et al (1999) Amiodarone for resuscitation after out-of-hospital cardiac arrest due to ventricular fibrillation. N Engl J Med 341:871–878
14. Singh BN, Vaughan Williams EM (1970) The effect of amiodarone, a new anti-anginal drug, on cardiac muscle. Br J Pharmacol 39:657–667
15. Pantazopoulos IN, Troupis GT, Pantazopoulos CN, Xanthos TT (2011) Nifekalant in the treatment of life-threatening ventricular tachyarrhythmias. World J Cardiol 3:169–176
16. Nakaya H, Tohse N, Takeda Y, Kanno M (1993) Effects of MS-551, a new class III antiarrhythmic drug, on action potential and membrane currents in rabbit ventricular myocytes. Br J Pharmacol 109:157–163
17. Kondoh K, Hashimoto H, Nishiyama H et al (1994) Effects of MS-551, a new class III antiarrhythmic drug, on programmed stimulation-induced ventricular arrhythmias, electrophysiology, and hemodynamics in a canine myocardial infarction model. J Cardiovasc Pharmacol 23:674–680
18. Sen L, Cui G, Sakaguchi Y, Singh BN (1998) Electrophysiological effects of MS-551, a new class III agent: comparison with dl-sotalol in dogs. J Pharmacol Exp Ther 285:687–694
19. Murakawa Y, Yamashita T, Kanese Y, Omata M (1997) Can a class III antiarrhythmic drug improve electrical defibrillation efficacy during ventricular fibrillation? J Am Coll Cardiol 29:688–692
20. Tsagalou EP, Anastasiou-Nana MI, Charitos CE et al (2004) Time course of fibrillation and defibrillation thresholds after an intravenous bolus of amiodarone – an experimental study. Resuscitation 61:83–89
21. Huang J, Skinner JL, Rogers JM, Smith WM, Holman WL, Ideker RE (2002) The effects of acute and chronic amiodarone on activation patterns and defibrillation threshold during ventricular fibrillation in dogs. J Am Coll Cardiol 40:375–383
22. Amino M, Yoshioka K, Opthof T et al (2010) Comparative study of nifekalant versus amiodarone for shock-resistant ventricular fibrillation in out-of-hospital cardiopulmonary arrest patients. J Cardiovasc Pharmacol 55:391–398
23. Harayama N, Nihei S, Nagata K et al (2014) Comparison of nifekalant and amiodarone for resuscitation of out-of-hospital cardiopulmonary arrest resulting from shock-resistant ventricular fibrillation. J Anesth 28:587–592
24. Ji XF, Li CS, Wang S, Yang L, Cong LH (2010) Comparison of the efficacy of nifekalant and amiodarone in a porcine model of cardiac arrest. Resuscitation 81:1031–1036
25. Amino M, Inokuchi S, Nagao K et al (2015) Nifekalant hydrochloride and amiodarone hydrochloride result in similar improvements for 24-hour survival in cardiopulmonary arrest patients: The SOS-KANTO 2012 Study. J Cardiovasc Pharmacol 66:600–609
26. SOS-KANTO_2012_study_group (2015) Changes in pre- and in-hospital management and outcomes for out-of-hospital cardiac arrest between 2002 and 2012 in Kanto, Japan: the SOS-KANTO 2012 Study. Acute Med Surg 2:225–233
27. Amino M, Inokuchi S, Yoshioka K et al (2016) Does antiarrhythmic drug during cardiopulmonary resuscitation improve the one-month survival: The SOS-KANTO 2012 Study. J Cardiovasc Pharmacol 68:58–66
28. Tagami T, Matsui H, Ishinokami S et al (2016) Amiodarone or nifekalant upon hospital arrival for refractory ventricular fibrillation after out-of-hospital cardiac arrest. Resuscitation 109:127–132

29. Tagami T, Matsui H, Tanaka C et al (2016) Amiodarone compared with lidocaine for out-of-hospital cardiac arrest with refractory ventricular fibrillation on hospital arrival: a nationwide database study. Cardiovasc Drugs Ther 30:485–491
30. Tagami T, Matsui H, Fushimi K, Yasunaga H (2016) Changes in therapeutic hypothermia and coronary intervention provision and in-hospital mortality of patients with out-of-hospital cardiac arrest: a nationwide database study. Crit Care Med 44:488–495
31. Huang Y, He Q, Yang M, Zhan L (2013) Antiarrhythmia drugs for cardiac arrest: a systemic review and meta-analysis. Crit Care 17:R173
32. Amino M, Yoshioka K, Kanda S et al (2014) Systematic review of the use of intravenous amiodarone and nifekalant for cardiopulmonary resuscitation in Japan. J Arrhyth 30:180–185
33. Sanfilippo F, Corredor C, Santonocito C et al (2016) Amiodarone or lidocaine for cardiac arrest: A systematic review and meta-analysis. Resuscitation 107:31–37
34. Laina A, Karlis G, Liakos A et al (2016) Amiodarone and cardiac arrest: Systematic review and meta-analysis. Int J Cardiol 221:780–788
35. Sugiyama K, Kashiura M, Hamabe Y (2016) Amiodarone and lidocaine for shock refractory ventricular fibrillation or ventricular tachycardia in out-of-hospital cardiac arrest: are they really effective? J Thorac Dis 8:E791–E793
36. Ho AF, Ong ME (2016) Antiarrhythmic drugs in out-of-hospital cardiac arrest-what does the Amiodarone, Lidocaine, or Placebo Study tell us? J Thorac Dis 8:E604–E606
37. Joglar JA, Page RL (2016) Out-of-hospital cardiac arrest – are drugs ever the answer? N Engl J Med 374:1781–1782
38. Kudenchuk PJ, Daya M, Dorian P, Resuscitation Outcomes Consortium I (2016) Amiodarone, lidocaine, or placebo in out-of-hospital cardiac arrest. N Engl J Med 375:802–803
39. Weisfeldt ML, Becker LB (2002) Resuscitation after cardiac arrest: a 3-phase time-sensitive model. JAMA 288:3035–3038

Airway and Ventilation During Cardiopulmonary Resuscitation

C. J. R. Gough and J. P. Nolan

Introduction

Intuitively, effective airway management and ventilation are essential components of effective cardiopulmonary resuscitation (CPR). However, studies have failed to show a benefit to early prioritization of ventilation, and international guidelines have reiterated the importance of effective, minimally-interrupted chest compressions [1]. There is no clear consensus on the best strategy for managing the airway during CPR, but at some stage in the resuscitation pathway an open airway, oxygenation and sufficient ventilation will be necessary. There is also the important step of isolating the lungs from the gastrointestinal tract and protecting them from aspiration of gastric contents. In this chapter, we will summarize the current approaches to airway and ventilation management during CPR, emphasizing the stepwise approach and highlighting ongoing research in this field.

Current Airway Options and the Concept of the Stepwise Approach

The ideal airway management strategy during CPR remains unclear. In practice, there is often a progression in complexity of airway management, from no intervention (compression-only CPR), mouth-to-mouth, and bag-mask ventilation, through to supraglottic airway (SGA) devices and tracheal intubation. The best airway is

C. J. R. Gough
Royal United Hospital
Bath, UK

J. P. Nolan (✉)
Resuscitation Medicine, University of Bristol
Bristol, UK
Anaesthesia and Intensive Care Medicine, Royal United Hospital
Bath, BA1 3NG, UK
e-mail: jerry.nolan@nhs.net

J.-L. Vincent (ed.), *Annual Update in Intensive Care and Emergency Medicine 2017*,
DOI 10.1007/978-3-319-51908-1_19

likely to vary depending on the time-point in the resuscitation process, and the skill set of the attending rescuers [2]. Ensure high quality chest compressions and minimize any interruptions for airway intervention.

Chest Compression-only and Mouth-To-Mouth Rescue Breathing

The current recommendation for the untrained bystander is for dispatcher-assisted chest compression-only CPR, while those trained in rescue breathing should perform this in addition to chest compressions if willing and able [3].

A meta-analysis of three randomized controlled trials showed that chest-compression-only CPR was associated with improved chance of survival (discharge or 30 days) compared with standard CPR (14 [211/1500]% versus 12 [178/1531]%; risk ratio 1.22, 95% CI 1.01–1.46) [4]. A more recent meta-analysis of two of these three trials has shown that the benefit of chest compression-only CPR was maintained for several years with a lower risk of death after adjustment for potential confounders (adjusted hazard ratio 0.91; 95% CI, 0.83–0.99; $p = 0.02$) [5].

Bag-mask Ventilation

Bag-mask ventilation with a self-inflating bag, often supplemented with an oropharyngeal or nasopharyngeal airway, is frequently used until advanced airway techniques such as SGA devices or tracheal intubation are undertaken. Several recent studies have supported the use of bag-mask ventilation in the pre-hospital setting, including a large national Japanese study of 649,654 adult patients which found that bag-mask ventilation was associated with better outcomes (return of spontaneous circulation [ROSC], one-month survival and neurological outcomes) when compared to the advanced airway techniques [6]. This was an observational study, with low rates of neurologically intact survival in both groups (1.1% versus 2.9% [odds ratio 0.38, 95% CI 0.36–0.39]). Observational studies like this are prone to selection bias – patients who recover rapidly from a cardiac arrest, and therefore likely to have a better outcome, are less likely to require advanced airway management. Conversely, those who require advanced airway management are already less likely to survive. Investigators often use propensity analysis to try to account for such confounders, but can only ever include data that have been collected and reported. There are likely to be other factors (hidden confounders) that may account for the apparent differences in outcome.

Although some patients achieve ROSC and regain consciousness without an advanced airway, many others will need an advanced airway at some stage during their pathway: this may be achieved before ROSC, directly after ROSC or after admission to hospital.

Supraglottic Airway Devices

SGA devices are an appealing alternative to tracheal intubation because they require less training for successful insertion, and may cause less interruption of chest compressions than tracheal intubation [7]. The most commonly used SGAs worldwide include the laryngeal tube, the laryngeal mask airway (LMA) and the i-gel.

Swine models raised concerns that SGAs could reduce carotid blood flow as a result of direct compression on the internal and external carotid arteries, but this is not apparent in the limited human studies [8–10]. The use of SGAs in situations where the skills for tracheal intubation are not immediately available has made their use widespread in both the pre-hospital and in-hospital setting; they have a documented high success rate in both settings [11, 12].

The ideal SGA for use during cardiac arrest is unclear, and a randomized controlled trial comparing SGA with tracheal intubation powered for long-term survival has not been done. A feasibility study has been conducted in Southwest England comparing cluster-randomization of two types of SGA (i-gel and LMA supreme) with usual practice, principally tracheal intubation, but also including bag-mask ventilation and LMA insertion [13]. As a feasibility study, it was not powered to detect statistical differences in outcome between groups, but it documented protocol adherence in 80% of patients and has led on to the AIRWAYS-2 trial (see below) [14]. Of note, in the feasibility study, the LMA supreme arm was discontinued in the final 2 months following three contamination incidents as a result of blood and gastric fluid being forcefully ejected from the gastric drainage port during CPR [15].

Tracheal Intubation

As with other emergency scenarios, intubation in cardiac arrest is not easy. The frequency of more difficult intubations (Cormack and Lehane grade 3 and above, or 3 or more intubation attempts) is roughly double during cardiac arrest in comparison with routine general anesthesia (10.3–13% versus 5.8% [95% CI 4.5–7.5]) [16, 17].

The risk of complications of tracheal intubation must be balanced against the risks associated with SGAs.

Advantages of Tracheal Intubation

Advantages of tracheal intubation include effective ventilation while minimizing interruptions to chest compressions, minimizing gastric insufflation and therefore reducing regurgitation, and protecting the pulmonary tree from aspiration of gastric contents.

Disadvantages of Tracheal Intubation

Disadvantages of tracheal intubation include interruptions to chest compressions (during insertion), delay to definitive care, endobronchial intubation and unrecognized esophageal intubation. Interruptions to chest compressions can be lengthy, and could outweigh any benefit of securing the airway. A study of 100 pre-hospital intubations by paramedics found the total duration of interruptions during CPR associated with tracheal intubation attempts was 110 (IQR 54–198) s, and in a quarter of cases the interruptions were over 3 min [18].

There is also a learning curve to successful intubation, and ongoing practice is required to retain this skill. A recent systematic review sought to determine the learning curve for tracheal intubation by direct laryngoscopy by healthcare professionals [19]. The authors identified 13 studies with a total of 1,462 students who had attempted to intubate 19,108, mostly elective, patients. At least 50 intubations with no more than two intubation attempts needed to be performed to reach a success rate of at least 90%. Given that intubation during cardiac arrest is likely to be more difficult than intubation for elective surgery it seems probable that considerably more than 50 intubations are required to exceed success rates of 90% during cardiac arrest. A study from the South of England showed that 75% of paramedics perform just one or no intubations a year [20]. There is therefore a training requirement to deliver successful intubation in the community.

Advantages of SGAs

SGAs are easier to insert than a tracheal tube, require less training for use, and can usually be inserted without interruption to chest compressions [21].

Disadvantages of SGAs

As yet, there is no randomized controlled trial that compares long-term survival between tracheal intubation and SGAs. Without a cuffed tube securing the trachea, the risk of pulmonary aspiration of gastric contents may be higher than with tracheal intubation. A recent small cadaver study, which compared a number of airway techniques, instilled 500 ml of colored solution into the stomachs of human cadavers, commenced 5 min of CPR, then used fiberoptic bronchoscopy to identify the presence of any colored solution below the vocal cords. Each group comprised five cadavers. Three cases of aspiration were identified with bag-mask ventilation, two cases of aspiration with the LMA and i-gel, one case with the laryngeal tube, and no cases of aspiration with tracheal intubation [22]. This high rate of aspiration with SGAs has not been a feature of many observational studies to date.

Videolaryngoscopy

Videolaryngoscopy is being implemented extensively in anesthetic practice and its contribution to ease of intubation in cardiac arrest has been evaluated recently. Two studies from Korea in 2015 assessed both out-of-hospital and in-hospital cardiac arrest; the first compared videolaryngoscopy with direct laryngoscopy for intubation by novice emergency physicians [23]. The videolaryngoscopy group had a greater success rate (92% versus 56%, $p<0.001$), was quicker (37 [CI: 29–55] s versus 62 [56–110] s, $p<0.001$), and had shorter median duration of interruption of chest compressions (0 [0–0] s versus 7 [3–16] s, $p<0.001$). The second study compared videolaryngoscopy with direct laryngoscopy for in-hospital cardiac arrest, and also found the first attempt success rate to be higher (72% versus 53%, $p = 0.003$), but mortality was no different between the groups [24]. A more recent study from the first group compared videolaryngoscopy with direct laryngoscopy undertaken by experienced intubators (> 50 intubations) [25]. Although there were no significant differences between success rates and median times to intubation, interruption of chest compressions was longer in the direct laryngoscopy group (median 4.0 [1.0–11.0] s versus 0.0 [0.0–1.0] s). The group also recorded episodes of "serious no-flow" (interruption > 10 s), which were dramatically more common with direct laryngoscopy (18/69 [26.1%]) compared with videolaryngoscopy (0/71) ($p < 0.001$), even for highly experienced intubators (14/55 [25.5%] versus 0/57 with videolaryngoscopy).

There is a challenge to implement videolaryngoscopy for all intubations, particularly within the pre-hospital setting. In addition to concerns about sterilization or use of disposable blades there are concerns about deskilling in direct laryngoscopy, which create problems at times when videolaryngoscopy is unavailable or not working. The additional equipment required for videolaryngoscopy is also a challenge to implementation in both the pre-hospital and ward-based areas.

Capnography

Continuous waveform capnography is recommended for all intubated patients, to confirm and continuously monitor the position of the tracheal tube [26]. Continuous capnography has several functions during CPR. The end-tidal carbon dioxide ($etCO_2$) value is associated with the quality of CPR (depth of compressions and ventilation rate) [27, 28]. It therefore could be used as a real time monitor of CPR quality and to guide effective CPR and identify tiring team members. These possibilities have yet to be proven in clinical trials.

Waveform capnography can also aid identification of ROSC: a sudden increase in $etCO_2$ can prompt a rhythm and pulse check [29]. An $etCO_2$ increase of $\geq$ 10 mmHg has good specificity (97% [95% CI 91–99]) but poor sensitivity (33% [95% CI 22–47]) for indicating ROSC [30]. Side effects of epinephrine can therefore be potentially avoided, or the epinephrine delayed until after the next rhythm check if still required.

Recent Systematic Reviews and Meta-Analyses

A meta-analysis of 17 observational studies included nearly 400,000 patients and compared the associated outcomes among those who received advanced airway intervention with those who received basic airway intervention [31]. Use of an advanced airway (either tracheal intubation or a SGA) was associated with reduced odds of long-term survival (advanced airway OR 0.49 [95% CI 0.37–0.65]).

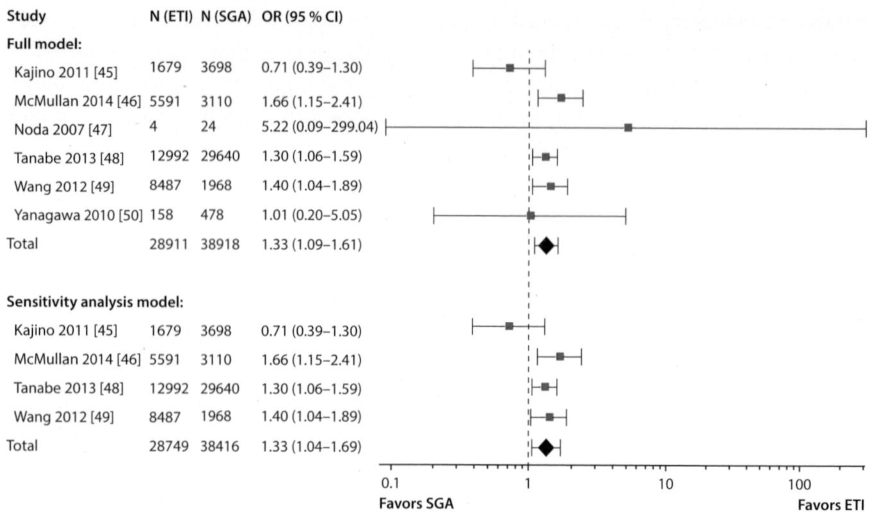

Fig. 1 Forest plot for neurologically intact survival to hospital discharge. *ETI*: endotracheal intubation; *SGA*: supraglottic airway; *OR*: odds ratio; *CI*: confidence interval; *full model*: random effects model with all studies included; *sensitivity analysis model*: random effects model excluding studies of 'very low' quality. Modified from [32] with permission

Another meta-analysis of 10 observational studies included 76,000 patients who were managed with either tracheal intubation or insertion of a SGA [32]. Four of these observational studies were also included in the previous meta-analysis. Tracheal intubation was associated with an increased rate of survival to hospital admission (OR 1.34, 95% CI 1.03–1.75), ROSC (OR 1.28, 95% CI 1.05–1.55) and neurologically intact survival (OR 1.33, 95% CI 1.09–1.61) (Fig. 1).

Propensity Analysis

Propensity analysis is used when two groups of patients have dissimilar characteristics that could affect any observed difference in outcome. A score is calculated that is the probability that a patient would receive the treatment of interest, based on characteristics of the patient, treating clinician and treating environment [33]. Many observational studies of airway management during CPR, such as some of those from the all-Japan out-of-hospital cardiac arrest registry, use propensity score matching, which involves creating two groups of study participants; one group that received the treatment of interest and the other that did not, while matching individuals with similar propensity scores. The two groups can then approximate those of a randomized trial, by comparing outcomes between matched individuals who received the intervention, and those who did not. There are several limitations to this approach. First, only the measured characteristics can be adjusted for, so any unmeasured confounders that affect treatment selection will not be corrected for.

Second, the quality of the propensity model used will affect its outcome, as will the size and quality of data included. Observational data cannot establish causal relationships or treatment effects, but appropriately used propensity analysis on a sufficient sample size, can provide a useful approximation of the effect of an intervention.

Ongoing Research

Cardiac Arrest Airway Management (CAAM)

In this French trial, patients with out-of-hospital cardiac arrest are being randomized to early tracheal intubation or bag-mask ventilation in the pre-hospital setting by physician-staffed emergency responders (clinicaltrials.gov NCT02327026). The primary outcome is 28-day survival with favorable neurological outcome. The primary hypothesis is that basic airway management is sufficient in cardiac arrest and avoids the risks of tracheal intubation. After randomization, patients whose lungs cannot be satisfactorily ventilated with a bag-mask device, or who have significant regurgitation, can be intubated. Those patients in the bag-mask device group will undergo tracheal intubation after ROSC. Thus this is really a study of early intubation versus intubation delayed until after ROSC. The study is due to complete enrolment by April 2017.

Pragmatic Airway Resuscitation Trial (PART)

In this North American trial, initial tracheal intubation is being compared with laryngeal tube insertion in patients with out-of-hospital cardiac arrest [34]. Participating EMS agencies (approximately 30) are clustered-randomized to airway management with primary tracheal intubation (control) or primary laryngeal tube insertion (intervention), with periodic crossover to the other arm twice per year. The trial authors opted for laryngeal tube insertion instead of other SGAs (such as laryngeal mask or i-gel) because the laryngeal tube is the most commonly used SGA out-of-hospital in the United States. If initial advanced airway insertion in either arm is unsuccessful the unrestricted use of other airway devices is allowed. The primary outcome is survival at 72 h; secondary outcomes include ROSC, survival to hospital discharge, and neurologically-intact survival at hospital discharge. The study is due to complete enrolment in October 2017.

AIRWAYS-2

This English multicenter cluster-randomized trial follows the feasibility study discussed earlier [13] and is comparing tracheal intubation with i-gel insertion as the initial advanced airway strategy in out-of-hospital cardiac arrest [14]. Paramedics will follow a standardized protocol for management of the airway, and the primary outcome measure is favorable neurological outcome at hospital discharge (or at 30 days if still hospitalized). In a sub-set of patients, from both arms of the trial, compression fraction will also be measured. This is the proportion of resuscitation time during which chest compressions are being delivered, with a higher fraction reflecting better quality CPR, and increased chance of survival [35]. The study is due to complete enrolment by June 2017.

Pragmatic Trials

These three ongoing airway trials in out-of-hospital cardiac arrest are all pragmatic clinical effectiveness trials. The need for pragmatic trials has arisen from the observation that relatively small trials with highly selected participants (optimized for efficacy) often conducted by experienced investigators tend to exaggerate the benefit of an intervention, and underestimate harm [36]. A pragmatic trial is one which aims to ascertain the real-world effectiveness of an intervention across a broad population. All aspects of the trial should relate as closely as possible to normal clinical practice, including recruitment of patients and investigators, the intervention and its delivery within the trial, the nature of follow up, and the nature, determination and analysis of outcomes. Some recent resuscitation trials have reflected this pragmatic approach [37] and the complex nature of airway management during cardiac arrest, which often involves several interacting components, will also be best investigated with a pragmatic trial [36].

Ventilation During and After CPR

Ventilation should be commenced as soon as possible in the apneic patient, either in a 30:2 ratio of chest compressions:ventilation breaths, or at a rate of roughly 10 breaths per minute in the intubated patient when chest compressions are delivered without pauses [3]. Hypercapnia occurs frequently both during and after cardiac arrest, but attempts to correct this can be detrimental. Hyperventilation leads to an increase in intrathoracic pressure and subsequent reduction in coronary perfusion pressure [38]. Although hyperventilation is frequently seen during cardiac arrest [39], a recent study of arterial blood gases taken during cardiac arrest or just after ROSC documented hypocapnia in only 6% of 115 patients [40]. Hypocapnia and hyperventilation should be avoided – there are several methods of achieving this, from retraining of personnel to metronomes and automated devices [41].

The optimal method of ventilation is still not clearly established. A recent pig study found that ventilation could lead to hypocapnia even if pre-arrest ventilator settings were maintained during the cardiac arrest [42]. Apneic oxygenation (100% oxygen at a pressure of 20 cmH_20) and constant oxygen flow (10 l/min via a 10 French catheter inserted down the tracheal tube), both via tracheal tubes, maintained PaO_2 values above 10 kPa up to 1 h after initiation of cardiac arrest. Median

$PaCO_2$ values were 12.3 and 6.2 kPa in the apneic oxygenation and constant oxygen flow groups respectively.

Maintenance of adequate cerebral perfusion after cardiac arrest will help to optimize neurological recovery. In a small ($n = 7$) interventional crossover trial, induction of mild hypercapnia ($PaCO_2$ 50–55 mmHg) increased cerebral tissue oxygen saturation values from 61% to 69–73 % ($p = 0.001$) [43]. In a phase two trial by the same group, targeted therapeutic mild hypercapnia ($PaCO_2$ 50–55 mmHg) was associated with a reduced increase in neuron specific enolase (NSE) values compared to targeted normocapnia ($PaCO_2$ 35–45 mmHg) [44]. Favorable neurological recovery occurred in 59% of the mild hypercapnia group and 46% of the normocapnia group ($p = 0.26$). Larger studies are needed to investigate further and monitor long-term outcomes.

The Future

Technology is advancing at a rapid pace, and this technology takes time to filter through to clinical applications. Developments in videolaryngoscopy technology should eventually enable widespread use of videolaryngoscopy in the pre-hospital setting, as well as across all hospital locations. The results of ongoing prospective trials comparing tracheal intubation and SGA insertion in cardiac arrest may provide us with the data to determine optimal airway management during cardiac arrest. Depending on the results of these studies it may then be appropriate to undertake a prospective comparison of videolaryngoscopy with either direct laryngoscopy or SGA insertion in cardiac arrest.

Conclusion

The ideal airway management strategy during CPR remains unclear. In practice, there is often a progression in complexity of airway management, from no intervention (compression only CPR), mouth-to-mouth, and bag-mask ventilation, through to SGA devices and tracheal intubation. The best airway is likely to vary depending on the time-point in the resuscitation process, and the skill set of the attending rescuers.

Observational studies of resuscitation are prone to a number of biases and cannot establish causal relationships or treatment effects. Appropriately used propensity analysis on a sufficient sample size, can provide a useful approximation of the effect of an intervention. The complex nature of airway management during cardiac arrest, which often involves several interacting components, will be best investigated with a pragmatic trial, three of which will finish enrolling in 2017.

References

1. Monsieurs KG, Nolan JP, Bossaert LL et al (2015) European Resuscitation Council Guidelines for Resuscitation 2015: Section 1. Executive summary. Resuscitation 95:1–80
2. Soar J, Nolan JP (2013) Airway management in cardiopulmonary resuscitation. Curr Opin Crit Care 19:181–187
3. Perkins GD, Handley AJ, Koster RW et al (2015) European Resuscitation Council Guidelines for Resuscitation 2015: Section 2. Adult basic life support and automated external defibrillation. Resuscitation 95:81–99
4. Hupfl M, Selig HF, Nagele P (2010) Chest-compression-only versus standard cardiopulmonary resuscitation: a meta-analysis. Lancet 376:1552–1527
5. Dumas F, Rea TD, Fahrenbruch C et al (2013) Chest compression alone cardiopulmonary resuscitation is associated with better long-term survival compared with standard cardiopulmonary resuscitation. Circulation 127:435–441
6. Hasegawa K, Hiraide A, Chang Y, Brown DF (2013) Association of prehospital advanced airway management with neurologic outcome and survival in patients with out-of-hospital cardiac arrest. JAMA 309:257–266
7. Kurz MC, Prince DK, Christenson J et al (2016) Association of advanced airway device with chest compression fraction during out-of-hospital cardiopulmonary arrest. Resuscitation 98:35–40
8. Segal N, Yannopoulos D, Mahoney BD et al (2012) Impairment of carotid artery blood flow by supraglottic airway use in a swine model of cardiac arrest. Resuscitation 83:1025–1030
9. Neill A, Ducanto J, Amoli S (2012) Anatomical relationships of the Air-Q supraglottic airway during elective MRI scan of brain and neck. Resuscitation 83:e231–e232
10. White JM, Braude DA, Lorenzo G, Hart BL (2015) Radiographic evaluation of carotid artery compression in patients with extraglottic airway devices in place. Acad Emerg Med 22:636–638
11. Roth D, Hafner C, Aufmesser W et al (2015) Safety and feasibility of the laryngeal tube when used by EMTs during out-of-hospital cardiac arrest. Am J Emerg Med 33:1050–1055
12. Duckett J, Fell P, Han K, Kimber C, Taylor C (2014) Introduction of the I-gel supraglottic airway device for prehospital airway management in a UK ambulance service. Emerg Med J 31:505–507
13. Benger J, Coates D, Davies S et al (2016) Randomised comparison of the effectiveness of the laryngeal mask airway supreme, i-gel and current practice in the initial airway management of out of hospital cardiac arrest: a feasibility study. Br J Anaesth 116:262–268
14. Benger J (2015) Cluster randomised trial of the clinical and cost effectiveness of the i-gel supraglottic airway device versus tracheal intubation in the initial airway management of out of hospital cardiac arrest. AIRWAYS-2. Protocol, version 5.0. http://www.nets.nihr.ac.uk/__data/assets/pdf_file/0003/130665/PRO-12-167-102.pdf. Accessed 10/11/16
15. Rhys M, Voss S, Benger J (2013) Contamination of ambulance staff using the laryngeal mask airway supreme (LMAS) during cardiac arrest. Resuscitation 84:e99
16. Breckwoldt J, Klemstein S, Brunne B, Schnitzer L, Mochmann HC, Arntz HR (2011) Difficult prehospital endotracheal intubation – predisposing factors in a physician based EMS. Resuscitation 82:1519–1524
17. Shiga T, Wajima Z, Inoue T, Sakamoto A (2005) Predicting difficult intubation in apparently normal patients: a meta-analysis of bedside screening test performance. Anesthesiology 103:429–437
18. Wang HE, Simeone SJ, Weaver MD, Callaway CW (2009) Interruptions in cardiopulmonary resuscitation from paramedic endotracheal intubation. Ann Emerg Med 54:645–652 (e1)
19. Buis ML, Maissan IM, Hoeks SE, Klimek M, Stolker RJ (2016) Defining the learning curve for endotracheal intubation using direct laryngoscopy: A systematic review. Resuscitation 99:63–71

20. Deakin CD, King P, Thompson F (2009) Prehospital advanced airway management by ambulance technicians and paramedics: is clinical practice sufficient to maintain skills? Emerg Med J 26:888–891
21. Gatward JJ, Thomas MJ, Nolan JP, Cook TM (2008) Effect of chest compressions on the time taken to insert airway devices in a manikin. Br J Anaesth 100:351–356
22. Piegeler T, Roessler B, Goliasch G et al (2016) Evaluation of six different airway devices regarding regurgitation and pulmonary aspiration during cardio-pulmonary resuscitation (CPR) – A human cadaver pilot study. Resuscitation 102:70–74
23. Park SO, Kim JW, Na JH et al (2015) Video laryngoscopy improves the first-attempt success in endotracheal intubation during cardiopulmonary resuscitation among novice physicians. Resuscitation 89:188–194
24. Lee DH, Han M, An JY et al (2015) Video laryngoscopy versus direct laryngoscopy for tracheal intubation during in-hospital cardiopulmonary resuscitation. Resuscitation 89:195–199
25. Kim JW, Park SO, Lee KR et al (2016) Video laryngoscopy vs. direct laryngoscopy: Which should be chosen for endotracheal intubation during cardiopulmonary resuscitation? A prospective randomized controlled study of experienced intubators. Resuscitation 105:196–202
26. Soar J, Nolan JP, Bottiger BW et al (2015) European Resuscitation Council Guidelines for Resuscitation 2015: Section 3. Adult advanced life support. Resuscitation 95:100–147
27. Murphy RA, Bobrow BJ, Spaite DW, Hu C, McDannold R, Vadeboncoeur TF (2016) Association between prehospital CPR quality and end-tidal carbon dioxide levels in out-of-hospital cardiac arrest. Prehosp Emerg Care 20:369–377
28. Sheak KR, Wiebe DJ, Leary M et al (2015) Quantitative relationship between end-tidal carbon dioxide and CPR quality during both in-hospital and out-of-hospital cardiac arrest. Resuscitation 89:149–154
29. Pokorna M, Necas E, Kratochvil J, Skripsky R, Andrlik M, Franek O (2010) A sudden increase in partial pressure end-tidal carbon dioxide (P(ET)CO(2)) at the moment of return of spontaneous circulation. J Emerg Med 38:614–621
30. Lui CT, Poon KM, Tsui KL (2016) Abrupt rise of end tidal carbon dioxide level was a specific but non-sensitive marker of return of spontaneous circulation in patient with out-of-hospital cardiac arrest. Resuscitation 104:53–58
31. Fouche PF, Simpson PM, Bendall J, Thomas RE, Cone DC, Doi SA (2014) Airways in out-of-hospital cardiac arrest: systematic review and meta-analysis. Prehosp Emerg Care 18:244–256
32. Benoit JL, Gerecht RB, Steuerwald MT, McMullan JT (2015) Endotracheal intubation versus supraglottic airway placement in out-of-hospital cardiac arrest: A meta-analysis. Resuscitation 93:20–26
33. Haukoos JS, Lewis RJ (2015) The propensity score. JAMA 314:1637–1638
34. Wang HE, Prince DK, Stephens SW et al (2016) Design and implementation of the Resuscitation Outcomes Consortium Pragmatic Airway Resuscitation Trial (PART). Resuscitation 101:57–64
35. Christenson J, Andrusiek D, Everson-Stewart S et al (2009) Chest compression fraction determines survival in patients with out-of-hospital ventricular fibrillation. Circulation 120:1241–1247
36. Ford I, Norrie J (2016) Pragmatic trials. N Engl J Med 375:454–463
37. Perkins GD, Lall R, Quinn T et al (2015) Mechanical versus manual chest compression for out-of-hospital cardiac arrest (PARAMEDIC): a pragmatic, cluster randomised controlled trial. Lancet 385:947–955
38. Aufderheide TP, Sigurdsson G, Pirrallo RG et al (2004) Hyperventilation-induced hypotension during cardiopulmonary resuscitation. Circulation 109:1960–1965
39. O'Neill JF, Deakin CD (2007) Do we hyperventilate cardiac arrest patients? Resuscitation 73:82–85

40. Spindelboeck W, Gemes G, Strasser C et al (2016) Arterial blood gases during and their dynamic changes after cardiopulmonary resuscitation: A prospective clinical study. Resuscitation 106:24–29
41. Nikolla D, Lewandowski T, Carlson J (2016) Mitigating hyperventilation during cardiopulmonary resuscitation. Am J Emerg Med 34:643–646
42. Kjaergaard B, Bavarskis E, Magnusdottir SO et al (2016) Four ways to ventilate during cardiopulmonary resuscitation in a porcine model: a randomized study. Scand J Trauma Resusc Emerg Med 24:67
43. Eastwood GM, Tanaka A, Bellomo R (2016) Cerebral oxygenation in mechanically ventilated early cardiac arrest survivors: The impact of hypercapnia. Resuscitation 102:11–16
44. Eastwood GM, Schneider AG, Suzuki S et al (2016) Targeted therapeutic mild hypercapnia after cardiac arrest: A phase II multi-centre randomised controlled trial (the CCC trial). Resuscitation 104:83–90
45. Kajino K, Iwami T, Kitamura T et al (2011) Comparison of supraglottic airway versus endotracheal intubation for the pre-hospital treatment of out-of-hospital cardiac arrest. Crit Care 15:R236
46. McMullan J, Gerecht R, Bonomo J et al (2014) Airway management and out-of-hospital cardiac arrest outcome in the CARES registry. Resuscitation 85:617–622
47. Noda E, Zaitsu A, Hashizume M, Takahashi S (2007) Prognosis of patient with cardiopulmonary arrest transported to kyushu university hospital. Fukuoka Igaku Zasshi 98:73–81
48. Tanabe S, Ogawa T, Akahane M et al (2013) Comparison of neurological outcome between tracheal intubation and supraglottic airway device insertion of out-of-hospital cardiac arrest patients: a nationwide, population-based, observational study. J Emerg Med 44:389–397
49. Wang HE, Szydlo D, Stouffer JA et al (2012) Endotracheal intubation versus supraglottic airway insertion in out-of-hospital cardiac arrest. Resuscitation 83:1061–1066
50. Yanagawa Y, Sakamoto T (2010) Analysis of prehospital care for cardiac arrest in an urban setting in Japan. J Emerg Med 38:340–345

Part VIII
Oxygenation and Respiratory Failure

High-Flow Nasal Cannula Support Therapy: New Insights and Improving Performance

G. Hernández, O. Roca, and L. Colinas

Introduction

Oxygen therapy is the first step in the prevention and treatment of hypoxemic respiratory failure and has traditionally been delivered using nasal prongs or masks. However, the maximal flow rates that these devices can deliver are limited because of the discomfort generated secondary to insufficient heat and humidity provided to the gas administered. Although high-flow oxygen therapy is currently defined as flows greater than 30 l/min, it is accepted that flows up to 15 l/min can be delivered using conventional nasal prongs or masks; this flow is far less than the peak inspiratory flow of a patient with dyspnea. In addition, flows exceeding 6 l/min can lead to insufficient humidification provided to the nasal mucosa, even when a cold bubble humidifier is used. Therefore, room air dilutes the supplemental oxygen, resulting in a significant decrease in the fraction of the inspired oxygen (FiO_2) that finally reaches the alveoli.

In recent years, new devices that deliver totally conditioned gas (37 °C containing 44 mg H_2O/l [100% relative humidity] using a heated humidifier and a heated inspiratory circuit) through a wide bore nasal cannula at very high flow (up to 60 l/min) at a predetermined constant oxygen concentration (21 to 100%) have emerged as a safe and useful supportive therapy in many clinical situations.

G. Hernández (✉) · L. Colinas
Dept of Critical Care Medicine, Virgen de la Salud University Hospital
Ave de Berber, 45005 Toledo, Spain
e-mail: ghernandezm@telefonica.net

O. Roca
Dept of Critical Care Medicine, Vall d'Hebron University Hospital
08035 Barcelona, Spain
Ciber Enfermedades Respiratorias (Ciberes), Instituto de Salud Carlos III
Madrid, Spain

J.-L. Vincent (ed.), *Annual Update in Intensive Care and Emergency Medicine 2017*,
DOI 10.1007/978-3-319-51908-1_20

High-flow nasal cannula (HFNC) supportive therapy exerts its potential benefits through a variety of mechanisms. In the literature this treatment strategy has been variously described as nasal high flow and high flow oxygen therapy, but we believe that the most appropriate term is heated and humidified HFNC supportive therapy. This term reflects the features that generate the technique's clinical effects (i. e., the delivery of warm and humidified air at high flows through a nasal cannula).

New Insights

Physiological Effects and Consequences

Heated and Humidified Oxygen

Inhaling dry and cold oxygen provokes upper airway dryness frequently leading to intolerance, and potentially impairing mucociliary functions, such as secretion clearance and airway defense. Results of studies demonstrate that HFNC reduces patient discomfort and upper airway dryness, although a potentially protective effect on mucociliary function requires further investigation. Another way in which HFNC improves extubation outcome and weaning is by conditioning the inspired gas. Various studies have demonstrated that HFNC improves the management of respiratory secretions and reported fewer reintubations secondary to upper airway obstruction and accelerated weaning in tracheostomy patients. These findings support the idea that gas conditioning probably alleviates inflammation of the tracheal mucosa after transglottic intubation, and a protocol that includes the use of HFNC prior to extubation, thereby preventing the administration of dry and cold air in the native airway of the patients, reinforces this approach [1].

Carbon Dioxide Clearance

There is still not much information about the role of HFNC in managing hypercapnia, except for the mechanism of dead-space washout. By providing a high flow of fresh air during expiration, HFNC may be able to more rapidly washout the carbon dioxide (CO_2) filling the nasopharyngeal cavity. Möller et al. constructed an airway model using a computed tomography (CT) scan, and analyzed the lavage of gas tracers under apneic conditions. The authors observed a linear positive correlation between tracer-gas clearance in the model and the flow rate of HFNC, approximately 1.8 ml/s increase in clearance for every 1.0 l/min increase in flow [2].

However, in recent years, new studies have highlighted some additional mechanisms affecting CO_2 clearance. Alveolar ventilation has been suggested by Patel et al., after obtaining a mean apnea time of 17 min in surgical patients [3]. The authors reported further evidence that classical apneic oxygenation provided little clearance of CO_2 apart from that obtained from limiting rebreathing. Continuous insufflation of a high-flow gas mixture facilitates oxygenation and CO_2 clearance through gaseous mixing. Evidence for the existence of flow-dependent, non-rhythmic ventilatory exchange can be provided by comparing the increase in rise of CO_2 under different continuous insufflation apneic conditions. While Rudolf and Hohenhorst [4] reported a rate of carbon dioxide increase of 0.24 kPa/min using a low-flow oxygen intratracheal cannula (0.5 l/min), Patel et al. [3] achieved a rate of carbon dioxide increase of 0.15 kPa/min and a steady-state carbon dioxide level was not reached. This result was improved only when using a high-flow oxygen intratracheal cannula (45 l/min), reaching a steady-state carbon dioxide level within 5 min of the start of the apnea [4].

Recently, Hernandez et al. [5] reported data supporting a possible role of HFNC in managing hypercapnia after extubation. The investigators compared non-invasive ventilation (NIV) to HFNC in a fixed 24 h protocol after extubation in high-risk for reintubation patients, using a non-inferiority randomized trial. There was a trend towards a higher rates of postextubation respiratory failure due to hypercapnia in the NIV group than in the HFNC group, although this difference was not translated to the rates of hypercapnia as the reason for reintubation. They argued that the real time under NIV, clearly inferior to the 24 h expected by protocol, suggests that discomfort could have been the reason for hypercapnic postextubation respiratory failure in some NIV patients, as $PaCO_2$ improved without any respiratory support in most patients. The reported rates of reintubation due to hypercapnia were similar in the two groups, as were the values of gasometric variables at reintubation, suggesting that high-flow is at least as good as NIV for managing postextubation hypercapnia in high-risk patients.

Positive Pharyngeal Pressure

HFNC can induce a positive pharyngeal pressure during expiration due to its constant ingoing flow, with the effect mainly determined by the flow rate provided by HFNC and the expiratory flow exhaled by the patient, with lower pressures when the patient keeps the mouth open.

Parke and McGuinness [6] reported that HFNC increased the mean pharyngeal pressure by about 1 cmH_2O per 10 l/min, within a range of 30–50 l/min, but more recently [7], the same group reported that the linear increase in the pharyngeal pressure was maintained when using extra high-flow with 100 l/min (combining two HFNC systems), obtaining pharyngeal pressures up to 11.9 cmH_2O. However, these values were obtained in healthy volunteers and extrapolation to the critical care arena may not be accurate.

Despite this uncertainty about how much positive end-expiratory pressure (PEEP) can really be offered by HFNC, studies [8] have demonstrated that end-expiratory lung impedance increases with rising flow rate of HFNC, suggesting an increase in end-expiratory lung volume. In addition, hemodynamic changes similar to those obtained in patients under NIV with pressure levels close to 10 cmH_2O have been reported [9]. Right atrial pressure has been considered as a surrogate of right ventricular preload and is most commonly estimated by inferior vena cava (IVC) diameter and the presence of inspiratory collapse. Changes in IVC diameter have been used to determine preload responsiveness in positive pressure ventilated patients. In a population of patients with New York Heart Association (NYHA) class III heart failure, treatment with HFNC at 20 and 40 l/min was associated with mean attributable reductions in the IVC inspiratory collapse of 20 and 53%

from baseline, respectively. These changes were reversible after HFNC withdrawal suggesting that HFNC therapy may modify the hemodynamic status in heart failure patients at the same rate as does NIV.

HFNC is, therefore, not entirely similar to applying continuous positive airway pressure (CPAP), which aims to maintain a steady level of positive pressure during the whole cycle of breath. The target of HFNC is flow instead of pressure, so the objective when applying HFNC should not be the pharyngeal pressure measured but the changes in hemodynamic status and the increase in lung aeration.

Clinical Data

Acute Hypoxemic Respiratory Failure

Effects of HFNC on Physiological Variables and Comfort

The first studies in patients with acute respiratory failure focused on the effects of HFNC therapy on physiological variables [10–12] and reported oxygenation enhancement with reductions in respiratory rate and no changes in $PaCO_2$ (Table 1). Moreover, HFNC appeared to be better tolerated and achieved a greater level of comfort than conventional oxygen devices [10, 12]. HFNC was also usually better tolerated than NIV, although NIV obtained greater improvements in oxygenation [13, 14].

In addition, HFNC has been used in small cohorts of patients with acute respiratory failure in the emergency department [15, 16] and even in 150 children less than 2 years old during interhospital transport [17]. The effects on oxygenation and rates of intubation reported in all these studies are similar to those found when HFNC has been used in patients with acute respiratory failure admitted to critical care areas, suggesting that, with adequate monitoring, HFNC can be safely used outside the critical care setting.

Effects on Intubation Rate and Mortality

These physiological studies provide the rationale for considering HFNC as a potentially useful tool for decreasing intubation rates and mortality in patients with acute respiratory failure. The first randomized controlled trial (RCT) included postoperative cardiac surgery patients with mild to moderate acute respiratory failure [18]. In that preliminary trial, HFNC patients were less likely to need escalation to NIV and had fewer desaturations than those treated using a standard humidified high flow face mask. In another retrospective analysis of a prospectively assessed cohort of 37 lung transplant patients readmitted to the ICU because of acute respiratory failure, HFNC therapy was the only variable at ICU admission associated with a decreased risk of mechanical ventilation in the multivariate analysis [19]. The absolute risk reduction for mechanical ventilation with HFNC was 29.8%, and only three patients needed to be treated with HFNC to prevent one intubation. Moreover, non-ventilated patients had an increased survival rate.

Table 1 Most relevant studies of high flow nasal cannula oxygen (HFNC)

Condition	Author [ref]	Design	Patients	Main results
Acute respiratory failure (ARF)	Roca et al. [19]	Retrospective cohort	37 lung transplant recipients readmitted to ICU due to ARF (40 episodes)	The absolute risk reduction for MV with HFNC was 29.8%, and the NNT to prevent one intubation with HFNC was 3. Multivariate analysis showed that HFNC therapy was the only variable at ICU admission associated with a decreased risk of MV (OR 0.11 [95% CI 0.02–0.69]; $p = 0.02$)
	Frat et al. [20]	Randomized controlled trial	313 ARF patients randomly assigned to HFNC, conventional oxygen therapy or NIV	The hazard ratio for death at 90 days was 2.01 (95% CI 1.01 to 3.99) with conventional oxygen therapy vs HFNC ($p = 0.046$) and 2.50 (95% CI, 1.31 to 4.78) with NIV vs HFNC ($p = 0.006$). In the subgroup of patients with a $PaO_2/F_iO_2 \leq 200$ mmHg, the intubation rate was significantly lower in the HFNC group
	Rello et al. [31]	Retrospective cohort	35 patients with ARF due to H1N1 viral pneumonia	After 6 h of HFNC, non-responders had a lower PaO_2/F_iO_2. All 8 patients on vasopressors required intubation
	Lemiale et al. [29]	Randomized controlled trial	100 immunocompromised patients with ARF randomized to a 2 h of HFNC vs conventional oxygen	No differences in NIV or invasive MV during the 2 h period were observed. No differences in secondary outcomes (RR, HR, comfort, dyspnea and thirst) were observed
	Mokart et al. [48]	Retrospective propensity-score analysis	178 cancer patients admitted to the ICU due to severe ARF	HFNC-NIV was associated with more VFD and less septic shock occurrence. Mortality of patients treated with HFNC 35 vs 57% for patients never treated with HFNC, $p = 0.008$
	Kang et al. [30]	Retrospective cohort	175 patients who failed on HFNC and required intubation	In propensity-adjusted and -matched analysis, early intubation (<48 h) was associated with better overall ICU mortality [adjusted OR = 0.317, $p = 0.005$; matched OR = 0.369, $p = 0.046$]
	Frat et al. [23]	Post-hoc analysis of a randomized controlled trial	82 immunocompromised patients of the FLORALI study	NIV was associated with higher risk of intubation and mortality
	Roca et al. [32]	Prospective cohort	157 patients with severe pneumonia	ROX index, defined as ratio of SpO_2/F_iO_2 to respiratory rate, ≥ 4.88 measured after 12 h of HFNC was significantly associated with lower risk for MV (HR 0.273 [95% CI 0.121–0.618])
	Coudroy et al. [25]	Retrospective cohort	115 immunocompromised patients	The rates of intubation and 28-day mortality were significantly higher in patients treated with NIV than with HFNC

Table 1 (Continued)

Condition	Author [ref]	Design	Patients	Main results
Cardiac surgery	Parke et al. [18]	Randomized	60 patients with non-severe hypoxemic ARF were randomized to receive HFNC or oxygen therapy	HFNC patients tended to need NIV less frequently (10 vs 30%; $p = 0.10$) and had significantly fewer desaturations ($p = 0.009$)
	Parke et al. [39]	Randomized controlled trial	340 patients after cardiac surgery randomized to HFNC vs conventional oxygen therapy for 48 h	No differences in oxygenation on Day 3 after surgery were observed, but HFNC did reduce the requirement for escalation of respiratory support (OR 0.47, 95% CI 0.29–0.7, $p = 0.001$)
	Corley et al. [40]	Randomized controlled trial	155 extubated patients with BMI $\geq 30\,kg/m^2$ received conventional oxygen therapy or HFNC	No difference was seen between groups in atelectasis. There was no difference in mean PaO_2/F_iO_2 ratio or RR. Five patients failed allocated treatment in the control group compared with three in the treatment group (OR 0.53; 95% CI 0.11, 2.24, $p = 0.40$)
	Stephan et al. [28]	Randomized non-inferiority trial	830 cardiothoracic surgical patients who developed ARF or were deemed at risk for respiratory failure after extubation. HFNC vs BiPAP	The treatment failed in 87 (21.0%) of 414 patients with HFNC and 91 (21.9%) of 416 patients with BiPAP ($p = 0.003$). No significant differences were found for ICU mortality (23 patients with BiPAP [5.5%] and 28 with HFNC [6.8%]; $p = 0.66$)
Pre-intubation	Vourc'h et al. [47]	Randomized controlled trial	124 patients with PaO_2/F_IO_2 ratio < 300 mmHg, RR ≥ 30 bpm and $F_IO_2 \geq 0.5$. Randomized to HFNC or facial mask	No differences in the lowest saturation was observed (HFNC 91.5% vs high flow facial mask 89.5%; $p = 0.44$). There was no difference in difficult intubation, VFD, intubation-related adverse events including desaturation < 80% or mortality

Table 1 (Continued)

Condition	Author [ref]	Design	Patients	Main results
Post-extubation	Maggiore et al. [38]	Randomized controlled trial	105 patients with $PaO_2/F_iO_2 \leq 300$ before extubation who were randomized to 48 h of conventional oxygen therapy or HFNC	HFNV improved the PaO_2/F_iO_2 ratio, comfort, airway dryness, episodes of interface displacements, oxygen desaturations, reintubation rate, or any form of ventilator support
	Rittayamai et al. [46]	Randomized crossover study	17 patients were randomized after extubation to sequential HFNC and conventional oxygen therapy for 30 min periods	At the end of the study, patients with HFNC reported less dyspnea and lower RR and HR. Most of the subjects (88.2%) preferred HFNC to conventional oxygen therapy
	Tiruvoipati et al. [37]	Randomized crossover study	50 patients were randomized to sequential HFNC and facial mask after extubation	There was no significant difference in gas exchange, RR or hemodynamics. HFNC was better tolerated ($p = 0.01$) and tended to be more comfortable ($p = 0.09$)
	Hernandez et al. [1]	Randomized controlled trial	527 extubated patients without any high-risk factor for reintubation were randomized to either HFNC or conventional oxygen therapy for 24 h	Reintubation within 72 h was less common in the high-flow group, 4.9 vs 12.2% in the conventional group ($p = 0.004$). Postextubation respiratory failure was less common in the high-flow group 8.3 vs 14.4% in the conventional group ($p = 0.03$)
	Hernandez et al. [5]	Randomized noninferiority trial	604 extubated patients with at least one high-risk factor for reintubation were randomized to either HFNC or NIV for 24 h	Reintubation within 72 h was noninferior in the HFNC group compared to the NIV group (22.8 vs 19.1%, absolute difference, −3.7%; 95% CI −9.1% to ∞); postextubation respiratory failure was lower in the HFNC group (26.9 vs 39.8%, risk difference, 12.9%; 95% CI 6.6% to ∞)

Table 1 (Continued)

Condition	Author [ref]	Design	Patients	Main results
Invasive procedures	Lucangelo et al. [45]	Randomized controlled trial	45 patients were randomly assigned to 3 groups: Venturi mask, nasal cannula, and HFNC during bronchoscopy	At the end of bronchoscopy, HFNC-treated patients had higher PaO_2/F_iO_2, and SpO_2
	Simon et al. [43]	Randomized controlled trial	40 patients with hypoxemic ARF received NIV or HFNC during bronchoscopy	NIV group had better oxygenation. Two patients with HFNC were unable to proceed to bronchoscopy due to progressive hypoxemia
Heart failure	Roca et al. [9]	Prospective cohort	10 adult patients with NYHA class III and left ventriclar ejection fraction 45% or less	Median inspiratory IVC collapse significantly ($p < 0.05$) decreased from baseline (37%) to HFNC with 20 l/min (28%) and HFNC with 40 l/min (21%). Changes in IVC inspiratory collapse were reversible
Emergency department	Rittayamai et al. [15]	Randomized comparative study	40 hypoxemic patients were randomized to receive HFNC or conventional oxygen for 1 h	HFNC improved dyspnea and comfort. No serious adverse events related to HFNC were observed
	Jones et al. [44]	Randomized controlled trial	303 hypoxemic and tachypneic patients admitted to the emergency department	5.5% of HFNC patients vs 11.6% of conventional oxygen therapy patients required MV within 24 h of admission ($p = 0.053$)

MV: mechanical ventilation; *RR*: respiratory rate; *ICU*: intensive care unit; *ARF*: acute respiratory failure; *VFD*: ventilator-free days; *NNT*: number needed to treat; *COT*: conventional oxygen therapy; *NIV*: non-invasive ventilation; *HR*: heart rate; *BMI*: body mass index; *IVC*: inferior vena cava

More recently, the results of the first large RCT to assess clinical outcomes with HFNC (50 l/min), conventional oxygen devices and NIV have been published [20]. The study included 310 patients with *de novo* hypoxemic acute respiratory failure, defined as PaO_2/FiO_2 ratio ≤ 300 mmHg or respiratory rate >25 bpm with 10 lpm of O_2. Patients with a history of chronic respiratory disease, including chronic obstructive pulmonary disease (COPD), as well as patients with acute cardiogenic pulmonary edema, severe neutropenia and hypercapnia ($PaCO_2 > 45$ mmHg) were excluded, as were patients with other organ failures, including hemodynamic instability or vasopressors at the time of inclusion. The most frequent cause of acute respiratory failure was pneumonia (75%) and 80% of the enrolled patients showed bilateral pulmonary infiltrates at study inclusion. The primary outcome (the rate of endotracheal intubation) did not differ significantly between the groups (HFNC 38% vs. standard oxygen 47% and NIV 50%; $p = 0.18$).

This negative result may be due to the fact that the observed rate of intubation with standard oxygen was lower than expected and, therefore, the study may have been underpowered. However, a *post hoc* adjusted analysis including the 238 patients with a PaO_2/FiO_2 ratio ≤ 200 mmHg found that HFNC reduced intubation rates ($p = 0.009$). In the entire cohort, HFNC increased ventilator-free days, reduced 90-day mortality and was associated with better comfort and lower dyspnea severity. In contrast, NIV patients had higher 90-day mortality rates than HFNC patients.

Mechanisms that may explain these findings are the small amount of positive airway pressure and increased CO_2 excretion with HFNC, the overall reduction in the need for intubation and the lower incidence of septic shock. Moreover, important concerns have been raised regarding how NIV was applied. First, half of the patients in the NIV group were treated with NIV for less than eight hours during the first two days of randomization and received HFNC between NIV sessions. Second, high tidal volumes (9.2 ± 3.0 ml/kg) were used, which may have aggravated the preexisting lung injury. In fact, patients with acute respiratory failure usually have high respiratory rates and minute volumes and are more likely to present patient-ventilator asynchronies. Third, relatively low levels of PEEP were used in potentially recruitable patients (5 ± 1 cmH_2O). Fourth, intermittent sessions of NIV may induce the phenomenon of recruitment/derecruitment, generating ventilator-induced lung injury (VILI). Finally, NIV was delivered through a face mask although it has later been shown that a helmet interface may be associated with better outcomes [21, 22]. Thus, the NIV protocol in this study could be assumed to be close to what is real practice at the bedside in many centers treating acute respiratory failure with NIV, so an underestimation of the NIV treatment effect in a pragmatic trial cannot be ruled out.

More recently, a *post hoc* subgroup analysis in a subset of immunocompromised patients was performed on the FLORALI study [23]. Thirty patients treated with standard oxygen therapy, 26 treated with HFNC, and 26 treated with NIV were included. The intubation and mortality rates were significantly higher in patients randomly assigned to NIV and, apart from age, the use of NIV as the first-line therapy was the only variable independently associated with a higher risk of endotracheal intubation and mortality in the multivariate logistic regression analysis.

Moreover, the expired tidal volume measured 1 h after NIV initiation was higher in the patients who died than in survivors (11.1 ± 2.6 ml/kg of predicted weight versus 7.6 ± 3.1 ml/kg; $p = 0.02$). Similarly, higher tidal volumes have been associated with NIV failure [24].

Thus, the high tidal volumes and high transpulmonary pressures obtained during NIV may induce VILI in a pre-injured lung and may be at least partially responsible for NIV failure and higher mortality. These results were similar to those observed in a recently published 8-year observational study of a cohort of 115 immunocompromised patients [25].

Two recent systematic reviews and meta-analyses have also been published that evaluated the effectiveness of HFNC [26, 27]. In the first study, no differences in terms of mortality or higher respiratory support requirement was observed [26]. Most recently, Monro-Somerville et al. [27] found that, although HFNC appears to be well tolerated, no difference in intubation rates or mortality was observed in patients treated with HFNC compared to those treated with usual care (conventional oxygen or NIV). However, the required information size was not reached: in fact, only 30.6 and 62.3% of the estimated needed patients were included for the primary (mortality) and secondary (intubation) outcomes, respectively. Moreover, HFNC was shown to have better survival and lower intubation rates than conventional oxygen and, although no differences were observed compared with NIV, HFNC was better tolerated. Finally, certain methodological issues regarding some of the studies included in both meta-analyses should be noted. First, a study by Stephan et al. [28] was a positive non-inferiority trial comparing HFNC and NIV; however, in the meta-analysis it appears as a negative trial as no differences were observed between HFNC and NIV. Second, in a study by Lemiale et al. [29], HFNC was only used for a 2 h-trial and in such a short period of time it would be difficult to observe any difference between treatments. Finally, and most importantly, studies included in both meta-analyses had very heterogeneous populations of acute respiratory failure patients in terms of severity with huge differences in risks of intubation.

Predictors of HFNC Success

The existence of accurate, early predictors of HFNC success is important. Indeed, a recent propensity-score analysis associated early intubation (within the first 48 h) with better ICU survival [30]. In spite of its limitations, the study by Kang et al. [30] raises an important issue – the fact that delayed intubation may worsen the prognosis of patients treated with HFNC. Therefore, the ability to describe accurate predictors of HFNC success that can allow timely endotracheal intubation in patients who are likely to fail is a point of special interest. Sztrymf et al. [12] reported that respiratory rate as well as the percentage of patients exhibiting thoraco-abdominal asynchrony as early as 30 and 15 min after the beginning of HFNC were significantly higher in patients who required endotracheal intubation. Moreover, the PaO_2/FiO_2 ratio 1 h after the start of HFNC was significantly lower in patients requiring invasive mechanical ventilation. Similarly, in a series of 20 patients with H_1N_1 infection treated with HFNC, worse PaO_2/FiO_2 ratios were observed in patients who required intubation after six hours of treatment [31]. Interestingly, a recent prospective study showed that patients with severe pneumonia who had a ROX index (defined as the ratio of SpO_2/FiO_2 to respiratory rate) ≥ 4.88 after 12 h of HFNC therapy were less likely to be intubated, even after adjusting for potential covariates [32]. Moreover, among patients who were still on HFNC after 18 h, the median change in the ROX index between 18 and 12 h was significantly higher in patients who did not require intubation. However, non-pulmonary severity has also been described as a good predictor of HFNC failure. Indeed, the presence of shock has been associated with a higher risk of mechanical ventilation [19, 23].

In a preliminary study by Hernandez et al. [33] titrating high-flow according to patient tolerance, a gas flow > 35 l/min 12 h after extubation predicted reintubation, suggesting that the flow tolerated by patients is a marker of severity; unfortunately, this result was not reproduced in the subsequent randomized trial [5].

ARDS Patients

Another controversial issue is whether patients with bilateral infiltrates treated with HFNC can be considered as having acute respiratory distress syndrome (ARDS). In fact, most patients included in studies have bilateral infiltrates [20, 32]. The Berlin definition of ARDS [34] requires a minimum of 5 cmH_2O of PEEP, and it has been shown that HFNC can provide a level of PEEP that is higher at peak expiratory pressure [35]. Moreover, ARDS does not begin at the time of mechanical ventilation onset. Therefore, it can be accepted that patients with a risk factor for ARDS, who are hypoxemic (PaO_2/FiO_2 ratio ≤ 300 mmHg) and have bilateral infiltrates not fully explained by cardiac failure or fluid overload, may be considered as ARDS patients. In these patients, HFNC may achieve success rates similar to those of NIV [36].

Prevention of Postextubation Respiratory Failure and Reintubation

Extubation failure is an independent predictor of mortality. The development of therapies to prevent this has been focused on specific causes of reintubation (corticoids for larynx edema and NIV for hypercapnic respiratory failure in patients with chronic pulmonary diseases) and in patients with risk factors associated with extubation failure. Usually, extubated patients receive conventional oxygen therapy for correcting the oxygenation impairment. This system provides low flow and does not guarantee the FiO_2.

Low-risk-of-reintubation Patients

Two preliminary physiological studies comparing HFNC with conventional oxygen devices using a crossover design and during a short period of time after extubation have confirmed the consistent benefit of HFNC in terms of overall comfort. Rittayamai et al. [15] observed a decrease in respiratory rate and heart rate when comparing HFNC therapy at 35 l/min vs conventional oxygen devices at 6–10 l/min in 17 patients during a 30 min period. In contrast, Tiruvoipati et al. [37] found no change in these physiological variables when comparing 30 l/min delivered through HFNC or 15 l/min through a high flow face mask. Shortly after this study, the first RCT comparing HFNC with conventional oxygen devices after extubation was published [38]. The study included patients with acute respiratory failure due to pneumonia and trauma who were mechanically ventilated for a mean of almost five days before extubation. In these patients, the use of HFNC was associated with better comfort, better oxygenation, fewer desaturations and interface displacements, and a lower reintubation rate.

Postoperative patients remain an important subgroup of patients with some differences related to the response to HFNC. The effectiveness of HFNC therapy during the extubation period in postoperative patients remains controversial; most studies on this issue have included patients after cardiothoracic surgery. Parke et al. [39] included a non-selected population of cardiac surgery patients with mild to moderate acute respiratory failure, observing that HFNC patients more frequently succeeded and could be weaned to conventional oxygen devices. In contrast, in patients randomized to conventional oxygen devices, acute respiratory failure was more likely to worsen and escalation to NIV or HFNC required. Corley et al. [40] included a population of cardiac surgery patients with body mass index (BMI) ≥ 30 who were randomly assigned to prophylactic HFNC therapy or conventional oxygen devices after extubation. The authors did not observe any difference in atelectasis formation, oxygenation, respiratory rate, or dyspnea. Finally, the BiPOP study [28], a multicenter, non-inferiority RCT, compared HFNC and NIV for preventing or resolving acute respiratory failure after cardiothoracic surgery. Three different types of patient were eligible: patients who failed after a spontaneous breathing trial; patients who succeeded but had a preexisting risk factor for postoperative acute respiratory failure (BMI >30, left ventricular ejection fraction $<40\%$, and failure of previous extubation); and patients who succeeded after a spontaneous breathing trial but then failed extubation (defined as at least one of the following: $PaO_2/FiO_2 < 300$, respiratory rate >25 bpm for at least 2 h, and use of accessory respiratory muscles or paradoxical respiration). After randomizing more than 800 patients, HFNC therapy did not increase the rate of treatment failure (defined as reintubation, switch to the other study treatment, or premature treatment discontinuation at the patient's request or due to an adverse event). Therefore, as HFNC therapy did not worsen outcomes, may be easier to administer, and requires lower nursing workload, the authors concluded that the results supported the use of HFNC in this subset of patients. Certain questions remain unanswered, however, such as the optimal flow and the subset of patients who would benefit the most from HFNC therapy.

Recently, Hernandez et al. [1] reported a multicenter randomized trial analyzing the effect of HFNC compared to conventional oxygen therapy in a population of low-risk-of-reintubation patients. In the study, the authors aimed to evaluate whether high flow oxygen therapy after planned extubation would reduce the need for reintubation compared with standard oxygen therapy. The all-cause reintubation within 72 h was lower in the high flow group (4.9 vs 12.2%). This difference was mainly attributable to a lower incidence of respiratory-related reintubations in the high flow group (1.5% vs 8.7%). The main benefit was observed on reducing reintubation secondary to hypoxemia and inability to clear secretions. These results agree with those obtained by Maggiore et al. [38].

The authors classified patients according to the criteria for risk of reintubation. They did not use the type of respiratory failure considering that the aim was to obtain the preventive effects of HFNC and not treatment once the failure was present. It is currently unclear how to identify at risk patients for extubation failure. Previous trials, like that of Thille et al. [41], have tried to identify the underlying risks of extubation outcome. In keeping with these studies, this trial included 10 risk factors, which can clearly select a low risk population.

High-risk-of-reintubation Patients

Simultaneously, Hernandez et al. [5] compared HFNC with NIV in patients at high risk for reintubation in a non-inferiority trial. While studies have suggested that prophylactic NIV could prevent postextubation respiratory failure, they appear inconsistent with regard to reintubation. However, Thille et al. [41] added new data supporting the benefit of NIV for this indication. In a general population of critical patients use of NIV has not been proved, for that reason in the low-risk group HFNC was compared to conventional oxygen therapy [1].

This study confirmed that the reintubation rate was non-inferior in the HFNC group compared to the NIV group within 72 h (22.8% vs 19.1%). For postextubation respiratory failure, the authors reported a lower rate in the HFNC group compared to the NIV group (26.9% vs 39.8%), suggesting that the postextubation respiratory failure rate could be even higher in the NIV group. This surprising result was explained by the significantly higher adverse event rate in the NIV group (43% vs 0%), mainly discomfort and subsequent early withdrawal of the therapy (mean real time under NIV 14 h, instead of the 24 h per protocol). This increased postextubation respiratory failure rate was not correlated with the reintubation rate, supporting a possible role of discomfort in NIV patients as the reason for the postextubation respiratory failure. In addition, the length of hospital stay was significantly reduced in the HFNC group [5].

Facilitating Weaning in Tracheostomized Patients

Weaning of tracheostomy patients is still a challenge. To our knowledge, only one randomized trial has included high flow therapy in the protocol [42]. This was a single-center study including 181 critically ill tracheostomy patients who were randomized to have the tracheal cuff deflated or not during spontaneous breathing trials. All patients received high-flow conditioned oxygen therapy through a direct tracheostomy connection to the maximum tolerated flow and conditioned up to 37 °C. Although that study was not specifically designed to assess the effectiveness of high flow through the trachea, the authors hypothesized that HFNC therapy may have some benefits in the weaning process of tracheostomy patients with a deflated tracheal cuff. Positive airway pressure may theoretically reduce microaspiration and, with a deflated cuff, a higher flow is conveyed through the pericannular space, allowing for better drainage of secretions.

Improving Performance

Regarding the methodology used in the protocol by Hernandez et al. [1], HFNC was applied before extubation to prevent the entrance of dry and cold air into the patient's native airway from the start of treatment. Although this is speculative, it could play a major role in the early benefit that was found in the lower rate of upper airway obstruction (laryngeal edema requiring reintubation was not observed in the HFNC group).

Flow was titrated according to patient tolerance; initially set at 10 l/min and titrated upward in 5 l/min steps until patients experienced discomfort. Twelve hours after extubation, a steady state is usually obtained. In that low-risk-of-reintubation study, authors observed a tolerated main gas flow of 31 l/min, a moderate flow as compared to the main flow tolerated in the high-risk-of-reintubation study (50 l/min), reinforcing the idea that under these conditions the flow tolerated is a marker of severity.

Another point of the protocol used by Hernandez et al. [1] deserves mention: patients who tolerated the spontaneous breathing trial were reconnected with the previous ventilator settings for rest and clinical evaluation of airway patency. Some preliminary studies suggest that spontaneous breathing trials could lead to mild respiratory muscle fatigue that could somehow influence extubation success. However, clinical evidence supporting this hypothesis is lacking.

After 24 h, high-flow therapy was stopped and, if necessary, patients received conventional oxygen therapy. Maggiore et al. [38] reported better results using high-flow for 48 h after extubation, with some of the variables showing significant improvement after 24 continuous hours of application, suggesting that some time-dependent effects could lead to improved performance of this therapy.

With this information in mind, clinicians should counterbalance efficacy and safety. On the one hand, the longer the duration of HFNC application, the greater the clinical efficacy. On the other hand, the longer the duration of HFNC, the greater the probability of delaying escalation of respiratory support when HFNC fails. In fact, as suggested by Kang et al. [30], applying HFNC in patients with respiratory failure according to clinical response could lead to delayed intubation. This could be associated with a worse outcome, as has been shown with NIV. This may be possible because HFNC increases comfort, oxygenation and may disguise respiratory distress. The results by Hernandez et al. [1], reinforce this idea; under a fixed 24-hour protocol after extubation, the time to reintubation was not increased, whether compared to conventional oxygen therapy in the low-risk-of-reintubation group or NIV in the high-risk-of-reintubation group. A 24-h limit probably helped physicians appreciate undertreated respiratory distress at an early stage and not delay reintubation. Nevertheless, the results confirmed that 24 h was enough to reduce the rate of reintubation.

HFNC does not delay reintubation under those conditions. This result can be attributed to the preventive intention, the fixed duration and to the predefined reintubation criteria.

Conclusion

Delivery of heated and humidified oxygen at high flow rates through nasal cannulas is now widely used in adult patients. Its mechanisms of action and potential clinical benefits can help to improve the management of patients with acute respiratory failure or during the weaning phase. With the currently available evidence, several questions still remain unanswered; there is strong evidence for some clinical indications, but for other situations without that evidence decisions on HFNC treatment should be individualized in each particular situation and institution, taking into account resources, and local and personal experience with all respiratory support therapies. However, HFNC therapy is an innovative and powerful technique that is currently changing the management of patients with respiratory failure.

References

1. Hernández G, Vaquero C, González P et al (2016) Effect of postextubation highflownasal cannula vs conventional oxygen therapy on reintubation in lowrisk patients. A randomized clinical trial. JAMA 315:1354–1361
2. Möller W, Celik G, Feng S et al (2015) Nasal high flow clears anatomical dead space in upper airway models. J Appl Physiol 118:1525–1532
3. Patel A, Nouraei SAR (2015) Transnasal Humidified Rapid Insufflation Ventilatory Exchange (THRIVE): a physiological method of increasing apnoea time in patients with difficult airways. Anaesthesia 70:323–329
4. Rudolf B, Hohenhorst W (2013) Use of apneic oxygenation for the performance of pan-endoscopy. Otolaryngol Head Neck Surg 149:235–239
5. Hernandez G, Vaquero C, Colinas L et al (2016) High flow conditioned oxygen therapy for prevention of reintubation in critically il patients at high risk for extubation failure: a multicenter randomised controlled trial. JAMA 316:1565–1574
6. Parke RL, McGuinness SP (2013) Pressures delivered by nasal high flow oxygen during all phases of the respiratory cycle. Respir Care 58:1621–1624
7. Parke RL, Bloch A, McGuinness SP (2015) Effect of very-high-flow nasal therapy on airway pressure and end-expiratory lung impedance in healthy volunteers. Respir Care 60:1397–1403
8. Riera J, Perez P, Cortes J et al (2013) Effect of high-flow nasal cannula and body position on end-expiratory lung volume: a cohort study using electrical impedance tomography. Respir Care 58:589–596
9. Roca O, Perez-Teran P, Masclans JR et al (2013) Patients with New York Heart Association class III heart failure may benefit with high flow nasal cannula supportive therapy: high flow nasal cannula in heart failure. J Crit Care 28:741–746
10. Roca O, Riera J, Torres F et al (2010) High-flow oxygen therapy in acute respiratory failure. Respir Care 55:408–413
11. Sztrymf B, Messika J, Mayot T et al (2012) Impact of high-flow nasal cannula oxygen therapy on intensive care unit patients with acute respiratory failure: a prospective observational study. J Crit Care 27:324e9–324e13
12. Sztrymf B, Messika J, Bertrand F et al (2011) Beneficial effects of humidified high flow nasal oxygen in critical care patients: a prospective pilot study. Intensive Care Med 37:1780–1786
13. Frat JP, Brugiere B, Ragot S et al (2015) Sequential application of oxygen therapy via high-flow nasal cannula and noninvasive ventilation in acute respiratory failure: an observational pilot study. Respir Care 60:170–178

14. Schwabbauer N, Berg B, Blumenstock G et al (2014) Nasal high-flow oxygen therapy in patients with hypoxic respiratory failure: effect on functional and subjective respiratory parameters compared to conventional oxygen therapy and non-invasive ventilation (NIV). BMC Anesthesiol 14:66–73
15. Rittayamai N, Tscheikuna J, Praphruetkit N et al (2015) Use of high-flow nasal cannula for acute dyspnea and hypoxemia in the emergency department. Respir Care 60:1377–1382
16. Lenglet H, Sztrymf B, Leroy C et al (2012) Humidified high flow nasal oxygen during respiratory failure in the emergency department: feasibility and efficacy. Respir Care 57:1873–1878
17. Schlapbach LJ, Schaefer J, Brady AM et al (2014) High-flow nasal cannula (HFNC) support in interhospital transport of critically ill children. Intensive Care Med 40:592–599
18. Parke RL, McGuinness SP, Eccleston ML (2011) A preliminary randomized controlled trial to assess effectiveness of nasal high-flow oxygen in intensive care patients. Respir Care 56:265–270
19. Roca O, de Acilu MG, Caralt B et al (2015) Humidified high flow nasal cannula supportive therapy improves outcomes in lung transplant recipients readmitted to the intensive care unit because of acute respiratory failure. Transplantation 99:1092–1098
20. Frat JP, Thille AW, Mercat A et al (2015) High-flow oxygen through nasal cannula in acute hypoxemic respiratory failure. N Engl J Med 372:2185–2196
21. Patel BK, Wolfe KS, Pohlman AS et al (2016) Effect of noninvasive ventilation delivered by helmet vs face mask on the rate of endotracheal intubation in patients with acute respiratory distress syndrome: a randomized clinical trial. JAMA 315:2435–2441
22. Liu Q, Gao Y, Chen R et al (2016) Noninvasive ventilation with helmet versus control strategy in patients with acute respiratory failure: a systematic review and meta-analysis of controlled studies. Crit Care 20:265–279
23. Frat JP, Ragot S, Girault C et al (2016) Effect of non-invasive oxygenation strategies in immunocompromised patients with severe acute respiratory failure: a post-hoc analysis of a randomised trial. Lancet Respir Med 4:646–652
24. Carteaux G, Millán-Guilarte T, De Prost N et al (2016) Failure of noninvasive ventilation for de novo acute hypoxemic respiratory failure: role of tidal volume. Crit Care Med 44:282–290
25. Coudroy R, Jamet A, Petua P et al (2016) High-flow nasal cannula oxygen therapy versus noninvasive ventilation in immunocompromised patients with acute respiratory failure: an observational cohort study. Ann Intensive Care 6:45–56
26. Maitra S, Som A, Bhattacharjee S et al (2016) Comparison of high-flow nasal oxygen therapy with conventional oxygen therapy and noninvasive ventilation in adult patients with acute hypoxemic respiratory failure: A meta-analysis and systematic review. J Crit Care 35:138–144
27. Monro-Somerville T, Sim M, Ruddy J et al (2016) The effect of high-flow nasal cannula oxygen therapy on mortality and intubation rate in acute respiratory failure: a systematic review and meta-analysis. Crit Care Med Sept 8, Epub ahead of print
28. Stéphan F, Barrucand B, Petit P et al (2015) High-flow nasal oxygen vs noninvasive positive airway pressure in hypoxemic patients after cardiothoracic surgery. JAMA 313:2331–2339
29. Lemiale V, Mokart D, Mayaux J et al (2015) The effects of a 2-h trial of high-flow oxygen by nasal cannula versus Venturi mask in immunocompromised patients with hypoxemic acute respiratory failure: a multicenter randomized trial. Crit Care 19:380–388
30. Kang BJ, Koh Y, Lim CM et al (2015) Failure of high-flow nasal cannula therapy may delay intubation and increase mortality. Intensive Care Med 41:623–632
31. Rello J, Pérez M, Roca O et al (2012) High-flow nasal therapy in adults with severe acute respiratory infection: a cohort study in patients with 2009 influenza A/H1N1v. J Crit Care 27:434–439
32. Roca O, Messika J, Caralt B et al (2016) Predicting success of high-flow nasal cannula in pneumonia patients with hypoxemic respiratory failure: The utility of the ROX index. J Crit Care 35:200–205

33. Hernández G, Vaquero C, García S et al (2015) High flow conditioned oxygen therapy for prevention of reintubation in critically ill patients: a preliminary cohort study. Int J Crit Care Emerg Med 1:2–9
34. Ranieri VM, Rubenfeld GD, Thompson BT et al (2012) Acute respiratory distress syndrome: the Berlin Definition. JAMA 307:2526–2533
35. Parke RL, Bloch A, McGuinness SP (2015) Effect of very-high-flow nasal therapy on airway pressure and end-expiratory lung impedance in healthy volunteers. Respir Care 60:1397–1403
36. Antonelli M, Conti G, Esquinas A et al (2007) A multiple-center survey on the use in clinical practice of noninvasive ventilation as a first-line intervention for acute respiratory distress syndrome. Crit Care Med 35:18–25
37. Tiruvoipati R, Lewis D, Haji K et al (2010) High-flow nasal oxygen vs high-flow face mask: a randomized crossover trial in extubated patients. J Crit Care 25:463–468
38. Maggiore SM, Idone FA, Vaschetto R et al (2014) Nasal highflow versus Venturi mask oxygen therapy after extubation. Effects on oxygenation, comfort, and clinical outcome. Am J Respir Crit Care Med 190:282–288
39. Parke R, McGuinness S, Dixon R et al (2013) Open-label, phase II study of routine high-flow nasal oxygen therpy in cardiac surgical patients. Br J Anaesth 111:925–931
40. Corley A, Bull T, Spooner AJ et al (2015) Direct extubation onto high-flow nasal cannulae post-cardiac surgery versus standard treatment in patients with a BMI >30: a randomized controlled trial. Intensive Care Med 41:887–894
41. Thille AW, Boissier F, BenGhezala H et al (2016) Easily identified at risk patients for extubation failure may benefit from noninvasive ventilation: a prospective beforeafter study. Crit Care 20:48–56
42. Hernandez G, Pedrosa A, Ortiz R et al (2013) The effects of increasing effective airway diameter on weaning from mechanical ventilation tracheostomized patients: a randomized controlled trial. Intensive Care Med 39:1063–1070
43. Simon M, Braune S, Frings D et al (2014) High-flow nasal cannula oxygen versus non-invasive ventilation in patients with acute hypoxaemic respiratory failure undergoing flexible bronchoscopy. A prospective randmised trial. Crit Care 18:712–721
44. Jones PG, Kimona S, Doran O et al (2015) Randomized controlled trial of humidified high-flow nasal oxygen for acute respiratory distress in the emergency department: the HOT-ER study. Respir Care 61:291–299
45. Lucangelo U, Vassallo FG, Marras E et al (2012) High-flow nasal interface improves oxygenation in patients undergoing bronchoscopy. Crit Care Res Pract 212:506–512
46. Rittayamai N, Tscheikuna J, Rujiwit P (2014) High-flow nasal cannula versus conventional oxygen therapy after endotracheal extubation: a randomized crossover physiologic study. Respir Care 59:485–490
47. Vourc´h M, Asfar P, Volteau C et al (2015) High-flow nasal cannula oxygen during endotracheal intubation in hypoxemic patients: a randomized controlled trial. Intensive Care Med 41:1538–1548
48. Mokart D, Geay C, Chow-Chine L et al (2015) High-flow oxygen therapy in cancer patients with acute respiratory failure. Intensive Care Med 41:2008–2010

Urgent Endotracheal Intubation in the ICU: Rapid Sequence Intubation Versus Graded Sedation Approach

G. Zaidi and P. H. Mayo

Introduction

Endotracheal intubation is a common procedure in the operating room (OR), which provides airway protection and safe delivery of anesthetic agents during surgery. In the OR, the complication rates of elective intubation performed by experienced anesthesiologists on fasting patients with good physiological reserve and prescreened airway are low [1]. On the contrary, urgent endotracheal intubation describes endotracheal intubation that occurs in critically ill patients in the intensive care unit (ICU), the emergency department (ED), or on the hospital wards. In contrast to the OR, patients requiring urgent endotracheal intubation are often unstable with limited physiological reserve due to the presence of cardiopulmonary failure. Potentially difficult airways and conditions that will complicate the procedure may go undetected before urgent endotracheal intubation. In addition, there is variation in the level of expertise of clinicians responsible for performing this high risk, low frequency event.

Several studies have reported a high rate of complications during urgent endotracheal intubation. Schwartz et al. [2] performed a prospective study to evaluate the complications of urgent endotracheal intubation in critically ill patients. In 297 consecutive intubations, they reported esophageal intubation in 8% of cases, aspiration in 4%, and a 3% incidence of death either during urgent endotracheal intubation or within 30 min of the procedure. More than one intubation attempt was required in 25% patients with an 8% rate of difficult intubation. These authors demonstrated a statistically significant correlation between the presence of hypotension during urgent endotracheal intubation and subsequent cardiac arrest. Similarly, in a multicenter prospective observational study, Jaber et al. [3] reported that at least one severe complication occurred in 28% of urgent endotracheal intubations, including

G. Zaidi (✉) · P. H. Mayo
Division of Pulmonary, Critical Care and Sleep Medicine, North Shore Long Island Jewish Medical Center, Northwell Health System, Hofstra-Northwell School of Medicine
New Hyde Park, New York, NY 11042, USA
e-mail: gzaidi@northwell.edu

J.-L. Vincent (ed.), *Annual Update in Intensive Care and Emergency Medicine 2017*,
DOI 10.1007/978-3-319-51908-1_21

severe hypoxemia in 26%, hemodynamic collapse in 25% and cardiac arrest in 2%. Griesdale et al. [4] examined the relationship between operator skill level during urgent endotracheal intubations in the ICU and the occurrence of serious complications. The overall risk of complications in this study was 39%. Difficult intubation occurred in 6.6% of cases, severe hypoxemia in 19.1%, esophageal intubation in 7.4%, aspiration in 5.9% and severe hypotension in 9.6%. In these three studies, anesthesiologists were the predominant clinicians performing urgent endotracheal intubation. However, in out-of-OR intubations, emergency medicine physicians or intensivists with significantly less experience in airway management than anesthesiologists, are often the primary providers of urgent endotracheal intubation.

These studies provide evidence that urgent endotracheal intubation in critically ill patients is a high-risk procedure that is complicated by hemodynamic instability, gas exchange failure, comorbidities, as well as suboptimal views on laryngoscopy. It is thus logical to standardize urgent endotracheal intubation with a combined team approach. In a prospective multicenter controlled study, Jaber et al. [5] reported a statistically significant reduction in life-threatening complications associated with intubation following the implementation of an intubation bundle protocol for all urgent endotracheal intubations in the ICU. Intensive simulation based training may also be useful in reducing risk of complications, as well as the use of videolaryngoscopy as the primary intubating device. Lakticova et al. [6] performed a prospective observational study comparing the rates of complications during videolaryngoscopy using standard direct laryngoscopy versus videolaryngoscopy in a medical ICU in which either the pulmonary and critical care fellows or the intensivists performed all intubations. In this study, they reported a reduction in the rates of esophageal intubation (0.4% using videolaryngoscopy vs 19% using direct laryngoscopy) as well as difficult intubation (7% using videolaryngoscopy vs 22% using direct laryngoscopy). In a systematic review and meta-analysis of videolaryngoscopy versus direct laryngoscopy for intubation in the ICU, De Jong et al. [7] concluded that in comparison to direct laryngoscopy, the use of videolaryngoscopy increased first pass success rates and reduced the risk of difficult intubation and esophageal intubation.

The pharmacologic agents that are chosen to facilitate urgent endotracheal intubation are selected to minimize risk and adverse effects. Currently practitioners have a choice between performing urgent endotracheal intubation using a rapid sequence intubation (RSI) technique or, alternatively, using sedation without paralytics, also known as graded sedation intubation (GSI). We review the evidence supporting each technique as well as the pros and cons of both approaches.

Rapid Sequence Intubation

RSI is a technique that requires the administration of an induction drug to be followed promptly by a neuromuscular blocking agent (NMBA) to induce paralysis. This technique originated in the OR and was designed to reduce the risk of aspiration in non-fasting patients. Although a large number of studies have reported out-of-OR RSI success rates as high as 98%, these results should be interpreted with caution [8–19], as most of these data originate from studies in which skilled operators performed the intubation on well-selected patients. The RSI strategy was not developed for urgent endotracheal intubation; rather, RSI was adapted from the controlled OR environment that is very different from that encountered in out-of-OR intubation sequence. Despite this, use of RSI has become widespread in the ED and in critical care units.

The goal of RSI is to increase the chances of first past success and to reduce the time to intubation by creating optimal intubating conditions. This multistep technique follows an algorithmic approach. The preparation phase involves developing an airway management plan by risk stratifying the patient's airway, deciding on a medication regimen, as well as ensuring that all required equipment is available. Following this, the patient undergoes a period of pre-oxygenation using high flow oxygen, with the option of using non-invasive ventilation (NIV). Once the patient is apneic, this will increase the duration of time before any significant desaturation occurs [20]. During intubation, manipulation of the oropharynx and the airway stimulates the autonomic nervous system. This results in activation of airway protection mechanisms, such as the cough and gag reflexes, which may cause tachycardia, hypertension and an increased intracranial pressure. The RSI sequence may include use of agents designed to attenuate response to airway manipulation, but these may be impractical in emergent cases.

The focus of RSI is the rapid induction of paralysis using a NMBA. Since NMBAs have no analgesic or sedative properties, their administration has to be preceded by an induction agent, such as a benzodiazepine, propofol, ketamine or etomidate. Neuromuscular blockade is then provided using either a depolarizing NMBA, such as succinylcholine, or a non-depolarizing NMBA, such as rocuronium. Succinylcholine mimics the effect of acetylcholine at the postsynaptic nicotinic receptors of the motor endplate. This results in a persistent state of depolarization of the neuromuscular junction. Non-depolarizing NMBAs inhibit all muscular function by competing with acetylcholine at the postsynaptic receptors of the motor endplate. Endotracheal tube insertion is performed immediately following adequate induction and paralysis. In order to avoid gastric insufflation, bag-mask ventilation is avoided and cricoid pressure may be applied in an attempt to prevent aspiration. A systematic review has questioned the effectiveness of cricoid pressure and it is considered optional during RSI [21].

While RSI is commonly used in the critical care setting, there is a lack of high quality evidence supporting this choice. It is not clear from the literature, whether the reported success of RSI in various studies was a result of a structured algorithmic approach to urgent endotracheal intubation as opposed to being related to the use of the specific pharmacological approach or intubation technique [22, 23]. Critically ill patients often have oxygen transport limitations due to alveolar volume loss and high shunt fraction, which may prevent an adequate response to pre-oxygenation efforts with little reserve to tolerate interruption of oxygen delivery. In the patient with hypoxemic respiratory failure, during apnea the time to oxyhemoglobin desaturation <85% is 23 versus 522 s in a healthy adult [24]. The successful use of RSI is predicated on the supposition that the patient will be easy to intubate on first pass. This is an uncertain proposition in the critically ill patient who has limited physiological reserve in combination with the challenge of identifying a difficult airway in this population. If the initial intubation attempt fails, the safety of RSI is further predicated on the supposition that the patient can be re-saturated using a bag-mask ventilation system. The paralyzed patient with sub-optimal facial anatomy or severe cardiopulmonary disease (e. g., pneumonia, acute respiratory distress syndrome [ARDS], pulmonary edema, or airway disease) may be difficult to re-oxygenate following failed intubation attempts. A potential failure point with RSI is that it may lead to a cannot intubate/cannot bag-mask ventilate scenario. RSI works well in the OR. It generally works well in the ICU; when it does not, the results may be catastrophic.

The rapid onset and short duration of action of succinylcholine makes it the NMBA of choice in RSI. However, succinylcholine may be associated with serious adverse effects including life-threatening hyperkalemia, bradycardia, malignant hyperthermia, and trismus-masseter muscle spasm. Rocuronium, a relatively short acting NMBA that lacks the risks of succinylcholine, is an alternative. However, its duration of action is sufficiently long that, if the intubation attempt fails, there may be need for prolonged bag-mask ventilation, which may be difficult to achieve in the patient with severe hypoxemic respiratory failure. A Cochrane review of the comparison of rocuronium to succinylcholine in order to facilitate RSI found that rocuronium is slightly less effective in creating acceptable intubation conditions [25], and its long duration of action leads to prolonged neuromuscular blockade.

The hyperkalemia associated with succinylcholine use is of particular concern in critically ill patients. Under normal circumstances, succinylcholine administration results in a 0 to 0.5 mEq/L increase in the serum potassium. However, patients can occasionally have a pathological response to succinylcholine with a sudden rise in serum potassium levels resulting in life-threatening arrhythmias or cardiac arrest [26–28]. An upregulation of nicotinic receptors at the motor endplate, as well as slow metabolism of succinylcholine results in sustained depolarization. Patients who have been immobilized due to casting or paralysis, or those who are immobilized with muscular dystrophy, neuropathy or cerebral injury will also have an upregulation of nicotinic receptors and are at risk of hyperkalemia with succinylcholine use. Renal failure, tumor lysis syndrome, and rhabdomyolysis are also associated with a risk of succinylcholine-induced hyperkalemia. Given the emergency nature of urgent endotracheal intubation, it may not always be possible for the clinical team to adequately identify risk factors for succinylcholine-induced hyperkalemia. Although a rare complication of RSI, the hyperkalemia may have lethal effect.

Malignant hyperthermia is a rare but life-threatening condition that can occur when individuals with abnormalities in the skeletal muscle ryanodine receptors are exposed to succinylcholine. An accumulation of intracellular calcium within the skeletal muscles following administration of succinylcholine results in a severe hypermetabolic crisis. Although this is a very rare complication, it is important for providers to screen patients as the mortality from malignant hyperthermia, despite treatment with dantrolene, ranges from 1% to 17% [29, 30].

Graded Sedation Intubation

Intubation without paralysis is an alternative strategy to facilitate urgent endotracheal intubation in critically ill patients and to avoid the risks associated with NMBAs. With GSI, the clinical team uses some combination of sedative and/or opiate agents to sedate the patient sufficiently to permit endotracheal intubation while allowing the patient to have spontaneous respiratory effort. In addition to a standard pre-oxygenation protocol (e. g., high flow, high fraction of inspired oxygen [FiO_2] systems or NIV), the patient receives high flow nasal oxygen throughout the laryngoscopy procedure. Because of maintenance of spontaneous respiration, the patient entrains the oxygen and maintains arterial saturation throughout the procedure. A variation of the GSI technique is to deliver oxygen thorough a nasal NIV mask with performance of the endotracheal intubation using a bronchoscopic approach. This is particularly suitable for the high-risk airway or for patients who cannot assume the supine position. The emphasis with GSI is on maintenance of oxygenation throughout the procedure rather than on the actual event of the endotracheal intubation. It avoids the risks intrinsic to use of succinylcholine and reduces the likelihood of conversion to a CI/CB event that may occur with RSI.

There are a number of agents that are suitable for use with GSI. Ketamine, fentanyl, midazolam, propofol or their congeners are effective agents for GSI. All are associated with hypotension. This is of concern with urgent endotracheal intubation, as the critically ill patient may be particularly susceptible to this complication by virtue of hemodynamic instability caused by their primary illness.

The use of propofol in critically ill patients is complicated by the risk of drug-induced hypotension occurring as a result of vasodilatation and possible negative inotropic effect [31]. However, studies have demonstrated that the hypotension resulting from propofol use can be reversed or prevented by intravascular volume expansion with fluid boluses and administration of vasopressors [32].

A study performed by Koenig et al. evaluated the safety of propofol as an induction agent for urgent endotracheal intubation in the medical ICU while performing GSI [33]. This study described 472 urgent endotracheal intubations performed in the medical ICU. Propofol was used as the sole induction agent in 409 patients. In all cases, endotracheal intubation was accomplished without the use of a paralytic agent. All urgent endotracheal intubations were performed using a standardized checklist-driven protocol using a combined team approach, crew resource communication protocol, and with the team leader pre-trained using scenario-based simulation methods. The team leader administered propofol to clinical effect. Propofol doses ranged between 0.5 and 1.0 mg/kg for initial bolus, with additional doses given as needed. In order to counteract the hypotensive effect of propofol, the team leader was trained in proactive use of vasopressors including their preemptive use, i. e., initiation before propofol was given. Complications of urgent endotracheal intubation in those patients who received propofol were as follows: desaturation 30 (7%), hypotension 19 (4%), difficult intubation 44 (10%), aspiration 6 (1%), and oropharyngeal injury 4 (1%). There were no deaths. Endotracheal intubation was successful on the first attempt in 303 (71%) cases, on second attempt in 80 (19%) cases. The rate of complication using propofol as the sole induction agent compares favorably with studies on urgent endotracheal intubation from the anesthesiology and emergency medicine literature.

Proponents of RSI argue that GSI provides sub-optimal intubating conditions with intact airway reflexes and that the sedation required results in apnea. Use of a NMBA may also reduce the risk of emesis during laryngoscopy in the event that the patient has fluid in their stomach. In an observational study of 80 urgent endotracheal intubations using left upper quadrant ultrasonography prior to intubation, Koenig et al. [34] reported that significant gastric fluid was identified and drained in 16% of patients prior to attempting intubation. No significant aspiration events were reported in this study. If ultrasonography examination for stomach contents is introduced as a standard part of the urgent endotracheal intubation sequence, the risk of unanticipated emesis can be reduced. GSI also obviates the risk of hyperkalemia, and conversion to a cannot intubate/cannot bag-mask ventilate scenario.

The advantages and disadvantages of the two techniques are summarized in Table 1.

Table 1 Advantages and disadvantages of rapid sequence induction (RSI) and graded sedation intubation (GSI) in urgent endotracheal intubation

GSI Advantages	RSI Advantages
– Maintenance of oxygenation function – No risk of hyperkalemia – Single center experience with results that compare favorably to RSI – Reduced risk of cannot intubate/cannot bag-mask ventilate – Better for ICU or ED staff who may lack high level airway management skills	– Extensive clinical experience in the OR – Provides excellent intubating conditions
GSI Disadvantages	**RSI Disadvantages**
– Risk of hypotension – Total duration of procedure likely longer than RSI	– Rare event of lethal hyperkalemia – Inability to perform intubation may result in cannot intubate/cannot bag-mask ventilate – Not designed for unstable patients in the ICU or ED – Not designed for intensivist or ED clinicians who may have non-expert level airway management skills

ICU: intensive care unit; *ED*: emergency department; *OR*: operating room

Conclusion

A randomized controlled trial comparing RSI to GSI is required in order to determine whether one method is superior to the other. Pending such a trial, the best approach is that of clinical equipoise. It is possible that the determinant of safety and outcome is not related to the pharmacological approach *per se*, but rather to the deployment of a well-organized combined team approach to urgent endotracheal intubation that utilizes simulation training, checklists, ultrasonography for detection of stomach contents, and the mandatory use of video laryngoscopy for all urgent endotracheal intubation.

References

1. Cheney FW, Posner KL, Lee LA, Caplan RA, Domino KB (2006) Trends in anesthesia-related death and brain damage: a closed claims analysis. Anesthesiology 105:1081–1086
2. Schwartz DE, Matthay MA, Cohen NH (1995) Death and other complications of emergency airway management in critically ill adults: a prospective investigation of 297 tracheal intubations. Anesthesiology 82:367–376
3. Jaber S, Amraoui J, Lefrant JY et al (2006) Clinical practice and risk factors for immediate complications of endotracheal intubation in the intensive care unit: a prospective, multiple-center study. Crit Care Med 34:2355–2361
4. Griesdale DE, Bosma TL, Kurth T, Isac G, Chittock DR (2008) Complications of endotracheal intubation in the critically ill. Intensive Care Med 34:1835–1842
5. Jaber S, Jung B, Corne P et al (2010) An intervention to decrease complications related to endotracheal intubation in the intensive care unit: a prospective, multiple-center study. Intensive Care Med 36:248–255
6. Lakticova V, Koenig SJ, Narasimhan M, Mayo PH (2015) Video laryngoscopy is associated with increased first pass success and decreased rate of esophageal intubations during urgent endotracheal intubation in a medical intensive care unit when compared to direct laryngoscopy. J Intensive Care Med 30:44–48
7. De Jong A, Molinari N, Conseil M et al (2014) Video laryngoscopy versus direct laryngoscopy for orotracheal intubation in the intensive care unit: a systematic review and meta-analysis. Intensive Care Med 40:629–639
8. Kovacs G, Law JA, Ross J et al (2004) Acute airway management in the emergency department by non-anesthesiologists. Can J Anaesth 51:174–180
9. Bair AE, Filbin MR, Kulkarni RG, Walls RM (2002) The failed intubation attempt in the emergency department: analysis of prevalence, rescue techniques, and personnel. J Emerg Med 23:131–140
10. Sakles JC, Laurin EG, Rantapaa AA, Panacek EA (1998) Airway management in the emergency department: a one-year study of 610 tracheal intubations. Ann Emerg Med 31:325–332
11. Tayal VS, Riggs RW, Marx JA, Tomaszewski CA, Schneider RE (1999) Rapid-sequence intubation at an emergency medicine residency: success rate and adverse events during a two-year period. Acad Emerg Med 6:31–37
12. Jones JH, Weaver CS, Rusyniak DE, Brizendine EJ, McGrath RB (2002) Impact of emergency medicine faculty and an airway protocol on airway management. Acad Emerg Med 9:1452–1456
13. Li J, Murphy-Lavoie H, Bugas C, Martinez J, Preston C (1999) Complications of emergency intubation with and without paralysis. Am J Emerg Med 17:141–143
14. Rose WD, Anderson LD, Edmond SA (1994) Analysis of intubations: before and after establishment of a rapid sequence intubation protocol for air medical use. Air Med J 13:475–478

15. Bernard S, Smith K, Foster S, Hogan P, Patrick I (2002) The use of rapid sequence intubation by ambulance paramedics for patients with severe head injury. Emerg Med (Fremantle) 14:406–411
16. Bozeman WP, Kleiner DM, Huggett V (2003) Intubating conditions produced by etomidate alone vs rapid sequence intubation in the prehospital aeromedical setting. Acad Emerg Med 10:445–446 (abst)
17. Pearson S (2003) Comparison of intubation attempts and completion times before and after the initiation of a rapid sequence intubation protocol in an air medical transport program. Air Med J 22:28–33
18. Bulger EM, Copass MK, Maier RV, Larsen J, Knowles J, Jurkovich GJ (2002) An analysis of advanced prehospital airway management. J Emerg Med 23:183–189
19. Davis DP, Ochs M, Hoyt DB, Bailey D, Marshall LK, Rosen P (2003) Paramedic-administered neuromuscular blockade improves prehospital intubation success in severely head-injured patients. J Trauma 55:713–719
20. Weingart SD, Levitan RM (2012) Preoxygenation and prevention of desaturation during emergency airway management. Ann Emerg Med 59:165
21. Ellis DY, Harris T, Zideman D (2007) Cricoid pressure in emergency department rapid sequence tracheal intubations: a risk-benefit analysis. Ann Emerg Med 50:653
22. Reynolds SF, Heffner J (2005) Airway management of the critically ill patient: rapid sequence intubation. Chest 127:1397–1412
23. Walls RM, Brown CA 3rd, Bair AE, Pallin DJ, NEAR II Investigators (2011) Emergency airway management: a multi-center report of 8937 emergency department intubations. J Emerg Med 41:347–354
24. Benumof JL, Dagg R, Benumof R (1997) Critical hemoglobin desaturation will occur before return to an unparalyzed state following 1 mg/kg intravenous succinylcholine. Anesthesiology 87:979–982
25. Tran DTT, Newton EK, Mount VAH, Lee JS, Wells GA, Perry JJ (2015) Rocuronium versus succinylcholine for rapid sequence induction intubation. Cochrane Database Syst Rev 10:CD002788
26. Markewitz BA, Elstad MR (1997) Succinylcholine-induced hyperkalemia following prolonged pharmacologic neuromuscular blockade. Chest 111:248–250
27. Schwartz DE, Kelly B, Caldwell JE, Carlisle AS, Cohen NH (1992) Succinylcholine-induced hyperkalemic arrest in a patient with severe metabolic acidosis and exsanguinating hemorrhage. Anesth Analg 75:291–293
28. Cowgill DB, Mostello LA, Shapiro HM (1974) Encephalitis and a hyperkalemic response to succinylcholine. Anesthesiology 40:409–411
29. Brandom BW, Larach MG, Chen MS, Young MC (2011) Complications associated with the administration of dantrolene 1987 to 2006: a report from the North American Malignant Hyperthermia Registry of the Malignant Hyperthermia Association of the United States. Anesth Analg 112:1115–1123
30. Rosero EB, Adesanya AO, Timaran CH, Joshi GP (2009) Trends and outcomes of malignant hyperthermia in the United States, 2000 to 2005. Anesthesiology 110:89–94
31. Angelini G, Ketzler JT, Coursin DB (2001) Use of propofol and other nonbenzodiazepine sedatives in the intensive care unit. Crit Care Clin 17:863–880
32. el-Beheiry H, Kim J, Milne B, Seegobin R (1995) Prophylaxis against the systemic hypotension induced by propofol during rapid-sequence intubation. Can J Anaesth 42:875–878
33. Koenig SJ, Lakticova V, Narasimhan M, Doelken P, Mayo PH (2015) Safety of propofol as an induction agent for urgent endotracheal intubation in the medical intensive care unit. J Intensive Care Med 30:499–504
34. Koenig SJ, Lakticova V, Mayo PH (2011) Utility of ultrasonography for detection of gastric fluid during urgent endotracheal intubation. Intensive Care Med 37:627–631

Sedation in ARDS: An Evidence-Based Challenge

D. Chiumello, O. F. Cozzi, and G. Mistraletti

Introduction

Sedation is of paramount importance in the management of patients with acute respiratory distress syndrome (ARDS). In this chapter, we will present the difficult balance that must be reached between the need to limit the potential harmful effects of mechanical ventilation (ventilation-induced lung injury [VILI], inflammation, asynchronies, lack of homogeneity) on the one hand and the need to limit the effects of prolonged deep sedation (hypotension, sepsis, weakness, delirium) on the other.

Ideally, there are two phases – without clear clinical cut-offs – that require different strategies for sedation targets and monitoring. First, supporting vital functions in the acute phase of acute respiratory failure management requires deep sedation, both to permit invasive procedures with the least iatrogenic damage and to control the body stress response. Analgesic and sedative drugs are necessary to permit pronation, for example, or to decrease work of breathing and respiratory asynchrony. In this phase, objective methods of monitoring sedation, such as the simplified electroencephalogram (EEG), should be used [1].

Once the patient is clinically stable and hypoxia is resolved, pain, agitation and delirium symptoms must be adequately controlled, while maintaining the lightest possible level of sedation [2]. Achieving compliance with mechanical ventilation, decreasing oxygen consumption, or controlling anxiety and agitation are some reasons justifying the use of sedative therapy in this phase.

D. Chiumello (✉) · O. F. Cozzi
Dipartimento di Scienze della Salute, A.S.S.T. dei Santi Paolo e Carlo, Ospedale San Paolo – Polo Universitario, Università degli Studi di Milano
Via A. Di Rudinì 8, 20142 Milan, Italy
e-mail: davide.chiumello@unimi.it

G. Mistraletti
Dipartimento di Fisiopatologia medico-chirurgica e dei trapianti, A.S.S.T. dei Santi Paolo e Carlo, Ospedale San Paolo – Polo Universitario, Università degli Studi di Milano
20142 Milan, Italy

J.-L. Vincent (ed.), *Annual Update in Intensive Care and Emergency Medicine 2017*,
DOI 10.1007/978-3-319-51908-1_22

Optimal sedation management should thus provide the best possible adjustment to the phase of critical illness while avoiding excessive depression of the conscious state [3]. In this context, the key intervention is to continuously monitor pain/agitation/delirium using validated tools [4], so that neurological dysfunction can be managed according to locally agreed protocols. Careful neurological status monitoring is even more important than the choice of a particular sedative agent, because the literature supports only modest differences in outcomes when using non-benzodiazepine-based sedation protocols [2]. During weaning from mechanical ventilation, in addition to early active physical mobilization and family engagement, intensivists should consider early sedation interruption, while maintaining a calm, conscious, and cooperative patient [5].

The Difficult Choice Between Deep and Light Sedation

Patients with ARDS need special management. From the start of treatment, many strategies have to be used, including protective ventilation with low tidal volume, use of high positive end-expiratory pressure (PEEP), prone positioning, use of neuromuscular blockers, and extracorporeal membrane oxygenation (ECMO) in the most severe cases. In these patients, administration of sedative agents is mandatory: they ensure compliance with these procedures and adjustment to the harsh ICU environment [6]. Moreover, ARDS has serious physical and psychological implications, and these patients need the most appropriate and individualized neurological treatment, because among many other vital organ failures, the early and long-term consequences of ARDS may lead to severe brain dysfunction [7].

Pain, agitation, delirium, anxiety, and alteration of consciousness are frequently triggered by treatable causes, such as hypoxemia, hypercarbia, acidosis, hypoglycemia, hypo- or hypernatremia, sepsis, hypovolemia, alcohol or drug withdrawal, or by life-saving medical treatments, including mechanical ventilation, invasive procedures, forced body postures, uninterrupted noise and light stimulation, or their consequences, such as sleep deprivation or the inability to communicate with the staff [1]. International guidelines recommend first treating all organic and metabolic causes of distress, and minimizing environment-linked stressors [2, 3]. As a second step, they suggest administration of analgesic, sedative and antipsychotic drugs to ensure comfort, at all stages of the illness. Adequate levels of sedation, therefore, represent a primary target for managing patients with ARDS, but these patients do not have a unique sedation target for their whole ICU stay; as soon as possible, the target sedative level should be changed from 'deep' to 'light'. Because sedative therapy has several important adverse effects, including hemodynamic instability and cardiac dysrhythmias [8], sepsis [9], ileus, delirium and prolonged respiratory weaning [10], it is important to titrate administration to the lowest effective amounts.

A conscious sedation target is an innovation particularly relevant to ARDS management. However, some intensivists tend to consider it unfeasible, considering the potential higher risk of ventilation-related lung damage, the risk of self-removal of invasive devices, and the possible stress/discomfort for patients. From an ICU staff perspective, it also raises the issue of increased workload. These beliefs are, however, at least partially unfounded [11]. Despite guidelines supporting minimal sedation and the fact that between 60 and 80% of ICUs use a specific score to evaluate the level of sedation [12], many physicians routinely maintain a deeper than desired level of sedation, likely causing avoidable adverse effects.

Although the clinical course of each ARDS patient is different, it is useful to distinguish at least two different scenarios leading to neuroactive drug prescription (Fig. 1). In the acute hypoxic phase, intubation, placement of vascular catheters and other maneuvers devoted to clinical stabilization require a deep sedation target, similar to general anesthesia. The use of protective ventilation strategies may necessitate the prolongation of this phase for several days. However, subsequent to this phase, it is important to change the target toward lighter sedation, using the small-

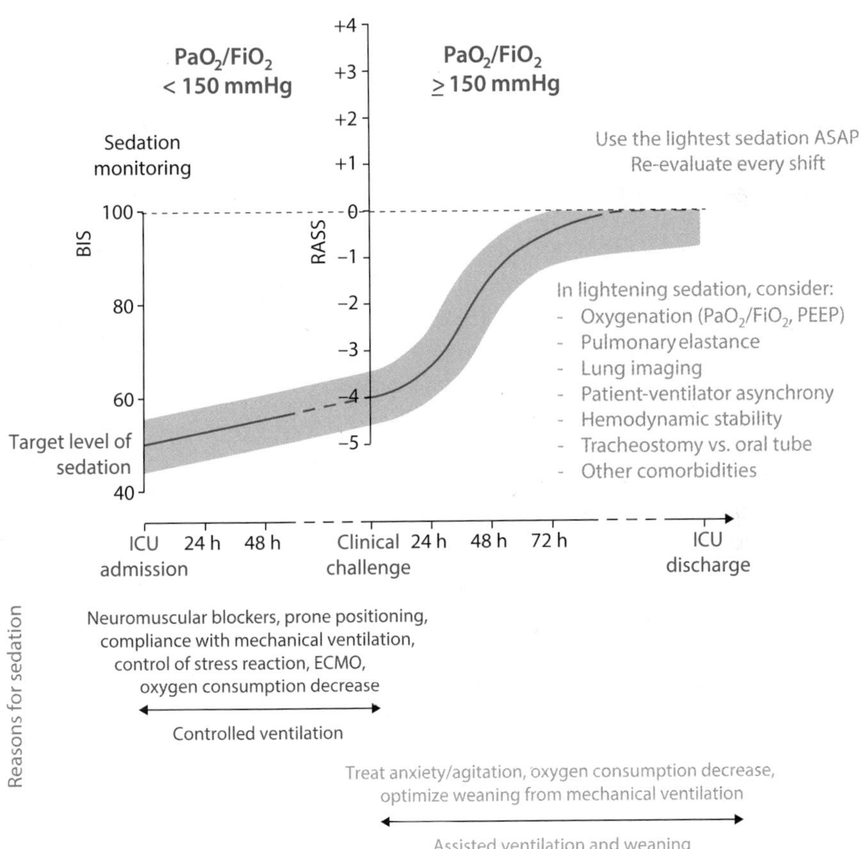

Fig. 1 Two scenarios requiring different sedative targets. *BIS*: bispectral index; *ASAP*: as soon as possible; *PEEP*: positive end-expiratory pressure; *ECMO*: extracorporeal membrane oxygenation

est possible amount of neuroactive drugs to ensure adequate patient adjustment to critical illness. This second phase should start as soon as possible, depending on the severity of pulmonary dysfunction. Other practices, such as adjustment of mechanical ventilation settings, of drug therapies and of the environment to the specific needs of each patient can help reduce discomfort.

Achieving the Sedative Target

The appropriate target level of sedation primarily depends on a patient's acute disease process and on the therapeutic and supportive interventions required. Generally, the use of deep levels of sedation to facilitate mechanical ventilation or painful procedures should be minimized with optimization of ventilation settings and adequate analgesia, rather than deepening unconsciousness [13, 14]. In any case, after hypoxia resolution, the sedation target should be a calm patient, awake during the day and asleep at night.

The appropriate balance of sedation and analgesia is difficult to achieve and maintain. Without a rational agreement on 'target levels' of sedation, different members of the healthcare team will have disparate treatment goals, increasing the risk of iatrogenic complications and potentially delaying recovery. The target level of sedation for each patient should thus be discussed between the different ICU staff members, defined at the beginning of each staff shift, and re-evaluated regularly as the clinical condition of the patient changes. The pharmacological treatment should be planned with sufficient flexibility to enable titration to the desired endpoint, anticipating fluctuations in sedation requirements throughout the day. Frequent monitoring with validated tools improves communication among clinicians and plays an important role in detecting and treating pain, agitation and delirium while avoiding excessive or prolonged sedation [12].

Continuous Neurological Assessment with Subjective, Validated Tools

Individual assessment of sedation, performed at the bedside by nurses or physicians, can be hampered by lack of objectivity. Guidelines recommend establishing a sedation target and regularly redefining it for each patient, using a validated sedation assessment scale [1–3]. These scales provide repeatable and comparable measurements, enabling adequate titration of analgesic, sedative and antipsychotic therapy and, as such, are a key component of sedation algorithms.

Among the validated tools, the scales with the highest psychometric properties [4] are the Verbal Numeric Rating (VNR), the Behavioral Pain Scale (BPS) [15] and the Critical-care Pain Observation Tool (CPOT) [16] for pain assessment; the Richmond Agitation-Sedation Scale (RASS) and the Sedation Agitation Scale (SAS) for agitation/sedation assessment; and the Confusion Assessment Method for the Intensive Care Unit (CAM-ICU) [17] and the Intensive Care Delirium Screening

Checklist (ICDSC) [18] for delirium assessment. Amongst these validated tools, each ICU should choose at least one for pain, one for agitation/sedation, and one for delirium.

Proper identification of pain symptoms in critically ill patients presents a challenge because of difficulty communicating with patients who have an endotracheal tube *in situ*, those with altered states of consciousness, and those receiving neuroactive drugs. To address these issues, specific behavioral scales have been designed and validated in unconscious/sedated and in conscious/awake patients, and established as valid, reliable, and simple tools to be used in clinical practice.

Under- or over-use of sedative drugs may compromise clinical stability. Potentially life-threatening adverse effects of untreated agitation and stress response are evident: self-removal of life-sustaining devices, tachypnea, tachycardia, hypertension, sustained hypoxemia and hypercarbia due to uncoordinated mechanical ventilation [3]. At the same time, deeper-than-necessary sedation may increase mortality [19], length of ICU stay [2], sepsis severity [9], and the onset of new neurological failure both during hospitalization and after discharge.

To obtain the best sedative titration, use of validated tools is mandatory. The RASS describes 10 levels of sedation/agitation using observation, verbal and physical stimulation. Scores range from −5 (unconscious, unresponsive to voice and physical stimuli) to +4 (overtly combative, violent, immediate danger to staff), adequately describing the possible neurological conditions that require immediate intervention. Interestingly, the RASS is also validated to assess degree of sedation over time, both in spontaneously breathing/mechanically ventilated and in sedated/not-sedated critically ill patients.

Although encouraging results regarding evaluation of pain and agitation have been reported in the literature, recognition and assessment of delirium [20] are more challenging, because they rely on effective and continuous staff education [21]. There is a direct relationship between increased morbidity and mortality and the duration (in days) of delirium [22]. The presence and duration of delirium also correlates with a significant deterioration in the quality of life after ICU discharge.

Assessments of sedation/agitation must be reported in the clinical chart at least once per shift, together with an evaluation of the adequacy of sedative treatment. Monitoring of neurological status plays a key role in patients with ARDS, and is easy and quick to perform: physicians should state the desired sedation target for the specific patient at the specific moment of their clinical course; nurses, for their part, should report the current neurological state, describing pain, anxiety, agitation, sleep, need for physical restraints, delirium, together with a comprehensive evaluation of sedative therapy, in order to achieve optimal treatment titration.

Teaching protocols used for implementation of sedation scales have shown good results among ICU caregivers. Different methods have been used to implement evaluation tools in clinical practice. Typically, they use an introductory in-service training for nurses and physicians followed by graded, staged educational interventions at regular intervals. Web-based, freely available teaching interventions have also been proposed (e. g., www.icudelirium.org, www.sedaicu.it).

Some problems remain, particularly regarding the fluctuation of consciousness. Patients with ARDS are prone to sudden changes in their state of consciousness as a result of effects of drugs, sleep disruption, organic and metabolic disease or delirium. Assessment of sedation once a shift is indispensable but not sufficient. Among the different possible values measured (minimal/maximal level, prevalent level, worst level), it is important to state the duration of each value within the observed shift. Sedation and agitation need to be reassessed on a regular basis and during any clinical modification, to promptly capture any changes requiring intervention. Moreover, it is relatively common for patients to manifest sudden aggressive behavior when recovering from sedation and without fully awakening. For this reason, it is important to encourage interdisciplinary communication between nurses and physicians in order to be aware of and prevent these problems.

Finally, assessing sedation during the night is frequently challenging. Most analgesics and sedatives are known to make patients sleepy, but without achieving restorative, physiological sleep [23]. If a critically ill patient appears calm and keeps his/her eyes closed during the night, he/she should not be stimulated just to make a sedation assessment. He/she could be observed during unavoidable procedures conducted during the night in the ICU, in order to discriminate normal sleep (with arousals due to noise or light) from sedation or coma.

Sedation Assessment Using Objective Methods

Several objective methods of sedation assessment have been proposed (e. g., bispectral index [BIS], entropy, auditory-evoked potentials [AEPs], actigraphy), but none is completely satisfactory [3].

The BIS is a four-channel EEG monitor that generates a single value correlated with the depth of consciousness during general anesthesia. The poor correlation between BIS and validated ICU sedation scales (Fig. 2) is related to BIS variability at awake/agitated levels and electromyography (EMG) interference [24]. Based on the analysis of EEG signal irregularity, the entropy monitor also uses the EMG signal, which may provide useful information for assessing whether a patient is responding to an external, painful stimulus, but provides no additional information on sedative level. In this context, the Responsiveness Index may offer some advantages [25]. AEPs are electrophysiological responses of the nervous system to standard sensory stimulation transmitted through headphones. These methods have a role in monitoring sedation levels only in patients needing deep sedation, or receiving neuromuscular blocking agents, as in this circumstance sedation scales cannot be used [24].

Actigraphy provides a continuous measure of body movements and was initially developed to measure sleep-wake cycles. This small electronic device, containing an accelerometer, continuously senses and records minimal movements, summarizing such data in numerical form. Although wrist actigraphy does not discriminate the effects of lack (or excess) of analgesics and sedatives from other acute neurological dysfunctions, preliminary observations suggest that the measurement of body

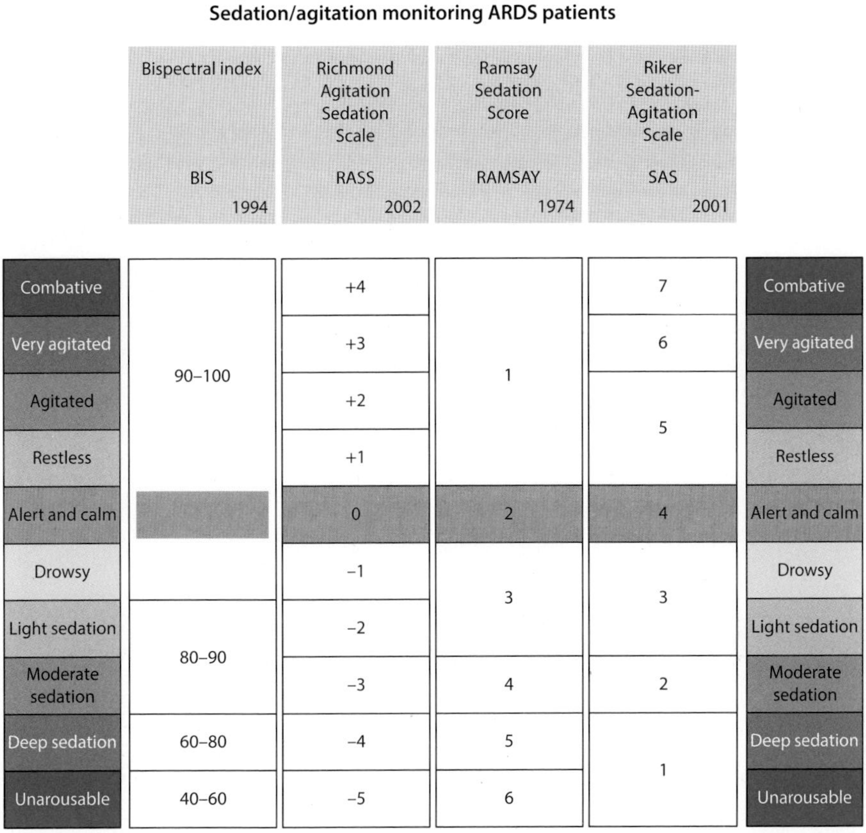

Sedation/agitation monitoring ARDS patients

<table>
<tr><th></th><th>Bispectral index
BIS
1994</th><th>Richmond Agitation Sedation Scale
RASS
2002</th><th>Ramsay Sedation Score
RAMSAY
1974</th><th>Riker Sedation-Agitation Scale
SAS
2001</th><th></th></tr>
<tr><td>Combative</td><td rowspan="6">90–100</td><td>+4</td><td rowspan="4">1</td><td>7</td><td>Combative</td></tr>
<tr><td>Very agitated</td><td>+3</td><td>6</td><td>Very agitated</td></tr>
<tr><td>Agitated</td><td>+2</td><td rowspan="2">5</td><td>Agitated</td></tr>
<tr><td>Restless</td><td>+1</td><td>Restless</td></tr>
<tr><td>Alert and calm</td><td>0</td><td>2</td><td>4</td><td>Alert and calm</td></tr>
<tr><td>Drowsy</td><td>−1</td><td rowspan="2">3</td><td rowspan="2">3</td><td>Drowsy</td></tr>
<tr><td>Light sedation</td><td rowspan="2">80–90</td><td>−2</td><td>Light sedation</td></tr>
<tr><td>Moderate sedation</td><td>−3</td><td>4</td><td>2</td><td>Moderate sedation</td></tr>
<tr><td>Deep sedation</td><td>60–80</td><td>−4</td><td>5</td><td rowspan="2">1</td><td>Deep sedation</td></tr>
<tr><td>Unarousable</td><td>40–60</td><td>−5</td><td>6</td><td>Unarousable</td></tr>
</table>

Fig. 2 Relationship between objective and subjective validated tools for sedation monitoring

movements could provide a timely indication of acute changes in neurological status generating motor agitation or hypoactive behavior [26]. This objective method is relatively new in this context. It presents interesting properties, worthy of future investigation [27].

Clinical Practice Flowchart for Sedation and Agitation Management in ARDS Patients

Recognition that inappropriately heavy sedation may increase mortality and morbidity has led to a new approach that maximizes patient comfort while they remain awake, interactive and oriented. This new approach relies on strategies, such as protocolized sedation, analgesia-based sedation, enteral sedation, avoidance of paralytic agents, early mobilization and use of validated tools for sedation assessment [28]. In recent years, many guidelines have been proposed [1–3], providing a guide

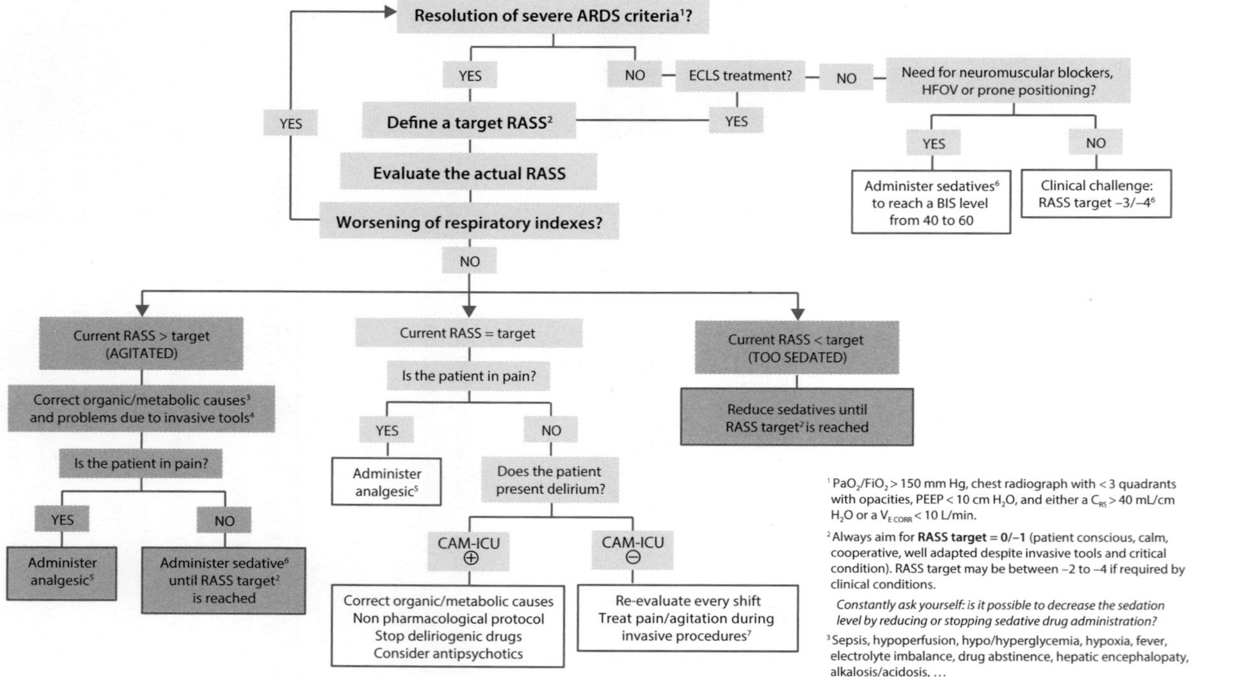

Fig. 3 Sedation management in ARDS. *ARDS*: acute respiratory distress syndrome; *ECLS*: extracorporeal life support; *HFOV*: high frequency oscillatory ventilation; *BIS*: bispectral index; *RASS*: Richmond Agitation-Sedation Scale; *CAM-ICU*: Confusion assessment method for the Intensive Care Unit; *PEEP*: positive end-expiratory pressure; C_{RS}: compliance of respiratory system; $V_{E\,CORR}$: corrected expiratory ventilation; *NGT*: nasogastric tube; *VNR*: verbal numeric rating; *BPS*: Behavioral Pain Scale

to symptom-oriented prevention, diagnosis, and treatment of delirium, anxiety and stress, and protocol-based analgesia, sedation, and sleep-management. These guidelines comprehensively describe all aspects that need to be considered in order to perform the optimal neurological management. Nevertheless, even in high quality guidelines, numerous recommendations are supported by only moderate or low levels of evidence [29].

The principal recommendation regarding analgesia is to evaluate pain and maintain its level at $\leq 4/10$, by beginning treatment early rather than late, and by using opioid drugs first, together with non-opioid and multimodal analgesic techniques. For sedation, a target RASS of 0/−1 is recommended once hypoxia is resolved, with the use of deep sedation reserved only for patients with specific indications (e. g., patients with early ARDS, requiring neuromuscular blockade or prone positioning). Intensivists should consider the specific indication and individual goal of sedation, and the pharmacokinetics/pharmacodynamics of each drug used. Non-benzodiazepine drugs, such as propofol or dexmedetomidine, are preferred. The need for sedation varies widely among different patients and with the course of illness, and should be defined as 'deep sedation', 'cooperative/awake sedation', and 'no sedation', always preferring superficial levels of sedation and promoting early mobilization. The use of containment measures in episodes of severe agitation should be performed in this order: first verbal, then pharmacological, and finally physical, considering that neuroactive drugs should not be administered in excess as a form of 'chemical immobilization'. In the sedation flowchart (Fig. 3), it is clear that defining a target and evaluating the current level of sedation or agitation using validated tools is an absolute priority. The choice of the specific sedative drug, albeit important, comes only after clinical reasoning focused on managing the organic/metabolic causes and the problems that may be caused by adjustable invasive devices.

Recommendations for delirium management suggest first that modifiable risk factors be identified and the presence of delirium assessed regularly using the CAM-ICU. If delirium occurs, a non-pharmacological protocol should be used first, while also stopping or decreasing any deliriogenic therapies; the most appropriate drug (haloperidol, atypical antipsychotics or dexmedetomidine; avoid the use of benzodiazepines) should then be chosen and titrated to the lowest effective dose.

Sedation Protocols in the Literature

Adoption of local sedation protocols is strongly advised by international guidelines [1–3]. The protocols should include daily interruption of short-term sedatives (propofol, dexmedetomidine), analgesia-based sedation (morphine, fentanyl or remifentanil), use of inhalational halogenated anesthetic agents in the early phase (e. g., sevoflurane) and use of an enteral approach during subsequent phases. Whichever the local protocol, international guidelines highlight the need to make mechanically ventilated patients "calm, conscious and cooperative" as soon as possible [5], while avoiding the iatrogenic risks associated with both under- and over-sedation.

Continuous intravenous infusion is the most frequently used method for administering sedatives, because of its pharmacokinetic properties. Intravenous infusions have predictable and easy to handle onset/offset properties, facilitating an early goal-directed sedation strategy. Although these characteristics are necessary for short ICU stays, they may be useless, or even dangerous, for patients requiring more than 3 days of mechanical ventilation [30]. When using potent drugs, it is easy to provide excessive doses even if appropriate goals are established [12]. Moreover, daily awakening trials produce far-from-physiological fluctuations in neurological state [31].

If continuous intravenous infusions of sedatives and/or analgesics are used, daily interruption may be recommended in order to reduce the total administered dosage and to enable spontaneous breathing trials to be performed if possible. The purpose is to reduce the development of complications and the duration of mechanical ventilation. This strategy may prove less effective if specific and ICU team-shared protocols are used [28].

Many different sedation protocols have been presented in the literature [10]; some rely essentially on the use of different drug doses [32], whereas others are based on nursing-implemented algorithms [33] or on analgesia-first sedation [19]. Tested methods to optimize sedation management in the ICU include patient-controlled sedation [34] or automated sedation in patients needing deep sedation [35], the use of inhaled halogenated anesthetic agents [36] and the enteral administration of drugs [37, 38]. All these protocols rely on continuous and adequate neurological assessment conducted with validated tools, in order to measure not only pain, agitation and delirium, but also level of consciousness and patient mobilization.

The most promising protocol, in terms of efficacy, recommends combining sedation strategies with early physiotherapy [39], mobilization [40] and occupational therapy [41], and also engaging patient families. Although implementing such protocols is not simple [42], it has offered the best results in terms of effectiveness [43]. Briefly, following the acronym ABCDEF, the authors make these suggestions: Assess, prevent and manage pain; Both spontaneous awakening trial and spontaneous breathing trial; Choice of analgesia and sedation; Delirium – assess, prevent and manage; Early mobility and exercise (goal-directed early mobilization); Family engagement and empowerment.

Special Circumstances

For patients with ARDS needing extracorporeal life support (ECLS), there is a gray area about sedation, in which safety aspects and the ability to positively influence recovery must be balanced. Patients on ECLS have numerous risk factors for developing delirium during the ICU stay and post-traumatic stress disorder (PTSD) after discharge. Hyperactive delirium or agitation can be life-threatening for these patients, so that effective monitoring and symptomatic therapy of stress, anxiety, delirium, pain and insomnia are essential to safely achieve a target RASS of 0. A higher level of alertness, enabling the patient to actively partake in physical exercise [44] is considered a feasible and safe goal [45, 46]. International guidelines recommend strict definition of sedation targets for patients on ECLS, including frequent clinical monitoring and continuous adjustment of the level of sedation required [1].

Positioning therapy has been shown to be effective in ameliorating the prognosis of patients with severe ARDS. It is used for prophylaxis and treatment of respiratory dysfunction, and requires an individualized sedation target. Changes in position frequently represent a challenge for the symptomatic treatment of anxiety, stress and pain. Therefore, a symptom-orientated therapy should be adapted to the changing demands during positioning therapy. Although deep sedation may be indicated for patient repositioning [47], excessive sedation should be avoided by using objective tools based on EEG analysis, as previously described.

The use of non-depolarizing neuromuscular blockers in patients with severe ARDS is suggested during the first 48 ICU hours. Once tracheostomy has been performed, it is advisable to consider a decrease in sedative and analgesic regimens. It is advisable not to use benzodiazepines for the withdrawal of mechanical ventilation. Dexmedetomidine is recommended in case of weaning difficulty, in patients with withdrawal syndrome, or after failed attempts at weaning secondary to agitation and delirium [48]. Low-dose remifentanil as a continuous infusion is another effective alternative during the weaning process. Music therapy is a possible non-pharmacological adjuvant to sedation [49]. Melatonin supplementation could be useful to decrease the need for sedative drugs, thus shortening the duration of mechanical ventilation [50], and to restore the sleep-wake rhythm.

Conclusion

Appropriate analgesic and sedative therapy plays a key role in the care of patients with ARDS. All available strategies must be used to avoid under- and over-sedation because they can affect morbidity and mortality. Among the many pharmacological strategies proposed in the literature, none has been clearly shown to be better than another. We therefore suggest that – irrespective of the local protocol used – intensivists should aim early and constantly to keep patients conscious, calm and cooperative, by titrating the therapy. To optimally guide sedation management, adequate validated assessment tools for analgesia (VNR and BPS), for sedation and agitation (BIS and RASS) and for delirium (CAM-ICU or ICDSC) must be used. The most crucial aspect in managing sedation in patients with ARDS remains the 'clinical challenge' of bridging the hyperacute phase, when evidence supports deep sedation, to the subsequent recovery phases, when it is recommended that sedation be kept as light as possible.

References

1. Baron R, Binder A, Biniek R et al (2015) Evidence and consensus based guideline for the management of delirium, analgesia, and sedation in intensive care medicine. Revision 2015 (DAS-Guideline 2015) – short version. Ger Med Sc 13:Doc19
2. Barr J, Fraser GL, Puntillo K et al (2013) Clinical practice guidelines for the management of pain, agitation, and delirium in adult patients in the intensive care unit. Crit Care Med 41:263–306
3. Celis-Rodriguez E, Birchenall C, de la Cal MA et al (2013) Clinical practice guidelines for evidence-based management of sedoanalgesia in critically ill adult patients. Med Intensiva 37:519–574
4. Robinson BR, Berube M, Barr J, Riker R, Gelinas C (2013) Psychometric analysis of subjective sedation scales in critically ill adults. Crit Care Med 41(9 Suppl 1):S16–29
5. Vincent JL, Shehabi Y, Walsh TS et al (2016) Comfort and patient-centred care without excessive sedation: the eCASH concept. Intensive Care Med 42:962–971
6. Sessler CN, Varney K (2008) Patient-focused sedation and analgesia in the ICU. Chest 133:552–565
7. Pandharipande PP, Girard TD, Jackson JC et al (2013) Long-term cognitive impairment after critical illness. N Engl J Med 369:1306–1316
8. Ice CJ, Personett HA, Frazee EN, Dierkhising RA, Kashyap R, Oeckler RA (2016) Risk factors for dexmedetomidine-associated hemodynamic instability in noncardiac intensive care unit patients. Anesth Analg 122:462–469
9. Nseir S, Makris D, Mathieu D, Durocher A, Marquette CH (2010) Intensive care unit-acquired infection as a side effect of sedation. Crit Care 14:R30
10. Jackson DL, Proudfoot CW, Cann KF, Walsh T (2010) A systematic review of the impact of sedation practice in the ICU on resource use, costs and patient safety. Crit Care 14:R59
11. Goodwin H, Lewin JJ, Mirski MA (2012) 'Cooperative sedation': optimizing comfort while maximizing systemic and neurological function. Crit Care 16:217
12. Martin J, Franck M, Fischer M, Spies C (2006) Sedation and analgesia in German intensive care units: how is it done in reality? Results of a patient-based survey of analgesia and sedation. Intensive Care Med 32:1137–1142
13. Cigada M, Corbella D, Mistraletti G et al (2008) Conscious sedation in the critically ill ventilated patient. J Crit Care 23:349–353
14. Strom T, Toft P (2011) Time to wake up the patients in the ICU: a crazy idea or common sense? Minerva Anestesiol 77:59–63
15. Payen JF, Bru O, Bosson JL et al (2001) Assessing pain in critically ill sedated patients by using a behavioral pain scale. Crit Care Med 29:2258–2263
16. Gelinas C, Fillion L, Puntillo KA, Viens C, Fortier M (2006) Validation of the critical-care pain observation tool in adult patients. Am Crit Care Nurs 15:420–427
17. Ely EW, Margolin R, Francis J et al (2001) Evaluation of delirium in critically ill patients: validation of the Confusion Assessment Method for the Intensive Care Unit (CAM-ICU). Crit Care Med 29:1370–1379
18. Bergeron N, Dubois MJ, Dumont M, Dial S, Skrobik Y (2001) Intensive Care Delirium Screening Checklist: evaluation of a new screening tool. Intensive Care Med 27:859–864
19. Strom T, Martinussen T, Toft P (2010) A protocol of no sedation for critically ill patients receiving mechanical ventilation: a randomised trial. Lancet 375:475–480
20. Morandi A, Pandharipande P, Trabucchi M et al (2008) Understanding international differences in terminology for delirium and other types of acute brain dysfunction in critically ill patients. Intensive Care Med 34:1907–1915
21. Spronk PE, Riekerk B, Hofhuis J, Rommes JH (2009) Occurrence of delirium is severely underestimated in the ICU during daily care. Intensive Care Med 35:1276–1280

22. Pisani MA, Kong SY, Kasl SV, Murphy TE, Araujo KL, Van Ness PH (2009) Days of delirium are associated with 1-year mortality in an older intensive care unit population. Am J Respir Crit Care Med 180:1092–1097
23. Brown EN, Lydic R, Schiff ND (2010) General anesthesia, sleep, and coma. N Engl J Med 363:2638–2650
24. Haenggi M, Ypparila-Wolters H, Buerki S et al (2009) Auditory event-related potentials, bispectral index, and entropy for the discrimination of different levels of sedation in intensive care unit patients. Anesth Analg 109:807–816
25. Walsh TS, Lapinlampi TP, Ramsay P, Sarkela MO, Uutela K, Viertio-Oja HE (2011) Responsiveness of the frontal EMG for monitoring the sedation state of critically ill patients. Br J Anaesth 107:710–718
26. Mistraletti G, Taverna M, Sabbatini G et al (2009) Actigraphic monitoring in critically ill patients: preliminary results toward an "observation-guided sedation". J Crit Care 24:563–567
27. Grap MJ, Hamilton VA, McNallen A et al (2011) Actigraphy: analyzing patient movement. Heart Lung 40:e52–59
28. Bein T, Grasso S, Moerer O et al (2016) The standard of care of patients with ARDS: ventilatory settings and rescue therapies for refractory hypoxemia. Intensive Care Med 42:699–711
29. Girardis M, Cantaroni C, Savoia G, Melotti R, Conti G (2016) A critical appraisal of the quality of analgosedation guidelines in critically ill patients. Minerva Anestesiol 82:230–235
30. Devlin JW (2008) The pharmacology of oversedation in mechanically ventilated adults. Curr Opin Crit Care 14:403–407
31. Svenningsen H, Egerod I, Videbech P, Christensen D, Frydenberg M, Tonnesen EK (2013) Fluctuations in sedation levels may contribute to delirium in ICU patients. Acta Anaesthesiol Scand 57(3):288–293
32. Zhou Y, Jin X, Kang Y, Liang G, Liu T, Deng N (2014) Midazolam and propofol used alone or sequentially for long-term sedation in critically ill, mechanically ventilated patients: a prospective, randomized study. Crit Care 18:R122
33. de Wit M, Gennings C, Jenvey WI, Epstein SK (2008) Randomized trial comparing daily interruption of sedation and nursing-implemented sedation algorithm in medical intensive care unit patients. Crit Care 12:R70
34. Chlan LL, Weinert CR, Skaar DJ, Tracy MF (2010) Patient-controlled sedation: a novel approach to sedation management for mechanically ventilated patients. Chest 138:1045–1053
35. Le Guen M, Liu N, Bourgeois E et al (2013) Automated sedation outperforms manual administration of propofol and remifentanil in critically ill patients with deep sedation: a randomized phase II trial. Intensive Care Med 39:454–462
36. Mesnil M, Capdevila X, Bringuier S et al (2011) Long-term sedation in intensive care unit: a randomized comparison between inhaled sevoflurane and intravenous propofol or midazolam. Intensive Care Med 37:933–941
37. Mistraletti G, Mantovani ES, Cadringher P et al (2013) Enteral vs. intravenous ICU sedation management: study protocol for a randomized controlled trial. Trials 14:92
38. Wanzuita R, Poli-de-Figueiredo LF, Pfuetzenreiter F, Cavalcanti AB, Westphal GA (2012) Replacement of fentanyl infusion by enteral methadone decreases the weaning time from mechanical ventilation: a randomized controlled trial. Crit Care 16:R49
39. Balas MC, Burke WJ, Gannon D et al (2013) Implementing the awakening and breathing coordination, delirium monitoring/management, and early exercise/mobility bundle into everyday care: opportunities, challenges, and lessons learned for implementing the ICU Pain, Agitation, and Delirium Guidelines. Crit Care Med 41(9 Suppl 1):S116–127
40. Morris PE, Goad A, Thompson C et al (2008) Early intensive care unit mobility therapy in the treatment of acute respiratory failure. Crit Care Med 36:2238–2243
41. Llano-Diez M, Renaud G, Andersson M et al (2012) Mechanisms underlying ICU muscle wasting and effects of passive mechanical loading. Crit Care 16:R209

42. Hodgson C, Bellomo R, Berney S et al (2015) Early mobilization and recovery in mechanically ventilated patients in the ICU: a bi-national, multi-centre, prospective cohort study. Crit Care 19:81
43. Balas MC, Vasilevskis EE, Olsen KM et al (2014) Effectiveness and safety of the awakening and breathing coordination, delirium monitoring/management, and early exercise/mobility bundle. Crit Care Med 42:1024–1036
44. Rahimi RA, Skrzat J, Reddy DR et al (2013) Physical rehabilitation of patients in the intensive care unit requiring extracorporeal membrane oxygenation: a small case series. Phys Ther 93:248–255
45. Del Sorbo L, Pisani L, Filippini C et al (2015) Extracorporeal Co2 removal in hypercapnic patients at risk of noninvasive ventilation failure: a matched cohort study with historical control. Crit Care Med 43:120–127
46. Fuehner T, Kuehn C, Hadem J et al (2012) Extracorporeal membrane oxygenation in awake patients as bridge to lung transplantation. Am J Respir Crit Care Med 185:763–768
47. Kredel M, Bischof L, Wurmb TE, Roewer N, Muellenbach RM (2014) Combination of positioning therapy and venovenous extracorporeal membrane oxygenation in ARDS patients. Perfusion 29:171–177
48. Riker RR, Shehabi Y, Bokesch PM et al (2009) Dexmedetomidine vs midazolam for sedation of critically ill patients: a randomized trial. JAMA 301:489–499
49. Chlan LL, Weinert CR, Heiderscheit A et al (2013) Effects of patient-directed music intervention on anxiety and sedative exposure in critically ill patients receiving mechanical ventilatory support: a randomized clinical trial. JAMA 309:2335–2344
50. Mistraletti G, Umbrello M, Sabbatini G et al (2015) Melatonin reduces the need for sedation in ICU patients: a randomized controlled trial. Minerva Anestesiol 81:1298–1310

Mechanical Ventilation in Obese ICU Patients: From Intubation to Extubation

A. De Jong, G. Chanques, and S. Jaber

Introduction

Obesity has become a worldwide health concern. The prevalence of obese adults in the United States of America has risen significantly over the last decade to 35% [1]. Bariatric surgery and complications associated with bariatric surgery are becoming increasingly frequent [2]. Obese patients represent a specific population in the intensive care unit [3]. Atelectasis formation is increased in obese patients, because of the negative effects of thoracic wall weight and abdominal fat mass on pulmonary compliance, leading to decreased functional residual capacity (FRC) and arterial oxygenation. These atelectases are further exacerbated by a supine position and further worsened after general anesthesia and mechanical ventilation. Atelectases contribute to hypoxemia during mechanical ventilation and after weaning from mechanical ventilation. More importantly, they persist after extubation in the obese patient in comparison with full resolution in non-obese patients [4], leading to pulmonary infections. Moreover, obese patients often present comorbidities, such as obstructive apnea syndrome or obesity hypoventilation syndrome. Obesity is a major risk factor for obstructive apnea syndrome (30 to 70% of subjects with obstructive apnea syndrome are obese). Many complications of respiratory care are directly related to the obstructive apnea syndrome: difficult airway management including difficult mask ventilation, difficult intubation and obstruction of the upper airway. The repetitive occurrence of rapid eye movement (REM) sleep, hypoventilation or obstructive sleep apnea with long-lasting apnea and hypopnea induces a secondary depression of respiratory drive with daytime hypercapnia, leading to obesity hypoventilation syndrome. Obesity hypoventilation syndrome is defined as

A. De Jong · G. Chanques · S. Jaber (✉)
Intensive Care Unit, Anesthesia and Critical Care Department, Saint Eloi Teaching Hospital, University Montpellier 1
80 avenue Augustin Fliche, 34295 Montpellier, Cedex 5, France
INSERM U1046, CNRS UMR 9214
Montpellier, France
e-mail: s-jaber@chu-montpellier.fr

J.-L. Vincent (ed.), *Annual Update in Intensive Care and Emergency Medicine 2017*,
DOI 10.1007/978-3-319-51908-1_23

Table 1 Pathophysiological specificities of the obese patient

1. Lung volume	– Atelectasis in the dependent pulmonary area – ↘ functional residual capacity (FRC) – ↗ intra-abdominal pressure – Diaphragm passively pushed cranially – ↘ thoracic and pulmonary compliance
2. Airway	– ↗ resistances (but normal after normalization to the functional lung volume) – ↗ work of breathing – ↗ risk factors for difficult mask ventilation (age >55 years old, snoring, beard, lack of teeth, obstructive apnea syndrome, associated congenital diseases) and difficult intubation (MACOCHA score: Mallampati III or IV, obstructive apnea syndrome, limited mouth opening, reduced cervical mobility, coma, hypoxemia, operator not trained, associated congenital diseases)
3. Ventilatory control	– ↘ ventilatory response to hypercapnia and hypoxia in case of obesity hypoventilation syndrome – ↗ breath rate
4. Pulmonary circulation	– Post-capillary pulmonary hypertension if associated cardiac dysfunction, pre-capillary if use of toxins (anorectics)
5. Blood gas exchange	– ↗ oxygen consumption – ↗ carbon dioxide production
6. Comorbidities	– Obstructive apnea syndrome – Obesity hypoventilation syndrome

a combination of obesity (body mass index [BMI] $\geq 30\,\text{kg/m}^2$), daytime hypercapnia ($PaCO_2$ >45 mm Hg), and disordered breathing during sleep (after ruling out other disorders that might cause alveolar hypoventilation) [5].

However, while obesity contributes to many diseases and is associated with higher all-cause mortality in the general population [6], obesity and mortality in the intensive care unit (ICU) are inversely associated as shown by meta-analyses [7, 8]. The "obesity paradox" phenomenon has recently become apparent in the ICU [9]. In particular, acute respiratory distress syndrome (ARDS) in obese patients, in whom diaphragmatic function is challenging, has a lower mortality risk when compared with non-obese patients [10, 11].

Obese patients can be admitted in a critical care setting for *de novo* acute respiratory failure, 'acute-on-chronic' respiratory failure with an underlying disease, such as an obesity hypoventilation syndrome, or in the perioperative period. The main challenges for ICU clinicians are to take into account the pulmonary pathophysiological specificities of the obese patient (detailed in Table 1) to optimize airway management and non-invasive or invasive mechanical ventilation.

Physiology

Oxygenation decreases with increase in weight, mostly because oxygen consumption and work of breathing are increased in obese patients [12]. At rest, oxygen consumption is 1.5 times higher in obese patients than in non-obese patients [12]. Obese patients have an excess production of carbon dioxide (CO_2), because of their increased oxygen consumption and increased work of breathing, especially when there is an associated obesity hypoventilation syndrome, including a decreased respiratory drive [13]. In several studies, the spontaneous breath rate was from 15 to 21 breaths per minute in morbidly obese patients ($BMI > 40\,kg/m^2$), whereas it was close to 10 to 12 in non-obese patients [14]. Moreover, abdominal pressure is increased because of increased abdominal and visceral adipose tissue deposition. The capacity of the chest is reduced compared to non-obese individuals, because the diaphragm is passively pushed cranially. Obese patients have decreased pulmonary and thoracic compliance, a reduction in FRC, and an increased work of breathing, compared to non-obese patients [15]. Airway resistance is increased, but not after normalization to the lung volume. The main change remains the decreased FRC, leading to more frequent atelectasis in obese than in non-obese patients after ventilation. Finally, as mentioned earlier, obesity is a major risk factor for obstructive apnea syndrome.

Noninvasive Respiratory Management

Non-invasive Ventilation

Non-invasive ventilation (NIV) may be applied to avoid intubation in obese patients with acute respiratory failure, without delaying intubation if needed. In hypercapnic obese patients, higher positive end-expiratory pressure (PEEP) might be used for longer periods to reduce the hypercapnia level below 50 mmHg [16]. NIV is as efficient in patients with obesity hypoventilation syndrome as in patients with chronic obstructive pulmonary disease (COPD), in case of acute hypercapnic respiratory failure [17].

High-Flow Nasal Cannula Oxygen

High flow nasal cannula oxygen (HFNC) could be particularly interesting in obese patients. HNFC permits continuously humidified and warmed oxygen to be delivered through nasal cannula, with an adjustable fraction of inspired oxygen (FiO_2). The flow administered can reach 60 l/min with 100% FiO_2 [18]. A moderate level of PEEP has been measured with this device [18] when the patient breaths with a closed mouth. In case of hypoxemia, HNFC could be performed between sessions of NIV.

Positioning

Optimization of body position can enhance respiratory function in patients requiring mechanical ventilation. In healthy spontaneously breathing obese subjects, a significant reduction in pulmonary compliance was shown in the supine position [19]. A sitting position should therefore be privilegied in case of respiratory failure.

Airway Management

Pre-oxygenation

Facial Mask

Following pre-oxygenation, there is a reduction in the non-hypoxic apnea time (length of apnea following anesthetic induction during which the patient has no oxygen desaturation) in obese patients [20]. Using classic bag-mask ventilation as a method of pre-oxygenation, desaturation during intubation thus occurs within 3 min on average, sometimes less than one minute in severe obesity. The end-expiratory volume is reduced by 69% after anesthetic induction in the supine position, compared with baseline values [21]. The main cause of this rapid desaturation is the decrease in the FRC.

Non-invasive Ventilation

Using a PEEP of 10 cmH_2O during pre-oxygenation is associated with a reduced atelectasis surface, improved oxygenation and increased time of apnea without hypoxemia by one minute on average [22]. Pre-oxygenation of 5 min with NIV, associating pressure support (PS) and PEEP, permits an exhaled fraction of oxygen (FeO_2) >90% to be reached more quickly [23]. In another study, the use of NIV limited the decrease in pulmonary volume and improved oxygenation compared to conventional pre-oxygenation with a face mask [24]. Continuous positive airway pressure (CPAP) or NIV are therefore the reference pre-oxygenation methods (Fig. 1).

High-flow Nasal Cannula Oxygen

HFNC may also be considered for pre-oxygenation of obese patients, including apneic oxygenation, enabling oxygen to be delivered during the apnea period (Fig. 1). This is particularly important in case of rapid sequence induction (RSI), where the obese patient does not receive oxygen between removal of the NIV mask and adequate positioning of the tracheal tube into the trachea.

Positioning

A sitting position during pre-oxygenation may decrease positional flow limitation and air trapping, limiting atelectasis and increasing oxygen desaturation during the intubation procedure (Fig. 1).

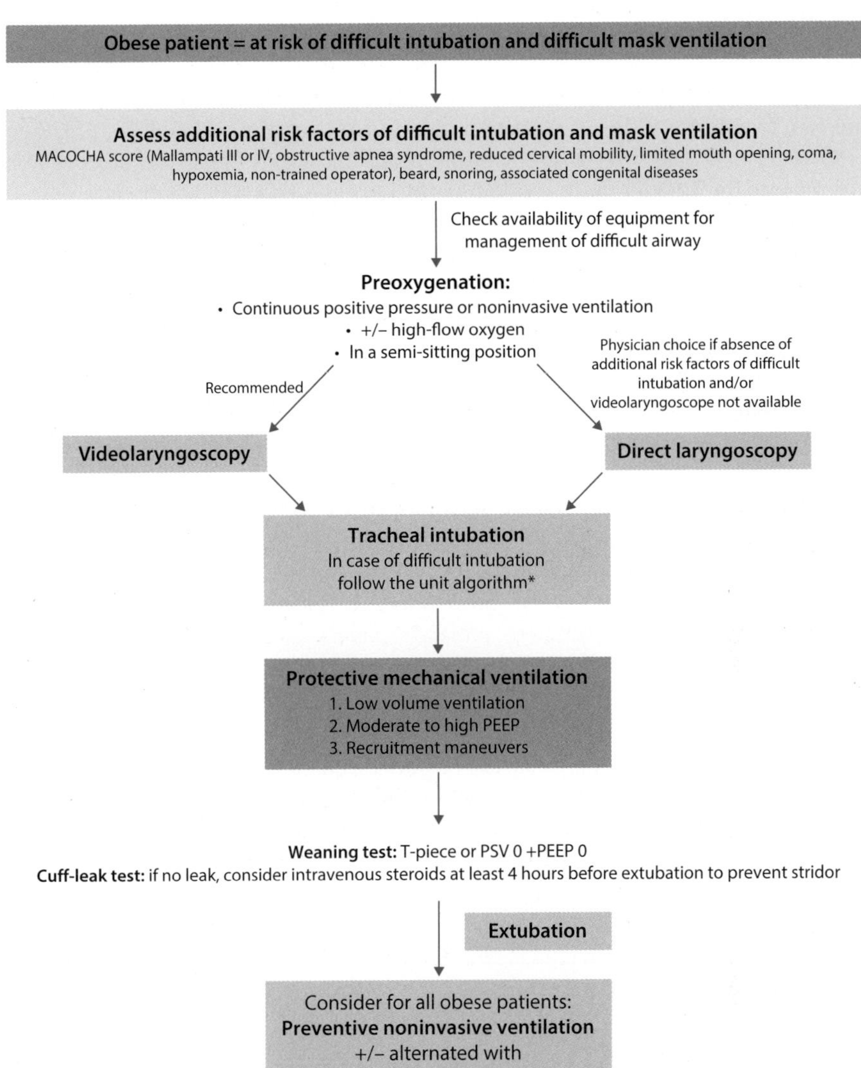

Fig. 1 Suggested airway and ventilation management algorithm in the obese patient in the intensive care unit. During the whole procedure, the patient should be ventilated in case of desaturation <80%. In case of non-adequate ventilation and unsuccessful intubation, emergency non-invasive airway ventilation (supraglottic airway) must be used. *In case of difficult intubation (multiple attempts), follow an intubation airway algorithm nonspecific to obese patients (for example see [50]). *PEEP*: positive end-expiratory pressure; *PSV*: pressure support ventilation

Intubation

Obesity and obstructive apnea syndrome, and *a fortiori* the combination of both, are risk factors for difficult intubation and difficult mask ventilation [3, 25]. Age >55 years old, BMI >26 kg/m^2, snoring, beard and lack of teeth are independent risk factors for difficult mask ventilation. Most of these factors are directly related to obesity. In the same way, tracheal intubation is more difficult in obese patients with obstructive apnea syndrome, with an incidence close to 15 to 20% (versus 2 to 5% in the general population), and associated with the severity of the obstructive apnea syndrome [26]. A recent study reported an increase in the incidence of difficult intubation in obese patients [3]. Moreover, in this study, elevated Mallampati score, limited mouth opening, reduced cervical mobility, presence of an obstructive apnea syndrome, coma and severe hypoxemia (risk factors included in the MACOCHA score [27]) were associated with difficult intubation in obese patients. Each intubation in a morbidly obese patient should be considered as difficult, and adequate preparation following an algorithm for difficult intubation performed (Fig. 1). Videolaryngoscopes are of particular interest in obese patients [28] and their use should be particularly emphasized when additional risk factors for difficult intubation are present.

Extubation

Obese patients are particularly at risk of post-extubation stridor [29]. A cuff-leak test [30] should be systematically performed in these patients, and in case of suspicion of laryngeal edema, prevention of stridor could be performed using a protocol of intravenous steroid administration, at least four hours before extubation, in the absence of contraindications [31].

Mechanical Ventilation

Protective Ventilation

Tidal Volume

In patients with pulmonary lesions, such as ARDS, the benefits of ventilation with low tidal volumes (6 ml/kg) has been widely demonstrated [32]. Since 2010, protective perioperative ventilation has been studied more closely. In the setting of abdominal surgery, the IMPROVE multicenter, randomized, double-blinded study [33], compared an "optimized" strategy of ventilation called "protective ventilation" (tidal volume 6–8 ml/kg of ideal body weight [IBW], PEEP 6–8 cmH_2O, systematic alveolar recruitment maneuvers every 30 min) with a "traditional" strategy called "non-protective ventilation" (tidal volume 10–12 ml/kg of IBW, without PEEP or recruitment maneuvers). The included patients had a moderate risk of postoperative pulmonary complications. Patients with a BMI >40 kg/m^2 were excluded. The main endpoint was a composite criterion including the onset of pulmonary complications (pulmonary infections or need for ventilation) and/or extrapulmonary complications (sepsis, septic shock, death) diagnosed by an observer blinded to the perioperative ventilator settings. Protective ventilation enabled a decrease in the global rate of complications from 27.5% to 10.5% and in the length of hospitalization by two days. In the randomized European PROVHILO study [34] including patients at risk of postoperative pulmonary complications after abdominal surgery, two ventilation strategies were compared. All the patients received a tidal volume of 8 ml/kg of IBW and were randomized into two groups: one group with low PEEP ($\leq 2\,cmH_2O$) without recruitment maneuvers and a group with high PEEP ($12\,cmH_2O$) with recruitment maneuvers. There was no significant difference between the two groups for the main endpoint, which was a composite of postoperative pulmonary complications in the five first days following surgery. There were significantly more cases of hemodynamic failure in the group with high PEEP. These two large randomized studies are complementary: while the first showed the usefulness of protective ventilation to decrease pulmonary and extrapulmonary postoperative complications, the second warns against the hemodynamic dangers of excessively high levels of PEEP for all patients, in particular when high PEEP levels are not associated with low tidal volume.

In obese patients, particularly at risk of atelectasis, the same rules can be applied. In spite of these recommendations, a recent study showed that obese patients were still ventilated in the perioperative period with tidal volumes that were too high [35]. In obese as in non-obese patients, the optimal tidal volume is between 6 to 8 ml/kg of IBW associated with PEEP to avoid atelectasis by alveolar closing (derecruitment). The tidal volume setting must be guided by the patient's height and not by his/her measured weight. The easiest formula for calculation of IBW to remember is the following: IBM (kg) = height (cm) – 100 for a man and height (cm) – 110 for a woman.

Positive End-expiratory Pressure

Given their decreased FRC, obese patients are more sensitive than non-obese patients to atelectasis and lack of PEEP. In several studies specifically performed in obese patients, respiratory mechanics and alveolar recruitment have been shown to be significantly improved by application of PEEP (improvement in compliance and decreased inspiratory resistance), as has gas exchange [36]. Moreover, the PEEP levels used help prevent derecruitment (alveolar closing) due to FRC decrease, but do not open alveoli once they are collapsed. It is consequently better to apply, from the start of mechanical ventilation and during the whole period of ventilation, a PEEP of $10\,cmH_2O$ associated with a tidal volume of 6 to 8 ml/kg of IBW [24, 37]. However, it is necessary to remain on guard and always assess the hemodynamic effects of high PEEP: risk of decreased oxygenation because of an impact on cardiac flow and of hypotension because of compromised venous drainage. In case of auto-PEEP, application of a PEEP will depend on the presence or not of a limitation in expiratory flow because of airway collapse during expiration. If this phenomenon exists, an extrinsic PEEP of 2/3 of the intrinsic PEEP should be applied.

The optimal level of PEEP in obese patients and the best means of titrating PEEP are still unknown. Some obese patients may benefit from higher levels of PEEP than others. Measuring transdiaphragmatic pressure seems crucial to determine the maximum pressure minimizing alveolar damage, taking into account that the plateau pressure is related to both transthoracic and transalveolar pressures.

Recruitment Maneuvers

To open alveoli once they are closed, recruitment maneuvers should be used, transitorily increasing the transpulmonary pressure. The impact of these maneuvers in the obese patient has been shown to improve arterial oxygenation and available lung volume [24].

The best recruitment maneuver has not been determined in the obese patient. Recruitment maneuvers are mandatory to fully reopen the lung after anesthesia induction and a PEEP must be applied to prevent the progressive closing of the lung leading to atelectasis. The optimal level of PEEP during protective ventilation remains to be determined, but many physiological studies suggest that PEEP levels of at least 5 cmH_2O are necessary, in particular in obese patients. Levels of pressure needed to open the alveoli seem to be higher than in the non-obese patient, mostly because of the increased transthoracic pressure. Questions persist regarding the type of recruitment maneuver to recommend. The reference method is an expiratory pause with a PEEP level of 40 cmH_2O during 40 s, but many alternatives exist, including progressive increase in PEEP until 20 cmH_2O with a constant tidal volume within 35 cmH_2O of plateau pressure, or a progressive increase in the tidal volume [38]. These recruitment maneuvers can be performed only if they are hemodynamically well tolerated. The ideal frequency for recruitment maneuvers has still not been determined.

Driving Pressure

Driving pressure is the difference between inspiratory plateau pressure and end-expiratory pressure. The concept of driving pressure assumes that functional lung size is better quantified by compliance than by predicted body weight. This concept explains why ventilator-induced lung injury (VILI), cyclic strain and survival may be better correlated with driving pressure than with tidal volume. Lower levels of driving pressure have been found to be associated with increased survival in ICU patients [39]. The ventilatory setting during mechanical ventilation, especially in obese patients, should be set to minimize driving pressure.

Respiratory Rate

Concerning the setting or respiratory rate, obese patients have an excess production of CO_2, because of their increased oxygen consumption and increased work of breathing, especially when there is an associated obesity hypoventilation syndrome, with a decreased respiratory drive [13]. In four studies, the spontaneous breath rate was from 15 to 21 breaths per minute in morbidly obese patients ($BMI > 40\ kg/m^2$), whereas it was close to 10 to 12 in non-obese patients [14]. Ventilation should, therefore, be adapted, essentially increasing breath rate.

Ventilatory Mode

Which ventilator mode is better in obese patients? The pressure modes deliver a constant pressure in the airway, decreasing the risk of barotrauma, with an insufflating pressure set at less than 30 cmH_2O. In case of increase in airway resistance (bronchospasm, obstructed tube) or decrease in compliance of the respiratory system (obesity, atelectasis, selective intubation, surgical pneumoperitoneum, pneumothorax ...), the tidal volume decreases, leading to hypercapnia acidosis if alveolar ventilation is too low. It is consequently important to carefully check tidal volume, minute ventilation and capnography when using a pressure mode. The use of a volume mode carries the risk of an increase in the insufflation pressure to deliver the required tidal volume (risk of barotrauma), hence the importance of checking the alveolar pressure at the end of inspiration, i. e., the plateau pressure.

In obese patients, some teams recommend the pressure controlled mode because the decelerating flow should allow a better distribution of the flow in the alveoli. However, studies comparing the two ventilatory modes report contradictory data: discordances can be explained by the different inclusion criteria and the methodological limitations of the studies [40]. In practice, the advantages and inconveniences of each mode must be known and the ventilatory mode that the physician prefers used.

Pressure support ventilation (PSV) seems very interesting in obese patients. In obese piglets, it was shown that PSV improved oxygenation and decreased inflammation [41]. In the obese patient, postoperative pulmonary complications were decreased by the use of PSV compared to pressure controlled ventilation [42]. In anesthesia as in the ICU, in obese ventilated patients, the scientific evidence is still weak and future studies are necessary to compare PSV, new ventilatory modes, such as neurally-adjusted ventilatory assist (NAVA), adaptive support ventilation (ASV), and proportional assist ventilation (PAV), with conventional pressure or volume controlled modes.

Positioning

In the supine position, positional flow limitation and air trapping impedes respiratory management particularly in obese patients [43]. A sitting position during mechanical ventilation is therefore advised. Prone positioning in obese ARDS patients enables an improvement in the partial arterial pressure of oxygen (PaO_2)/FiO_2 ratio more than in the non-obese patient, and is not associated with more complications [10].

Weaning from Mechanical Ventilation

A recent physiological study specifically investigated the inspiratory effort during weaning of mechanical ventilation in a population of critically ill, morbidly obese patients [44]. The main result of this study was that for obese patients, T-piece and PSV 0 + PEEP 0 cmH_2O weaning tests were the tests that best predicted post-extubation inspiratory effort and work of breathing ([44]; Fig. 1). Following extubation, positive protective ventilation should be pursued, both in the ICU and in the recovery room. Postoperative CPAP or NIV might be extended to all obese patients, even those without obstructive apnea syndrome.

Specific Settings

Acute-on-chronic Respiratory Failure

Prevention of relapses of acute-on-chronic respiratory failure are essential and should be ensured by the intensivist. Positive airway pressure therapies can be implemented in the ICU and continued at home, with the support of home therapists. Sleep-related breathing disorders, including obesity hypoventilation syndrome, should be followed by a specialist after ICU discharge, ideally in the setting of a multidisciplinary obesity team.

Perioperative Management

In obese patients with obstructive apnea syndrome, nocturnal CPAP should be initiated before surgery, especially if the apnea hypopnea index (AHI) is more than 30 events per hour or if there is severe cardiovascular comorbidity. If CPAP or NIV were used prior to surgery, they should be pursued throughout the perioperative period, including the postoperative period.

The risk factors for postoperative respiratory failure include the severity of obstructive apnea syndrome, the intravenous administration of opioids, the use of sedatives, the site (close to the diaphragm) and the invasive nature of the surgical procedure, and the apnea onset during paradoxical sleep on the third or fourth postoperative day.

Some postoperative interventions that can decrease the risk of respiratory failure are a postoperative analgesia strategy sparing opioids, oxygenation by CPAP or NIV, careful patient positioning and monitoring. CPAP or NIV must be resumed in the recovery room [45]. Compliance to CPAP or NIV will be better if the patients bring their own equipment to the hospital. In case of frequent or severe hypoxemias, start of CPAP or NIV should not be delayed. If possible, the supine position should be avoided in patients with an obstructive apnea syndrome at risk of postoperative pulmonary complications, and a sitting position adopted. The prophylactic application of NIV after extubation decreases the risk of acute respiratory failure by 16% and reduces length of stay [45]. Moreover, in obese hypercapnic patients, the use of NIV following extubation is associated with decreased mortality [46]. A randomized controlled trial performed in morbidly obese patients after bariatric surgery reported an improvement in ventilatory function when CPAP was immediately implemented after extubation compared to CPAP started 30 min following extubation [47]. Hence, NIV associating pressure support and PEEP or CPAP alone must be used liberally in the postoperative period, in order to reduce the aggravation of atelectasis, a long period of oxygen dependence and consequently the patients' length of stay in the post-surgical unit and in the hospital [45]. Among patients with hypoxemic respiratory failure following abdominal surgery, use of NIV compared with standard oxygen therapy reduced the risk of tracheal reintubation within 7 days [48]. These findings support the use of NIV in this setting.

Oxygen supplementation should be administered continuously to all patients with obstructive apnea syndrome at increased perioperative risk until they are able to maintain their baseline oxygen saturation on ambient air; oxygen saturations should be monitored after leaving the recovery room [49].

Respiratory physiotherapy and patient education of exercises, such as incentive spirometry or high volume respiration, also limit the reduction in lung volume induced by surgery.

Conclusion

Obese patients admitted to the ICU are at risk of atelectasis, which is associated with pulmonary complications. NIV can be safely and efficiently used to prevent and/or treat acute respiratory failure, without delaying intubation if needed. HNFC enable continuously humidified and warmed oxygen to be delivered through nasal cannula, with an adjustable FiO_2, with a flow reaching 60 l/min and providing a moderate level of PEEP. Because of the increased incidence of difficult mask ventilation and intubation in obese patients, a protocol of difficult airway-management should be systematically applied to prevent the complications related to the intubation-procedure (severe hypoxemia, arterial hypotension and cardiac arrest). Pre-oxygenation should be optimized using positive-pressure ventilation (CPAP or NIV) in a semi-sitting position, eventually added to apneic oxygenation using HFNC in the more severely obese patients. After tracheal intubation, to avoid both baro-volutrauma and atelecto-biotrauma, association of low tidal volume, moderate to high PEEP and recruitment maneuvers (lung protective ventilation) should be applied. The height of the lung being correlated to the height of the patient, tidal volume should be set according to IBW and not actual body weight, between 6 and 8 ml/kg IBW. In patients with ARDS, prone position is a safe procedure which permits respiratory mechanic improvements and oxygenation. Obstructive-apnea syndrome and obesity-hypoventilation syndrome should be investigated to introduce appropriate treatment, including implementation of positive airway pressure at home.

References

1. NCD Risk Factor Collaboration (NCD-RisC) (2016) Trends in adult body-mass index in 200 countries from 1975 to 2014: a pooled analysis of 1698 population-based measurement studies with 19.2 million participants. Lancet 387:1377–1396
2. Montravers P, Ribeiro-Parenti L, Welsch C (2015) What's new in postoperative intensive care after bariatric surgery? Intensive Care Med 41:1114–1117
3. De Jong A, Molinari N, Pouzeratte Y et al (2015) Difficult intubation in obese patients: incidence, risk factors, and complications in the operating theatre and in intensive care units. Br J Anaesth 114:297–306
4. Eichenberger A, Proietti S, Wicky S et al (2002) Morbid obesity and postoperative pulmonary atelectasis: an underestimated problem. Anesth Analg 95:1788–1792
5. Pepin JL, Timsit JF, Tamisier R, Borel JC, Levy P, Jaber S (2016) Prevention and care of respiratory failure in obese patients. Lancet Respir Med 4:407–418
6. Flegal KM, Kit BK, Orpana H, Graubard BI (2013) Association of all-cause mortality with overweight and obesity using standard body mass index categories: a systematic review and meta-analysis. JAMA 309:71–82
7. Hogue CW, Stearns JD, Colantuoni E et al (2009) The impact of obesity on outcomes after critical illness: a meta-analysis. Intensive Care Med 35:1152–1170
8. Akinnusi ME, Pineda LA, El Solh AA (2008) Effect of obesity on intensive care morbidity and mortality: a meta-analysis. Crit Care Med 36:151–158
9. De Jong A, Jung B, Chanques G, Jaber S, Molinari N (2012) Obesity and mortality in critically ill patients: another case of the simpson paradox? Chest 141:1637–1638
10. De Jong A, Molinari N, Sebbane M et al (2013) Feasibility and effectiveness of prone position in morbidly obese patients with ARDS: A case-control clinical study. Chest 143:1554–1561
11. O'Brien JM Jr, Philips GS, Ali NA, Aberegg SK, Marsh CB, Lemeshow S (2012) The association between body mass index, processes of care, and outcomes from mechanical ventilation: a prospective cohort study. Crit Care Med 40:1456–1463
12. Kress JP, Pohlman AS, Alverdy J, Hall JB (1999) The impact of morbid obesity on oxygen cost of breathing (VO(2RESP)) at rest. Am J Respir Crit Care Med 160:883–886
13. Pepin J, Borel JC, Janssens JP (2012) Obesity hypoventilation syndrome: an underdiagnosed and undertreated condition. Am J Respir Crit Care Med 186:1205–1207
14. Chlif M, Keochkerian D, Choquet D, Vaidie A, Ahmaidi S (2009) Effects of obesity on breathing pattern, ventilatory neural drive and mechanics. Respir Physiol Neurobiol 168:198–202
15. Pelosi P, Croci M, Ravagnan I, Vicardi P, Gattinoni L (1996) Total respiratory system, lung, and chest wall mechanics in sedated-paralyzed postoperative morbidly obese patients. Chest 109:144–151
16. Gursel G, Aydogdu M, Gulbas G, Ozkaya S, Tasyurek S, Yildirim F (2011) The influence of severe obesity on non-invasive ventilation (NIV) strategies and responses in patients with acute hypercapnic respiratory failure attacks in the ICU. Minerva Anestesiol 77:17–25
17. Carrillo A, Ferrer M, Gonzalez-Diaz G et al (2012) Noninvasive ventilation in acute hypercapnic respiratory failure caused by obesity hypoventilation syndrome and chronic obstructive pulmonary disease. Am J Respir Crit Care Med 186:1279–1285
18. Chanques G, Riboulet F, Molinari N et al (2013) Comparison of three high flow oxygen therapy delivery devices: a clinical physiological cross-over study. Minerva Anestesiol 79:1344–1355
19. Naimark A, Cherniack RM (1960) Compliance of the respiratory system and its components in health and obesity. J Appl Physiol 15:377–382
20. De Jong A, Futier E, Millot A et al (2014) How to preoxygenate in operative room: Healthy subjects and situations "at risk". Ann Fr Anesth Reanim 33:457–461
21. Futier E, Constantin JM, Petit A et al (2010) Positive end-expiratory pressure improves end-expiratory lung volume but not oxygenation after induction of anaesthesia. Eur J Anaesthesiol 27:508–513

22. Gander S, Frascarolo P, Suter M, Spahn DR, Magnusson L (2005) Positive end-expiratory pressure during induction of general anesthesia increases duration of nonhypoxic apnea in morbidly obese patients. Anesth Analg 100:580–584
23. Delay JM, Sebbane M, Jung B et al (2008) The effectiveness of noninvasive positive pressure ventilation to enhance preoxygenation in morbidly obese patients: a randomized controlled study. Anesth Analg 107:1707–1713
24. Futier E, Constantin JM, Pelosi P et al (2011) Noninvasive ventilation and alveolar recruitment maneuver improve respiratory function during and after intubation of morbidly obese patients: a randomized controlled study. Anesthesiology 114:1354–1363
25. Langeron O, Masso E, Huraux C et al (2000) Prediction of difficult mask ventilation. Anesthesiology 92:1229–1236
26. Siyam MA, Benhamou D (2002) Difficult endotracheal intubation in patients with sleep apnea syndrome. Anesth Analg 95:1098–1102
27. De Jong A, Molinari N, Terzi N et al (2013) Early identification of patients at risk for difficult intubation in the intensive care unit: development and validation of the MACOCHA score in a multicenter cohort study. Am J Respir Crit Care Med 187:832–839
28. Andersen LH, Rovsing L, Olsen KS (2011) GlideScope videolaryngoscope vs. Macintosh direct laryngoscope for intubation of morbidly obese patients: a randomized trial. Acta Anaesthesiol Scand 55:1090–1097
29. Frat JP, Gissot V, Ragot S et al (2008) Impact of obesity in mechanically ventilated patients: a prospective study. Intensive Care Med 34:1991–1998
30. Jaber S, Chanques G, Matecki S et al (2003) Post-extubation stridor in intensive care unit patients. Risk factors evaluation and importance of the cuff-leak test. Intensive Care Med 29:69–74
31. Jaber S, Jung B, Chanques G, Bonnet F, Marret E (2009) Effects of steroids on reintubation and post-extubation stridor in adults: meta-analysis of randomised controlled trials. Crit Care 13:R49
32. Petrucci N, De Feo C (2013) Lung protective ventilation strategy for the acute respiratory distress syndrome. Cochrane Database Syst Rev CD003844
33. Futier E, Constantin JM, Paugam-Burtz C et al (2013) A trial of intraoperative low-tidal-volume ventilation in abdominal surgery. N Engl J Med 369:428–437
34. Hemmes SN, Gama de Abreu M, Pelosi P, Schultz MJ (2014) High versus low positive end-expiratory pressure during general anaesthesia for open abdominal surgery (PROVHILO trial): a multicentre randomised controlled trial. Lancet 384:495–503
35. Jaber S, Coisel Y, Chanques G et al (2012) A multicentre observational study of intra-operative ventilatory management during general anaesthesia: tidal volumes and relation to body weight. Anaesthesia 67:999–1008
36. Pelosi P, Croci M, Ravagnan I et al (1997) Respiratory system mechanics in sedated, paralyzed, morbidly obese patients. J Appl Physiol 82:811–818
37. Talab HF, Zabani IA, Abdelrahman HS et al (2009) Intraoperative ventilatory strategies for prevention of pulmonary atelectasis in obese patients undergoing laparoscopic bariatric surgery. Anesth Analg 109:1511–1516
38. Constantin JM, Jaber S, Futier E et al (2008) Respiratory effects of different recruitment maneuvers in acute respiratory distress syndrome. Crit Care 12:R50
39. Amato MB, Meade MO, Slutsky AS et al (2015) Driving pressure and survival in the acute respiratory distress syndrome. N Engl J Med 372:747–755
40. Aldenkortt M, Lysakowski C, Elia N, Brochard L, Tramer MR (2012) Ventilation strategies in obese patients undergoing surgery: a quantitative systematic review and meta-analysis. Br J Anaesth 109:493–502
41. Spieth PM, Carvalho AR, Güldner A et al (2011) Pressure support improves oxygenation and lung protection compared to pressure-controlled ventilation and is further improved by random variation of pressure support. Crit Care Med 39:746–755

42. Zoremba M, Kalmus G, Dette F, Kuhn C, Wulf H (2010) Effect of intra-operative pressure support vs pressure controlled ventilation on oxygenation and lung function in moderately obese adults. Anaesthesia 65:124–129
43. Lemyze M, Mallat J, Duhamel A et al (2013) Effects of sitting position and applied positive end-expiratory pressure on respiratory mechanics of critically ill obese patients receiving mechanical ventilation. Crit Care Med 41:2592–2599
44. Mahul M, Jung B, Galia F et al (2016) Spontaneous breathing trial and post-extubation work of breathing in morbidly obese critically ill patients. Crit Care 20:346
45. Jaber S, Chanques G, Jung B (2010) Postoperative noninvasive ventilation. Anesthesiology 112:453–461
46. El-Solh AA, Aquilina A, Pineda L, Dhanvantri V, Grant B, Bouquin P (2006) Noninvasive ventilation for prevention of post-extubation respiratory failure in obese patients. Eur Respir J 28:588–595
47. Neligan PJ, Malhotra G, Fraser M et al (2009) Continuous positive airway pressure via the Boussignac system immediately after extubation improves lung function in morbidly obese patients with obstructive sleep apnea undergoing laparoscopic bariatric surgery. Anesthesiology 110:878–884
48. Jaber S, Lescot T, Futier E et al (2016) Effect of noninvasive ventilation on tracheal reintubation among patients with hypoxemic respiratory failure following abdominal surgery: a randomized clinical trial. JAMA 315:1345–1353
49. Bolden N, Smith CE, Auckley D, Makarski J, Avula R (2007) Perioperative complications during use of an obstructive sleep apnea protocol following surgery and anesthesia. Anesth Analg 105:1869–1870
50. De Jong A, Jung B, Jaber S (2014) Intubation in the ICU: we could improve our practice. Crit Care 18:209

Novel Insights in ICU-Acquired Respiratory Muscle Dysfunction: Implications for Clinical Care

A. Jonkman, D. Jansen, and L. M. A. Heunks

Introduction

The respiratory muscles drive ventilation. Under normal conditions, the diaphragm is the main muscle for inspiration, whereas expiration is largely passive, driven by relaxation of the inspiratory muscles and elastic recoil pressure of the lung. A disturbance in the balance between capacity and loading of the inspiratory muscles will result in respiratory failure. This may occur in the course of numerous disorders that increase loading of the diaphragm, such as pneumonia, acute respiratory distress syndrome (ARDS), acute exacerbation of chronic obstructive pulmonary disease (COPD) and trauma. On the other hand, capacity of the respiratory muscles may be impaired due to congenital myopathies or acquired muscle dysfunction (e. g., in COPD or cancer cachexia). Mechanical ventilation can partially or completely unload the respiratory muscles. Despite being life-saving, studies published in the last decade have demonstrated that respiratory muscle function may further deteriorate in ventilator bound intensive care unit (ICU) patients. Respiratory muscle weakness in ventilated ICU patients is associated with prolonged duration of ventilator weaning [1] and increased risk of ICU and hospital readmission [2]. Therefore, it seems of crucial importance to limit the detrimental effects of critical illness, and in particular mechanical ventilation, on the respiratory muscles. The aim of this chapter is to describe recent insights into the pathophysiology of diaphragm dysfunction in ICU patients and how these new findings may affect clinical care for our patients. We will focus on studies performed in humans.

A. Jonkman · L. M. A. Heunks (✉)
Department of Intensive Care Medicine, VU University Medical Center
1007 MB Amsterdam, Netherlands
e-mail: l.heunks@vumc.nl

D. Jansen
Department of Anesthesiology, Radboudumc
Nijmegen, Netherlands

J.-L. Vincent (ed.), *Annual Update in Intensive Care and Emergency Medicine 2017*,
DOI 10.1007/978-3-319-51908-1_24

Effects of Critical Illness on Diaphragm Structure and Function

Effects of Critical Illness on Diaphragm Structure

Less than a decade ago, Levine et al. were the first to describe a rapid loss of diaphragm muscle mass in patients on controlled mechanical ventilation [3]. Biopsies were obtained from 14 brain-dead organ donors on controlled mechanical ventilation for 18 to 69 h before organ harvest. The cross-sectional area (CSA) of diaphragm fibers was significantly lower (53% and 57% for fast- and slow-twitch fibers respectively) compared to fibers obtained from patients referred for elective lung cancer surgery. Interestingly, the severity of atrophy was less pronounced in the pectoralis muscle, indicating that the diaphragm is much more sensitive to the effects of disuse. In subsequent studies, it was demonstrated that the decrease in diaphragm fiber CSA was proportional to the duration of mechanical ventilation (Pearson $r^2 = 0.28$) [4]. Diaphragm inactivity was associated with oxidative stress, active caspase-3 expression and upregulation of mRNAs coding for ligands related to the proteolytic ubiquitin-proteasome pathway (muscle atrophy F-box [MAFBx] and muscle ring finger 1 [MuRF-1]). In addition, activation of the lysosomal-autophagy pathway was demonstrated in the diaphragm of these brain-dead patients ventilated for ±60 h [5]. Very recently, Matecki et al. demonstrated increased oxidation, nitrosylation and phosphorylation of the diaphragm sarcoplasmic reticulum ryanodine calcium release channel in ventilated brain-dead patients [6]. These molecular modifications were associated with enhanced calcium leak from the channel (increased open probability). Additional experiments in mice indicated that leaky ryanodine channels are associated with diaphragm weakness.

Collectively, these data demonstrate that inactivity of the diaphragm under controlled mechanical ventilation is associated with rapid posttranslational protein modifications, activation of proteolytic pathways and muscle fiber atrophy. However, these early studies used biopsies of the diaphragm of brain-dead patients. This might be an excellent model for diaphragm disuse associated with mechanical ventilation, but differences in treatment and underlying pathophysiology in more representative ICU patients should be recognized. Hooijman et al. were the first to study structural, biochemical and functional modifications of biopsies obtained from the diaphragm of ventilated ICU patients (n = 22, mean duration on the ventilator: 7 days, range 14 to 607 h) [7]. These authors found that both fast- and slow-twitch diaphragm fibers had a CSA that was approximately 25% smaller than that of fibers from the diaphragm of patients referred for elective surgery. Biochemical analysis revealed activation of the proteolytic ubiquitin-proteasome pathway. Histological analysis demonstrated that the number of inflammatory cells, including neutrophils and macrophages, was significantly increased in the diaphragm of ICU patients; this supports a role for inflammatory mediators in the development of atrophy or injury. Interestingly, van Hees et al. demonstrated that plasma from septic shock patients, but not from healthy subjects, induced atrophy in (healthy) cultured skeletal muscle myotubes [8]. This indicates that plasma from septic shock patients contains molecules with catabolic properties. Additional experiments presented in that paper suggest that interleukin (IL)-6 plays a role in the development of muscle atrophy in sepsis.

Effect of Critical Illness on Diaphragm Function

Structural modifications of the respiratory muscles as described above may have functional implications. Single muscle fibers isolated from the diaphragm provide an excellent model to study contractile protein function. The force generated by single fibers from the diaphragm of ICU patients was significantly reduced compared to fibers from non-ICU patients [7]. Reduction in force resulted from loss of contractile proteins (atrophy) and contractile protein dysfunction.

The gold standard to evaluate *in vivo* diaphragm contractile function in ventilated patients is to assess the change in endotracheal tube pressure induced by magnetic stimulation of the phrenic nerves during airway occlusion (Ptr,magn). The major advantage of this technique is that it can be performed at the bedside and does not require patient cooperation. Demoule et al. measured Ptr,magn within 24 h of mechanical ventilation in a population of 85 critically ill patients [9]. Of this group, 54 (64%) patients were diagnosed with diaphragm dysfunction defined as a Ptr,magn $< 11\ cmH_2O$. More recently, the same investigators confirmed these earlier findings in 43 ventilated patients [10]; 23 (53%) of these patients exhibited diaphragm dysfunction at ICU admission. These are important findings, as they indicate that other factors besides disuse play a role in the pathophysiology of respiratory muscle weakness in ICU patients. In fact, in their earlier study [9], the authors reported that diaphragm dysfunction was independently associated with sepsis. Consistent with that study, Supinski et al. [11] found that measures for *in vivo* contractile force were affected more in ventilated patients with infection than in ventilated patients without infection.

In a follow up study, Jaber et al. measured Ptr,magn every 24 to 36 h in ICU patients (n = 6) ventilated for > 5 days [4]. Ptr,magn rapidly declined by approximately 30% in the first 5 to 6 days of controlled mechanical ventilation. The recent study by Demoule et al. [10] also assessed Ptr,magn during the ICU stay. In that study, 61% of patients fulfilling criteria for diaphragm dysfunction at admission had persistent respiratory muscle weakness while in the ICU. Of the patients with normal diaphragm function at ICU admission, 55% developed weakness while on the ventilator. This study demonstrates that 80% of all patients fulfilling their inclusion criteria (i. e., > 5 days on mechanical ventilation), develop respiratory muscle weakness at some time while on the ventilator.

Goligher et al. described the evolution of diaphragmatic thickness during mechanical ventilation and its impact on diaphragm function, assessed with ultrasound [12]. Changes in diaphragm thickness were found in 56% of the study population (n = 128). Both loss and gain of diaphragm thickness were observed during the first week of ventilation, in 44% and 12% of the patients, respectively. Contractile activity of the diaphragm was estimated as the diaphragm thickening fraction during maximal inspiratory effort. There was a significant correlation between the mean diaphragm thickening fraction during the first 3 days of ventilation and changes in diaphragm thickness ($p = 0.01$): a loss of diaphragm muscle mass was associated with lower contractile activity, while higher contractile activity was found for patients exhibiting increases in diaphragm thickness. Both increased and decreased diaphragm thickness seemed to be modulated by the intensity of respiratory muscle work performed by the patient, because the change in diaphragm thickness was inversely correlated with the driving pressure applied by the ventilator over the first 72 h of ventilation ($p = 0.04$, after removal of one outlier).

In conclusion, in the last decade our knowledge of the effects of critical illness and mechanical ventilation on respiratory muscle function has markedly improved. We have gained more insight into the pathophysiology, including molecular pathways, associated with dysfunction. In addition, it appears that the most important clinical risk factors for development of dysfunction include disuse and inflammation/sepsis.

Clinical Implications of Current Knowledge

Monitoring Diaphragm Function in the ICU

As described above, disuse is proposed to be an important risk factor for the development of atrophy and dysfunction of the diaphragm in ventilated patients. Therefore, a reasonable clinical goal is to limit the duration of respiratory muscle inactivity by using partially assisted modes, such as pressure support ventilation as soon as feasible and safe (fulfilling criteria for lung-protective ventilation). It should be recognized that even in partially assisted modes, full unloading of the diaphragm may occur ([13]; Fig. 1). Moreover, this study demonstrated that clinicians are often unable to recognize diaphragm inactivity based on pressure and flow signals on the ventilator screen. Therefore, there may be a role for more advanced respiratory muscle monitoring techniques [14, 15]. Recently, we reviewed clinically available methods to monitor respiratory muscle function in ventilated ICU patients [14].

Today, the state of the art technique for monitoring diaphragm activity is assessment of the transdiaphragmatic pressure (Pdi). This can be estimated by simultaneous measurement of esophageal pressure (Pes) and gastric pressure (Pga) as surrogates for the pleural and abdominal pressures, respectively. Recently, recommendations for the use of Pes monitoring in ICU patients were published [16, 17]. Although no reference values for Pdi are available for critically ill patients, monitoring will prevent unwanted periods of diaphragm inactivity due to over-assist in partially supported modes. In addition, Pes monitoring enables the clinician to detect patient-ventilator asynchronies.

Binding of acetylcholine to the skeletal muscle acetylcholine receptor will result in depolarization of the plasma membrane, which in turn opens calcium release channels that activate contractile proteins, resulting in the generation of force. Depolarization of the plasma membranes can be visualized by electromyography

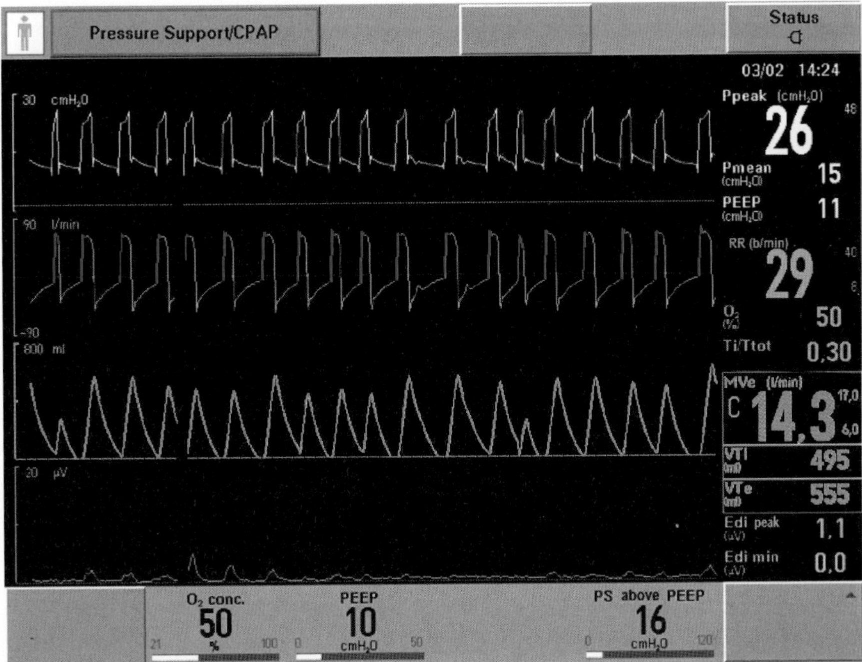

Fig. 1 Ventilator screen of a patient in pressure support mode. Despite the fact that this patient was in a partial assist mode, the diaphragm was inactive as demonstrated by the absence of diaphragm electrical activity (lower tracing). Technical issues for absence of diaphragm electrical activity were excluded

(EMG). Recently, continuous monitoring of diaphragm electrical activity (EAdi) has become available for ICU patients. Neurally-adjusted ventilator assist (NAVA) is a relatively new mode for partially assisted ventilation that uses EAdi to control the ventilator. EAdi is acquired using a dedicated nasogastric feeding tube with nine electrodes positioned at the level of the diaphragm muscle. The electrical activity is shown real-time on the ventilator screen (Servo-i/U, Maquet Sweden), even when the patient is ventilated in another mode than NAVA. Therefore, EAdi may be an alternative to esophageal and gastric balloons to monitor diaphragm activity (Fig. 2). Indeed, absence of EAdi is consistent with inactivity of the diaphragm, when technical issues have been excluded. However, conversion of EAdi (in microvolt) into pressure has not yet been well validated. Bellani et al. proposed a proportionality coefficient (pressure-electrical activity index, PEi) that allows calculation of pressure generated by the diaphragm from EAdi [18]. Another index derived from the EAdi is the patient-ventilator breath contribution (PVBC) index, which provides an estimation of the fraction of breathing effort that is generated by the patient compared to the total work of breathing (ventilator + patient). Liu et al. demonstrated in 12 patients ventilated using the NAVA mode that PVBC predicts the contribution of the inspiratory muscles versus the pressure delivered by the ventilator [19]. Al-

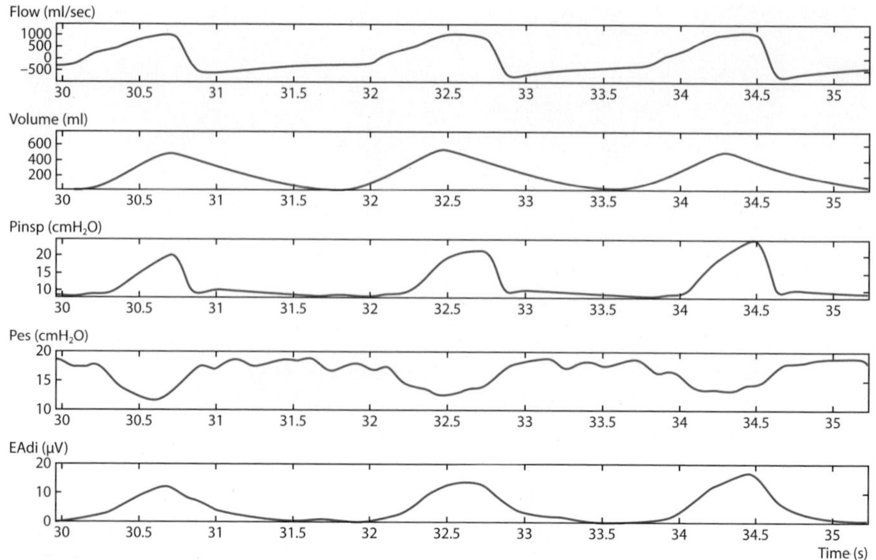

Fig. 2 Physiological tracings of a patient ventilated in partially assisted mode. The electrical activity of the diaphragm (EAdi, lower tracing) reflects inspiratory effort, as shown by a decrease in esophageal pressure (Pes)

though both PEi and PVBC may be helpful to limit the risk of ventilator over-assist, additional studies are required before clinical implementation is justified.

Strategies to Prevent Diaphragm Dysfunction

Although respiratory muscle weakness may already be present at ICU admission [9], many patients develop weakness while in the ICU [10]. Sepsis is a recognized risk factor for development of respiratory muscle weakness [10], but apart from appropriate treatment of sepsis, no specific interventions can be applied to protect the respiratory muscles. Certain drugs have been associated with the development of respiratory muscle weakness, in particular corticosteroids and neuromuscular blockers. The effect of both drugs, together or separately, on muscle dysfunction is complex and beyond the scope of this paper. We refer to an excellent recent review on this subject [20]. However, it should be noticed that short periods (48 h) of full neuromuscular blockade are not associated with the development of clinically relevant respiratory muscle weakness, because ARDS patients treated with a neuromuscular blocker were liberated faster from mechanical ventilation than patients in a placebo group [21].

As discussed earlier, inactivity appears to be an important risk factor for the development of respiratory muscle dysfunction. No clinical studies have compared the effects of controlled and partially supported modes on the development of respiratory muscle dysfunction in humans. Sassoon et al. [22] investigated the effect of controlled mechanical ventilation or partially supported modes of mechanical ventilation on diaphragm force-velocity relationships *in vitro* in rabbits. The loss of diaphragmatic force-generating capacity was significantly less in rabbits on partially supported modes compared to those receiving controlled mechanical ventilation. Despite the absence of evidence in humans, from a physiological perspective it is reasonable to apply partially assisted ventilator modes when feasible and safe. Recently, it was demonstrated that assisted ventilation in patients with mild-to-moderate ARDS improved patient-ventilator interaction and preserved respiratory variability, while maintaining lung-protective ventilation in terms of tidal volume and lung-distending pressure [23].

Nevertheless, in some critically ill patients admitted to the ICU partially assisted modes are not feasible, for instance due to very high respiratory drive. In these patients, high levels of sedation may be required, resulting in full unloading of the respiratory muscles. An interesting hypothesis is that in these patients electrical activation of the muscles ('pacing') may limit development of dysfunction. Pavlovic and Wendt were the first to hypothesize that electrical pacing of the diaphragm may prevent disuse atrophy and contractile dysfunction in mechanically ventilated patients [24]. This hypothesis was based on evidence that electrical pacing of limb skeletal muscle is an effective therapy to maintain muscle activity without patient cooperation. For example, multiple studies have shown that non-invasive pacing of the quadriceps in COPD patients improves muscle performance and exercise capacity [25–27]. Based on the effectiveness of these studies, there is a growing interest for pacing the respiratory muscles in the critically ill ventilated patient.

Today, the major clinical application of non-invasive pacing of the phrenic nerve has been as a diagnostic tool, using brief transcutaneous stimuli at the neck for the evaluation of phrenic nerve conduction time, diaphragm contractility and fatigue [28, 29]. However, this method is not feasible for therapeutic purposes, because prolonged transcutaneous pacing is uncomfortable for patients and correct positioning of the stimulator (coil) is cumbersome in an ICU setting because of its selectiveness: minor changes in the location of the stimulus can result in submaximal activation of the phrenic nerve and co-activation of other anatomically related nerves.

Although there is no clinical evidence for therapeutic pacing to reduce diaphragm atrophy and dysfunction during mechanical ventilation, a few studies have been conducted. A very novel technique, using transvenous phrenic nerve pacing, has been investigated recently [30]. To activate the phrenic nerves bilaterally, a pacing catheter is introduced in the left subclavian vein and advanced into the superior vena cava. The preclinical study in mechanically ventilated pigs showed that loss of diaphragm muscle mass was attenuated in pigs subjected to phrenic nerve pacing. Future studies should evaluate the feasibility of this device in humans.

Strategies to Restore Respiratory Muscle Dysfunction

ICU-acquired respiratory muscle weakness may prolong duration of mechanical ventilation. Therefore, in difficult-to-wean patients, strategies that improve respiratory muscle strength are of potential clinical importance. Surprisingly, very few studies have evaluated strategies to enhance respiratory muscle function in these patients. We will discuss the role of inspiratory muscle training and pharmacological interventions.

Inspiratory Muscle Training

We have recently discussed the rationale for inspiratory muscle training in ICU patients [31]. Briefly, few studies have evaluated the effects of inspiratory muscle training in ICU patients. In the largest trial [32], 69 patients admitted to a long-term weaning facility were randomized to inspiratory muscle strength training or sham training. In both groups, endurance training was accomplished by progressive spontaneous breathing trials. Inspiratory muscle strength training significantly improved inspiratory muscle strength and facilitated weaning from the ventilator. Importantly, no adverse effects of inspiratory strength training were reported.

Inspiratory muscle weakness after extubation is associated with increased risk of ICU and hospital readmission within 6 weeks after ICU discharge [2]. Therefore, the recently published trial by Bissett and colleagues [33], in which 70 ICU patients ventilated for >7 days were randomized to inspiratory muscle strength training or usual care after successful extubation (>48 h), is of particular relevance. Training was performed five days/week for two weeks. The primary endpoint, respiratory muscle strength, was significantly improved in the training group (training: 17% versus control: 6%, $p=0.02$), but this did not result in clinical benefits, such as length of stay or risk of readmission.

In conclusion, based on these preliminary studies, inspiratory muscle strength training appears to be effective in enhancing inspiratory muscle strength and is safe in ICU patients. Future studies are required to determine the optimal moment to start inspiratory muscle training (early versus late in ICU admission) and to investigate the optimal training protocol.

Pharmacotherapy

In contrast to cardiac muscle dysfunction, surprisingly no drug is approved to improve respiratory muscle function. We briefly discuss the role of anabolic hormones and of the cardiac inotrope, levosimendan. For more extensive discussion we refer to an earlier review by our group [31].

Anabolic steroids increase bodyweight, fat-free mass and muscle strength in healthy people [34]. Although many clinical trials have assessed the effects of anabolic steroids in patients with chronic diseases, they do not have sufficient statistical power for clinically relevant endpoints. Pan et al. [35] conducted a meta-analysis and selected eight randomized controlled trials investigating the effects of anabolic steroids in patients with COPD. They concluded that anabolic steroids improve fat-free mass and quality of life, but do not influence inspiratory muscle strength, although some high quality studies did demonstrate that anabolic hormones improved inspiratory muscle strength when administered during a rehabilitation program [36]. No randomized studies have been performed in weak difficult-to-wean ICU patients. Notably, Takala et al. reported that early administration of growth hormone increased mortality in ICU patients [37]. In conclusion, anabolic hormones should not be routinely used in ICU patients to enhance muscle strength. Whether they may have a role for difficult-to-wean patients with severe respiratory muscle weakness remains to be investigated.

Levosimendan is a relatively novel cardiac inotrope, which enhances the binding of calcium to troponin and improves contractile efficiency of the muscle fibers. It is approved for the treatment of heart failure, but exerts effects in other organs as well [38]. Levosimendan has been shown to enhance contractile efficiency of muscle fibers isolated from the diaphragm of healthy subjects and patients with COPD [39]. Doorduin et al. demonstrated in healthy subjects that levosimendan reversed fatigue and improved neuromechanical efficiency of the diaphragm *in vivo* [40]. Future studies should evaluate the effects of levosimendan on respiratory muscle function in difficult to wean patients.

Conclusion

In the last decade, our understanding of the pathophysiology of ICU-acquired respiratory muscle weakness has improved considerably. Molecular mechanisms include activation of different proteolytic pathways and posttranslational protein modifications, in particular of calcium release channels. This results in atrophy of respiratory muscle fibers and dysfunction of the remaining contractile proteins. Weakness is associated with prolonged mechanical ventilation and increased risk of ICU and hospital readmission. Risk factors for the development of respiratory muscle weakness include sepsis and disuse. In particular, duration of disuse can be limited in selected patients by applying appropriate monitoring techniques that help reduce over-assist by the ventilator. Future studies should reveal the optimal monitoring techniques and the precise goals of monitoring. In patients who have developed ICU-acquired respiratory muscle weakness, no intervention has been shown to improve outcome. Nevertheless, several studies have demonstrated that inspiratory muscle strength training improves strength. No drug has been approved to improve respiratory muscle function. As respiratory muscle weakness has detrimental effects on patient outcomes, clinically effective treatment strategies are urgently needed.

References

1. De Jonghe B, Bastuji-Garin S, Durand MC et al (2007) Respiratory weakness is associated with limb weakness and delayed weaning in critical illness. Crit Care Med 35:2007–2015
2. Adler D, Dupuis-Lozeron E, Richard JC, Janssens JP, Brochard L (2014) Does inspiratory muscle dysfunction predict readmission after intensive care unit discharge? Am J Respir Crit Care Med 190:347–350

3. Levine S, Nguyen T, Taylor N et al (2008) Rapid disuse atrophy of diaphragm fibers in mechanically ventilated humans. N Engl J Med 358:1327–1335
4. Jaber S, Petrof BJ, Jung B et al (2011) Rapidly progressive diaphragmatic weakness and injury during mechanical ventilation in humans. Am J Respir Crit Care Med 183:364–371
5. Hussain SN, Mofarrahi M, Sigala I et al (2010) Mechanical ventilation-induced diaphragm disuse in humans triggers autophagy. Am J Respir Crit Care Med 182:1377–1386
6. Matecki S, Dridi H, Jung B et al (2016) Leaky ryanodine receptors contribute to diaphragmatic weakness during mechanical ventilation. Proc Natl Acad Sci U S A 113:9069–9074
7. Hooijman PE, Beishuizen A, Witt CC et al (2015) Diaphragm muscle fiber weakness and ubiquitin-proteasome activation in critically ill patients. Am J Respir Crit Care Med 191:1126–1138
8. van Hees HW, Schellekens WJ, Linkels M et al (2011) Plasma from septic shock patients induces loss of muscle protein. Crit Care 15:R233
9. Demoule A, Jung B, Prodanovic H et al (2013) Diaphragm dysfunction on admission to the intensive care unit. Prevalence, risk factors, and prognostic impact – a prospective study. Am J Respir Crit Care Med 188:213–219
10. Demoule A, Molinari N, Jung B et al (2016) Patterns of diaphragm function in critically ill patients receiving prolonged mechanical ventilation: a prospective longitudinal study. Ann Intensive Care 6:75
11. Supinski GS, Westgate P, Callahan LA (2016) Correlation of maximal inspiratory pressure to transdiaphragmatic twitch pressure in intensive care unit patients. Crit Care 20:77
12. Goligher EC, Fan E, Herridge MS et al (2015) Evolution of diaphragm thickness during mechanical ventilation. Impact of inspiratory effort. Am J Respir Crit Care Med 192:1080–1088
13. Colombo D, Cammarota G, Alemani M et al (2011) Efficacy of ventilator waveforms observation in detecting patient-ventilator asynchrony. Crit Care Med 39:2452–2457
14. Doorduin J, van Hees HW, van der Hoeven JG, Heunks LM (2013) Monitoring of the respiratory muscles in the critically ill. Am J Respir Crit Care Med 187:20–27
15. Heunks LM, Doorduin J, van der Hoeven JG (2015) Monitoring and preventing diaphragm injury. Curr Opin Crit Care 21:34–41
16. Akoumianaki E, Maggiore SM, Valenza D et al (2014) The application of esophageal pressure measurement in patients with respiratory failure. Am J Respir Crit Care Med 189:520–531
17. Mauri T, Eronia N, Turrini C et al (2016) Bedside assessment of the effects of positive end-expiratory pressure on lung inflation and recruitment by the helium dilution technique and electrical impedance tomography. Intensive Care Med 42:1576–1587
18. Bellani G, Mauri T, Coppadoro A et al (2013) Estimation of patient's inspiratory effort from the electrical activity of the diaphragm. Crit Care Med 41:1483–1491
19. Liu L, Liu S, Xie J et al (2015) Assessment of patient-ventilator breath contribution during neurally adjusted ventilatory assist in patients with acute respiratory failure. Crit Care 19:43
20. Annane D (2016) What Is the evidence for harm of neuromuscular blockade and corticosteroid use in the intensive care unit? Semin Respir Crit Care Med 37:51–56
21. Papazian L, Forel JM, Gacouin A et al (2010) Neuromuscular blockers in early acute respiratory distress syndrome. N Engl J Med 363:107–116
22. Sassoon CS, Zhu E, Caiozzo VJ (2004) Assist-control mechanical ventilation attenuates ventilator-induced diaphragmatic dysfunction. Am J Respir Crit Care Med 170:626–632
23. Doorduin J, Sinderby CA, Beck J et al (2015) Assisted ventilation in patients with acute respiratory distress syndrome: Lung-distending pressure and patient-ventilator interaction. Anesthesiology 123:181–190
24. Pavlovic D, Wendt D (2003) Diaphragm pacing during prolonged mechanical ventilation of the lungs could prevent from respiratory muscle fatigue. Med Hypotheses 60:398–403
25. Maddocks M, Nolan CM, Man WD et al (2016) Neuromuscular electrical stimulation to improve exercise capacity in patients with severe COPD: a randomised double-blind, placebo-controlled trial. Lancet Respir Med 4:27–36

26. Zanotti E, Felicetti G, Maini M, Fracchia C (2003) Peripheral muscle strength training in bed-bound patients with COPD receiving mechanical ventilation: effect of electrical stimulation. Chest 124:292–296
27. Abdellaoui A, Prefaut C, Gouzi F et al (2011) Skeletal muscle effects of electrostimulation after COPD exacerbation: a pilot study. Eur Respir J 38:781–788
28. Luo YM, Lyall RA, Lou HM, Rafferty GF, Polkey MI, Moxham J (1999) Quantification of the esophageal diaphragm electromyogram with magnetic phrenic nerve stimulation. Am J Respir Crit Care Med 160:1629–1634
29. Cattapan SE, Laghi F, Tobin MJ (2003) Can diaphragmatic contractility be assessed by airway twitch pressure in mechanically ventilated patients? Thorax 58:58–62
30. Reynolds SC, Meyyappan R, Thakkar V et al (2016) Mitigation of ventilator-induced diaphragm atrophy by transvenous phrenic nerve stimulation. Am J Respir Crit Care Med Aug 8, Epub ahead of print
31. Schellekens WJ, van Hees HW, Doorduin J et al (2016) Strategies to optimize respiratory muscle function in ICU patients. Crit Care 20:103
32. Martin AD, Smith BK, Davenport PD et al (2011) Inspiratory muscle strength training improves weaning outcome in failure to wean patients: a randomized trial. Crit Care 15:R84
33. Bissett BM, Leditschke IA, Neeman T, Boots R, Paratz J (2016) Inspiratory muscle training to enhance recovery from mechanical ventilation: a randomised trial. Thorax 71:812–819
34. Bhasin S, Storer TW, Berman N et al (1996) The effects of supraphysiologic doses of testosterone on muscle size and strength in normal men. N Engl J Med 335:1–7
35. Pan L, Wang M, Xie X, Du C, Guo Y (2014) Effects of anabolic steroids on chronic obstructive pulmonary disease: a meta-analysis of randomised controlled trials. PLoS One 9:e84855
36. Schols AM, Soeters PB, Mostert R, Pluymers RJ, Wouters EF (1995) Physiologic effects of nutritional support and anabolic steroids in patients with chronic obstructive pulmonary disease. A placebo-controlled randomized trial. Am J Respir Crit Care Med 152:1268–1274
37. Takala J, Ruokonen E, Webster NR et al (1999) Increased mortality associated with growth hormone treatment in critically ill adults. N Engl J Med 341:785–792
38. Farmakis D, Alvarez J, Gal TB et al (2016) Levosimendan beyond inotropy and acute heart failure: Evidence of pleiotropic effects on the heart and other organs: An expert panel position paper. Int J Cardiol 222:303–312
39. van Hees HW, Dekhuijzen PN, Heunks LM (2009) Levosimendan enhances force generation of diaphragm muscle from patients with chronic obstructive pulmonary disease. Am J Respir Crit Care Med 179:41–47
40. Doorduin J, Sinderby CA, Beck J et al (2012) The calcium sensitizer levosimendan improves human diaphragm function. Am J Respir Crit Care Med 185:90–95

Part IX
Neurological Conditions

Neuroanatomy of Sepsis-Associated Encephalopathy

N. Heming, A. Mazeraud, and F. Verdonk

Introduction

Sepsis is defined as a life-threatening organ dysfunction caused by a non-homeostatic response of the host to an infection [1]. Sepsis associated encephalopathy (SAE) is a transient and reversible brain dysfunction, occurring when the source of sepsis is located outside of the central nervous system. SAE affects approximately a third of septic patients [2] and is a risk factor for long term disability and mortality [2, 3]. SAE is characterized by an altered mental status, which may range from delirium to coma. Electrophysiological and brain imaging anomalies may be present [4, 5]. The electroencephalogram (EEG) anomalies of SAE were described and classified by Young et al., including, from the most benign to the most severe, excessive theta rhythms, predominant delta rhythms, triphasic waves and burst suppression [6]. A recent study reported that seizures were recorded in up to 15% of patients [4]. However, the exact place of EEG monitoring in sepsis remains to be defined. Evoked potentials, when investigated in sepsis, show evidence of increased latencies and decreased amplitudes. Cerebral imaging shows various patterns of brain injury during SAE. Brain magnetic resonance imaging (MRI) can be normal or show focal injuries, such as white matter hyperintensities or ischemic stroke, in the presence of disseminated intravascular coagulation (DIC) or of cardiac arrhythmia [5]. Although there is no hallmark biomarker for SAE, elevated plasma levels of S100β or neuron-specific enolase (NSE) have been reported. Their exact significance, however remains unclear [7].

N. Heming (✉)
Réanimation Médicale, Hôpital Raymond Poincaré, Assistance Publique Hôpitaux de Paris AP-HP
104 boulevard Raymond-Poincaré, 92380 Garches, France
e-mail: nicholas.heming@aphp.fr

A. Mazeraud · F. Verdonk
Human Histopathology and Animal Models Institut Pasteur
75015 Paris, France

J.-L. Vincent (ed.), *Annual Update in Intensive Care and Emergency Medicine 2017*,
DOI 10.1007/978-3-319-51908-1_25

Syndromes

The neurological anomalies associated with sepsis include, from the least to the most severe, sickness behavior, delirium and coma (Fig. 1). The most common physiological and behavioral modifications associated with any viral or bacterial infection are called "sickness behavior". This condition is characterized clinically by reduced attention and alertness, as well as by eating and drinking disorders, anxiety and social withdrawal [8]. Biological characteristics include activation of the adrenal axis and the adrenergic system. Sickness behavior relates to the general feeling of being unwell. These modifications result from the action of proinflammatory cytokines (interleukin [IL]-1α and IL-1β, tumor necrosis factor (TNF)-α and IL-6) on centers controlling the behavioral, neuroendocrine and autonomic responses. Sickness behavior is considered to be a physiological reaction to an infectious insult, enabling subjects to better cope with the disease and to protect them from a dangerous environment. Sickness behavior can be maladaptive when its intensity or duration does not correlate with the intensity of the insult [8].

A more severe form of neurological impairment occurring during sepsis is delirium [9]. Delirium is defined by the DSM-5 as an acute and fluctuating disturbance in attention and awareness that is not explained by a preexisting neurological condition and does not occur in the context of a severely reduced level of arousal such as coma [10]. Standardized tools for assessing delirium in the ICU have been developed, such as the Confusion Assessment Method for the ICU (CAM-ICU). Using such a score, delirium occurs in up to 80% of critically ill patients [9]. Two major forms of delirium are described – hypoactive and hyperactive – with a range of possible forms in between. Delirium is associated with prolonged mechanical ventilation, increased ICU length of stay and death [11]. An imbalance between

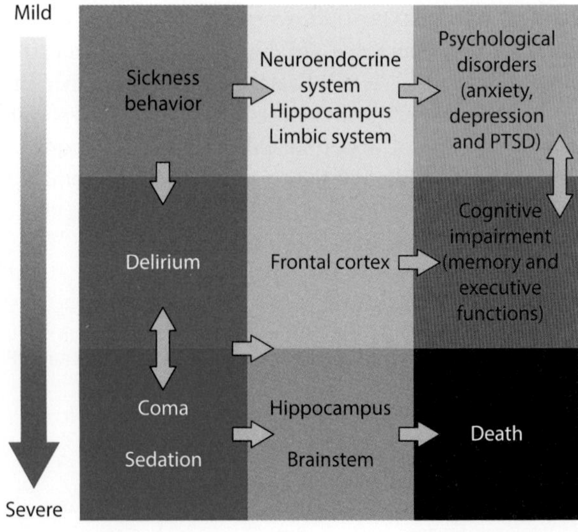

Fig. 1 Schematic representation of the interaction between sepsis-associated neurological syndromes, the affected structures and clinical outcomes. Modified from [15] with permission

neurotransmitters is implicated in the pathophysiology of delirium in the critically ill [12]. However, randomized trials assessing the neuromodulatory effects of psychotropes in the critically ill failed to show benefit and even suggested worsened outcomes [3, 13, 14]. Finally, substance withdrawal, kidney or liver failure, electrolyte anomalies as well as the toxic effect of drugs may all be implicated in the genesis of delirium [15].

The most severe form of neurological impairment during the course of sepsis is the occurrence of coma. Coma may in part be linked to the administration of sedative drugs in a critically ill patient. The depth of coma may easily be assessed using the Glasgow Coma Scale score or the FOUR score [16] and is associated with mortality [2]. The FOUR score adds an additional layer of sophistication to the assessment of coma by scoring brainstem reflexes in addition to the classical eye, motor and verbal responses elicited spontaneously or in response to a nociceptive stimuli. For example, an absent cough reflex is associated with 28-day mortality in sedated critically ill patients [17].

Long-term neuropsychological sequelae, including memory, attention, verbal fluency and executive function impairment, are frequent in the critically ill [18]. Sepsis is a major risk factor for long-term cognitive impairment [3]. Hospitalization for severe sepsis increases the prevalence of moderate to severe cognitive decline by more than 10% [19]. An episode of acute brain dysfunction may lead to anxiety, depression, post-traumatic stress disorders [20] and self-harm [21]. Two out of five patients who have had sepsis are subsequently unable to return to full-time employment [22].

Structures

Two distinct pathways transmit inflammatory signals to the brain in the absence of blood brain barrier disruption: (1) the vagal nerve senses local inflammation and transfers the information to the medullary autonomic nuclei [23, 24]; and (2) circumventricular organs allow the trafficking of inflammatory mediators into the brain [25]. The vagal nerve is stimulated shortly after a lipopolysaccharide (LPS) challenge [24]. The vagal nerve reaches the autonomic and neuroendocrine systems [23, 24]. Deprived of a blood brain barrier, the circumventricular organs are located in the vicinity of the third ventricle and include the area postrema, which controls nausea and transmits peripheral vagal nerve information to the rest of the central nervous system (CNS). Sickness behavior is induced by the action of pro-inflammatory cytokines on the brain. In rodents, the systemic or central administration of IL-1β induces all the behavioral, endocrine and autonomic features of sickness behavior [26]. The other proinflammatory cytokines that affect the brain are IL-1α, TNF-α and IL-6.

Brainstem

A host of arguments point to the existence of brainstem dysfunction during sepsis, which may be the consequence of neuroinflammation. The area postrema allows the passage of circulating inflammatory mediators into the brainstem. Its surgical ablation in rats is equivalent to a central vagotomy [27]. Therefore, it is conceivable that excessive inflammatory signaling can be deleterious. Experimentally, injecting endotoxin in rodents models the apoptosis of autonomic centers that is induced by oxidative stress. We have reported multifocal necrotizing leukoencephalopathy in a septic shock patient, characterized by an intense expression of inflammatory cytokines and neuronal apoptosis within the pons [28]. Neuronal apoptosis within autonomic centers has also been described [29]. The brainstem is involved in three general functions: arousal, brainstem reflexes, and control of vital functions and modulation of the immune response [23]. Brainstem dysfunction might result in impaired alertness and impaired cardiovascular and immune controls, thereby leading to increased mortality. We found that the early abolition of the cough reflex and oculocephalogyric response was independently associated with increased ICU mortality in sedated critically ill patients [17]. Decreased heart rate variability, reflecting an impaired sympathetic activity originating from the brainstem autonomic centers, is also associated with a worse outcome in sepsis [30]. Absent EEG reactivity, indicating a dysfunction of the reticular activating ascending substance, is a predictor of death in septic patients [4].

Hypothalamus and Pituitary Axis

Sepsis is associated with multiple neuroendocrine disorders [23, 25, 31–35]. While the initial stage of sepsis is marked by increased secretion of pituitary hormones notably in response to a decreased sensitivity in peripheral hormonal receptors, prolonged sepsis is characterized by a decrease in pituitary hormone release [36]. For example, septic shock is associated with relative adrenal insufficiency and increased mortality, responding favorably to substitutive opotherapy [33, 37]. Septic shock may also be associated with impaired production of vasopressin [31, 34, 38] due to hyperpolarization of neurons of the organum vasculosum lamina terminalis (OVLT) region [38].

Amygdala

Psychological consequences of sepsis include anxiety, depression and post-traumatic stress disorder (PTSD) [39] all of which involve the amygdala and its network with the prefrontal cortex, hypothalamus or brainstem. The amygdala is particularly affected by microglial activation during sepsis [29, 39]. Studies in military personnel presenting with PTSD showed that the amygdala was desensitized in response to stressful stimuli. The incriminated mechanism is a dampened response to corticosteroids which could be overcome by direct corticosterone administration [40]. A recent study translated these findings in order to prevent PTSD in sepsis patients [41]. Such a beneficial effect of corticosteroids may involve non-genetic or epigenetic effects of these drugs [42], inducing a major modulation of aversive memory formation [43].

Hippocampus

Memory impairment can be induced by insults to the hippocampus or the frontal cortex. Hippocampal atrophy is associated with loss of memory, such as in Alzheimer's disease. In rodents, sepsis is also associated with hippocampal dysfunction and subsequent spatial memory alterations evidenced by the Morris Water Maze test [44], which are correlated with long term potentiation, late neuronal death, gliosis and increased production of reactive oxygen species (ROS). TNF-α, caspase 1 and hypoxia seem to be implicated in the pathogenesis of this hippocampal dysfunction [45].

Frontal Cortex

The prefrontal cortex and other sensorimotor areas constitute the frontal cortex. Cognitive defects occurring after frontal cortex injuries include mainly impaired memorization, attention and executive functions. Ultrastructural neuronal anomalies were shown within the sensorimotor cortex in a dog model of endotoxic shock. Pre-frontal cortex-related cognitive functions including memorization and verbal fluency are frequently affected after sepsis [19]. Neuroinflammation within the frontal cortex results in cognitive impairment [46].

White Matter

As shown by MRI studies, sepsis can induce axonal damage; which may contribute to the cognitive decline [46].

Processes

Three major processes are involved in the pathophysiology of SAE including diffuse neuroinflammation, ischemic processes and excitotoxicity.

Neuroinflammation

Microglial cells are the mononuclear phagocytes of the brain, implicated in immune defense and synaptic plasticity. Microglia express membrane-bound receptors that are able to detect endogenous or exogenous danger signals. Microglial activation implies a level of blood brain barrier disruption or the local release of proinflammatory mediators. Microglial activity ranges from proinflammatory to anti-inflammatory. Microglial activation is a frequent neuropathological feature of SAE [29, 47]. The modulation of microglial activity, although still in the pre-clinical phase, may be an interesting option for treating SAE [48].

Astrocytes are supportive glial cell components. Astrocytes are involved in neuroinflammation as they are reactive and able to secrete various mediators [49]. Astrocytes are thus involved in cerebral blood flow control through the release of mediators, such as nitric oxide (NO), prostaglandins and arachidonic acid [50]. Astrocytes regulate the concentration of neurotransmitters, such as glutamate, GABA, and glycine, in the synaptic space by taking up any excess neurotransmitter, preventing their potential for accumulation [51]. Animal studies consistently report the presence of astrogliosis during SAE. By contrast, no such finding has been reported in man, possibly due to technical issues.

Neuroinflammation affects cellular metabolism, potentially leading to oxidative stress and mitochondrial dysfunction [52]. Mitochondrial dysfunction has been found in the brain of septic animals, associated with the production of oxygen/nitrogen reactive species [53].

Ischemic Processes

The gliovascular unit associates endothelial cells, astrocytes and pericytes [54]. Exchanges between the brain and components of the blood occur through endothelial cells. Astrocytes regulate water and ionic homeostasis through the transmembrane channel aquaporin 4 (AQP4). Gliovascular units are implicated in adjusting blood flow at the arteriolar and capillary levels in order to provide the energetic requirement of a given cerebral area [54].

Ischemia can result from macrocirculatory dysfunction, including hypotension, decreased cerebral flow and impaired autoregulation. Sepsis induces activation of cerebral endothelial cells which, by impairing microvascular tone and activating coagulation, promotes ischemic and/or hemorrhagic lesions of the brain [55]. Some experimental data indicate that during the early stages of sepsis, there is an increased expression of endothelial NO synthase (eNOS), which causes additional NO release and enhances the activation of cerebral endothelial cells [56]. This endothelial activation, coupled with the neuroinflammation process, can result in impaired blood brain barrier permeability, upregulated AQP4, parenchymal infiltration by neutrophils, and the activation of astrocytes [57]. MRI studies have shown blood brain barrier breakdown in patients with septic shock [58], possibly originating from the perivascular spaces of Wirchow-Robin, which may go on to involve the whole white matter. It has to be noted that posterior reversible encephalopathy syndromes have been reported in septic patients [59]. Experimental studies confirm that blood brain barrier impairment relates to a dysfunction of tight junction proteins, such as occludin, ZO-1, ZO-2, claudin-3 and claudin-5 [60].

Neurovascular coupling is a specific brain mechanism of vasoregulation that adapts local cerebral blood flow to the neural metabolic needs. SAE is associated with neurovascular uncoupling due to microcirculatory dysfunction and low blood flow. In septic patients, a discrepancy between neuronal activation, increased metabolic needs and vascular reactivity is observed [61].

The combination of macro- and micro-circulatory defects, endothelial dysfunction and neurovascular uncoupling contribute to ischemic lesions, which were constantly observed in a post-mortem study of patients who died of septic shock. These ischemic lesions were found in brain areas sensitive to ischemia (i. e., the hippocampus, the basal ganglia, frontal cortex, dentate gyrus and the bulbar olive) but also, and specifically to sepsis, in the nuclei of the autonomic nervous system (i. e., amygdala, anterior and posterior hypothalamus, locus coeruleus). Similarly, pronounced neuronal apoptosis was observed in these areas. Furthermore, brain hemorrhages were found in 17–26% of these neuropathological cases [47].

Neurotransmitter Dysfunction

A small number of brain structures, namely the amygdala, nucleus tractus solitarii and locus coeruleus, are particularly vulnerable to sepsis and liable to neuronal apoptosis [29]. Glutamate plays a role in neuronal apoptosis during sepsis, through excitoxicity [62]. For example, the recycling and glutamate-stimulated export of ascorbate by astrocytes are inhibited during sepsis [63]. Interestingly, analysis of the cerebrospinal fluid of patients with SAE showed a decrease in the levels of ascorbate, an anti-oxidant produced by astrocytes that plays a role in neuroprotection [64]. When activated, microglia cells also release large amounts of glutamate [65].

The dopaminergic, β-adrenergic [66], the GABA receptor [67], and the cholinergic [52] systems are all impaired during sepsis. An imbalance between dopaminergic and cholinergic neurotransmission might be particularly involved in delirium [12]. However, cholinergic drugs, such as rivastigmine [13] as well as anti-dopaminergic drugs, such as haloperidol [14], do not reduce the incidence or duration of delirium. The use of GABA-agonists, such as benzodiazepines, actually increases the risk of delirium [3], which is reduced by noradrenergic drugs, such as dexmedetomidine [68]. Impaired neurotransmission might result from the production of NO [69], but also from circulating neurotoxic amino-acids (ammonium, tyrosine, tryptophan and phenylalanine) that are released in excess by the liver and muscles during sepsis [70]. Metabolic disorders and drug toxicity (e. g., sedatives, analgesics, antibiotics ...) contribute to neurotransmitter dysfunction.

Conclusion

The clinical spectrum of SAE includes sickness behavior, delirium, focal deficits and coma associated or not with brainstem reflex loss. It is associated with increased mortality and long-term psychocognitive impairment. SAE results from inflammatory, ischemic and neurotoxic processes that affect, in particular, the frontal cortex, the hippocampus, the amygdala and the brainstem. Its diagnosis essentially relies on neurological examination and EEG findings, which may indicate the need for brain imaging. In daily clinical practice, brain infection has to be ruled out whenever suspected, as well as drug toxicity or metabolic disturbances. There is no specific treatment for SAE, apart from resolution of the underlying sepsis.

Acknowledgment

We would like to acknowledge the help of Drs Fernando Bozza and Fabrice Chrétien from, respectively, the Evandro Chagas National Institute of Infectious Diseases, Fiocruz, Rio de Janeiro, Brazil and the Unit of Neuropathology, Saint Anne Hospital in Paris, France and of Dr Tarek Sharshar from the General ICU, Raymond Poincaré Hospital in Garches, France in drafting this manuscript.

References

1. Singer M, Deutschman CS, Seymour CW et al (2016) The Third International Consensus Definitions for Sepsis and Septic Shock (Sepsis-3). JAMA 315:801–810
2. Eidelman LA, Putterman D, Putterman C, Sprung CL (1996) The spectrum of septic encephalopathy. Definitions, etiologies, and mortalities. JAMA 275:470–473
3. Pandharipande PP, Girard TD, Jackson JC et al (2013) Long-term cognitive impairment after critical illness. N Engl J Med 369:1306–1316
4. Azabou E, Magalhaes E, Braconnier A et al (2015) Early standard electroencephalogram abnormalities predict mortality in septic intensive care unit patients. PLoS One 10:e0139969
5. Polito A, Eischwald F, Maho AL et al (2013) Pattern of brain injury in the acute setting of human septic shock. Crit Care 17:R204
6. Young GB, Bolton CF, Archibald YM, Austin TW, Wells GA (1992) The electroencephalogram in sepsis-associated encephalopathy. J Clin Neurophysiol 9:145–152
7. Grandi C, Tomasi CD, Fernandes K et al (2011) Brain-derived neurotrophic factor and neuron-specific enolase, but not S100β, levels are associated to the occurrence of delirium in intensive care unit patients. J Crit Care 26:133–137
8. Dantzer R (2004) Cytokine-induced sickness behaviour: a neuroimmune response to activation of innate immunity. Eur J Pharmacol 500:399–411
9. Ely EW, Inouye SK, Bernard GR et al (2001) Delirium in mechanically ventilated patients: validity and reliability of the confusion assessment method for the intensive care unit (CAM-ICU). JAMA 286:2703–2710
10. American Pychatric Association (2013) Diagnostic and statistical manual of mental disorders: DSM-5. American Psychiatric Association Publishing, Arlington
11. Ely EW, Shintani A, Truman B et al (2004) Delirium as a predictor of mortality in mechanically ventilated patients in the intensive care unit. JAMA 291:1753–1762

12. van Gool WA, van de Beek D, Eikelenboom P (2010) Systemic infection and delirium: when cytokines and acetylcholine collide. Lancet 375:773–775
13. van Eijk MM, Roes KC, Honing ML et al (2010) Effect of rivastigmine as an adjunct to usual care with haloperidol on duration of delirium and mortality in critically ill patients: a multicentre, double-blind, placebo-controlled randomised trial. Lancet 376:1829–1837
14. Page VJ, Ely EW, Gates S et al (2013) Effect of intravenous haloperidol on the duration of delirium and coma in critically ill patients (Hope-ICU): a randomised, double-blind, placebo-controlled trial. Lancet Respir Med 1:515–523
15. Annane D, Sharshar T (2015) Cognitive decline after sepsis. Lancet Respir Med 3:61–69
16. Wijdicks EF, Bamlet WR, Maramattom BV, Manno EM, McClelland RL (2005) Validation of a new coma scale: The FOUR score. Ann Neurol 58:585–593
17. Sharshar T, Porcher R, Siami S et al (2011) Brainstem responses can predict death and delirium in sedated patients in intensive care unit. Crit Care Med 39:1960–1967
18. Jackson JC, Hart RP, Gordon SM et al (2003) Six-month neuropsychological outcome of medical intensive care unit patients. Crit Care Med 31:1226–1234
19. Iwashyna TJ, Ely EW, Smith DM, Langa KM (2010) Long-term cognitive impairment and functional disability among survivors of severe sepsis. JAMA 304:1787–1794
20. Wintermann GB, Brunkhorst FM, Petrowski K et al (2015) Stress disorders following prolonged critical illness in survivors of severe sepsis. Crit Care Med 43:1213–1222
21. Lund-Sørensen H, Benros ME, Madsen T et al (2016) A nationwide cohort study of the association between hospitalization with infection and risk of death by suicide. JAMA Psychiatry 73:912–919
22. Rothenhäusler HB, Ehrentraut S, Stoll C, Schelling G, Kapfhammer HP (2001) The relationship between cognitive performance and employment and health status in long-term survivors of the acute respiratory distress syndrome: results of an exploratory study. Gen Hosp Psychiatry 23:90–96
23. Carlson DE, Chiu WC, Fiedler SM, Hoffman GE (2007) Central neural distribution of immunoreactive Fos and CRH in relation to plasma ACTH and corticosterone during sepsis in the rat. Exp Neurol 205:485–500
24. Reyes EP, Abarzúa S, Martin A, Rodríguez J, Cortés PP, Fernández R (2012) LPS-induced c-Fos activation in NTS neurons and plasmatic cortisol increases in septic rats are suppressed by bilateral carotid chemodenervation. Adv Exp Med Biol 758:185–190
25. Sharshar T, Hopkinson NS, Orlikowski D, Annane D (2005) Science review: The brain in sepsis – culprit and victim. Crit Care 9:37–44
26. Anforth HR, Bluthe RM, Bristow A et al (1998) Biological activity and brain actions of recombinant rat interleukin-1alpha and interleukin-1beta. Eur Cytokine Netw 9:279–288
27. Skoog KM, Blair ML, Sladek CD, Williams WM, Mangiapane ML (1990) Area postrema: essential for support of arterial pressure after hemorrhage in rats. Am J Physiol 258:R1472–8
28. Sharshar T, Gray F, Poron F, Raphael JC, Gajdos P, Annane D (2002) Multifocal necrotizing leukoencephalopathy in septic shock. Crit Care Med 30:2371–2375
29. Sharshar T, Gray F, Lorin de la Grandmaison G et al (2003) Apoptosis of neurons in cardiovascular autonomic centres triggered by inducible nitric oxide synthase after death from septic shock. Lancet 362:1799–1805
30. Annane D, Trabold F, Sharshar T et al (1999) Inappropriate sympathetic activation at onset of septic shock: a spectral analysis approach. Am J Respir Crit Care Med 160:458–465
31. Siami S, Bailly-Salin J, Polito A et al (2010) Osmoregulation of vasopressin secretion is altered in the postacute phase of septic shock. Crit Care Med 38:1962–1969
32. Sonneville R, Guidoux C, Barrett L et al (2010) Vasopressin synthesis by the magnocellular neurons is different in the supraoptic nucleus and in the paraventricular nucleus in human and experimental septic shock. Brain Pathol 20:613–622
33. Aboab J, Polito A, Orlikowski D, Sharshar T, Castel M, Annane D (2008) Hydrocortisone effects on cardiovascular variability in septic shock: a spectral analysis approach. Crit Care Med 36:1481–1486

34. Siami S, Polito A, Porcher R et al (2013) Thirst perception and osmoregulation of vasopressin secretion are altered during recovery from septic shock. PLoS One 8:e80190
35. Escartin C, Rouach N (2013) Astroglial networking contributes to neurometabolic coupling. Front Neuroenergetics 5:1
36. Schroeder S, Wichers M, Klingmüller D et al (2001) The hypothalamic-pituitary-adrenal axis of patients with severe sepsis: altered response to corticotropin-releasing hormone. Crit Care Med 29:310–316
37. Annane D, Sébille V, Charpentier C et al (2002) Effect of treatment with low doses of hydrocortisone and fludrocortisone on mortality in patients with septic shock. JAMA 288:862–871
38. Stare J, Siami S, Trudel E, Prager-Khoutorsky M, Sharshar T, Bourque CW (2015) Effects of peritoneal sepsis on rat central osmoregulatory neurons mediating thirst and vasopressin release. J Neurosci 35:12188–12197
39. Muscatell KA, Dedovic K, Slavich GM et al (2015) Greater amygdala activity and dorsomedial prefrontal-amygdala coupling are associated with enhanced inflammatory responses to stress. Brain Behav Immun 43:46–53
40. Henckens MJ, van Wingen GA, Joels M, Fernandez G (2010) Time-dependent effects of corticosteroids on human amygdala processing. J Neurosci 30:12725–12732
41. Schelling G, Stoll C, Kapfhammer HP et al (1999) The effect of stress doses of hydrocortisone during septic shock on posttraumatic stress disorder and health-related quality of life in survivors. Crit Care Med 27:2678–2683
42. Hunter RG (2012) Epigenetic effects of stress and corticosteroids in the brain. Front Cell Neurosci 6:18
43. Steckert AV, Comim CM, Igna DM et al (2015) Effects of sodium butyrate on aversive memory in rats submitted to sepsis. Neurosci Lett 595:134–138
44. Liu L, Xie K, Chen H et al (2014) Inhalation of hydrogen gas attenuates brain injury in mice with cecal ligation and puncture via inhibiting neuroinflammation, oxidative stress and neuronal apoptosis. Brain Res 1589:78–92
45. Di Paola M, Caltagirone C, Fadda L, Sabatini U, Serra L, Carlesimo GA (2008) Hippocampal atrophy is the critical brain change in patients with hypoxic amnesia. Hippocampus 18:719–728
46. Sonneville R, Derese I, Marques MB et al (2015) Neuropathological correlates of hyperglycemia during prolonged polymicrobial sepsis in mice. Shock 44:245–251
47. Sharshar T, Annane D, de la Grandmaison GL, Brouland JP, Hopkinson NS, Françoise G (2004) The neuropathology of septic shock. Brain Pathol 14:21–33
48. Adembri C, Selmi V, Vitali L et al (2014) Minocycline but not tigecycline is neuroprotective and reduces the neuroinflammatory response induced by the superimposition of sepsis upon traumatic brain injury. Crit Care Med 42:e570–82
49. Retamal MA, Froger N, Palacios-Prado N et al (2007) Cx43 hemichannels and gap junction channels in astrocytes are regulated oppositely by proinflammatory cytokines released from activated microglia. J Neurosci 27:13781–13792
50. Iadecola C, Nedergaard M (2007) Glial regulation of the cerebral microvasculature. Nat Neurosci 10:1369–1376
51. Seifert G, Schilling K, Steinhäuser C (2006) Astrocyte dysfunction in neurological disorders: a molecular perspective. Nat Rev Neurosci 7:194–206
52. Semmler A, Frisch C, Debeir T et al (2007) Long-term cognitive impairment, neuronal loss and reduced cortical cholinergic innervation after recovery from sepsis in a rodent model. Exp Neurol 204:733–740
53. Comim CM, Rezin GT, Scaini G et al (2008) Mitochondrial respiratory chain and creatine kinase activities in rat brain after sepsis induced by cecal ligation and perforation. Mitochondrion 8:313–318
54. Abbott NJ, Rönnbäck L, Hansson E (2006) Astrocyte-endothelial interactions at the blood-brain barrier. Nat Rev Neurosci 7:41–53

55. Khakpour S, Wilhelmsen K, Hellman J (2015) Vascular endothelial cell Toll-like receptor pathways in sepsis. Innate Immun 21:827–846
56. Handa O, Stephen J, Cepinskas G (2008) Role of endothelial nitric oxide synthase-derived nitric oxide in activation and dysfunction of cerebrovascular endothelial cells during early onsets of sepsis. Am J Physiol Hear Circ Physiol 295:H1712–1719
57. Alexander JJ, Jacob A, Cunningham P, Hensley L, Quigg RJ (2008) TNF is a key mediator of septic encephalopathy acting through its receptor, TNF receptor-1. Neurochem Int 52:447–456
58. Sharshar T, Carlier R, Bernard F et al (2007) Brain lesions in septic shock: a magnetic resonance imaging study. Intensive Care Med 33:798–806
59. Bartynski WS (2008) Posterior reversible encephalopathy syndrome, part 1: fundamental imaging and clinical features. Am J Neuroradiol 29:1036–1042
60. Luissint AC, Artus C, Glacial F, Ganeshamoorthy K, Couraud PO (2012) Tight junctions at the blood brain barrier: physiological architecture and disease-associated dysregulation. Fluids Barriers CNS 9:23
61. Rosengarten B, Krekel D, Kuhnert S, Schulz R (2012) Early neurovascular uncoupling in the brain during community acquired pneumonia. Crit Care 16:R64
62. Viviani B, Boraso M, Marchetti N, Marinovich M (2014) Perspectives on neuroinflammation and excitotoxicity: A neurotoxic conspiracy? Neurotoxicology 43:10–20
63. Korcok J, Wu F, Tyml K, Hammond RR, Wilson JX (2002) Sepsis inhibits reduction of dehydroascorbic acid and accumulation of ascorbate in astroglial cultures: intracellular ascorbate depletion increases nitric oxide synthase induction and glutamate uptake inhibition. J Neurochem 81:185–193
64. Voigt K, Kontush A, Stuerenburg HJ, Muench-Harrach D, Hansen HC, Kunze K (2002) Decreased plasma and cerebrospinal fluid ascorbate levels in patients with septic encephalopathy. Free Radic Res 36:735–739
65. Takeuchi H, Jin S, Wang J et al (2006) Tumor necrosis factor-alpha induces neurotoxicity via glutamate release from hemichannels of activated microglia in an autocrine manner. J Biol Chem 281:21362–21368
66. Kadoi Y, Saito S, Kunimoto F, Imai T, Fujita T (1996) Impairment of the brain beta-adrenergic system during experimental endotoxemia. J Surg Res 61:496–502
67. Kadoi Y, Saito S (1996) An alteration in the gamma-aminobutyric acid receptor system in experimentally induced septic shock in rats. Crit Care Med 24:298–305
68. Pandharipande PP, Pun BT, Herr DL et al (2007) Effect of sedation with dexmedetomidine vs lorazepam on acute brain dysfunction in mechanically ventilated patients: the MENDS randomized controlled trial. JAMA 298:2644–2653
69. Jacob A, Brorson JR, Alexander JJ (2011) Septic encephalopathy: inflammation in man and mouse. Neurochem Int 58:472–476
70. Basler T, Meier-Hellmann A, Bredle D, Reinhart K (2002) Amino acid imbalance early in septic encephalopathy. Intensive Care Med 28:293–298

Clinical Utility of Blood-Based Protein Biomarkers in Traumatic Brain Injury

S. Mondello, A. I. R. Maas, and A. Buki

Introduction

Biomarkers are defined as "a characteristic that is objectively measured and evaluated as an indicator of normal biological processes, pathogenic processes or pharmacological responses to a therapeutic intervention" [1]. Traumatic brain injury (TBI) is a complex disorder that is characterized by substantial injury-specific and patient-specific variability. In particular, its clinical, radiological and pathological heterogeneity is considered one of the greatest obstacles to optimizing diagnosis and emergency management, to developing a reliable, efficient and valid classification and prognostic system, and to finding effective targeted therapeutic interventions [2]. Therefore, blood biomarkers that reliably capture the different aspects of interindividual pathophysiological TBI heterogeneity are urgently needed [3]. Such biomarkers may allow more timely and accurate diagnosis, as well as improved characterization of TBI, assessment of disease progression and outcome prediction in individual patients with TBI, conveying information beyond that obtained from clinical evaluation and current neuroimaging techniques. Furthermore, by reflect-

S. Mondello (✉)
Department of Biomedical and Dental Sciences and Morphofunctional Imaging, University of Messina, A.O.U. "Policlinico G. Martino"
Via Consolare Valeria, 98125 Messina, Italy
e-mail: stm_mondello@hotmail.com

A. I. R. Maas
Department of Neurosurgery, Antwerp University Hospital and University of Antwerp
2650 Edegem, Belgium

A. Buki
Department of Neurosurgery, University of Pécs
7623 Pécs, Hungary
János Szentágothai Research Center, University of Pécs
7624 Pécs, Hungary
MTA-PTE Clinical Neuroscience MR Research Group
7623 Pécs, Hungary

J.-L. Vincent (ed.), *Annual Update in Intensive Care and Emergency Medicine 2017*,
DOI 10.1007/978-3-319-51908-1_26

ing ongoing molecular mechanisms and pathological pathways, biomarkers might provide opportunities for individualized, targeted interventions and may be incorporated in clinical trials, ultimately moving the concept of precision medicine into clinical TBI management [4].

During the past decades, great efforts have been undertaken to translate biomarkers for TBI into clinical practice. In this chapter, we discuss the strength of evidence for biomarkers in TBI as diagnostic, prognostic and predictive parameters. We specifically focus on questions of particular clinical interest in which biomarkers might assist in clinical decision making: to distinguish between patients with and without computed tomography (CT)-detectable intracerebral lesions following mild TBI, to predict outcome after injury, and to explore the potential of biomarkers in clinical trials.

Early Diagnosis of Mild TBI

Of all TBIs, more than 90% are considered mild, with an annual incidence of 100–550/100,000 making it one of the most common neurological disorders [5] and one of the most common reasons for emergency department (ED) care [6].

Although most cases can be discharged without sequelae, a small proportion of patients with mild TBI will have intracranial pathology and a minority of those (~ 1%) will develop a potential life-threatening condition that requires neurosurgical intervention [7]. The key to managing these patients is early diagnosis of intracranial injuries using CT [7]. Unfortunately, although various clinical decision rules based upon medical history and clinical examination are available for more selective use of CT scans, their low efficiency results in over 90% of CTs being negative for clinically important brain injury [8]. In addition to unnecessary exposure to potentially harmful ionizing radiation, this inefficient use of CT adds significantly to health care costs and to the burden of overcrowding in the ED [9].

Biomarkers capable of reliably and objectively identifying those patients who have post-traumatic lesions following mild head injuries would be highly valuable. The ultimate goal would be to use these biomarkers as a reliable screening tool in the ED to optimize clinical decision rules for the initial management of mild head injuries and eliminate a large number of unnecessary CT scans without compromising patient care. However, to enable adoption and use in the emergency setting, these biomarkers should be reproducible, stable over time, inexpensive, and thoroughly validated. Ultimately, short turnaround times and highly sensitive assays might be particularly relevant to aid in clinical decision making in terms of triage for CT scans, hospital admissions and/or need for structured follow-up.

Diagnostic Biomarkers

Numerous studies have explored the diagnostic performance of blood-based biomarkers in predicting intracranial injury in adult patients following mild head trauma in the acute setting. In terms of diagnostic application, the most substantial research has focused on S100B. S100B is an astrocyte-enriched Ca^{2+}-binding protein, mainly expressed in astrocytes [3] but that can also be detected in extracerebral tissues, such as adipose tissue, cartilage and bone marrow [10]. The serum half-life of S100B is about 30 to 90 min and it can be detected soon after injury [11].

A number of studies have consistently demonstrated that initial circulating levels of S100B are strong predictors of an absence of CT pathology with high individual sensitivities (75%–100%) and very high individual negative predictive values (NPVs, 90%–100%) [12–14]. As a result, S100B has recently been introduced for the first time into clinical practice guidelines [15]. Using a low cutoff of 0.10 µg/l, analysis of S100B within 6 h following trauma, should safely reduce the number of unnecessary CT scans by up to 30% in adult patients with low risk for intracranial complication and/or neurosurgical intervention after mild head injury. However, as S100B is not brain-specific and has a short half-life, patients with polytrauma and those who sustained trauma more than 6 h prior to testing have a substantial risk of false positive and negative results, respectively, and thus are not considered suitable for S100B sampling.

Importantly, data from a study by Thaler and colleagues showed that older age and platelet aggregation inhibitors did not appear to affect the diagnostic accuracy of S100B [16]. Given the changing patterns in the epidemiology of TBI [17], this is of substantial relevance. Nonetheless, future larger studies confirming these findings are needed.

At present, data are insufficient to recommend the introduction of S100B into pediatric head injury guidelines [18] considering also the age-dependent liabilities. Further studies are needed to determine the value and validity in pediatric TBI settings.

Glial fibrillary acidic protein (GFAP) is a brain-specific intermediate filament protein found in astrocytes. It was recently identified as a biomarker candidate indicative of intracranial lesions after head trauma [19, 20]. In their study including 94 patients with mild brain injury (Glasgow Coma Scale [GCS] score 13 to 15), Metting and colleagues [20] reported significantly higher GFAP levels within 3 h after injury in patients with an abnormal admission CT compared to those with a normal CT. In 108 patients with mild to moderate TBI, GFAP serum concentrations within 4 h of injury were significantly higher in patients with intracranial injury evident on CT scan. In particular, a cutoff level of 0.035 ng/ml yielded a sensitivity of 97%, a specificity of 18%, and a NPV of 94% to rule out intracranial lesions on CT. Furthermore, using a cutoff value of 0.17 ng/ml, GFAP was also able to identify patients requiring neurosurgical intervention with a sensitivity of 100%, a specificity of 42% and a NPV of 100% [19].

Based on these encouraging results, shortly thereafter the same group published data on 209 mild to moderate TBI patients enrolled within 4 h of injury and 188 trauma patients with no TBI [21]. A sensitivity of 81%, a specificity of 70% and NPV of 70% to rule out intracranial lesions on CT were reported. A blind comparison of GFAP and S100B was also carried out demonstrating that GFAP outperformed S100B in detecting traumatic intracranial lesions on CT, particularly in the presence of fractures and extracranial lesions (area under the receiver operating characteristics curve [AUC] 0.93 versus 0.75, respectively). The authors concluded that GFAP might be a more accurate and valuable diagnostic tool in the acute real world emergency setting. Similarly, GFAP appeared to out-perform S100B in detecting traumatic intracranial lesions on CT in children and youths with mild head trauma and has been proposed as a potentially valuable tool for the diagnosis and clinical management of pediatric TBI [22]. Further prospective studies with larger numbers of patients will be required to assess the reproducibility of these findings and to establish meaningful thresholds.

Of the neuronal protein markers evaluated, only the neuronal ubiquitin C-terminal hydrolase-L1 (UCH-L1) has been found to be promising as a pre-head CT screening test. UCH-L1 is a highly enriched and abundant neuronal protein that is stable and able to diffuse rapidly into the circulation after brain injury. It is known to be involved in either the addition or removal of ubiquitin from metabolic proteins via the ATP-dependent pathway, thereby playing a critical role in removal of damaged, misfolded or over-expressed proteins in neurons both under normal conditions and in response to pathological insults. UCH-L1 was shown to be 100% sensitive for detecting intracranial lesions on CT scan in two different studies by the same group [23, 24]. Although promising, these initial studies require independent verification and rigorous validation. To gain definitive evidence for its clinical utility, it will be essential to establish meaningful thresholds.

The diagnostic value of neuron-specific enolase (NSE), a glycolytic enzyme enriched in neuronal cell bodies, remains uncertain, as there are important variations and contrasting results among studies. No evidence of a significant association between initial circulating concentrations of the microtubule-associated protein, Tau, and CT findings was found. Finally, the use of phosphorylated NF (pNF-H) – the extensively phosphorylated, axon-specific form of the NF-H subunit of neurofilament – for detecting intracranial lesions on CT scan was evaluated in a single study reporting encouraging sensitivity (87.5%) and specificity (70%) [25]. However, the results have been difficult to replicate.

Taken together, although these studies and findings support the concept that biomarker assessment on ED admission may be highly relevant to the routine clinical diagnosis of patients who have sustained a mild head injury, they point to the difficulty of using a snapshot of a single marker at one moment in time to predict or rule out intracranial lesions, given the complexity of the pathobiological cascade of events triggered by TBI, heterogeneity of type of injuries, as well as patient characteristics including genetics, comorbid conditions, and medications. More accurate prediction enabling more selective use of CT likely depends on a more 'holistic' approach consisting of a multimarker strategy of complementary markers reflecting different pathogenic mechanisms and brain damage patterns and with distinct temporal profiles and release dynamics in conjunction with relevant demographic and clinical factors.

Outcome Prediction After TBI

Early determination of prognosis after TBI remain a priority for relatives and physicians involved in the care of these patients. Despite international management guidelines for severe head injury [26], recent meta-analyses have highlighted no clear reduction in TBI-related mortality over the past two decades or improvement in overall outcome following severe TBI [17], with approximately 30% of patients dying and 50% remaining disabled as a consequence of their brain injury. Indeed, the incidence of complications and poor outcomes is rising, owing to the emergent epidemiological transition characterized by an increase in TBI among elderly individuals.

Although mild TBI has historically been considered a benign entity, a nontrivial subset of patients (~ 15%) develops persistent dysfunction affecting many domains of a person's life, including physical functions, cognitive and psychosocial abilities, and it may even prove fatal [27]. Although clinical descriptors are helpful and widely used to assess patients with mild TBI, they are not objective and provide little information on the underlying TBI pathophysiology. Routine CT imaging studies, on the other hand, have suboptimal sensitivities in detecting the subtle structural damage and changes that occur after mild TBI, and do not provide insight into the complex cascade of molecular events triggered by the injury that are considered the main contributors to long-term complication, and, thus are not closely correlated with long-term neurocognitive and neuropsychiatric disabilities.

Over the past 20 years, biochemical markers of brain damage have been increasingly studied as potential tools to improve the prognostic assessment of patients who sustain TBI. There is an emerging recognition that biomarkers represent sensitive and objective indicators of brain injury and yield important additional information on injury-specific and patient-specific variability, and disease mechanisms. As such, they are the ideal complement to clinical risk factors and imaging-based assessments to help strengthen prognostic accuracy and lead to more precise outcome prediction. There is now substantial evidence that a multimodal strategy that categorizes patients based on a combination of biomarker levels and traditional clinical predictors enables more accurate risk stratification over a broad range of short- and long-term outcomes [28]. However, to date, no blood-based brain injury markers have been integrated into validated prognostic algorithms.

Prognostic Biomarkers

There are numerous reviews on the diagnostic performance of the blood-based protein biomarkers. In particular, a growing body of evidence suggests that high blood concentrations of S100B are associated with increased mortality and poorer outcomes in moderate to severe TBI patients. Studies evaluating the accuracy of a single baseline determination of S100B for prediction of mortality indicated that thresholds to attain 100% specificity ranged from 1.38 to 10.50 μg/l, with a sensitivity ranging from 14% to 60%. On the other hand, the accuracy of circulating

S100B for prediction of poor outcome as defined by the Glasgow Outcome Score (GOS < 4 or GOS-E < 5) indicated that threshold values for 100% specificity ranged from 2.16 to 14.0 μg/l, with sensitivity ranging from 9% to 50% [29]. The different assays and reagents used to measure S100B levels as well as the heterogeneity in study populations can in part explain the substantial differences in the cut-off values identified across the studies. The optimal prognostic threshold values for S-100B therefore remain uncertain.

Data across prognostic studies of GFAP are also encouraging. Most studies reported fairly similar findings and a similar cut-off, albeit they were conducted by different groups and using different assays and reagents by different manufacturers. Specifically, at a cut-off value of ~ 1.5 ng/ml, individual sensitivity and specificity in predicting death ranged from 66% to 85% and from 52% to 93%, respectively. Conversely, for unfavorable neurological prognosis (GOS < 4 or GOS-E < 5), threshold values varied widely (0.22 to 1.5 μg/l) and yielded specificities between 59% [30] and 100% [31]. Nonetheless, reliable and valid thresholds remain elusive for research and clinical practice.

While the prognostic value of NSE remains uncertain, UCH-L1 has consistently shown high specificity in predicting death (96%) [32].

Taken together, these data provide evidence that biomarker assessment could potentially play a role in the prognostic evaluation of patients with moderate to severe TBI and improve discriminative capacity to inform clinical decision-making. Yet, no specific recommendations on the optimal prognostic threshold values or sampling time have been developed. This should be an important avenue for future investigation. Moreover, studies exploring the added value of biomarkers over clinical predictors are limited in number and size.

Biomarkers able to identify early after injury those patients with mild TBI who are likely to experience long-term complications would be of great value and are essential to facilitate treatment and maximize benefit to subjects enrolled in clinical trials.

Evidence of the ability of S100B to evaluate prognosis of patients with mild TBI is conflicting. A few studies found a correlation between S100B levels and persistent cognitive abnormalities or post-concussive symptoms after mild TBI [33, 34]. Nonetheless, these findings were not replicated in later studies [35, 36].

Recent studies have also evaluated the ability of serum tau proteins to predict prolonged post-concussive symptoms after mild TBI. Neither cleaved nor total-tau appeared to provide any prognostic information related to persistent post-concussive symptoms [35]. However, a recent study showed that levels of tau-A, a newly discovered tau fragment, correlated with the duration of post-concussive symptoms and may play a role in the setting of mild TBI [37]. Future studies are needed.

NSE does not provide significant prognostic data in mild TBI. To date, only a single small prospective study has shown that initial GFAP levels were associated with initial and follow-up symptom burden up to 1 month after injury in children after concussion [38].

Overall, at present there is no sufficient evidence to support the prognostic value of biomarkers after mild TBI.

Clinical Trials in TBI

In the last decade, there have been intensive efforts to develop neuroprotective and disease-modifying agents to improve patient outcomes after TBI. Among the several factors which have contributed to the long history of failed TBI trials, clinical trial design ignoring substantial interindividual pathological heterogeneity has played a major role. Current patient enrollment criteria are, indeed, mainly unidimensional (based on GCS score or imaging classification) and do not permit appropriate and accurate characterization of the complexity and variability of TBI patients [39]. This means that the populations included in these trials is highly heterogeneous in terms of brain pathology and underlying pathophysiological mechanisms and, thus, a large proportion of individuals do not have the specific molecular pathways that drive disease or represent targets for which the drug is to be tested, adversely affecting the ability to identify a beneficial effect of the treatment. The diagnostic accuracy is probably even lower when considering patients with mild TBI who will develop long-term complications (e. g., post-concussive syndrome).

Consequently, there is a critical need for further progress in the development and validation of diagnostic tools that can accurately identify patients for inclusion in TBI clinical trials and stratify them according to the magnitude of injury, pathoanatomic features and pathophysiological molecular mechanisms. Biomarkers informing clinical trial design and determining the targeted patient population of likely responders are likely to greatly increase the possibility of assessing drug efficacy while holding promise for personalized (precision) medicine [40].

Furthermore, the absence of reliable biomarkers to identify and monitor the biochemical effects of drugs (theranostic markers) and the lack of validated effective 'endpoints' of brain injury and recovery are considered to be additional major obstacles to the development of neuroprotective agents for TBI. To this end, the FDA has recently recommended that development of a companion diagnostic be performed in concert with clinical drug development to improve delivery of safe and effective therapies, and the Traumatic Brain Injury Endpoints Development (TED) Initiative has begun "to assess the regulatory readiness of a variety of clinical outcome assessments (COAs), blood-based biomarkers, and neuroimaging biomarkers that may be used as tools for TBI clinical trials" [41].

The ultimate goal will be to develop and qualify appropriate biomarker signatures for use during a clinical trial, and then move from clinical trials toward the real world to guide patient management in routine clinical practice.

TBI Biomarkers: Role in Clinical Trials

Combinations of serum levels of glial and neuronal markers have been shown to have a high predictive value for characterizing the initial type of injury and have been increasingly incorporated in clinical trials [32]. However, at present, only preliminary evidence exists.

Evidence of the utility of S100B in the assessment of therapeutic effects, dose optimization and as a safety marker has been provided by a recent pilot study comparing administration of different hyperosmotic agents (mannitol versus hypertonic saline) after TBI [42]. The study found a decrease in serum S100B levels during treatment with both osmotic agents, which was dose-dependent and linked to the mechanism of action of the drugs and the clinical outcome. In summary, these findings support the concept that brain damage biomarkers could be valuable tools to monitor biochemical drug effects in clinical trials.

Large multicenter clinical trials that have been recently completed, including the EPO-TBI (Erythropoietin in Traumatic Brain Injury, NCT00987454), BioProTECT (Blood Tests to Study Injury Severity and Outcome in Traumatic Brain Injury Patients, NCT01730443) and INTREPID2566 (NCT00805818), have assessed biomarker levels as a secondary endpoint. The initial results of INTREPID2566 demonstrated that serum levels of UCH-L1, GFAP, and SBDP150 on admission as well as their change over time were strongly associated with clinical outcomes, suggesting that biomarker determination may be useful to improve characterization and stratification of trial participants. The results of these trials will hopefully provide support for the application of biomarkers as proof of disease-modifying effects of neuroprotective compounds and their adoption as surrogate endpoints for clinical outcomes, thereby facilitating their qualification and implementation into clinical practice.

Additional support is coming from the Operation Brain Trauma Therapy (OBTT), a multicenter preclinical drug screening consortium for TBI. Incorporation of circulating brain injury biomarker assessments into these preclinical studies has provided substantial evidence of the diagnostic and theranostic utility of GFAP as well as its considerable potential to serve as a substitute for clinically relevant endpoints. These findings are accelerating the development and the ultimate translation of therapies to the human condition while supporting the adoption of biomarkers in clinical trials of TBI [43, 44].

Conclusion

The translation of biomarkers from bench tools to bedside aids in clinical decision-making is ongoing. The evidence for the benefit of biomarkers in TBI is compelling as many studies have demonstrated the spectrum of potential clinical applications and indicated that biomarkers can be crucial to bringing personalized medicine to TBI patients (Table 1). However, there are still many unresolved issues and no universally validated tests are currently available. It is, therefore, essential to accelerate the validation process through standardization efforts with established standard operating procedures, well-validated cutoff values and rigorous quality control programs, as well as well-designed studies. Development of fully automated enzyme assay systems would also be instrumental in reducing interlaboratory and analytical variation. Finally, large, concerted, international collaborative efforts involving all the key-stakeholders (governmental, academia, industry and commu-

Table 1 Traumatic brain injury (TBI) biomarkers in clinical practice

Biomarker	Location	Function/pathogenic process	Clinical application			Comment
			Early diagnosis	Prognosis (stratification)	Role in clinical trials	
Neuronal and axonal markers						
UCH-L1	Neuronal cell body (perikaryon)	Protein de-ubiquitinization/indicative of neuronal damage and/or death	+	+ in severe TBI	+	UCH-L1 levels in blood are increased by compromised BBB integrity
NSE	Neuronal cytoplasm	Upregulated release from damaged axons to maintain cellular homeostasis	–/+	–/+ in severe TBI – in mild TBI	–/+	Also present in erythrocytes and platelets causing false positive results in the setting of hemolysis
pNF-H	Axon/large-caliber myelinated axons	Main component of the axonal cytoskeleton Indicative of axonal injury	–/+	–/+	–/+	Gradual serum increase likely resulting from secondary axonal damage and/or axonal degeneration after a primary injury
Tau	Axon/thin, nonmyelinated axons of cortical interneurons	Binds to and stabilizes microtubules in axons ensuring axonal transport Indicative of injury to thin nonmyelinated axons (grey matter neurons) or axonal degeneration	–	–/+ in severe TBI – in mild TBI	–/+	Ultrasensitive assays are needed for accurate quantification of protein in serum
Glial markers						
S100B	Astroglial cells	Ca^{2+}-binding protein	++	++ in severe TBI – in mild TBI	–/+	Established cut-off to rule out intracranial lesions on CT (0.10 µg/l) Sensitivities: 75–100% NPV: 90–100%
GFAP	Major protein constituent of glial filaments in astrocytes	Cytoskeleton support	+	+ in severe TBI + in mild TBI	+	In clinical trials, GFAP demonstrated potential as theranostic, risk stratification and surrogate endpoint marker

BBB: blood brain barrier; *CT*: computed tomography; *NPV*: negative predictive value; *NSE*: neuron specific enolase; *UHC-L1*: ubiquitin C-terminal hydrolase-L1; *GFAP*: glial fibrillary acidic protein; – not useful; –/+ utility not demonstrated; + potentially useful, but limited evidence; ++ useful, strong evidence nities) are highly desirable for the further valorization of biomarkers in TBI and for their implementation into clinical practice.

References

1. Biomarkers Definitions Working Group (2001) Biomarkers and surrogate endpoints: preferred definitions and conceptual framework. Clin Pharmacol Ther 69:89–95
2. Saatman KE, Duhaime AC, Bullock R, Maas AI, Valadka A, Manley GT (2008) Classification of traumatic brain injury for targeted therapies. J Neurotrauma 25:719–738
3. Mondello S, Muller U, Jeromin A, Streeter J, Hayes RL, Wang KK (2011) Blood-based diagnostics of traumatic brain injuries. Expert Rev Mol Diagn 11:65–78
4. Mondello S, Hayes RL (2015) Biomarkers. Handb Clin Neurol 127:245–265
5. Katz DI, Cohen SI, Alexander MP (2015) Mild traumatic brain injury. Handb Clin Neurol 127:131–156
6. Cassidy JD, Carroll LJ, Peloso PM et al (2004) Incidence, risk factors and prevention of mild traumatic brain injury: results of the WHO Collaborating Centre Task Force on Mild Traumatic Brain Injury. J Rehabil Med 43:28–60
7. Haydel MJ, Preston CA, Mills TJ, Luber S, Blaudeau E, DeBlieux PM (2000) Indications for computed tomography in patients with minor head injury. N Engl J Med 343:100–105
8. Stiell IG, Wells GA, Vandemheen K et al (2001) The Canadian CT Head Rule for patients with minor head injury. Lancet 357:1391–1396
9. Stiell IG, Clement CM, Rowe BH et al (2005) Comparison of the Canadian CT Head Rule and the New Orleans Criteria in patients with minor head injury. JAMA 294:1511–1518
10. Donato R (2001) S100: a multigenic family of calcium-modulated proteins of the EF-hand type with intracellular and extracellular functional roles. Int J Biochem Cell Biol 33:637–668
11. Jonsson H, Johnsson P, Hoglund P, Alling C, Blomquist S (2000) Elimination of S100B and renal function after cardiac surgery. J Cardiothorac Vasc Anesth 14:698–701
12. Biberthaler P, Linsenmeier U, Pfeifer KJ et al (2006) Serum S-100B concentration provides additional information fot the indication of computed tomography in patients after minor head injury: a prospective multicenter study. Shock 25:446–453
13. Unden J, Romner B (2010) Can low serum levels of S100B predict normal CT findings after minor head injury in adults?: an evidence-based review and meta-analysis. J Head Trauma Rehabil 25:228–240
14. Zongo D, Ribereau-Gayon R, Masson F et al (2012) S100-B protein as a screening tool for the early assessment of minor head injury. Ann Emerg Med 59:209–218
15. Unden J, Ingebrigtsen T, Romner B, Scandinavian Neurotrauma Committee (2013) Scandinavian guidelines for initial management of minimal, mild and moderate head injuries in adults: an evidence and consensus-based update. BMC Med 50
16. Thaler HW, Schmidsfeld J, Pusch M et al (2015) Evaluation of S100B in the diagnosis of suspected intracranial hemorrhage after minor head injury in patients who are receiving platelet aggregation inhibitors and in patients 65 years of age and older. J Neurosurg 123:1202–1208
17. Roozenbeek B, Maas AI, Menon DK (2013) Changing patterns in the epidemiology of traumatic brain injury. Nat Rev Neurol 9:231–236
18. Astrand R, Rosenlund C, Unden J, Scandinavian Neurotrauma Committee (2016) Scandinavian guidelines for initial management of minor and moderate head trauma in children. BMC Med 14:33
19. Papa L, Lewis LM, Falk JL et al (2012) Elevated levels of serum glial fibrillary acidic protein breakdown products in mild and moderate traumatic brain injury are associated with intracranial lesions and neurosurgical intervention. Ann Emerg Med 59:471–483
20. Metting Z, Wilczak N, Rodiger LA, Schaaf JM, van der Naalt J (2012) GFAP and S100B in the acute phase of mild traumatic brain injury. Neurology 78:1428–1433

21. Papa L, Silvestri S, Brophy GM et al (2014) GFAP out-performs S100beta in detecting traumatic intracranial lesions on computed tomography in trauma patients with mild traumatic brain injury and those with extracranial lesions. J Neurotrauma 31:1815–1822
22. Papa L, Zonfrillo MR, Ramirez J et al (2015) Performance of glial fibrillary acidic protein in detecting traumatic intracranial lesions on computed tomography in children and youth with mild head trauma. Acad Emerg Med 22:1274–1282
23. Papa L, Lewis LM, Silvestri S et al (2012) Serum levels of ubiquitin C-terminal hydrolase distinguish mild traumatic brain injury from trauma controls and are elevated in mild and moderate traumatic brain injury patients with intracranial lesions and neurosurgical intervention. J Trauma Acute Care Surg 72:1335–1344
24. Welch RD, Ayaz SI, Lewis LM et al (2016) Ability of serum glial fibrillary acidic protein, ubiquitin c-terminal hydrolase-L1, and S100B to differentiate normal and abnormal head computed tomography findings in patients with suspected mild or moderate traumatic brain injury. J Neurotrauma 33:203–214
25. Gatson JW, Barillas J, Hynan LS et al (2014) Detection of neurofilament-H in serum as a diagnostic tool to predict injury severity in patients who have suffered mild traumatic brain injury. J Neurosurg 121:1232–1238
26. Brain Trauma Foundation (2007) Guidelines for the management of severe traumatic brain injury. J Neurotrauma 24(Suppl 1):S1–S106
27. Carroll LJ, Cassidy JD, Cancelliere C et al (2014) Systematic review of the prognosis after mild traumatic brain injury in adults: cognitive, psychiatric, and mortality outcomes: results of the International Collaboration on Mild Traumatic Brain Injury Prognosis. Arch Phys Med Rehabil 95(3 Suppl):S152–S173
28. Steyerberg EW, Moons KG, van der Windt DA et al (2013) Prognosis Research Strategy (PROGRESS) 3: prognostic model research. PLoS Med 10:e1001381
29. Mercier E, Boutin A, Lauzier F et al (2013) Predictive value of S-100beta protein for prognosis in patients with moderate and severe traumatic brain injury: systematic review and meta-analysis. BMJ 346:f1757
30. Vos PE, Lamers KJ, Hendriks JC et al (2004) Glial and neuronal proteins in serum predict outcome after severe traumatic brain injury. Neurology 62:1303–1310
31. Czeiter E, Mondello S, Kovacs N et al (2011) Brain injury biomarkers may improve the predictive power of the IMPACToutcome calculator. Acta Neurochir (Wien) 153:1882
32. Mondello S, Papa L, Buki A et al (2011) Neuronal and glial markers are differently associated with computed tomography findings and outcome in patients with severe traumatic brain injury: a case control study. Crit Care 15:R156
33. De Kruijk JR, Leffers P, Menheere PP, Meerhoff S, Rutten J, Twijnstra A (2002) Prediction of post-traumatic complaints after mild traumatic brain injury: early symptoms and biochemical markers. J Neurol Neurosurg Psychiatry 73:727–732
34. Savola O, Hillbom M (2003) Early predictors of post-concussion symptoms in patients with mild head injury. Eur J Neurol 10:175–181
35. Bazarian JJ, Zemlan FP, Mookerjee S, Stigbrand T (2006) Serum S-100B and cleaved-tau are poor predictors of long-term outcome after mild traumatic brain injury. Brain Inj 20:759–765
36. Begaz T, Kyriacou DN, Segal J, Bazarian JJ (2006) Serum biochemical markers for post-concussion syndrome in patients with mild traumatic brain injury. J Neurotrauma 23:1201–1210
37. Shahim P, Linemann T, Inekci D et al (2016) Serum tau fragments predict return to play in concussed professional ice hockey players. J Neurotrauma 33:1995–1999
38. Mannix R, Eisenberg M, Berry M, Meehan WP 3rd, Hayes RL (2014) Serum biomarkers predict acute symptom burden in children after concussion: a preliminary study. J Neurotrauma 31:1072–1075
39. Skolnick BE, Maas AI, Narayan RK et al (2014) A clinical trial of progesterone for severe traumatic brain injury. N Engl J Med 371:2467–2476

40. Mattes WB, Walker EG, Abadie E et al (2010) Research at the interface of industry, academia and regulatory science. Nat Biotechnol 28:432–433
41. Traumatic Brain Injury Endpoints Development (TED) Initiative Seed Project Awards. https://tbiendpoints.ucsf.edu/seed-projects. Accessed November 2016
42. Hendoui N, Beigmohammadi MT, Mahmoodpoor A et al (2013) Reliability of calcium-binding protein S100B measurement toward optimization of hyperosmolal therapy in traumatic brain injury. Eur Rev Med Pharmacol Sci 17:477–485
43. Mondello S, Shear DA, Bramlett HM et al (2016) Insight into pre-clinical models of traumatic brain injury using circulating brain damage biomarkers: Operation Brain Trauma Therapy. J Neurotrauma 33:595–605
44. Kochanek PM, Bramlett HM, Shear DA et al (2016) Synthesis of findings, current investigations, and future directions: Operation Brain Trauma Therapy. J Neurotrauma 33:606–614

Novel Metabolic Substrates for Feeding the Injured Brain

H. White, P. Kruger, and B. Venkatesh

Introduction

Brain injury is common with high mortality and morbidity, with implications for both society and individuals in terms of cost, loss of production and long-term impairment [1]. The cellular and molecular events initiated by cerebral injury are complex, restricting the precision of characterization into primary, secondary and long term as the durations of pathogenic events are variable and can overlap. Following injury, cellular energetics play a vital role in maintaining cerebral homeostasis [2]. A better understanding of the impact of substrate supply on the injured brain may help improve management following brain injury and provide novel therapeutic options.

The adult brain consumes approximately 20% of basal metabolism, most of which is provided by the oxidation of 100–120 g of glucose/24 h [3]. However, in times of starvation or injury, the primary cerebral metabolic substrates may alter. Following traumatic brain injury (TBI), a number of biochemical changes take place in the brain, which diverts the processing of glucose via the normal pathways.

The purpose of this chapter is to examine cerebral energetics and alternative substrates capable of supplying cerebral energy requirements (Table 1).

H. White
Department of Intensive Care, Logan Hospital, Griffiths University
Meadowbrook, QLD 4131, Australia

P. Kruger · B. Venkatesh (✉)
Critical Care Medicine, Wesley & Princess Alexandra Hospitals, University of Queensland
Brisbane, QLD 4102, Australia
e-mail: bala.venkatesh@health.qld.gov.au

J.-L. Vincent (ed.), *Annual Update in Intensive Care and Emergency Medicine 2017*,
DOI 10.1007/978-3-319-51908-1_27

Table 1 Potential substrates for enhancing cerebral energy supply

Substrate	Proposed mechanism of action
Ketones	BHB is more energy efficient then glucose Increase in free energy of ATP hydrolysis Increase in intermediary metabolites delivered to citric acid cycle Protect against glutamate mediated apoptosis by attenuation of reactive oxidant species Enhancement of GABA mediated inhibition Increase in cerebral blood flow
Lactate	Sparing of cerebral glucose metabolism Regulation of cerebral blood flow Protects neural tissue against excitotoxicity as it attenuates neuronal death
BCAAs	Limited protein loss from skeletal muscle Contribute to synthesis of both inhibitory and stimulatory neurotransmitters Lower cerebral levels of serotonin and catecholamines Supplement intermediates in TCA cycle
Triheptanoin	Replenish TCA cycle intermediates Improvement in cerebral energetics

BHB: beta-hydroxybutyrate; *GABA*: gamma-aminobutyric acid; *BCAA*: branch chain amino acids; *TCA*: tricarboxylic acid

Cerebral Metabolism

Despite comprising only 2% of total body weight, the brain receives 15% of the cardiac output and can use up to 20% of total body oxygen [4]. The main cerebral energy source is derived from ATP produced almost completely from the oxidative metabolism of glucose. As such, 25% of total glucose is metabolized by the brain. During starvation however, hepatic glycogen stores rapidly become exhausted. After several days, brain glucose is produced as a result of gluconeogenesis from amino acids derived from muscle metabolism [5]. From a week onward however, hepatic gluconeogenesis decreases and ketone bodies become the dominant fuel source for the brain (Fig. 1).

The Injured Brain

Disruption of ionic equilibrium shortly following TBI requires energy to correct, reflected by an initial increase in cerebral glucose uptake [6]. This is followed by a prolonged period of glucose metabolic depression. Further disruptions include shunting of glucose through the pentose phosphate pathway, increase in production of reactive oxidant species and DNA damage and inhibition of glycolytic processing of glucose (see Fig. 2; [2]). As such, other substrates including ketones may provide the injured brain with much needed energy.

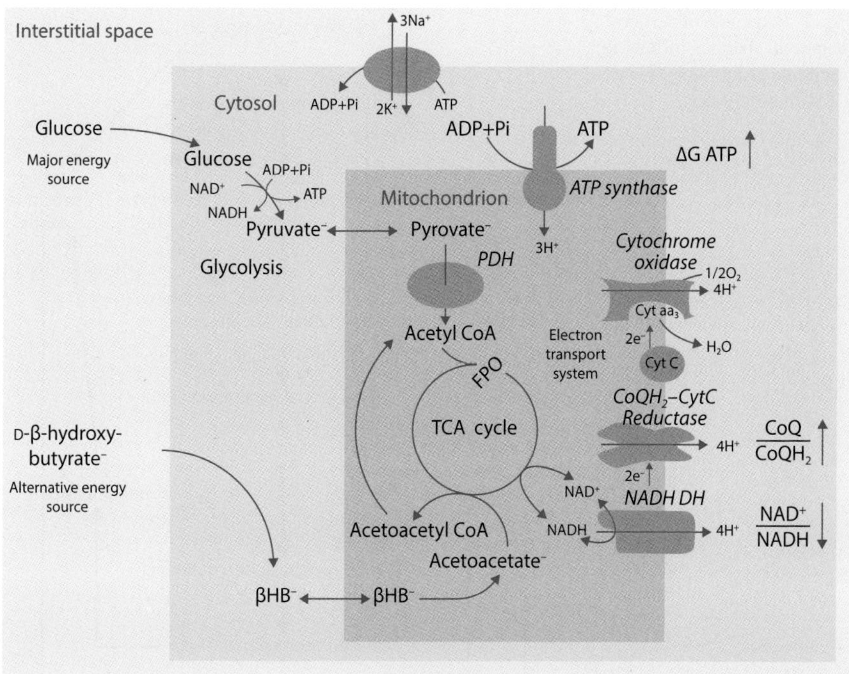

Fig. 1 Cerebral metabolic substrate use in health and during starvation. Ketone bodies added to glucose fundamentally alter mitochondrial metabolism. When added to glucose, a physiological level of ketone bodies reduces the mitochondrial NAD couple, oxidizes the co-enzyme Q couple, and increases metabolic efficiency. These changes are shown on the right side of the figure. The arrows illustrate the effects of ketone bodies compared to glucose alone. Ketone bodies provide an alternative metabolic fuel which can act during blockade of glycolysis. *TCA*: tricarboxylic acid. From [23] with permission

Studying Cerebral Metabolic Dysfunction

The metabolic dysfunction resulting from TBI has been extensively studied. In general, injury is still classified as primary, occurring at the time of injury, and secondary, a result of complex pathological processes occurring hours to days post-injury. Experimental studies have revealed a number of changes including disruption to cellular membranes and homeostasis, release of excitatory neurotransmitters including glutamate, impaired mitochondrial function and generation of free radicals [4, 7–9]. Mitochondrial failure further exacerbates the cerebral energy deficit leading ultimately to apoptosis and cellular death. Much of the current research is aimed at restoring failing cerebral metabolic pathways and providing supplements to augment cerebral energy supply.

Various techniques have been employed to investigate the underlying metabolic perturbations following TBI and the impact of substrate supplementation in these patients [6]. Arteriovenous gradient studies have investigated the cerebral metabolic

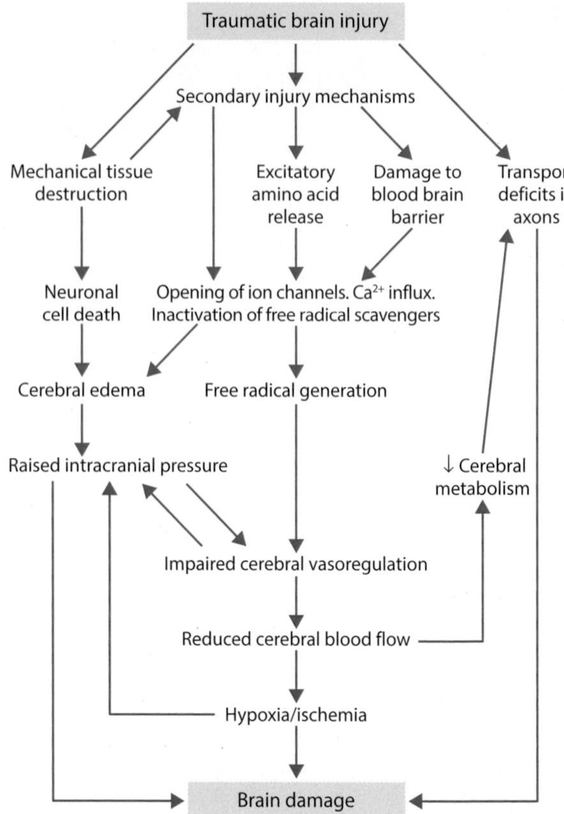

Fig. 2 Sequence of cerebral metabolic changes following traumatic brain injury. From [2] with permission

rate of glucose, the uptake of a number of precursors including lactate, fatty acids, essential amino acids and ketones [10–12]. Although simple to perform, these tests lack the precision and the ability to differentiate between injured from normal cerebral tissues. Microdialysis improves upon these limitations providing continuous sampling from localized areas of interest with the opportunity to analyze a variety of molecules [12]. Features associated with adverse outcomes include high concentrations of lactate, high lactate/pyruvate ratio and both high and low glucose concentrations [13, 14]. Despite these findings, microdialysis is still an experimental technique. Parameters may be difficult to interpret and owing to the focal nature of the findings, their impact on treatment options is uncertain.

Positron emission tomography (PET) scanning has the advantage of being non-invasive, quantitative and dynamic. PET imaging studies using labeled substrates, including 2-deoxy-D-glucose, have provided valuable information regarding glucose metabolism, confirming the relative depression in glucose utilization post TBI [15]. Newer techniques, however, allow PET studies of labeled β-hydroxybutyrate (BHB) and acetoacetate to determine the metabolic fate of ketone bodies in the brain and other tissues [16]. To date studies have confirmed that, in the brain, ketosis reduces glucose utilization and increases ketone oxidation. With the steady increase in the availability of tracers, more research into cerebral metabolism will improve our understanding of these pathways.

Magnetic resonance imaging (MRI) techniques (such as magnetic resonance spectroscopy [MRS]) can be useful in detecting the uptake and metabolism of a number of substrates including N-acetylaspartate, choline-containing phospholipids, creatine and phosphocreatine, lactate, myoinositol, glutamate, ketones, gamma-aminobutyric acid (GABA), and lipids [17]. An important advantage is their ability to provide biochemical information non-invasively and without the need for tracers. A number of studies has utilized MRS to provide data on cerebral metabolism of both lactate and BHB during starvation and following TBI [18]. The main limitation of the technique is the need to transfer critically ill patients to the MRI scanner and the associated risks.

Potential Substrates Capable of Maintaining Cerebral Energetics

Neuroprotective Effects of Ketones

Ketogenesis is the process by which ketone bodies are produced via fatty acid metabolism in the liver [19]. Ketones or ketone bodies are by-products of fat metabolism. They consist of four carbon units with part of the molecule containing a carbon-oxygen bond (C=O). They provide an alternative pathway for the metabolism of acetyl CoA through the ß-oxidation of free fatty acids. Acetoacetate is the central ketone body. Subsequently acetoacetate can be reduced to BHB by β-hydroxybutyrate dehydrogenase in a NADH-requiring reaction.

In health, glucose is the major fuel for human brains. During times of starvation however, the brain has the capacity to adapt to the use of ketones as its major energy source. Once glucose stores are depleted, supplying sufficient glucose to support brain metabolic requirements from protein alone would lead to death in about 10 days. However, there are reports of survival for 50–70 days in people undergoing prolonged fasting and ketones play a key role [5]. During periods of ongoing starvation, an average size person produces about 150 g of ketone bodies per day, capable of supplying 70% of cerebral metabolic requirements [20]. Ketones therefore play a critical role in human evolution.

Aside from their evolutionary benefits, ketones may have neuroprotective effects as they represent an alternative fuel for both the normal and the injured brain [21–23]. There are unique properties of ketone metabolism that may make it a more suitable cerebral fuel under various neuropathologic conditions:

1. Ketones are more energy efficient than glucose.
2. Ketones protect against glutamate-mediated apoptosis.
3. Ketones enhance GABA-mediated inhibition.
4. Cerebral ketone metabolism alters cerebral blood flow.

Exogenous ketone supplementation has been examined in a wide range of animal and human models of neurological disorders including autism, Alzheimer's disease, migraine, strokes, hypoxic-ischemic encephalopathy, Parkinson disease, amyotrophic lateral sclerosis, epilepsy and TBI [24, 25]. More recent studies have examined the use of these diets in the management of brain tumors based on the fact that altered glucose metabolism may have anti-tumor effects [26]. Most human research has looked at ketone supplementation in children for the management of refractory epilepsy. Although initially contentious, there is now good evidence supported by two randomized controlled trials that ketogenic diets in children improve seizure control [27, 28]. The evidence in adults is less compelling but no good studies exist.

Non-Esterified Fatty Acids (NEFA) as a Cerebral Energy Supplement

The ability of ketones to improve cerebral energy metabolism is not shared by other fatty acid containing compounds. Despite being hydrogen rich, fatty acids are utilized poorly by the brain as fuel and may have a number of deleterious properties including the induction of apoptotic pathways [29]. Although highly protein bound, the slow passage of NEFA across the blood brain barrier does not appear to be the cause of poor fatty acid oxidation. Certainly, there is evidence that NEFA may actually damage the blood brain barrier by enhancing oxidative stress in endothelial cells. Furthermore, despite rapid oxidation in peripheral tissues, NEFA is metabolized slowly by the brain and appears to require more oxygen than glucose, further exacerbating the hypoxic environment of the injured brain [30]. The poor anti-oxidative defenses in neurons may be considerably overwhelmed by the rapid accumulation of superoxides following β-oxidation of NEFA. Thus the many benefits associated with ketone supplementation are not shared by free fatty acids which may prove detrimental in the TBI population.

Lactate as a Glucose Sparing Fuel

Lactate is a dead-end metabolite of its redox partner, pyruvate [31]. In mammals, physiological levels may vary between 0.05–5 mmol/l. Lactate is metabolized via lactate dehydrogenase with the extent and direction of the reaction determined by the NAD/NADH(H) ratio. Along with pyruvate, it forms the initial substrate for the tricarboxylic acid (TCA) cycle and subsequently is critical for cellular energetics [32]. Lactate has two optically active forms, L(–) and D(+). The predominant physiological form is L(–) and the metabolic effects resulting from metabolism of the two forms differ significantly. Lactate is actively transported across plasma membranes including red cells, kidney and liver and somewhat slower in the heart skeletal muscle and the brain.

Evidence suggests that lactate can act as an energy source for the brain, especially during periods of substrate deficiency. Data confirm a significant increase in brain lactate following 2–3 days of fasting [18]. This may arise from a shift in lactate metabolism following the shift toward ketone oxidation. Others suggest a continuous production of lactate through glycolysis possibly via a complex interaction between astrocytes and oligodendrocytes (the so call astrocyte-neuron lactate shuttle) [33].

Studies in TBI patients seem to support a role for hypertonic lactate solution in reducing intracranial pressure (ICP) and demonstrate positive effects on cerebral energetics. However, this may depend on the baseline cerebral metabolic state [34]. Studies in animals confirm the supposition that lactate may improve outcomes in TBI. Animal models of both trauma and hypoxic injury have demonstrated a reduction in functional deficits, decrease in lesion volumes and cerebral blood flow augmentation [35, 36]. Only a small number of studies have involved humans. Glenn et al. demonstrated that peripheral lactate production accounted for approx. 70% of carbohydrate consumed for energy production by the traumatized brain and suggested lactate should be supplemented to compensate for decrease in glucose cerebral metabolism [37]. To assess the impact of exogenous lactate on cerebral energy metabolism, Bouzat et al. administered hypertonic lactate to 15 patients with TBI [38]. Using cerebral microdialysis, they demonstrated an increase in lactate, pyruvate and glucose and noted a concomitant decrease in glutamate and ICP. They concluded that hypertonic lactate solution had a positive effect on cerebral energetics and may be a useful therapeutic intervention. Similarly, Ichai et al. demonstrated that hypertonic lactate was more effective at lowering and maintaining ICP when compared with other hypertonic solutions [39]. By sparing cerebral glucose and decreasing ICP, hypertonic lactate may provide an alternative means of controlling ICP while improving cerebral energy metabolism.

Branch-chain Amino Acids and Recovery Post-TBI

The branch-chain amino acids consist of leucine, isoleucine and valine. They account for approximately 35% of essential amino acids and 14% of amino acids in skeletal muscle. Branch-chain amino acids, while nutritionally essential, cannot be synthesized by humans and must be supplied in the diet. They have been demonstrated to impact positively on protein metabolism by inhibiting muscle breakdown and promoting muscle and hepatic protein synthesis [40]. They are essential in the nutritional support of the critically ill. Branch-chain amino acids impact on the production of cerebral neurotransmitters in several ways and contribute to the synthesis of both inhibitory and stimulatory amino acids [41]. They are essential for synthesis of glutamate, which has been implicated in excess cellular damage following TBI, but also of GABA, considered to be an inhibitory neurotransmitter and therefore potentially neuroprotective [42]. Furthermore, by competing for transport across the blood brain barrier, branch-chain amino acids lower cerebral levels of tryptophan, tyrosine and phenylalanine and therefore, indirectly, levels of serotonin and catecholamines. They can also supplement intermediates in the citric acid cycle, potentially improving cerebral energetics.

Branch-chain amino acids have been shown to improve cognitive function in a number of conditions. In animal studies, supplementation with branch-chain amino acids provided a sustained improvement in cognitive function in a mouse model of TBI [43]. In healthy, exercising people, branch-chain amino acids reduce exertional and mental fatigue. Patients with hepatic encephalopathy benefit from branch-chain amino acid supplementation, with improved mental status, asterixis orientation, speech and writing. In an observational study of the TBI population, Vuille-Dit-Bille et al. demonstrated that raised levels of the aromatic amino acids were associated with decreased ICP and increased jugular venous oxygen saturation as compared to branch-chain amino acids [42]. One small study ($n = 20$) demonstrated that TBI patients administered branch-chain amino acids maintained a positive nitrogen balance but data on morbidity and mortality were not provided [44]. Aquilani et al. conducted two small studies (total of 42 patients in the intervention group and 39 control patients) examining the benefits of branch-chain amino acid supplementation on cognitive function in the recovery period post-TBI [45, 46]. They were able to demonstrate a significant improvement in the Disability Rating Scale in patients receiving the supplements. However, the branch-chain amino acids were administered anywhere from 19–140 days following injury and, therefore, the studies do not address their use in the acute setting. There is currently no strong evidence supporting branch-chain amino acid use following acute brain injury.

Triheptanoin and Anaplerosis

Anaplerosis is the process by which intermediates in the TCA cycle are replenished involving the carboxylation of pyruvate and propionyl-CoA. Anaplerotic molecules may include amino acids and odd chain fatty acids. Pyruvate carboxylase appears to be the main anaplerotic enzyme in the brain. Cerebral ATP production is largely dependent on a functioning TCA cycle. Evidence suggests that during neurological injury, including seizures, energy production may be compromised. Therefore, improving cerebral energetics may be an effective therapeutic target.

Triheptanoin was discovered by Roe et al. as an oral anaplerotic treatment for metabolic disorders [47]. It is a triglyceride of heptanoate (C7 fatty acid) capable of being metabolized by β-oxidation to provide propionyl-CoA, which can subsequently be carboxylated to produce succinyl-Coa, and enter the TCA cycle. Triheptanoin is a tasteless oil, which may enter the brain directly or following metabolism in the liver to C5 ketone bodies β-hydroxypentanoate and β-ketopentanoate. These may subsequently be taken up in the brain through monocarboxylate transporters (MCTs) [48]. The result is an increase in acetyl-CoA and ATP production.

Triheptanoin has proven effective in patients with different metabolic problems, including cardiomyopathy and rhabdomyolysis in acyl-CoA dehydrogenase deficiency, pyruvate carboxylase deficiency and carnitine-palmitoyltransferase II deficiency. Several studies involving animal models of epilepsy found triheptanoin to be effective as an anticonvulsant [49, 50]. Adenyeguh et al. reported that triheptanoin administered to patients with early stage Huntington's disease was able to partially correct the abnormal brain energy profile noted in these patients [51]. Efforts are underway to further evaluate the anticonvulsant effects of triheptanoin and to understand its clinical potential for management of epilepsy and other brain disorders [49, 52].

Challenges in Developing New Fuel Substrates for the Injured Brain

While several examples exist that might make metabolic sense in the injured brain, the impact of their therapeutic use and other aspects of systemic metabolism remain to be seen. Probably the most researched substrates are ketones. Adverse effects related to chronic oral intake are well described in the pediatric literature. Less is known about the consequences of administering high doses in the acute brain injury population. Furthermore, there are a number of potential routes of administration which may present their own challenges. Several papers have looked at the administration of BHB as a sodium salt via the intravenous route [53–55]. This allows for a rapid increase in peripheral BHB levels although long-term infusions lead to an increase in pH. The effects of this on ICP have not been investigated to date. Other potential routes of administration include various ketogenic enteral formulations, the commercial product, KetoCal®, and more recently, as a ketone monoester [56].

Lactate can be administered as an iso or hypertonic formulation. The benefits of hypertonic solutions in the head injury population are well described [57]. In general, the likelihood of potential adverse effects, including hypernatremia, increased osmolality and metabolic alkalosis will depend on the formulation provided and the duration. Bouzat et al. administered a hypertonic solution of lactate to head injury patients and did not find any change in physiological variables including $PaCO_2$ however, the infusion only ran for 3 h [38].

The impact on systemic glucose metabolism is variable. Ketone administration is associated with decreased glucose concentration [58]. Lactate is thought to produce a glucose sparing effect in the brain while NEFA may actually lead to hyperglycemia [59]. Branch-chain amino acids seem to stimulate insulin production in the short-term but may lead to insulin resistance following long-term administration [46].

Consideration should also be given to the impact of organ dysfunction such as liver or renal failure when considering substrate supplementation. Branch-chain amino acids have been extensively studied in critically ill patients and appear to be well tolerated and certainly have been demonstrated to be protein sparing [55]. Similarly, NEFA may have a positive impact in critical illness although, as previously noted, may be deleterious in the brain injury population [59, 60]. Ketones and lactate may accumulate and potentially lead to metabolic derangements such as systemic acidemia if liver/renal function is markedly impaired, leading to an inability to metabolize these substrates.

It is therefore necessary to consider the implications of supplementing substrates in terms of other potential metabolic effects and in the setting of major metabolic derangements.

Conclusion

In healthy individuals, glucose is the main substrate for cerebral energy production. However, it is clear that in the damaged brain a significant alteration takes place in metabolic pathways and other substrates may become more important. Of the various potential substances investigated, ketones have received the most in-depth study and would appear to be an excellent alternative to glucose. Research into the field of cerebral energetics however, is still in its infancy. More effort is required to determine which metabolic substrate or combinations of these might provide the damaged brain with the optimum energy requirements.

References

1. Ponsford JL, Downing MG, Olver J et al (2014) Longitudinal follow-up of patients with traumatic brain injury: outcome at two, five, and ten years post-injury. J Neurotrauma 31:64–77
2. Jain KK (2008) Neuroprotection in traumatic brain injury. Drug Discov Today 13:1082–1089
3. Cahill GF Jr, Veech RL (2003) Ketoacids? Good medicine? Trans Am Clin Climatol Assoc 114:149
4. Reilly P, Bullock R (1997) Head Injury: Pathophysiology and Management of Severe Closed Injury. Chapman & Hall Medical, London
5. Owen OE, Caprio S, Reichard GA et al (1983) Ketosis of starvation: a revisit and new perspectives. Clin Endocrinol Metab 12:359–379
6. Jalloh I, Carpenter KLH, Helmy A et al (2015) Glucose metabolism following human traumatic brain injury: methods of assessment and pathophysiological findings. Metab Brain Dis 30:615–632
7. Dash PK, Zhao J, Hergenroeder G et al (2010) Biomarkers for the diagnosis, prognosis, and evaluation of treatment efficacy for traumatic brain injury. Neurother J Am Soc Exp Neurother 7:100–114
8. Andriessen TMJC, Jacobs B, Vos PE (2010) Clinical characteristics and pathophysiological mechanisms of focal and diffuse traumatic brain injury. J Cell Mol Med 14:2381–2392
9. Cederberg D, Siesjö P (2010) What has inflammation to do with traumatic brain injury? Childs Nerv Syst 26:221–226
10. Meierhans R, Brandi G, Fasshauer M et al (2012) Arterial lactate above 2 mM is associated with increased brain lactate and decreased brain glucose in patients with severe traumatic brain injury. Minerva Anestesiol 78:185–193
11. Glenn TC, Kelly DF, Boscardin WJ et al (2003) Energy dysfunction as a predictor of outcome after moderate or severe head injury: indices of oxygen, glucose, and lactate metabolism. J Cereb Blood Flow Metab 23:1239–1250
12. Jalloh I, Helmy A, Shannon RJ et al (2013) Lactate uptake by the injured human brain: evidence from an arteriovenous gradient and cerebral microdialysis study. J Neurotrauma 30:2031–2037
13. Vespa PM, McArthur D, O'Phelan K et al (2003) Persistently low extracellular glucose correlates with poor outcome 6 months after human traumatic brain injury despite a lack of increased lactate: a microdialysis study. J Cereb Blood Flow Metab 23:865–877

14. Stein NR, McArthur DL, Etchepare M et al (2012) Early cerebral metabolic crisis after TBI influences outcome despite adequate hemodynamic resuscitation. Neurocrit Care 17:49–57
15. Nortje J, Coles JP, Timofeev I et al (2008) Effect of hyperoxia on regional oxygenation and metabolism after severe traumatic brain injury: preliminary findings. Crit Care Med 36:273–281
16. Bouteldja N, Andersen LT, Møller N et al (2014) Using positron emission tomography to study human ketone body metabolism: A review. Metabolism 63:1375–1384
17. Marino S, Ciurleo R, Bramanti P et al (2011) 1H-MR spectroscopy in traumatic brain injury. Neurocrit Care 14:127–133
18. Pan JW, Rothman DL, Behar KL et al (2000) Human brain β-hydroxybutyrate and lactate increase in fasting-induced ketosis. J Cereb Blood Flow Metab 20:1502–1507
19. Fukao T, Lopaschuk GD, Mitchell GA (2004) Pathways and control of ketone body metabolism: on the fringe of lipid biochemistry. Prostaglandins Leukot Essent Fatty Acids 70:243–251
20. Owen OE, Morgan AP, Kemp HG et al (1967) Brain metabolism during fasting. J Clin Invest 46:1589–1595
21. Veech RL (2004) The therapeutic implications of ketone bodies: the effects of ketone bodies in pathological conditions: ketosis, ketogenic diet, redox states, insulin resistance, and mitochondrial metabolism. Prostaglandins Leukot Essent Fatty Acids 70:309–319
22. Prins ML (2008) Cerebral metabolic adaptation and ketone metabolism after brain injury. J Cereb Blood Flow Metab 28:1–16
23. Veech RL, Chance B, Kashiwaya Y, Lardy HA, Cahill GF Jr (2001) Ketone bodies, potential therapeutic uses. IUBMB Life 51:241–247
24. Paoli A, Bianco A, Damiani E et al (2014) Ketogenic diet in neuromuscular and neurodegenerative diseases. Biomed Res Int 2014:474296
25. Stafstrom CE, Rho JM (2012) The ketogenic diet as a treatment paradigm for diverse neurological disorders. Front Pharmacol 3:59
26. Otto C, Kaemmerer U, Illert B et al (2008) Growth of human gastric cancer cells in nude mice is delayed by a ketogenic diet supplemented with omega-3 fatty acids and medium-chain triglycerides. BMC Cancer 8:122
27. Freeman JM, Vining EPG, Pillas DJ et al (1998) The efficacy of the ketogenic diet – 1998: A prospective evaluation of intervention in 150 children. Pediatrics 102:1358–1363
28. Neal EG, Chaffe H, Schwartz RH et al (2008) The ketogenic diet for the treatment of childhood epilepsy: a randomised controlled trial. Lancet Neurol 7:500–506
29. Schönfeld P, Reiser G (2013) Why does brain metabolism not favor burning of fatty acids to provide energy? – Reflections on disadvantages of the use of free fatty acids as fuel for brain. J Cereb Blood Flow Metab 33:1493–1499
30. Schönfeld P, Wojtczak L (2008) Fatty acids as modulators of the cellular production of reactive oxygen species. Free Radic Biol Med 45:231–241
31. Veech RL (1991) Metabolism of lactate. NMR Biomed 4:53–58
32. Bouzat P, Oddo M (2014) Lactate and the injured brain: friend or foe? Curr Opin Crit Care 20:133–140
33. Barros LF (2013) Metabolic signaling by lactate in the brain. Trends Neurosci 36:396–404
34. Quintard H, Patet C, Zerlauth J-B et al (2016) Improvement of neuroenergetics by hypertonic lactate therapy in patients with traumatic brain injury is dependent on baseline cerebral lactate/pyruvate ratio. J Neurotrauma 33:681–687
35. Pinto FCG, Capone-Neto A, Prist R et al (2006) Volume replacement with lactated Ringer's or 3% hypertonic saline solution during combined experimental hemorrhagic shock and traumatic brain injury. J Trauma 60:758–763
36. Rice AC, Zsoldos R, Chen T et al (2002) Lactate administration attenuates cognitive deficits following traumatic brain injury. Brain Res 928:156–159
37. Glenn TC, Martin NA, Horning MA et al (2015) Lactate: brain fuel in human traumatic brain injury: a comparison with normal healthy control subjects. J Neurotrauma 32:820–832

38. Bouzat P, Sala N, Suys T et al (2014) Cerebral metabolic effects of exogenous lactate supplementation on the injured human brain. Intensive Care Med 40:412–421
39. Ichai C, Payen J-F, Orban J-C et al (2013) Half-molar sodium lactate infusion to prevent intracranial hypertensive episodes in severe traumatic brain injured patients: a randomized controlled trial. Intensive Care Med 39:1413–1422
40. Elkind JA, Lim MM, Johnson BN et al (2015) Efficacy, dosage, and duration of action of branched chain amino Acid therapy for traumatic brain injury. Front Neurol 6:73
41. Jeter CB, Hergenroeder GW, Ward NH et al (2013) Human mild traumatic brain injury decreases circulating branched-chain amino acids and their metabolite levels. J Neurotrauma 30:671–679
42. Vuille-Dit-Bille RN, Ha-Huy R, Stover JF (2012) Changes in plasma phenylalanine, isoleucine, leucine, and valine are associated with significant changes in intracranial pressure and jugular venous oxygen saturation in patients with severe traumatic brain injury. Amino Acids 43:1287–1296
43. Cole JT, Mitala CM, Kundu S et al (2010) Dietary branched chain amino acids ameliorate injury-induced cognitive impairment. Proc Natl Acad Sci USA 107:366–371
44. Ott LG, Schmidt JJ, Young AB et al (1988) Comparison of administration of two standard intravenous amino acid formulas to severely brain-injured patients. Drug Intell Clin Pharm 22:763–768
45. Aquilani R, Boselli M, Boschi F et al (2008) Branched-chain amino acids may improve recovery from a vegetative or minimally conscious state in patients with traumatic brain injury: a pilot study. Arch Phys Med Rehabil 89:1642–1647
46. Aquilani R, Iadarola P, Contardi A et al (2005) Branched-chain amino acids enhance the cognitive recovery of patients with severe traumatic brain injury. Arch Phys Med Rehabil 86:1729–1735
47. Borges K, Sonnewald U (2012) Triheptanoin – A medium chain triglyceride with odd chain fatty acids: A new anaplerotic anticonvulsant treatment? Epilepsy Res 100:239–244
48. Mochel F, DeLonlay P, Touati G et al (2005) Pyruvate carboxylase deficiency: clinical and biochemical response to anaplerotic diet therapy. Mol Genet Metab 84:305–312
49. Kim TH, Borges K, Petrou S et al (2013) Triheptanoin reduces seizure susceptibility in a syndrome-specific mouse model of generalized epilepsy. Epilepsy Res 103:101–105
50. Willis S, Stoll J, Sweetman L et al (2010) Anticonvulsant effects of a triheptanoin diet in two mouse chronic seizure models. Neurobiol Dis 40:565–572
51. Adanyeguh IM, Rinaldi D, Henry P-G et al (2015) Triheptanoin improves brain energy metabolism in patients with Huntington disease. Neurology 84:490–495
52. Schwarzkopf TM, Koch K, Klein J (2015) Reduced severity of ischemic stroke and improvement of mitochondrial function after dietary treatment with the anaplerotic substance triheptanoin. Neuroscience 300:201–209
53. Suzuki M, Suzuki M, Sato K et al (2001) Effect of beta-hydroxybutyrate, a cerebral function improving agent, on cerebral hypoxia, anoxia and ischemia in mice and rats. Jpn J Pharmacol 87:143–150
54. White H, Venkatesh B, Jones M et al (2013) Effect of a hypertonic balanced ketone solution on plasma, CSF and brain beta-hydroxybutyrate levels and acid-base status. Intensive Care Med 39:727–733
55. Smith SL, Heal DJ, Martin KF (2005) KTX 0101: a potential metabolic approach to cytoprotection in major surgery and neurological disorders. CNS Drug Rev 11:113–140
56. Clarke K, Tchabanenko K, Pawlosky R et al (2012) Kinetics, safety and tolerability of (R)-3-hydroxybutyl (R)-3-hydroxybutyrate in healthy adult subjects. Regul Toxicol Pharmacol 63:401–408
57. White H, Cook D, Venkatesh B (2006) The use of hypertonic saline for treating intracranial hypertension after traumatic brain injury. Anesth Analg 102:1836–1846
58. Ritter AM, Robertson CS, Goodman JC et al (1996) Evaluation of a carbohydrate-free diet for patients with severe head injury. J Neurotrauma 13:473–485

59. Hall TC, Bilku DK, Neal CP et al (2016) The impact of an omega-3 fatty acid rich lipid emulsion on fatty acid profiles in critically ill septic patients. Prostaglandins Leukot Essent Fatty Acids 112:1–11
60. De Bandt JP, Cynober L (2006) Therapeutic use of branched-chain amino acids in burn, trauma, and sepsis. J Nutr 136:308S–313S

Part X
Burn Patients

Fluid Therapy for Critically Ill Burn Patients

A. Dijkstra, C. H. van der Vlies, and C. Ince

Introduction

Burn injuries continue to pose significant medical and surgical challenges in both military and civilian injuries due to limitations of autogenous skin, wound infection, severe metabolic deregulation and other associated injuries. Annually more than 500,000 people seek medical attention, resulting in 40,000 hospitalizations and 4,000 deaths in the United States.

Additionally, burn injuries have a considerable health-economic impact. The annual cost for the medical treatment of burn injuries is estimated to be more than 1 billion dollars in the US, excluding the costs for rehabilitation, chronic disability or other quality of life indices. Because of the high morbidity and mortality rate of burn injuries, numerous studies have been conducted to uncover the complex pathophysiology of burns. Clinical improvements in the critical care management of severely burned patients have led to a decrease in length of hospitalization and mortality over the years [1]. Adequate fluid resuscitation in the acute phase remains critical in terms of survival and overall outcome. However, excessive fluid resuscitation has become a widespread problem in the management of severely burned patients. The primary objective during this phase includes the restoration and preservation of tissue perfusion in order to prevent ischemia from hypovolemic shock. Despite the availability of large data sets in the field of fluid resuscitation,

A. Dijkstra (✉)
Department of Intensive Care and Burn Care, Maasstad Hospital
Maasstadweg 21, 3079 DZ Rotterdam, Netherlands
e-mail: DijkstraA@maasstadziekenhuis.nl

C. H. van der Vlies
Department of Trauma and Burn Surgery, Maasstad Hospital
3079 DZ, Rotterdam, Netherlands

C. Ince
Department of Intensive Care, Erasmus MC, University Medical Center
3015 CE Rotterdam, Netherlands

J.-L. Vincent (ed.), *Annual Update in Intensive Care and Emergency Medicine 2017*,
DOI 10.1007/978-3-319-51908-1_28

there is no international consensus regarding the appropriate type or quantity of fluid for resuscitation. This overview provides insights into the complex pathophysiological process of burn injuries, and the importance and various options of targeting adequate fluid resuscitation.

The Pathophysiology of Burns

Understanding the pathophysiology of burn injuries is crucial for appropriate measures of action. Different types of burn require specific treatment strategies. Therefore, it is necessary to evaluate the mechanism of injury and understand the subsequent physiological response. Irradiation, thermal, electrical and chemical injuries can lead to burns. Thermal burns are responsible for approximately 80% of all reported burns. Burn injuries may result in a local or systemic response depending on the severity of the injury.

The three zones of burn wounds as described by Jackson include: the zones of coagulation, stasis and hyperemia. The different zones divide the burn wound based on the severity of tissue destruction and altered blood perfusion. The coagulation zones represent the area that was destroyed during the injury, which is surrounded by the stasis zone with relatively less perfusion and inflammation. The outermost layer consists of the hyperemia zone, where microvascular perfusion is still ongoing. Burn injuries involving more than 15–20% of the total body surface area (TBSA) may lead to hypovolemic, cardiogenic and distributive shock because of the massive release of cytokines and inflammatory mediators [2]. Interleukins, histamines, prostaglandins, bradykinins, serotonins and catecholamines induce a hypermetabolic state that often leads to organ malfunction. Shock represents an abnormal physiological state in which ischemia occurs due to insufficient tissue perfusion and oxygenation. Burn shock is a complex process of hemodynamic instability and microvascular dysfunction. Increased fluid permeability because of capillary leak leads to a decrease in the intravascular plasma oncotic pressure and to an increase in the interstitial oncotic pressure and subsequent volume depletion. Compensatory vasoconstriction occurs. Because of the massive loss of fluids, proteins and electrolytes, this state may lead to hypoperfusion (Fig. 1) and systemic hypotension. Movement of the intravascular volume into the interstitium causes edema formation. This edema increases rapidly within the acute phase of the injury. Edema formation occurs when the lymph vessels draining a specific tissue mass are overloaded with fluid leaking from microvessels. The amount of edema formation is dependent on the type and severity of the injury. The edema reaches its maximum between 12–24 h in the acute phase [3]. Because of the acute release of inflammatory mediators, edema formation will not stop and may lead to increased tissue pressure and hypoperfusion. Clinically these changes lead to hypotension and a decrease in urinary output. Adequate fluid resuscitation remains the cornerstone treatment for burn shock patients in order to restore tissue perfusion and oxygenation.

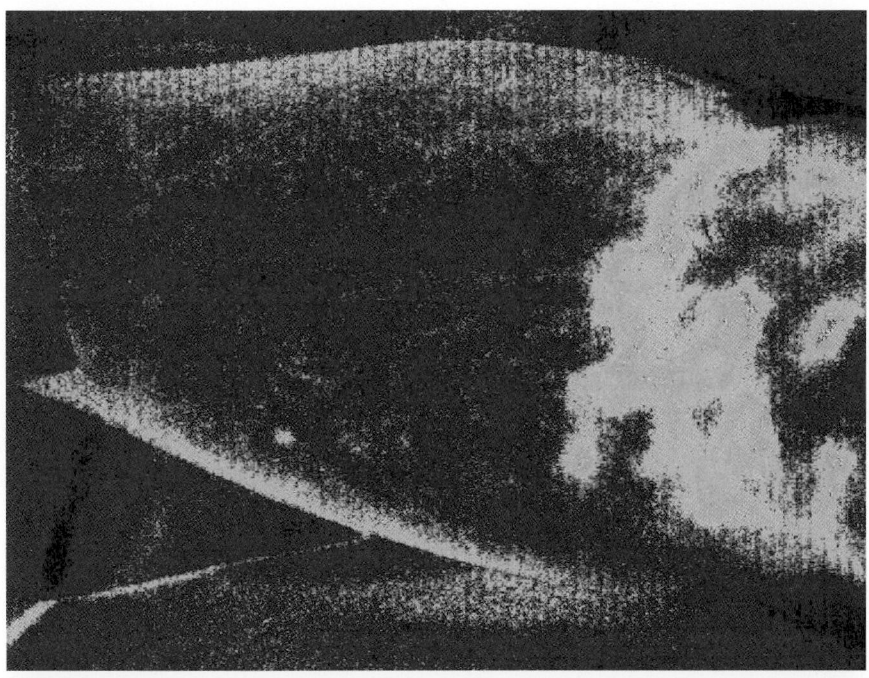

a

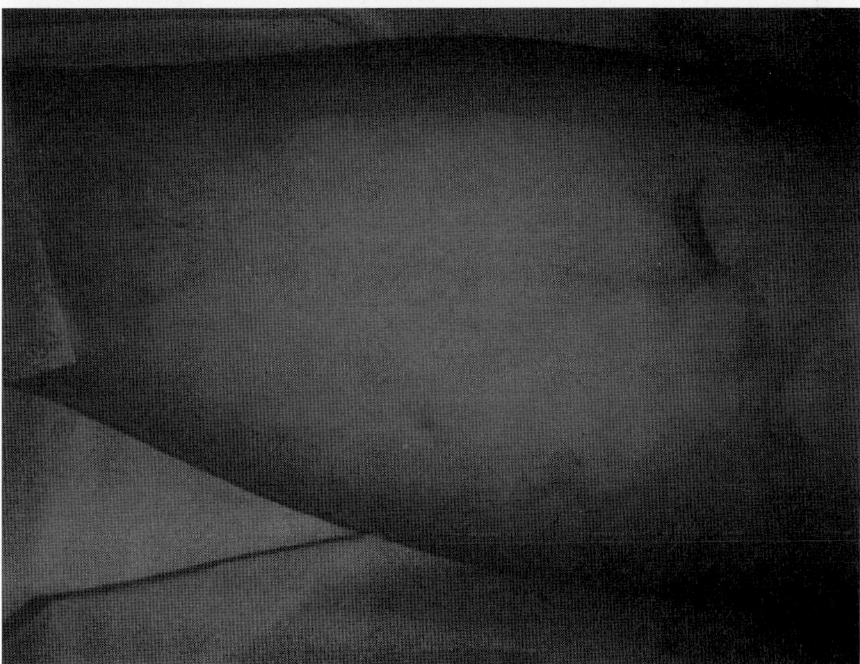

b

Fig. 1 A laser speckle image of the leg of a burn patient, identifying perfused (*green/yellow*) and non-perfused tissue (*blue*) areas (**a**). In (**b**) the black and white video image of the same location is shown

Tissue Oxygenation and Wound Healing

A burn is considered as a complex trauma that needs continuous and multidisciplinary care. The main objective of this complex care is to ensure optimal resuscitation in the acute period and then achieve re-epithelialization of injured or destroyed skin either by support of endogenous healing or by surgical necrectomy and grafting with split skin grafts. Poor wound healing, contraction and scar formation pose significant challenges for clinicians in burn patients. It is, therefore, necessary to understand the process and determinants of wound healing in burn patients that are different from other types of wound healing. Burn injuries are clinically categorized into superficial, superficial-partial, deep-partial, and full-thickness burns corresponding to the depth of the injury. Superficial wounds heal within 21 days, whereas deep and full thickness injuries require surgical therapy and lead to scarring of the skin. The healing process of burns involves three phases: the inflammatory phase, the proliferative phase and the remodeling phase. Superficial burns tend to heal relatively rapidly as the epidermis has regenerative healing capabilities in itself. Deep tissue burns heal slowly and are dependent on various factors. After the acute inflammatory response, the burn wound harbors different cell types that contribute to healing. Platelets, neutrophils, macrophages, lymphocytes and fibroblasts directed by cytokines and chemokines move into the burn wound. Growth factors, such as vascular endothelial growth factor (VEGF), platelet-derived growth factor (PDGF) and transforming growth factor-β (TGF-β), are major regulators that contribute to angiogenesis and fibroblast proliferation.

An important prerequisite in all these phases of healing is that of a preserved microcirculation, which is crucial in regulating the blood flow and tissue perfusion, mediating the delivery of oxygen and nutrients to living parts of the wound and in so doing sustaining the newly formed granulation tissue [4]. Burn injuries not only cause damage to the vessels in the injured areas but also alter blood flow in the surrounding areas (Jackson model). Hypoxia in the injured areas induces angiogenesis to reconstruct the microcirculation, which includes small arteries, arterioles, capillaries and the venules that can be observed in several ways [5]. The relationship between the depth of burn and the microcirculation has been the focus of attention for many years with recent technological developments to visualize the dynamics of the microcirculatory environment. In 1974, Bruce Zawacki concluded that capillary stasis could be reversed and necrosis avoided in the zone of stasis by appropriate prevention of dehydration of the wound [6]. The deeper the burn, the less reversal of capillary stasis and more necrosis was observed in the induced wounds in guinea pigs. Altintas et al. observed microcirculatory disturbances and histomorphological alterations during burn shock treatment using *in vivo* laser-scanning microscopy [7]. Ten burn shock patients underwent measurements prior to and after 24 h of resuscitation using confocal-laser scanning microscopy. Ten matched hemodynamically stable burn intensive care unit (ICU) patients served as controls. At baseline, hemodynamically unstable burn shock patients showed a significant reduction in microvascular blood flow compared to hemodynamically stable burn patients. After 24 h of fluid resuscitation, microvascular blood flow was significantly improved in the burn shock group but there was no significant change in the control group compared to baseline. Post-resuscitation, the granular cell size, basal layer thickness and epidermal thickness increased significantly in burn shock group, but there was a non-significant difference in the control group. Adequate fluid resuscitation in burn shock patients was able to improve the microcirculatory environment leading to restoration of blood flow and enhanced wound healing compared to the control group. Microcirculatory alterations are key determinants of tissue perfusion, oxygenation and capillary leak, which in turn have enormous impact on wound healing after a burn injury. The goal of fluid resuscitation in critically ill burn patients is to maintain key organ perfusion and avoid shock by replacing intravascular fluid losses.

Resuscitation fluids and protocols that restore intravascular volume losses are continuously being investigated in terms of efficacy and outcome. Choosing the appropriate fluid for resuscitation and protocol remains a topic of discussion.

Why Burn Victims Need Fluid Therapy

In 1930, Underhill described studies on patients burned in the Rialto theatre in New Haven [8]. These studies described how systemic shock in these severely burned patients was related to initial fluid losses. This finding was based on the understanding that the origin of the large amounts of accumulated fluids in blisters was filtrate of circulating plasma. Prior to these studies almost no documentation was available relating to burn resuscitation. In a publication from Blalock in 1931, hemodynamic parameter alterations, specifically blood pressure, were related to edema found in burnt tissue. One of the first specific recommendations regarding burn resuscitation using clinical indices to direct fluid therapy was initiated during World War II. Blood values, such as hematocrit and hemoglobin levels, were used to detect hemoconcentration at different time points in severe burn patients during resuscitation.

However, this approach led to inappropriate resuscitation. From that time on, it was acknowledged that a standardized formula of resuscitation was warranted to improve patient outcome. This led to various burn resuscitation formulas being developed including the Wallace rule of nines [9], the rule of the surface of the hand and the Lund and Browder Chart rule. Finally, the Parkland formula was developed by Baxter and Shires [10]. This formula is based on percentage TBSA (%TBSA) burned and is currently the most used algorithm worldwide. Fewer patients now die in the initial 24–48 h because of implementation of immediate fluid resuscitation.

The main goal of fluid resuscitation in severe burn patients is to preserve organ perfusion and prevent ischemia. Different guidelines and protocols use different degrees of TBSA burned for initiation of resuscitation. It is common practice to resuscitate in patients having burns greater than 15–20% TBSA. The main immediate hemodynamic consequences of severe burns greater than 15% TBSA is hypovolemic shock with severe organ damage, increased burn depth or death if not immediately and adequately treated. Inflammatory mediators released by the burn induce an overwhelming systemic inflammatory response that causes capillary leak. At 12–24 h post burn, profound intravascular hypovolemia develops. During this phase, fluid resuscitation is of utmost importance. Fluid needs can be extreme due to proteins and plasma leaking into the interstitium. Because of the large amounts of fluids administered in this phase, a daily positive fluid balance can result in complications, including renal, respiratory (acute respiratory distress syndrome [ARDS]), gastrointestinal dysfunction, abdominal hypertension and compartment syndrome. Excessive use of narcotics and opioids during the first day of the burns injury can be part of the cause of excessive fluid administration. As systemic inflammation is resolved, polyuria occurs to excrete the initial resuscitation fluids. Despite many publications regarding burn resuscitation, there still is no consensus on the optimal resuscitation fluid, nor the endpoints that need to be targeted to avoid fluid-overload. Since the development of the Parkland Formula, almost no progress has been made in the field of fluid resuscitation for severe burns in critically ill patients. Recent years have seen a tendency to over-resuscitate patients in the first 24 h, a phenomenon referred to as "fluid creep". The next section describes the most appropriate solutions for burn patient resuscitation, how to quantify the amounts of fluids needed and to what target based on current knowledge.

Which Type of Fluid, How Much and to What Target

Fluid resuscitation is the cornerstone in the immediate care of the severely burned critically ill patient to preserve organ perfusion. The ideal resuscitation solution to achieve this aim has, however, not yet been identified. The amount of fluid to be administered is directly related to the severity of the injury based on TBSA, the patient's age, the amount of smoke inhalation and electrical injury. A TBSA of > 15% is considered as a major burn and requires strict intravenous resuscitation. The primary endpoint in burn care to guide resuscitation is a urine output of > 0.5 ml/kg/h in adults and 1 ml/kg/h in children. However, some studies have questioned this endpoint because no correlation between urine output and invasively derived hemodynamic parameters has been found [11]. Some studies even suggest that targeting urine output contributes to the phenomenon of fluid creep [12]. The reader is referred to two recent reviews on this topic [13, 14].

Crystalloids

Administration of large volumes of 0.9% NaCl (normal saline) solutions can result in adverse conditions like the development of hyperchloremic metabolic acidosis. Because large amounts of fluid are needed in burn resuscitation, the recommendation is that normal saline should be avoided as a first choice in burn resuscitation protocols in favor of balanced crystalloids [15]. Literature discussing the most appropriate type of crystalloid for burn resuscitation, however, is scarce. In the Parkland formula, Ringers lactate (RL) is used, which is the reason why RL is the fluid of choice in the resuscitation of burn patients. To date only two observational studies have been reported regarding crystalloid resuscitation in burn patients. Oda et al.

[16] described an observational cohort study of 36 burn patients with TBSA >40% and compared the development of abdominal compartment syndrome (ACS) in burn patients resuscitated with hypertonic lactated saline (HLS) versus RL. They found that resuscitations with HLS resulted in a lower fluid volume compared to RL and suggested that this could reduce the risk of secondary ACS. In 2013, Gille et al. [17] performed an observational case control retrospective (RL) and prospective (Ringers acetate [RA]) study in 80 burn patients with a TBSA of 20–70%. They compared fluid resuscitation with RL (n = 40) to RA (n = 40), based on the Parkland formula and targeting an hourly urine output of 0.5–1.0 ml/kg/h. They found lower SOFA (Sequential Organ Failure Assessment) scores for RA solution versus RL. Based on current available knowledge, balanced crystalloid solutions would seem to be the most appropriate resuscitation fluid for large volume replacement. RA has been shown to have a favorable profile in trauma patients; however, the evidence for its use in burn patients is limited. Further studies comparing RL and RA for burn resuscitation are needed.

Colloids

The use of colloids in burn management remains controversial. Colloids contain high molecular weight molecules that increase intravascular plasma oncotic pressure. Theoretically, this enhances intravascular volume expansion by a factor of 1.5 compared to crystalloids. The use of synthetic colloids in the first 24 h of burn resuscitation has been controversial from the beginning because of the idea that an existing capillary leak will allow large molecules to leak into the interstitium leading to the formation of edema [18]. However, Vlachou et al. demonstrated that capillary leakage and endothelial dysfunction were present within 2 h post burn with a median duration of only 5 h [19]. During the last 15 years, a renewed interest in colloids has developed. These colloids can have synthetic (hydroxyethyl starch [HES] and gelatin) or natural (albumin and plasma) components. HES molecules are metabolized slowly, give a longer intravascular volume expansion, but have the potential to accumulate in liver, kidney and skin and can interfere with blood coagulation. Since the recent reluctance to use HES, gelatins are the only synthetic colloids used in burns, although their efficacy is less than that of HES [20]. The reluctance to use HES has, however, been questioned, because some of the studies on which this reluctance was based have been criticized for being methodologically questionable [21]. Some studies were carried out with starches of the first and second generation, which are no longer used for this goal, and not applied to burn patients. These studies were, however, the basis that HES should not be used in burn resuscitation leading to the recommendation from the Parmacovigilance Risk Assessment Committee (PRAC) against the use of HES in critically ill patients with burns. Nowadays, the indication for HES solutions in acute hypovolemic shock has been suggested by the CRISTAL study [22].

The safety of gelatin is unclear. Two meta-analyses found no advantage of gelatins over crystalloids, and older generation gelatins have been associated with anaphylaxis. Their safety cannot be ascertained in a systematic review of randomized controlled trials, and no studies guaranteeing their safety in burn patients are available. The current recommendation is that colloids, especially HES, cannot be recommended for the resuscitation of critically ill burn patients.

Albumin

Albumin is a plasma protein contributing to the intravascular oncotic pressure. As with all colloids, questions regarding safety and efficacy have been ongoing. In 1998, one meta-analysis showed increased mortality in the group receiving albumin, however the small size of the studies included limited the conclusions [23]. After this study the SAFE-trial was conducted [24]. In this randomized controlled trial, 7,000 critically ill patients were included and a comparison made between albumin 4% and normal saline. There were no differences in mortality or organ failure. However, no burn patients were included. In 2007, in a case-control study, Cochran et al. studied patients receiving albumin during resuscitation and reported decreased mortality compared to patients who did not received albumin [25]. Lawrence et al. reported that colloid administration ameliorated fluid creep and normalized the resuscitation ratio [26]. Albumin 20%, based on the available evidence, can be recommended in severe burns, especially in the de-resuscitation phase after 24 h if guided by indices of capillary leak, fluid balance, extravascular lung water, intraabdominal pressure, fluid overload and cumulative fluid balance.

Hypertonic Saline

Hypertonic saline expands the circulating volume by attracting water to the intravascular compartment. In 1973, studies showed that hypertonic saline reduced the amount of fluid needed for burn resuscitation [27]. When large amounts of hypertonic saline are used, hypernatremia, associated with acute cerebral fluid shift and renal failure can occur [28]. In 1995, a study comparing hypertonic saline versus controls who received crystalloids showed a significantly higher rate of acute kidney injury (AKI) and mortality in the hypertonic saline group. In 2006, however, Oda et al. reported a significantly reduced risk of secondary ACS in patients receiving hypertonic saline [15]. At the moment, no consensus can be reached regarding the use of hypertonic saline in burn resuscitation. When hypertonic saline is used, close monitoring of sodium levels is strongly advised.

Quantification of Amount of Fluid Needed

Large amounts of fluids are administered during the first 24 h in burn patients. Initial resuscitation is usually started with crystalloids. Most burns units worldwide have been using the Parkland formula as the gold standard for fluid resuscitation in acute burns for many decades [29]. Since its introduction, under-resuscitation has become rare and it has revolutionized acute burn care management by reducing mortality and morbidity during the last 50 years. In the formula, 4 ml/kg/%TBSA crystalloid (mostly RL) is given for the first 24 h of which half is given over the first 8 h. Resuscitation fluids traditionally target an hourly urine output of 0.5–1 ml/kg/h. As a resuscitation endpoint, this is far from ideal, because urine output may not reflect end-organ or tissue hypoperfusion at the microvascular level. In 1991, Dries and Waxman found that fluid resuscitation guided by vital signs may be inadequate [30]. Urine output and vital signs showed little variation after fluid replacement, whereas significant alterations were observed in parameters measured by the pulmonary artery catheter (PAC). Since then, one of the most important measures to guide volume therapy has been cardiac output, but only 8% of burn units base their resuscitation plan on it because of the need for a PAC initially. A publication in 2005 by Holm et al. [31] showed the reproducibility of transpulmonary thermodilution measurements in patients with hypothermia and burn shock. All studies of goal-directed therapy in major burn patients reported similar results where the directed therapy group received more fluid than those treated with the Parkland formula. Curiously, only the study of Tokarik et al. [32] showed results incongruent with those reported earlier. After reviewing the results of all the goal-directed therapy studies, it seems reasonable to say that goal-directed therapy using transpulmonary thermodilution has a role in burn resuscitation. However, it must be kept in mind that these studies included small numbers of patients and the effect of goal-directed therapy on patient survival has not yet been shown. Multicenter studies with large number of patients are needed to obtain a good level of evidence.

What Target?

The optimal amount of fluid to be administered when resuscitating burn patients has to be evaluated. The interpretation of the hemodynamic status can be very difficult in burn patients. Despite advances in hemodynamic monitoring and the goal-directed therapy concept, most burn care providers still base their practice with regard to resuscitation on formulas developed 40 years ago. Resuscitation formulas can be seen as guidelines for initiating fluid resuscitation. Infusion rates need to be adjusted to physiological endpoints, which can be obtained by minimally invasive monitoring methods. These endpoints, such as systemic blood pressure, mean arterial pressure (MAP), lactate levels, cardiac output, global end-diastolic index, and urine output, all have their own limitations. Every severely burned patient (TBSA > 20%) should be monitored adequately. As diuresis is a poor endpoint and leads to under- or over-resuscitation, diuresis is no longer recommended as a target parameter. In situations where there is limited monitoring, however, it can be used with support of a urine output algorithm [33]. Fluid resuscitation should only be given when tissue hypoperfusion is present as indicated by increasing base deficit, increasing lactate etc. Burn patients receiving fluids for resuscitation should be guided by physiological parameters or tests that are able to predict fluid responsiveness. From this perspective, the use of microcirculatory monitoring may provide a guide to optimizing the amount of administered fluids [34]. As barometric preload parameters, such as central venous pressure (CVP) and pulmonary artery occlusion pressure (PAOP) are inferior to volumetric preload parameters, these are not recommended to guide fluid resuscitation in burn patients. Volumetric preload variables like global end-diastolic volume (GEDV) and intrathoracic blood volume (ITBV) have been shown in numerous studies to represent preload more precisely than urine output [35] or cardiac filling pressure.

Challenges for Fluid Therapy

Our understanding of the pathophysiology of burn shock has improved. The development of fluid resuscitation strategies has led to dramatic outcome improvement. Over-resuscitation, which occurs more frequently than under-resuscitation, is related to more morbidity and mortality and leads to complications such as compartment syndrome and respiratory failure.

To prevent these complications all efforts should be made to resuscitate organ perfusion with the least amount of fluids. There is a need to redefine endpoints in burn resuscitation. Advanced hemodynamic monitoring with transpulmonary hemodilution and pulse contour analysis can provide superior endpoints to avoid over-resuscitation and guide the de-resuscitation process [35]. However, this personalized care using a stepwise approach in predefined algorithms, has to be established by more studies in the severely burned patient. Furthermore, in the context of fluid resuscitation, it is important to establish whether the resuscitation procedure under investigation effectively improves tissue perfusion and oxygenation because it is clear that the ultimate aim of resuscitation is the restoration of perfusion of vital organs and tissues where oxygen supply to the tissues is compromised due to shock. To accomplish this end-point, oxygen-carrying red blood cells must successfully enter the microcirculation and deliver oxygen to the tissues. In burn resuscitation, conventional procedures, such as administering fluids, are applied to accomplish this aim.

Most clinicians aim at normalizing physiological and systemic hemodynamic variables of pressure, flow and/or oxygen delivery. Whether these procedures are successful in achieving adequate perfusion and oxygen transport to tissues in the burn patient is unknown at the bedside, and relies on the assumption that there is a hemodynamic coherence between the macro- and microcirculations. Hemodynamic coherence is the condition where resuscitation targeting correction of systemic hemodynamic variables is effective in correcting microcirculatory and tissue perfusion and oxygenation so that the parenchymal cells are able to perform their functional activities in support of organ function [34]. Many studies have described the presence of a loss of hemodynamic coherence in which resuscitation based on the normalization of systemic hemodynamic variables did not lead to a parallel improvement in microcirculatory perfusion and oxygenation [34]. Two of the four types of microcirculatory condition in which there is a loss of hemodynamic coherence are of specific relevance to burn patients, namely the presence of hemodilution and the presence of tissue edema [34]. Taking this into consideration, monitoring of the microcirculation may be advised to ensure that fluid resuscitation is effective in improving tissue perfusion. An optimal microcirculatory perfusion by monitoring perfusion at the bedside could contribute to the administration of the optimal amount of resuscitation fluids thereby preventing complications of under- and over resuscitation [36]. With the introduction of hand held microscopy at the bedside [37], the nature of microcirculatory alterations during burn shock resuscitation can be elucidated. An alternative technique, which could be of use to identify areas of hypoperfusion, is laser speckle imaging [38]. This modality allows microcirculatory imaging of large areas of tissue and can be readily used at the bedside and during surgery [39]. At the moment, little is known about fluid therapy and its effectiveness in recruiting the microcirculation in burn shock patients. In 2014, Altintas et al. studied the effect of cold therapy on histomorphology, edema formation and microcirculation in superficial burn. They found that these variables were significantly influenced by local cold application, however these alterations were transient and ineffective after 30 min [40]. In 2016, Medved et al. determined that the best reconstructive approach for an outer ear reconstruction after a severe burn injury was by means of analyzing the microcirculation. Pedicled flaps were most similar to healthy ear tissue. Although the external validity is suboptimal because of the small number of patients, these results improve the knowledge of soft tissue viability. It also facilitates the process of reconstruction of the burned auricle [41]. Several studies have demonstrated that fluids can improve microvascular perfusion by increasing the proportion of perfused capillaries and decreasing perfusion heterogeneity. The greatest effect on microcirculatory perfusion alterations is in the early phase of resuscitation. The type of fluid and its impact on the microcirculation is also a source of ongoing investigation. Recently, there has been a proposal for the microcirculation to guide fluid resuscitation [36]. This could be very interesting in severe burn patients as the optimal amount of fluids to be administered is still an area of uncertainty.

Conclusion

Burn injuries continue to pose significant medical and surgical challenges and have considerable health-economic impact. Due to a better understanding of burn shock pathophysiology, dramatic improvements in outcome have been achieved. This is mainly caused by development of fluid resuscitation strategies. Organ hypoperfusion has become rare and there is growing concern that over-resuscitation is occurring more frequently. In an attempt to prevent over resuscitation and its associated complications, new targets and endpoints of resuscitation have to be defined. As many studies have described that resuscitation based on normalization of systemic hemodynamic variables does not lead to a parallel improvement in microcirculatory perfusion and oxygenation, a microcirculatory-guided approach could be helpful to determine the optimal amounts and types of fluids to be administered to critically ill burn patients.

Acknowledgements

We thank Dr. Servet Duran and Yasin Ince for providing the laser speckle image shown in Fig. 1.

References

1. Brusselaers N, Monstrey S, Vogelaers D, Hoste E, Blot S (2010) Severe burn injury in Europe: a systematic review of the incidence, etiology, morbidity, and mortality. Crit Care 14:R188
2. Mitra B, Fitzgerald M, Cameron P, Cleland H (2006) Fluid resuscitation in major burns. ANZ J Surg 76:35–38
3. Infanger M, Schmidt O, Kossmehl P, Grad S, Ertel W, Grimm D (2004) Vascular endothelial growth factor serum level is strongly enhanced after burn injury and correlated with local and general tissue edema. Burns 30:305–311
4. Schreml S, Szeimies RM, Prantl L, Karrer S, Landthaler M, Babilas P (2010) Oxygen in acute and chronic wound healing. Br J Dermatol 163:257–268
5. Eriksson S, Nilsson J, Sturesson C (2014) Non-invasive imaging of microcirculation: a technology review. Med Devices (Auckl) 7:445–452
6. Zawacki BE (1974) Reversal of capillary stasis and prevention of necrosis in burns. Ann Surg 180:98–102
7. Altintas MA, Altintas AA, Guggenheim M et al (2010) Insight in microcirculation and histomorphology during burn shock treatment using in vivo confocal-laser-scanning microscopy. J Crit Care 25:173 (e1–7)
8. Underhill F (1930) The significance of anhydremia in extensive surface burn. JAMA 95:852–857
9. Evans EI, Purnell OJ, Robinett PW, Batchelor A, Martin M (1952) Fluid and electrolyte requirements in severe burns. Ann Surg 135:804–817
10. Baxter C (1979) Fluid resuscitation, burn percentage, and physiological age. J Trauma 19:864–865
11. Dries DJ, Waxman K (1991) Adequate resuscitation of burn patients may not be measured by urine output and vital signs. Crit Care Med 19:327–329
12. Shah A, Kramer GC, Grady JJ, Herndon DN (2003) Meta-analysis of fluid requirements for burn injury 1980–2002. J Burn Care Rehabil 152:S118
13. Peeters Y, Vandervelden S, Wise R, Malbrain M (2015) An overview on fluid resuscitation and resuscitation endpoints in burns: Past, present and future. Part 1 – historical background, resuscitation fluid and adjunctive treatment. Anaesthesiol Intensive Ther 47:s6–s14
14. Guilabert P, Usua G, Martin N, Abarca L, Barret JP, Colomina MJ (2016) Fluid resuscitation management in patients with burns:update. Br J Anaesth 117:284–296
15. Marik PE (2014) Iatrogenic salt water drowning and the hazards of a high central venous pressure. Ann Intensive Care 4:21
16. Oda J, Ueyama M, Yamashita K et al (2006) Hypertonic lactated saline resuscitation reduces the risk of abdominal compartment syndrome in severely burned patients. J Trauma 60:64–71
17. Gille J, Klezcewski B, Malcharek M et al (2014) Safety of resuscitation with Ringer's acetate solution in severe burn (VolTRAB) – an observational trial. Burns 40:871–880
18. Baxter CR (1974) Fluid volume and electrolyte changes of the early postburn period. Clin Plast Surg 1:693–703
19. Vlachou E, Gosling P, Moiemen NS (2006) Microalbuminuria: a marker of endothelial dysfunction in thermal injury. Burns 32:1009–1016
20. Coriat P, Guidet B, de Hert S et al (2014) Counter statement to open letter to the Executive Director of the European Medicines Agency concerning the licensing of hydroxyl ethyl starch solutions for fluid resuscitation. Br J Anesth 113:194–195

21. Van der Linden P, James M, Mythen M, Weiskopf RB (2013) Safety of modern starches used during surgery. Anesth Analg 116:35–48
22. Annane D, Siami S, Jaber S et al (2013) Effects of fluid resuscitation with colloids vs crystalloids on mortality in critically ill patients presenting with hypovolemic shock: the CRISTAL randomized trial. JAMA 310:1809–1817
23. Cochrane Injuries Group Albumin Reviewers (1998) Human albumin administration in critically ill patients: systematic review of randomised controlled trials. BMJ 317:235–240
24. Finfer S, Bellomo R, Boyce N et al (2004) A comparison of albumin and saline for fluid resuscitation in the intensive care unit. N Engl J Med 350:2247–2256
25. Cochran A, Morris SE, Edelman LS, Saffle JR (2007) Burn patient characteristics and outcomes following resuscitation with albumin. Burns 33:25–30
26. Lawrence A, Faraklas I, Watkins H et al (2010) Colloid administration normalizes resuscitation ratio and ameliorates "fluid creep". J Burn Care Res 31:40–47
27. Moylan JA Jr., Reckler JM, Mason AD Jr (1973) Resuscitation with hypertonic lactate saline in thermal injury. Am J Surg 125:580–584
28. Shimazaki S, Yoshioka T, Tanaka N, Sugimoto T, Onji Y (1977) Body fluid changes during hypertonic lactated saline solution therapy for burn shock. J Trauma 17:38–43
29. Greenhalgh DG (2010) Burn resuscitation: The results of the ISBI/ABA survey. Burns 36:176–182
30. Dries DJ, Waxman K (1991) Adequate resuscitation of burn patients may not be measured by urine output and vital signs. Crit Care Med 19:327–329
31. Holm C, Mayr M, Hörbrand F et al (2005) Reproducibility of transpulmonary thermodilution measurements in patients with burn shock and hypothermia. J Burn Care Rehabil 26:260–265
32. Tokarik M, Sjoeberg F, Balik M, Pafcuga I, Broz L (2013) Fluid therapy LiDCO controlled trial-optimization of volume resuscitation of extensively burned patients through non invasive continuous real-time hemodynamic monitoring LiDCO. J Burn Care Res 34:537–542
33. Peeters Y, Lebeer M, Wise R, Malbrain ML (2015) An overview on fluid resuscitation and resuscitation endpoints in burns: Past, present and future. Part 2 – avoiding com plications by using the right endpoints with a new personalized protocolized approach. Anaesthesiol Intensive Ther 47:s15–s26
34. Ince C (2015) Hemodynamic coherence and the rationale for monitoring the microcirculation. Crit Care 19:S8–S13
35. Sanchez M, Garcia-de-Lorenzo A, Herrero E et al (2013) A protocol for resuscitation of severe burn patients guided by transpulmonary thermodilution and lactate levels: a 3-year prospective cohort study. Crit Care 17:R176
36. Ince C (2014) The rationale for microcirculatory guided fluid therapy. Curr Opin Crit Care 20:301–308
37. Aykut G, Veenstra G, Scorcella C, Ince C, Boerma C (2015) Cytocam-IDF (incident dark field illumination) imaging for bedside monitoring of the microcirculation. Intensive Care Med Exp 3:40
38. Bezemer R, Klijn E, Khalilzada M et al (2010) Validation of near-infrared laser speckle imaging for assessing microvascular (re)perfusion. Microvasc Res 79:139–143
39. Klijn E, Hulscher HC, Balvers RK et al (2013) Laser speckle imaging identification of increases in cortical microcirculatory blood flow induced by motor activity during awake craniotomy. J Neurosurg 118:280–286
40. Altintas B, Altintas AA, Kramer R, Sorg H, Vogt PM, Altintas MA (2014) Acute effects of local cold therapy in superficial burns on pain, in vivo microcirculation, edema formation and histomorphology. Burns 40:915–921
41. Medved F, Medesan R, Rothenberger JM et al (2016) Analysis of the microcirculation after soft tissue reconstruction of the outer ear with burns in patients with severe burns injuries. J Plast Reconstr Aesthet Surg 69:988–993

Burn Patients and Blood Product Transfusion Practice: Time for a Consensus?

A. Holley, A. Cook, and J. Lipman

Introduction

Severe burn injury commonly leads to anemia and coagulopathy [1–3]. This results from the underlying injury, as well as the subsequent treatment [1, 2]. An appreciation of the pathophysiology driving these changes is important in guiding both preventative and targeted treatment strategies. There is increasing evidence from observational studies to support a more restrictive blood transfusion target in burn patients, however high quality multicenter randomized controlled trials in this cohort are lacking [4, 5]. The clinician must consider the evidence for restrictive blood utilization balanced against the unique hematological changes and perfusion requirements in burn patients. Currently, there are no formal recommendations in regard to transfusion strategies and targets specific to patients with severe burns and, therefore, practice among burns units remains very diverse [1, 5].

Mechanism of Anemia in Burns Patients

Anemia associated with severe burns is a common finding, with a multitude of potential causes, including decreased erythropoiesis, direct red cell injury, erythrocyte sequestration in burn tissue, hemodilution, blood loss from debridement, donor site bleeding, and recurrent phlebotomy over the duration of an often prolonged admission [1] (Fig. 1).

A. Holley (✉) · A. Cook
Department of Intensive Care Medicine, Royal Brisbane Hospital
Herston, QLD 4029, Australia
e-mail: anthony.d.holley@gmail.com

J. Lipman
Department of Intensive Care Medicine, Royal Brisbane & Women's Hospital
Herston, QLD 4029, Australia
Burns, Trauma and Critical Care Research Centre, The University of Queensland
Herston, QLD 4029, Australia

J.-L. Vincent (ed.), *Annual Update in Intensive Care and Emergency Medicine 2017*,
DOI 10.1007/978-3-319-51908-1_29

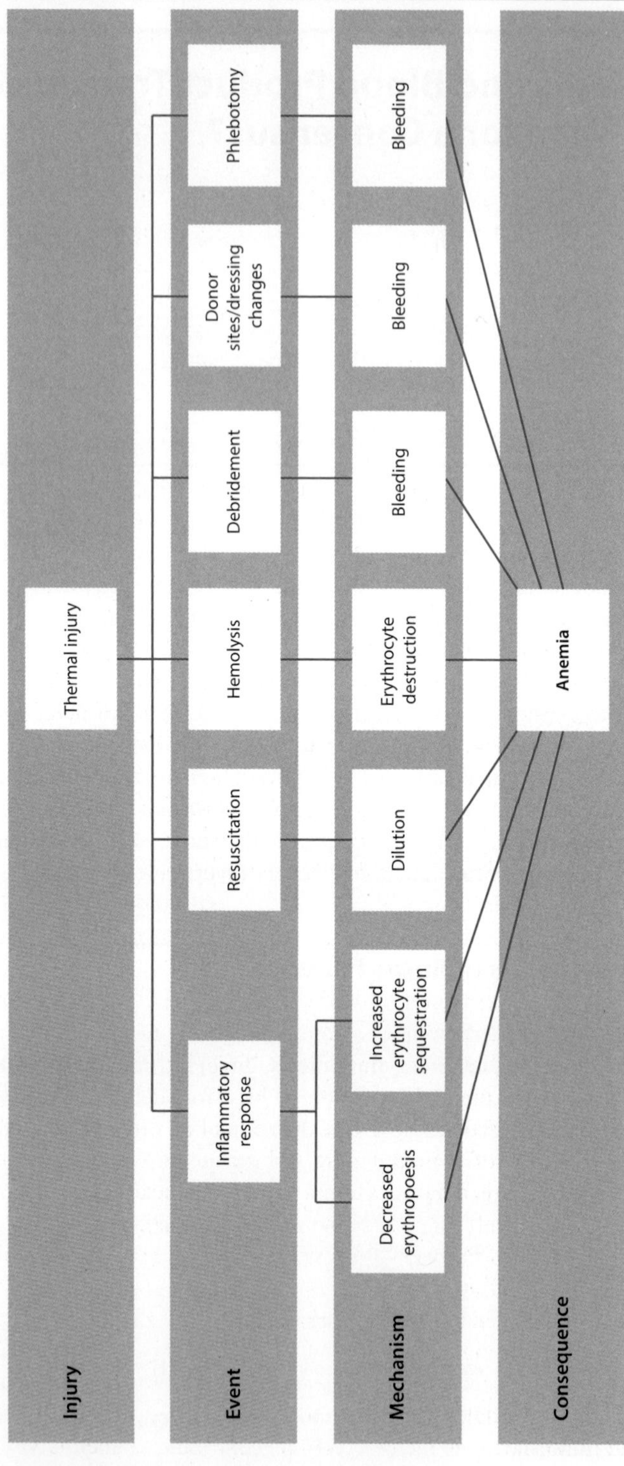

Fig. 1 Proposed mechanisms in the development of burn anemia

An understanding of the pathophysiology and timing of this anemia should lead to improved prevention and targeted treatment. It is important to distinguish between anemia that occurs due to acute blood loss after a burn injury, and the anemia that occurs in the setting of critical illness and persists despite wound healing [2]. The anemia needs to be interpreted in the context of the adequacy of organ perfusion, rather than simply as an isolated hemoglobin value.

Acute anemia secondary to blood loss may occur as a result of the thermal injury as well as due to the subsequent surgical management. Excision of burn wounds mandates debridement down to viable bleeding tissue. There is further potential blood loss from skin donor sites. As a result, significant amounts of blood can be lost during surgical management [2]. Chronic blood loss due to iatrogenic factors, such as phlebotomy, minor procedures, and dressing changes, are also likely to contribute to the persistent and delayed anemia that characterizes major burns [2, 6].

An additional form of acute blood loss anemia is postulated to occur as a direct result of the thermal injury with subsequent accelerated erythrocyte destruction [7–9]. There is evidence that heating of erythrocytes directly to 50 °C, then performing an autologous transfusion leads to alterations in the red cell morphology resulting in a significant reduction in the erythrocyte half-life [7].

Aside from the direct thermal damage to the red cells, there appears to be a process of active red cell lysis in burn patients [8]. Loebl et al. demonstrated this process by transfusing red blood cells derived from healthy volunteers into patients with severe thermal injuries, which led to a significantly shortened lifespan of the transfused cells [8]. The pathophysiology of this was investigated in a rodent model that appeared to demonstrate complement-mediated intravascular hemolysis in response to thermal injury [9]. There appears to be burn-induced complement stimulation of neutrophil free radical production, although additional proposed processes include C5b-9 mediated membrane attack complex lysis or C3b-mediated opsonization and erythrocyte sequestration in the reticuloendothelial system [9]. A small case series also demonstrated similar early intravascular hemolysis in human burns patients [10]. The magnitude of these early effects may be insufficient to warrant red blood cell transfusion in the first few days post-injury, as highlighted by Palmieri et al. who demonstrated that the average timing of first transfusion among burn patients was five days post-admission [4].

Burn patients are also particularly prone to anemia of critical illness as a result of the prolonged duration of hemodynamic and metabolic stress associated with a major burn injury [6]. This delayed anemia is not specifically related to surgical debridement, may occur well into the phase of wound healing, and appears to be responsible for a significant number of transfusions in severely burned patients [4, 6]. Based on our understanding of anemia of critical illness in general intensive care unit (ICU) patients, shortened red cell lifespan, red cell loss, and diminished red cell production are all contributing factors [11].

Blunted erythropoiesis seen in burn patients is likely secondary to systemic inflammation and nutritional deficiencies. Circulating cytokines, including interleukin (IL)-1, IL-6 and tumor necrosis factor (TNF)-α, contribute to anemia via reduced transcription of the erythropoietin gene and inhibited erythropoietin production, a direct effect on erythroid progenitor cells to inhibit red blood cell production, and by their effect on iron metabolism via upregulation of hepcidin, which impairs duodenal iron absorption and macrophage release of iron [11]. It is known that severe burn injury leads to a 'hyper-inflammatory' state, with a similar pattern of circulating proinflammatory cytokines [12] and it is, therefore, likely that severe burn injury contributes to impaired red cell formation via the above mechanisms [11, 13].

The specific role that nutritional deficiencies play in impaired erythropoiesis in the critically ill is not entirely clear [13] although one study demonstrated that up to 13% of patients can have deficiencies that may contribute (9% iron deficient, 2% folate deficient, 2% B12 deficient) [14].

The link between burn injuries and the blunted erythropoiesis of critical illness is highlighted by the work of Wallner et al. [15, 16]. Autopsy studies have demonstrated a reduced percentage of erythroblasts, yet preserved numbers of granulocytes and megakaryocytes in the bone marrow of patents who died of burn injury when compared with controls, indicative of retarded red cell production [15]. An elegant murine model has also demonstrated severely blunted erythropoiesis in the bone marrow of burned mice, with evidence of markedly depleted erythroid stem cells. This effect was most pronounced at day 21, and persisted for as long as 40 days, highlighting the delayed and persistent nature of the anemia related to burn injuries [16].

Mechanism of Coagulopathy in Burn Patients

The exact pathophysiology of the entity we refer to as burn-induced coagulopathy remains relatively undefined, although is likely to share common mechanisms with acute traumatic coagulopathy (Fig. 2). Acute traumatic coagulopathy is now a well-recognized phenomenon, commonly present on admission to hospital prior to resuscitation and is associated with subsequent organ dysfunction, mortality and increased transfusion requirement [3, 17–20]. The pathophysiology of this entity is multifactorial, with contributions from a consumptive coagulopathy, systemic endogenous anticoagulants, such as activated protein C, and enhanced fibrinolysis [19, 20].

Tissue injury due to trauma or burns leads to subendothelial tissue factor exposure, and localized coagulation and platelet activation [20]. This sequence of events, combined with widespread cellular hypoperfusion and circulating proinflammatory cytokines disrupts both the pro- and anticoagulant pathways and contributes to widespread coagulation system dysfunction [3, 18, 21]. It is well recognized that the severity of coagulopathy correlates with the severity of the burn injury as well as the serum lactate, providing further evidence that the coagulopathy can be attributed to direct endothelial injury and hypoperfusion respectively [3]. A contribution from either localized coagulation factor consumption or the subsequent development of disseminated intravascular coagulopathy (DIC) may also provide a plausible explanation. Inflammation associated with major burns leads to early and widespread

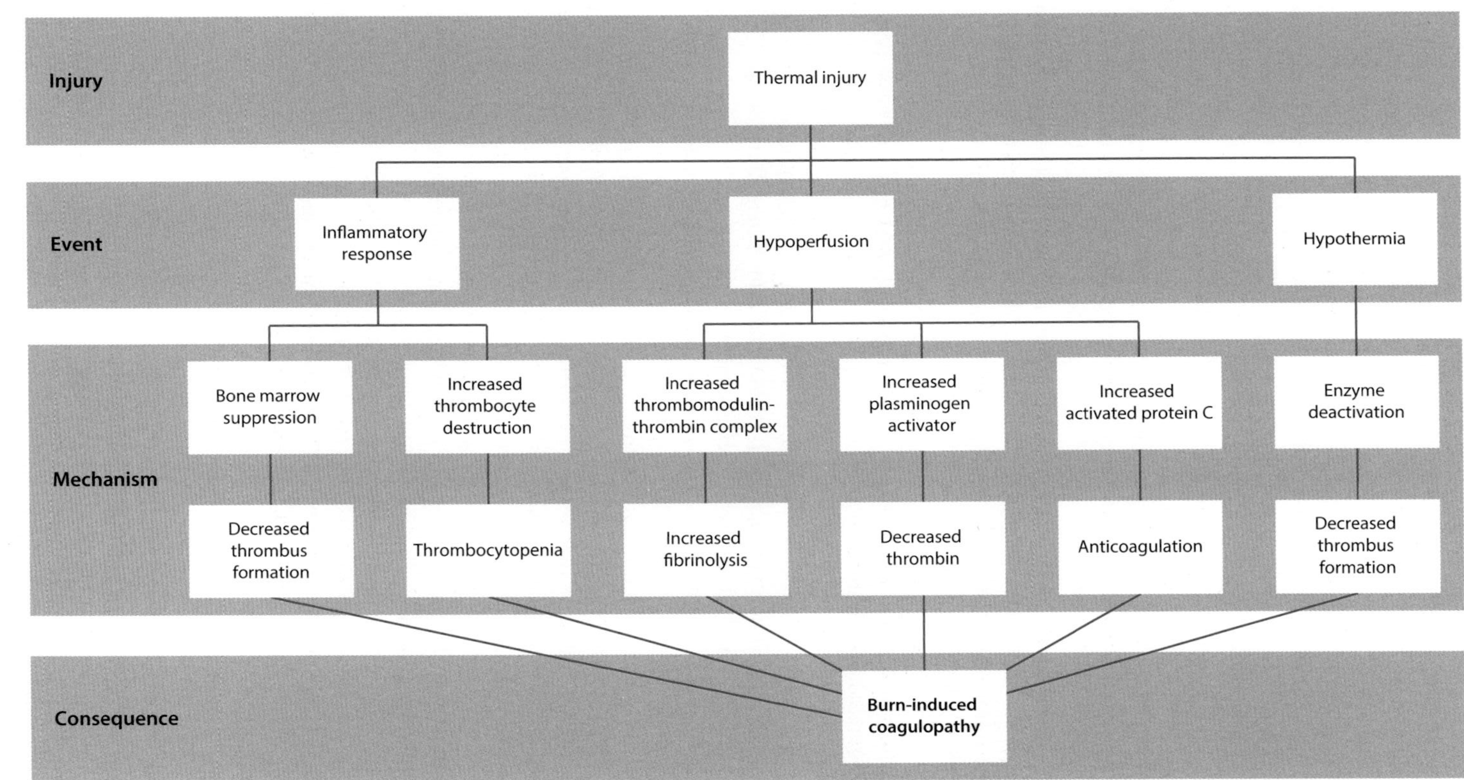

Fig. 2 Proposed mechanisms in the development of burn-induced coagulopathy

coagulation system activation, consumption of endogenous coagulation factors, and enhanced fibrinolytic activity [22]. Two studies, in particular, illustrate this concept. A small case series by King et al. demonstrated a hypercoagulable state proportional to the size of the burn up to 40% total body surface are (TBSA), after which point a hypocoagulable state developed as fibrinolysis exceeded thrombosis, as measured by high D-dimer titers [23]. Garcia-Avello et al. also demonstrated marked concurrent hypercoagulability and hyperfibrinolysis, and also demonstrated that the severity of this effect was related to the extent of the burn and correlated with organ failure and poor prognosis [24].

An additional mechanism contributing to burn-induced coagulopathy relates to circulating systemic anticoagulants, such as activated protein C, as well as hyperfibrinolysis due to dysregulated tissue plasminogen activator [19, 20].

Tissue injury and endothelial activation enhances thrombin-thrombomodulin binding, which accelerates protein C activation [25]. A systemic anticoagulation effect can ultimately develop via this mechanism, as activation of protein C contributes to inactivation of coagulation factors Va and VIIIa [19]. This endothelial activation is actively triggered by inflammatory cytokines such as TNF and IL-1 [20], which are present in increased concentrations in patients with large burns [21]. Exaggerated fibrinolysis also occurs in this setting, as thrombin, produced as a result of tissue injury, as well as circulating catecholamines and vasopressin are associated with systemic illness and contribute to increased production of endogenous tissue plasminogen activator (t-PA) and subsequent fibrinolysis [20]. Abnormal inhibition of t-PA may further contribute to exaggerated fibrinolysis, as activated protein C consumes the serine protease plasminogen activator inhibitor-1, which typically has a regulatory effect on t-PA [19].

The impact of dilutional coagulopathy in severe burns should not be underestimated. Hemodilution in the setting of burns occurs due to fluid shifts from the interstitial compartment to the vascular compartment in response to changed Starling forces, as well as potentially large volumes of exogenous resuscitation fluid administration [20]. A large retrospective analysis interrogating the German Trauma Registry demonstrated a positive correlation between the amount of intravenous fluid administered and the incidence of coagulopathy in trauma patients [26]. One recent study on patients with major burns presenting to a tertiary burns referral center similarly demonstrated an association between the presence of coagulopathy and the volume of intravenous fluid administered [17]. This study interestingly observed that the majority of patients did not present with an established coagulopathy, but rather developed a coagulopathy within 24 h of presentation, suggesting the underlying mechanism is not identical to the acute coagulopathy of trauma and that dilutional coagulopathy, in the setting of large volume resuscitation, may be a significant contributing factor [17].

The presence of hypothermia, either due to heat loss from damaged tissue, or as a result of aggressive fluid resuscitation, may also exacerbate coagulopathy [18]. *In vitro* studies suggest that this is predominately due to impaired platelet function, although impaired clotting enzyme function becomes apparent in moderate hypothermia with core temperatures below 33 °C [27].

Mechanism of Thrombocytopenia of Burn Patients

Thrombocytopenia is a common finding in burn patients. The predominant mechanism for this finding is probably platelet consumption in the setting of activation of the coagulation cascade, with a possible contribution from dilution from resuscitation fluids, bone marrow suppression from critical illness, or exposure to certain medications such as heparin [28]. A distinct pattern of thrombocytopenia has been observed following a burn injury, with a nadir at day 3, followed by a return to normal value and subsequent thrombocytosis at day 15. Although the effect that this thrombocytopenia has on bleeding is unclear, a large retrospective observational study demonstrated that a low thrombocyte trough was predictive for mortality [29].

Current Evidence and Practice

Despite the well-recognized anemia and coagulopathy associated with thermal injury there is a remarkable paucity of information in the medical literature to guide therapy.

There is no high quality evidence to guide clinical practice in acute burn transfusion care. The majority of evidence derives from retrospective observational studies [5]. Significantly, there are no specific recommendations for transfusion practice in burn patients in the European Transfusion Guidelines [30], The Canadian National Advisory Committee on Blood and Blood Products [31] or the Australian National Blood Authority guidelines [32].

Several studies have attempted to quantify the frequency and volume of blood product transfusion in burns patients (Table 1). A universal finding is that transfusion requirement is significant, and consistently related to size and severity of the burn [4, 33–37]. The largest of these studies demonstrated that patients with >20% TBSA burn received 13.7 units on average during their admission, whereas those with >50% TBSA burn received more than 30 units during their admission [4]. There may be a developing trend in burn centers to transfuse to lower hemoglobin targets than in previous years, likely as a result of evidence in favor of restrictive transfusion targets for general ICU patients [1].

There is substantial evidence from large multicenter transfusion trials in favor of a restrictive red cell transfusion strategy demonstrating a mortality benefit. It is important however to note that burn patients were specifically excluded from these studies [38, 39]. A large retrospective multicenter cohort study conducted in the USA and Canada, specifically looking at transfusions in burn patients (outside of the operating room) showed that, on average, a transfusion trigger greater than 9 g/dl was employed although there existed substantial variation among the institutions. Importantly, this study also demonstrated that increasing mortality was related to the number of blood transfusions, even when corrected for the severity of the burns [4]. A single center observational study compared outcomes after adopting a restrictive transfusion trigger of 7 g/dl among their burn patients and this study also demonstrated significantly better mortality outcomes in its restrictive group, when

Table 1 Burn transfusion literature

Author	Year	Patients	Study	Transfusion rates per admission	Patient outcomes
Graves [33]	1989	594	Retrospective analysis	Mean 19.7 transfusions/patient/admission	Significant correlation between number of transfusions and infection
Yogore [34]	2006	1,615 admitted 180 transfused	Retrospective analysis	< 10% TBSA: 4 units 11–19% TBSA: 8 units 20–40% TBSA: 12 units >40% TBSA: 20 units	Morbidity/mortality outcomes not assessed
Palmieri [4]	2006	666	Multicenter retrospective cohort analysis	79% of patients with burns > 20% TBSA received RBCs Mean units per patient >20% TBSA: 13.7 units >50% TBSA: >30 units	Number of transfusions associated with mortality. Number of transfusions associated with infection
Kwan [40]	2006	172	Retrospective analysis	Transfusion triggers: Liberal group: 9.2 g/dl Restrictive group: 7 g/dl	30-day mortality and overall in-hospital mortality lower in the restrictive group
Jeschke [42]	2007	277 pediatric patients	Retrospective cohort study	Stratified into high (>20 units) and low (<20 units) blood transfusion groups	Pediatric patients with 60% TBSA burns and concomitant inhalation injury more likely to develop sepsis if given high amounts of blood products
Boral [41]	2009	1,615	Retrospective analysis	Mean units among patients with comorbidities: – who required grafting: 12 units RBC, 19 units FFP, 19 doses of platelets – who did not require grafting: 5 units RBC, 8 units FFP, 13 doses of platelets	5× mortality in transfused patients with comorbidities than in non-transfused group. Patients with comorbidities more likely to be transfused in the <20% TBSA group
Fuzaylov [37]	2015	928	Multicenter retrospective study	30.5% of transfusions were given in patients with TBSA < 10% All patients (regardless of TBSA) transfused to a hemoglobin target of close to 9 g/dl	Not specifically assessed

Table 1 (Continued)

Author	Year	Patients	Study	Transfusion rates per admission	Patient outcomes
Wu [35]	2016	133	Retrospective analysis	97.7% of patients with > 40% TBSA burns received blood products. Median 19 units of RBCs and 28.5 units of plasma per patient	Factors associated with significantly increased consumption of RBCs: age, total TBSA, full thickness TBSA, coagulopathy, patient transfer, tracheostomy, escharotomy, number of operations
Koljonen [36]	2016	558	Retrospective analysis of registry data	180 pts received RBC transfusions. Mean 12.6 units per patient	Association between transfusions and mortality

TBSA: total body surface area; *RBC*: red blood cell; *FFP*: fresh frozen plasma

compared to the unit's previous practice of transfusing to higher targets (9.2 g/dl in this study) [40]. There is a suggestion that transfusions in patients with smaller burns, or those in patients without comorbidities are also associated with higher mortality [41].

Multiple potential harmful effects of blood transfusions are well recognized and there is specific evidence among the burns population that the risk of infection is increased, probably secondary to an immunomodulatory effect [4, 34]. Palmieri et al. remarkably demonstrated that the patient's risk of infection increased by 13% per unit of blood transfused [4]. There exists compelling evidence in the pediatric population that the risk of sepsis is increased by the number of transfusion events [42].

In regard to coagulopathy, specific recommendations are also lacking. Rational prescription of blood products, including fresh frozen plasma (FFP), should possibly be best guided by functional tests, such as rotational thromboelastometry (ROTEM), where available. This approach may provide more reliable and clinically relevant information than traditional measures, such as prothrombin time or partial thromboplastin time [43]. Other pharmacological agents targeting hemostasis are also available. Recombinant factor VIIa has been successful in case reports [44] although, overall, its efficacy remains unproven and it is associated with an increased risk of thrombotic arterial events [45].

Prothrombin complex concentrate (PCC) can be considered as an adjunct in the resuscitation of trauma patients who require massive transfusion, although its use has not been thoroughly evaluated outside of vitamin K antagonist-associated coagulopathy, let alone burn patients [46]. The anti-fibrinolytic agent, tranexamic acid, has been demonstrated to improve mortality in trauma patients with, or at risk of, significant bleeding [47] although evidence for its use in patients with coagulopathy associated with burns is lacking [48].

Table 2 Suggested trigger thresholds for transfusion

Product	Stable patient	Actively bleeding patient	Neuroaxial/ocular or risk of neuroaxial bleeding	Pre-surgery
Packed red blood cells	Target Hb ≥ 7 g/dl	Target Hb ≥ 10 g/dl	Target Hb ≥ 8 g/dl	Target Hb ≥ 9 g/dl
Fresh frozen plasma	Target INR ≤ 2.5	Target INR ≤ 2	Target INR ≤ 1.5	Target INR ≤ 2
Platelets	Target platelets $\geq 30 \times 10^9$/l	Target platelets $\geq 50 \times 10^9$/l	Target platelets $\geq 100 \times 10^9$/l	Target platelets $\geq 50 \times 10^9$/l
Cryoprecipitate	Target INR ≤ 2.5 or aPTT ≤ 60 s	Target INR ≤ 2 or aPTT ≤ 50 s	Target INR ≤ 1.5 or aPTT ≤ 45 s	Target INR ≤ 2 or aPTT ≤ 50 s

Hb: hemoglobin; *INR*: International Normalized Ratio; *aPTT*: activated partial thromboplastin time

We suggest normalization of coagulopathy in burns patients as a potential therapeutic target, given the association between burns coagulopathy and mortality. However practice among burns units both nationally and internationally remains diverse [19].

Our Recommendations

It is important that well designed studies are undertaken to better inform our transfusion practice in the thermal injury population. Ideally, national transfusion guidelines and Burn Societies should promulgate this information. Until then, general preventative measures are reasonable, including prevention of hypoperfusion via adequate fluid resuscitation and avoidance of hypothermia. Also important is employing strategies to minimize blood loss, including rationalization of blood tests, venesecting smaller volume samples, meticulous surgical technique in early wound debridement, the use of minimally invasive surgical procedures and the use of topical hemostatic techniques [1, 2]. Until further evidence is available, we suggest the 'trigger thresholds' shown in Table 2. While high quality evidence is lacking, this would appear to provide a rational approach in the interim.

Conclusion

Anemia and coagulopathy in patients with severe burns is a common, yet incompletely understood process. Contributing factors to anemia include blood loss, direct thermal injury and impaired erythropoiesis, and factors implicated in coagulopathy include consumption of procoagulant factors, endogenous anticoagulants, dilutional effects, and hypothermia; each of these represents a potential preventative treatment target. There is evidence in burn patients that the presence of coagulopathy is associated with higher mortality, whereas this is less evident with anemia, which can be managed with more restrictive transfusion targets, although evidence from multicenter randomized controlled trials to guide practice is lacking. Although a strategy of rational blood product use seems logical, there are no clear, established guidelines from national blood authorities to guide blood utilization practices in the management of burns patients, and current practice remains diverse.

References

1. Curina G, Jain A, Feldman M, Prosciak M, Phillips B, Milner S (2011) Red blood cell transfusion following burn. Burns 37:742–752
2. Posluszny JA, Gamelli RL (2010) Anemia of thermal injury: combined blood loss anemia and anemia of critical illness. J Burn Care Res 31:229–242
3. Sherren PB, Hussey R, Martin R, Kundishora T, Parker M, Emerson B (2013) Acute burn induced coagulopathy. Burns 39:1157–1161
4. Palmieri T, Caruso D, Foster K et al (2006) Effect of blood transfusion on outcome after major burn injury: a multicentre study. Crit Care Med 34:1602–1007
5. Henschke A, Lee R, Delany A (2016) Burns management in ICU: quality of evidence; a systematic review. Burns 42:1173–1182
6. Poluszny JA, Conrad P, Halerz M et al (2011) Classifying transfusions related to anemia of critical illness in burn patients. J Trauma 71:26–31
7. Kimber RJ, Lander H (1964) The effect of heat on human red cell morphology, fragility, and subsequent survival in vivo. J Lab Clin Med 64:922–933
8. Loebl EC, Marvin JA, Curreri W, Baxter CR (1974) erythrocyte survival following thermal injury. J Surg Res 16:96–101
9. Hatherill JR, Till GO, Bruner LH, Ward PA (1986) Thermal injury, intravascular hemolysis, and toxic oxygen products. J Clin Invest 78:629–636
10. Lawrence C, Atac B (1992) Hematologic changes in massive burn injury. Crit Care Med 20:1284–1288
11. Hayden SJ, Albert TJ, Watkins TR, Swenson ER (2012) Anemia in critical illness: insights into etiology, consequences and management. Am J Respir Crit Care Med 185:1049–1057
12. Mace JE, Park MS, Mora AG et al (2012) Differential expression of the immunoinflammatory response in trauma patients: burn vs non-burn. Burns 38:599–606
13. Walsh TS, Saleh EE (2006) Anaemia during critical illness. Br J Anaesth 97:278–291
14. Rodriguez RM, Corwin HL, Gettinger A, Corwin MJ, Gubler D, Pearl RG (2001) Nutritional deficiencies and blunted erythropoietin response as causes of the anaemia of critical illness. J Crit Care 16:36–41
15. Wallner SF, Warren GH (1985) The haematopoietic response to burning: an autopsy study. Burns Incl Therm Inj 12:22–27
16. Wallner SF, Vautrin R, Murphy J, Anderson S, Peterson V (1984) The haemoatopoietic response to burning: studies in animal model. Burns Incl Therm Inj 10:236–251
17. Mitra B, Wasiak J, Cameron PA, O'Reilly G, Dobson H, Cleland H (2012) Early coagulopathy of major burns. Injury 44:40–43
18. Glas GJ, Levi M, Schultz MJ (2016) Coagulopathy and its management in patients with severe burns. J Thromb Haemost 14:865–874
19. Firth D, Davenport R, Brohi K (2012) Acute traumatic coagulopathy. Current Opin Anaesthesiol 25:229–234
20. Cap A, Hunt B (2014) Acute traumatic coagulopathy. Curr Opin Crit Care 20:638–645
21. Vindenes HA, Ulvestad E, Bjerknes R (1988) Concentration of cytokines in plasma of patients with large burns: their relation to time after injury, burn size, inflammatory variables, infection, and outcome. Eur J Surg 164:647–652

22. Lavrentieva A, Kontakiotis T, Bitzani M (2008) Early coagulation disorders after severe burn injury: impact on mortality. Intensive Care Med 34:700–706
23. King D, Namias N, Andrews D (2010) Coagulation abnormalities following thermal injury. Blood Coag Fibrin 21:666–669
24. Garcia-Avello A, Lorente JA, Cesar-Perez J et al (1998) Degree of hypercoagulability and hyperfibrinolysis is related to organ failure and prognosis after burn trauma. Thromb Res 89:59–64
25. Holley AD, Reade MC (2013) The 'procoagulopathy' of trauma: too much, too late? Curr Opin Crit Care 19:578–586
26. Maegele M, Lefering R, Yucel N et al (2006) Early coagulopathy in multiple injury: an analysis from the German trauma registry on 8724 patients. Injury 38:298–304
27. Wolberg AS, Meng ZH, Monroe DM, Hoffman MD (2004) A systematic evaluation of the effect of temperature on coagulation enzyme activity and platelet function. J Trauma 56:1221–1228
28. George A, Bang RL, Lari AR, Gang RK (2001) Acute thrombocytopenic crisis following burns complicated by staphylococcal septicemia. Burns 27:84–88
29. Marck RE, Montagne HL, Tuinebreijer WE, Breederveld RS (2013) Time course of thrombocytes in burn patients and its predictive value for outcome. Burns 39:714–722
30. Spahn DR, Bouillon B, Cerny V et al (2013) Management of bleeding and coagulopathy following major trauma: an updated European guideline. Crit Care 17:R76
31. Dzik WH, Blajchman MA, Fergusson D et al (2011) Clinical review: Canadian National Advisory Committee on Blood and Blood Products – Massive transfusion consensus conference 2011: report of the panel. Crit Care 15:242
32. National Blood Authority Australia (2016) Patient blood management guidelines. Available at www.blood.gov.au/pbm-guidelines Accessed November 10, 2016
33. Graves TA, Cioffi WG, Mason AD, McManus WF, Pruitt BA (1989) Relationship of transfusion and infection in burns population. J Trauma 29:948–952
34. Yogore MG 3rd, Boral L, Kowal-Vern A, Patel H, Brown S, Latenser BA (2006) Use of blood bank services in a burn unit. J Burn Care Res 27:835–841
35. Wu G, Zhuang M, Fan X et al (2016) Blood transfusions in severe burns patients: epidemiology and predictive factors. Burns 42:1721–1727
36. Koljonen V, Tuimala J, Haglund C (2016) The use of blood products in adult patients with burns. Scand J Surg 105:178–185
37. Fuzaylov G, Anderson R, Lee J (2015) Blood transfusion trigger in burns: a four year retrospective analysis of blood transfusions in eleven burn centres in Ukraine. Ann Burns Fire Disasters 28:178–182
38. Hébert PC (1998) Transfusion requirements in critical care (TRICC): a multicentre, randomized, controlled clinical study. Br J Anaesth 81(Suppl 1):25–33
39. Corwin HL, Gettinger A, Pearl RG et al (2004) The CRIT study: Anemia and blood transfusion in the critically ill – current clinical practice in the United States. Crit Care Med 32:39–52
40. Kwan P, Gomez M, Carlotto R (2006) Safe and successful restriction of transfusion in burn patients. J Burn Res 27:826–834
41. Boral L, Kowal-Vern A, Yogore M, Patel H, Latenser B (2009) Transfusion in burn patients with/without comorbidities. J Burn Care Res 30:268–273
42. Jeschke MD, Chinkes DL, Finnerty CC, Przkora R, Pereira CT, Herndon DN (2007) Blood transfusions are associated with increased risk for development of sepsis in severely burned pediatric patients. Crit Care Med 35:579–583
43. Davenport R, Manson J, De'Ath H et al (2011) Functional definition and characterization of acute traumatic coagulopathy. Crit Care Med 39:2652–2658
44. Martin JT, Alkhoury F, McIntosh BC, Fidler P, Schulz J (2009) Recombinant factor VIIa: haemostatic adjunct in the coagulopathic patient. Eplasty 09:e27

45. Simpson E, Lin Y, Stanworth S, Birchall J, Doree C, Hyde C (2012) Recombinant factor VIIa for the prevention and treatment of bleeding in patients without haemophilia. Cochrane Database Syst Rev CD005011
46. Matsushima K, Benjamin E, Demetriades D (2015) Prothrombin complex concentrate in trauma patients. Am J Surg 209:413–417
47. Shakur H, Roberts I, Bautista R (2010) Effects of Tranexamic acid on death, vascular occlusive events, and blood transfusion in trauma patients with significant haemorrhage (CRASH-2): a randomized, placebo-controlled trial. Lancet 376:23–32
48. Walsh K, Nikkhah D, Dheansa B (2014) What is the evidence for tranexamic acid in burns? Burns 40:1055–1057

Part XI

Drug Development and Pharmaceutical Issues

Bridging the Translational Gap: The Challenges of Novel Drug Development in Critical Care

S. Lambden and C. Summers

Introduction

During the last 30 years, intensive care medicine has seen a progressive improvement in patient outcomes [1], which has largely been achieved through reductions in iatrogenic injury associated with interventions such as fluid therapy [2] and invasive mechanical ventilation [3]. Over this time, numerous therapeutic agents have been examined in large randomized controlled trials, involving tens of thousands of patients and costing many millions of dollars. Of those agents, none has been shown to improve survival in patients with sepsis, and both of the agents that were licensed for use in sepsis, HA-1A [4] and activated protein-C [5], have subsequently been withdrawn amid concerns regarding efficacy and safety. Table 1 summarizes the phase III trials of novel therapeutics undertaken in sepsis and their outcomes since 1990.

Sepsis remains a syndrome that is associated with a huge healthcare, social and economic burden, which results in the loss of an estimated 5.3 million lives worldwide every year [6]. Demand for therapeutic intervention remains considerable, and in developing new treatments careful consideration must be given to each stage of the drug development pathway in order to maximize the likelihood of success. In this chapter, we will address each stage of the drug development pathway – basic science, animal models and clinical studies – and, using examples from the field, consider how study design could be optimized to maximize the likelihood of the next generation of therapies being successful.

S. Lambden · C. Summers (✉)
Cambridge Critical Care Research Group, University of Cambridge
Cambridge, UK
Department of Medicine, Addenbrooke's Hospital
Hills Road, Cambridge, CB2 0QQ, UK
e-mail: cs493@medschl.cam.ac.uk

J.-L. Vincent (ed.), *Annual Update in Intensive Care and Emergency Medicine 2017*,
DOI 10.1007/978-3-319-51908-1_30

Table 1 Selection of completed phase III trials of novel therapeutic agents in sepsis

Study	Date	Intervention	Outcome	Reference
CHESS	1994	HA-1A (monoclonal antibody binding to LPS)	No effect	[45]
Opal et al.	1997	Anakinra (recombinant human IL-1ra)	No effect	[46]
NORASEPT II	1998	BAYX-1351 (TNF specific monoclonal antibody)	No effect	[36]
Angus et al.	2000	E5 (monoclonal antibody binding to LPS)	No effect	[47]
MONARCS	2001	Afelimomab (fragment of TNF specific monoclonal antibody)	Benefit	[37]
PROWESS	2001	Drotrecogin alfa (activated protein C)	Benefit	[38]
OPTIMIST	2003	Tifacogin (recombinant human tissue factor pathway inhibitor)	No effect	[48]
Opal et al.	2004	Pafase (recombinant human platelet-activating factor acetylhydrolase)	No effect	[49]
Lopez et al.	2004	546C88 (inhibitor of nitric oxide synthase)	Harm	[7]
PROWESS-SHOCK	2012	Drotrecogin alfa (activated protein C)	No effect	[5]
ACCESS	2013	Eritoran (TLR4 antagonist)	No effect	[19]
OASIS	2015	Talactoferrin (recombinant human lactoferrin)	Possible harm	[50]

TNF: tumor necrosis factor; *TLR*: Toll-like receptor; *LPS*: lipopolysaccharide; *IL-1ra*: interleukin-1 receptor antagonist

Building on Basic Science: Understanding the Pathway Is Crucial to Therapeutic Plausibility

Understanding 'On-Target' Effects

One of the main challenges that must be considered when developing a new therapeutic agent is the detailed understanding of the pathway that is to be targeted. Sepsis is a multisystem disorder with complex pathophysiological responses, some essential to mounting an appropriate response, others deleterious. As much as the avoidance of unexpected off-target effects is a critical part of drug design, a comprehensive understanding of the biology may help to avoid unwanted 'on target' effects. An example of this is the development of the therapeutic inhibitor of nitric oxide synthase (NOS), L-NMMA (546C88®) [7]. NO was only definitively identified in 1987, although its actions had been recognized for over a century. The discovery of the enzymatic system that synthesizes NO, the NOS, and their role in sepsis-induced vasodilatation led to considerable interest in modulation of this pathway as a potential therapy. Within just 10 years of its discovery, a phase III trial of a global inhibitor of NOS activity in septic shock was underway. As predicted, 546C88 had a significant impact on systemic vascular resistance, unfortunately it was also associated with increased mortality [7]. Over succeeding years, as understanding of the biology of NO synthesis has evolved, it has become clear that in addition to modulating the synthesis of NO in the vasculature, NO plays a dynamic role in a diverse range of tissues. As a result, global inhibition of NOS activity leads to impaired cardiac and immune cell responses to infection that are critical to an appropriate response to infection [8]. Detailed understanding of the biological system offers the opportunity to develop compounds that target elements of a pathway that are harmful, whilst leaving appropriate responses unimpaired. In the case of NO, it has become possible to target excessive vascular NO synthesis without causing unwanted immune and cardiac dysfunction [9].

Human Target Validation

An alternative approach to discovery of potential therapeutic targets is through the identification of potentially important pathways in human studies, and then developing modulatory agents which may be experimentally tested. This approach typically relies on studies of genetic polymorphisms in critically ill populations to identify pathways in which a change in function mediated by genetic predisposition confers a protective or deleterious effect. An example of this approach comes from the development of PCSK9 inhibitors as a potential therapeutic agent in sepsis. Walley et al. [10] used data from two clinical cohorts to demonstrate that loss of function of the PCSK9 gene, caused by the presence of a number of polymorphisms, was associated with improved sepsis survival, whereas gain of function in the same gene was associated with an increased risk of death from septic shock. This offered valuable human target validation that the improvement in survival observed in septic animals treated with a PSCK9 inhibitor may be conserved across species.

Animal Models of Sepsis: Matching Experiments to the Clinical Paradigm

Bridging the gap from basic science to clinical utility necessitates the use of whole animal models to explore the therapeutic potential and safety of new drugs. The failure in human clinical trials of many compounds previously shown to be efficacious in animal models has led to concern regarding whether it is possible to reproduce the apparent benefits seen in pre-clinical models of disease in human clinical studies. A number of features of conventional animal models of sepsis may limit their potential for translation into therapeutic efficacy, including choice of species, type of infective stimulus, the timing of administration of the therapeutic intervention, and the impact of other therapies upon the treatment response.

Mammalian Models of Sepsis: Animal Selection

The animals most commonly employed in pre-clinical studies of septic shock therapies are rodents, which have been extensively used as a model of the response to infection. A number of techniques are available to induce infection, and it is possible to monitor the hemodynamic response in real time, as well as to deliver conventional therapies in order to understand both the evolution of the septic response and the impact of treatment. Concern has been expressed for some time that there are significant inter-species differences in the physiological responses to infection, which may reduce the ability to translate observations made in rodents to humans with sepsis. In particular, it has been established for some time that the immune response of the mouse differs both in profile and systemic impact to that of humans; for example, murine monocyte NO production may be one or two orders of magnitude greater than in the equivalent cell type in humans [11]. Hence, therapies targeting the NO pathway may have a different magnitude of effect across the two species, and beneficial effects seen in the mouse may not be reproduced in humans.

In addition to specific differences in certain parts of the immune response, in a landmark paper, Seok et al. explored the genomic responses to burns, trauma and endotoxemia in mice and humans, demonstrating that there was an almost total absence of correlation between the human and murine responses to endotoxin administration [12]. This finding validated the observation that the murine physiological response to infection differs significantly from the human response, with hypothermia and a hibernation phenotype predominating in murine septic shock [13]. By contrast, the rat demonstrates a hyperdynamic response to infection, with cardiovascular failure only observed in the immediate period prior to death, a pattern more consistent with the human clinical phenotype [14].

Careful consideration should therefore be given to the demonstration of therapeutic efficacy in a species other than mouse prior to progression to human sepsis trials. Whilst relatively low cost and well established models will make mice a continued part of sepsis drug development, there is increasing use of larger mammals to test therapeutic potential, rather than merely for the assessment of potential toxicity. Porcine and ovine models offer the ability to deliver complex critical care interventions, including ventilation, sedation, fluids and vasopressor therapy, over clinically relevant time periods [15]. In addition, use of these models means that it is possible to undertake more invasive monitoring of cardiovascular parameters, organ perfusion and treatment response than is possible in rodent studies.

There is recognition that a further limitation of traditional models is the use of juvenile/young adult animals, which may be less representative of the clinical population with sepsis, which is largely from an older age group. As a result, aging animals for longer prior to experimentation is increasingly undertaken [16, 17]. Although the optimum age of animals included in these experimental models has yet to be defined, and therapies have yet to be evaluated in this way, it may be that this approach should be considered as a routine component of animal models moving forward.

Mammalian Models of Sepsis: The Septic Insult

The nature of the septic insult is an important determinant of the validity of an animal model. Both the form and the timing of the chosen model of infection are likely to be critical in determining the reproducibility of data in subsequent human trials.

Two models of sepsis predominate in early trials of the efficacy of novel therapeutic agents: bacterial endotoxin (lipopolysaccharide [LPS]) and single live bacterial injection. LPS is a product of the cell wall of Gram-negative bacteria and is not a true infective stimulus. It delivers a specific Toll-like receptor 4 (TLR4) mediated inflammatory stimulus, rather than the simultaneous activation of multiple pathways typically seen in microbial infections, and traditionally forms a major part of efficacy studies of novel compounds [18].

The second most common model of infection used is a single injection of live bacteria. The clinical pattern of severe infection is typically one of continuing exposure to an infective and inflammatory stimulus for an often indeterminate period until appropriate antimicrobial therapy and source control are delivered. This contrasts with a single injection of live bacteria in animal models, where the insult delivers a sudden onset of profound bacteremia. This produces a severe model of infection, but one that may not be representative of the clinical course of sepsis. An example of this is in the development of E5564 (Eritoran®), a TLR4 antagonist that ultimately showed no mortality benefit in a randomized controlled trial in patients with severe sepsis [19]. Published pre-clinical models used LPS or a single bolus of Gram-negative bacteria as the infection model [20]. Other examples of these approaches dominating pre-clinical development include the development phases of interleukin-1 receptor antagonist (IL-1ra) therapy in sepsis [21] and Lenercept®, an inhibitor of tumor necrosis factor (TNF) receptor-mediated inflammatory signaling [22].

Alternative infective models are available, such as cecal ligation and puncture (CLP) and intraperitoneal slurry administration [23, 24]. These produce a more heterogeneous response when compared to the injection of a single kind of bacteria; however they offer a persistent polymicrobial infective source that drives pro- and anti-inflammatory signaling in a manner consistent with a specific human disease state. In addition to polymicrobial, largely Gram-negative infective models of fecal peritonitis, there is increasing interest in the development of other techniques that may recapitulate other common primary modes of infection. It is now possible to model pneumonia with Gram-negative microorganisms, such as *Pseudomonas aeruginosa*, Gram-positive organisms, such as *Staphylococcus aureus,* and a range of viral stimuli [25, 26]. This may offer an additional route for the validation of novel therapies, where increased confidence may be generated that the treatment may have broad applicability through the use of different infection models. Alternatively, it may aid in the identification of patient populations likely to benefit from therapy and facilitate clinical trial design.

Mammalian Models of Sepsis: The Timing of Treatment Initiation

The timing of administration of the therapeutic agent being tested is also of relevance when designing drug development studies. It is well established that the time of presentation of patients with sepsis is highly variable, and it is rarely the case that patients are identified at the moment of infection. One of the characteristics of agents that have failed to demonstrate benefit in human clinical trials is that in early phase studies the therapeutic tested has been administered either simultaneous with, or even before, the induction of sepsis. This is of particular relevance in immunomodulatory therapies, where preventing the initial proinflammatory signaling cascade may be an effective strategy in pre-clinical models. By contrast, in patient populations, by the time a treatment is initiated a more complex interaction of pro- and anti-inflammatory activation is usually well established, which may impair the efficacy of these therapies. An example of this comes from the study of Eritoran® in which pre- or simultaneous treatment models dominated the early-phase development, and showed positive effects on survival. However, the first animal study of Eritoran® in which the therapy was delayed until just one hour after the administration of an infective insult showed that delay significantly reduced the beneficial effects of therapy on outcome. This study was not published until after the human phase II study in severe sepsis was already underway [27, 28]. Critical primate trials of a number of agents have used simultaneous or pre-treatment models, including Lenercept® [22] and activated protein C [29]. Given that the delivery of any treatment for sepsis is determined largely by the development of clinical indices of illness, some studies are now using the development of clinically relevant hemodynamic compromise following the onset of sepsis to determine the timing of therapy [9, 30]. This may better represent the clinical context in which these therapies would be employed, and may improve the likelihood of successful translation.

Mammalian Models of Sepsis: The Use of Conventional Therapies in Animal Studies

Critical care for the patient with severe sepsis or septic shock includes a broad array of supportive therapies. The traditional model of drug development has used only simple treatments, such as intermittent fluid boluses and in some cases antibiotic therapy. However, mortality in these models is extremely high, and a therapy that shows promise may not offer the same positive results in clinical practice, where supportive therapies demonstrably reduce the risk of death. Therefore, animal models of sepsis that include the co-administration of clinically relevant treatments may give greater insight into the therapeutic potential of agents. A number of approaches exist to address this challenge, for example using a rat model in which a tether can be implanted facilitating continuous central venous and arterial monitoring. Through this it is possible to deliver titratable infusions of fluids and vasopressors to maintain blood pressure in polymicrobial septic shock [9]. In larger mammals, more complex strategies can be employed. In their study of angiotensin II therapy in sepsis, Correa et al. used a delayed treatment model in ventilated pigs. In their experiments, designed to reflect the clinical time course, the therapeutic intervention followed the onset of fecal peritonitis by 12 h, and included both appropriate fluid resuscitation and either norepinephrine or angiotensin II targeted to maintain blood pressure [15].

There has been considerable progress in the development of animal models that more closely represent the clinical course of sepsis. These models are costly, technically demanding, and more time consuming than some more traditional models, but may offer increased confidence that a compound may have clinical utility. In the future, these approaches may form part of the novel drug development pathway after initial rodent models have proved promising. However, until a model is developed in which outcomes correlate with those seen in human trial populations, questions will continue to be asked about the validity of animal studies in this area.

Clinical Trial Design

Sepsis Definitions

Sepsis has recently been defined as the "life-threatening organ dysfunction caused by a dysregulated host response to infection" [31]. This definition represents patients presenting with a clinical syndrome associated with an increased risk of death from an invading pathogen; however, within it falls the impact of a broad range of organisms, sites of infection and host responses. This, coupled with the observation that the application of the definition of sepsis in clinical trials is variable [1], means that populations recruited into clinical trials are diverse. Whilst this confers the advantage that findings from these trials may be applicable to a range of clinical cohorts, there is also a risk that subgroups of patients within the trial may experience benefit, but that this signal may be lost amongst the noise generated by a heterogeneous population.

Clinical Trial Enrichment

The challenge of identifying appropriate patient populations may be addressed through 'enrichment' of inclusion criteria. This may include selection of patients with a specific illness severity, or the use of biomarkers to identify a target population.

Retrospective analysis of clinical cohorts has suggested that patients with a higher risk of death, as opposed to the whole patient population that meet the definition of sepsis, may benefit from specific therapies [32]. This is not true in all cases, but the recruitment of more severely ill populations with a higher risk of death may be a valuable approach in drug trials in this area. Caution must be employed, however, as setting too high a threshold of illness severity could lead to the selection of patients for whom no therapy will be effective [33].

An alternative to using clinical indices as the sole inclusion criteria for patients with septic shock is the use of biomarker driven approaches to recruitment. Whilst no tool exists that will detect sepsis in an infected patient cohort with perfect sensitivity and specificity, a number of assays have offered promise in this area [34, 35]. Of these, procalcitonin (PCT) is the best studied [35], and although an imperfect discriminator, may alone or in combination with other tools make it possible to identify patients suitable for clinical trials of novel agents. For this approach to be effective, rapid or point-of-care testing must be available to facilitate timely study recruitment.

In addition to the identification of patients with sepsis, biomarkers may allow the identification of subgroups who may benefit from a specific therapy. For example, TNF-α release is a common feature of sepsis pathophysiology and levels of TNF-α expression in the plasma have been associated with poor outcome. However, observational data from clinical cohorts suggest that increased TNF-α is not a universal feature of severe disease, with a proportion of patients showing no elevation at any stage of the disease course. This suggests that there may be some patients in whom an anti-TNF therapy may be beneficial, and others in whom it may have little effect. This variability in response is one of the potential explanations for a number of therapies targeting this pathway proving unsuccessful [36]. It is also important to note that using a biomarker of this kind to guide therapy is only a valid approach if it represents both the true activity of the pathway in the target tissue and also a clinically important target. An example of a potentially successful use of this approach comes from the phase III MONARCS trial of a novel anti-TNF therapy. A rapid assay of IL-6 levels was undertaken and patients stratified according to the result. The *a priori* primary analysis of this trial was of the group of patients with high plasma IL-6 concentrations, and after adjustment this study showed a statistically significant improvement in 28-day mortality following treatment [37]. A number of factors have led to this treatment not becoming a standard of care; however, it did demonstrate that biomarker-driven selection of patients is feasible and may offer advantages in therapeutic trials.

A further use of robust biomarkers of therapeutic effect is in the duration of treatment. The duration of most drug courses used in clinical trials of novel therapies is determined during the course of pre-clinical and early phase dose finding studies. This approach has led to a standard duration of therapy being the norm in phase III trials of new drugs [38]. Future therapies may use readily measurable markers of target engagement to determine individualized durations of therapy, which may offer either improved efficacy or a lower toxicity profile.

Alternative Study Designs: The Choice of Primary Outcome

Opportunities to change the design of clinical trials to offer an increased chance of successful translation can be broadly divided into the choice of clinical outcome, and the design of the trial itself. The gold standard primary outcome in clinical trials of novel therapeutic agents undertaken to date has been a change in 28-day or 90-day mortality, with many trials aiming to detect a 5–10% reduction in absolute mortality following treatment, compared to placebo treated patients. It is now well established, despite the absence of a therapy that increases survival in sepsis, that improvements in supportive care have led to a reduction in sepsis mortality to around 20% (from more than 30% a decade ago [1]). This means that to demonstrate efficacy, a new agent must achieve at least a 25% relative reduction in the risk of death. This may be a difficult goal to achieve given the illness severity of this population, and so two alternatives approaches are possible. The first is to accept a less dramatic improvement in mortality, although designing studies to detect very subtle treatment effects is challenging and may require both increased sample size and narrower inclusion criteria. An alternative is to consider other clinical outcomes that are important both to the patient and the clinician. Recent work has confirmed that many patients view persistent disability as an outcome they consider worse than death [39], and so composite outcomes including measures of disability/function and overall mortality may provide a greater insight into the efficacy of a novel therapy. In their published analysis plan for The Augmented versus Routine approach to Giving Energy Trial (TARGET) by the Australian and New Zealand Intensive Care Society Clinical Trials Group, Iwahsyna and Deane have proposed a novel approach to analysis of a 4,000 patient randomized controlled trial of enteral feeding approaches in ventilated patients on the intensive care unit (ICU) [40]. In addition to the primary outcome of a reduction in absolute mortality at 90 days, the study will pilot individualized outcomes in this clinical trial population. By determining the functional status of patients prior to the development of illness, and allocating them to one of eight categories, the trial will explore whether the intervention is more effective at returning each patient to a category-specific endpoint assessment of function. This may offer a new strategy for measuring outcome, in which returning patients to their pre-morbid state is the therapeutic target.

In addition to patient-centered outcomes, the impact of a novel therapy on the overall length of stay in the ICU or number of supportive therapies patients require may be a clinically relevant outcome for clinicians and patients. Given the extremely high costs of delivering critical care, a treatment that is safe and reduces duration of ventilation, length of ICU stay or requirement for renal replacement therapy may be recommended on a health economic basis. For example, the recent Vasopressin vs Norepinephrine as Initial Therapy in Septic Shock (VANISH) trial suggested that although the use of vasopressin as a first line agent did not lead to improvements in the primary composite outcome of kidney failure free days, it did report a significant reduction in the requirement for hemofiltration [41]. This may make vasopressin a potential first line therapy on the grounds that it will provide a net saving on the cost of an ICU admission, a question that remains to be definitively answered.

Alternative Study Designs: The Design of Clinical Trials

The design of clinical trials in critical care has focused on the traditional randomized controlled trial, in which patients with a broad range of disease are recruited and randomized to receive either the novel therapy or placebo. To date, this approach has not proven successful, and there is now considerable interest in adaptive trial designs as an alternative, which can facilitate more efficient dose response studies, and also potentially improve the conduct, patient selection and recruitment of late stage clinical trials. Adaptive designs are now increasingly used in randomized trials in other areas of medicine [42].

Efficacy trials with an adaptive design can be divided into two categories, 'response adapting' and sample size modifying trials [43]. In essence, the response adapting trial relies on Bayesian approaches in which at the beginning of a trial, multiple treatment or patient selection arms begin simultaneously, and the assumptions regarding outcomes and target populations can be modified at interim analysis as the study continues (Fig. 1). Following interim review of the data, recruitment of patients to arms of the study that show no benefit for a particular group or from a specific therapy can be stopped, and randomization tools revised to exclude that arm from recruitment to the study. Through this technique and repeated interim analysis, trial design becomes dynamic with changes in patient selection and end point possible in the context of the available data. The second type of adaptive design acknowledges the challenge of sample size calculation in clinical trials. This is often an issue, and a number of recent clinical trials in critical care have produced results that – had they been adequately powered – may have suggested clinically important benefits [44]. However, these trials were undersized in terms of recruitment due to sample size calculations that were made on the basis of pilot data from

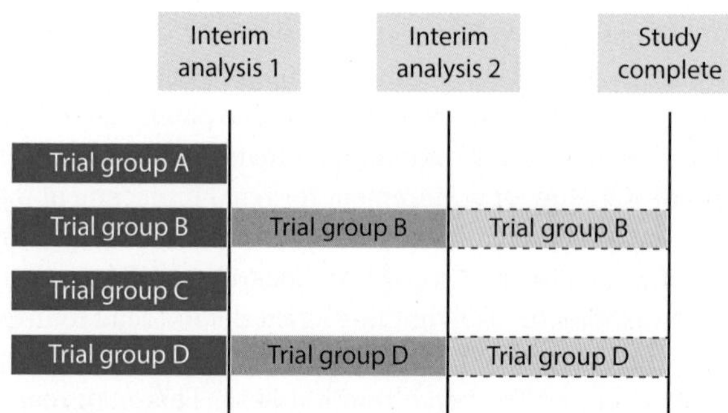

Fig. 1 Adaptive clinical trial design. This image depicts the stylized course of an adaptive randomized clinical trial of a novel therapeutic agent involving four groups. At the first interim analysis, groups A and C display no evidence of improved outcome and randomization is focused on groups B and D. At the second interim analysis, a signal to benefit is seen for treatment over control, sample size calculations are repeated and additional recruitment undertaken prior to study completion and final analysis

small preliminary studies. By recalculating sample size at interim analysis, it is possible to recruit more patients if the study appears underpowered, but also stop a study if an experimental therapy proves unsuccessful. Adaptive trial designs can potentially offer insights into the effectiveness or otherwise of a therapy, and also explore simultaneously which subgroups of patients benefit most, more rapidly than in traditional randomized trials. Limitations may include dependence on surrogates for outcome at the interim stage, which may not correlate strongly with the primary outcome at the final analysis, and issues regarding the traditional tools available for the interpretation of results. If these issues are addressed, critical care may be well suited to the conduct of this kind of trial.

Conclusion

In summary, the search for a therapeutic agent that improves survival in the critically ill septic patient has to date proven unsuccessful, and there must be a limit to how far improvements in supportive care delivery will be able to reduce mortality. Basic science is identifying novel pathways and exciting potential therapeutic avenues for the treatment of life-threatening infection on a regular basis. As we enter an era of burgeoning antimicrobial resistance, the development and validation of novel supportive therapies will become increasingly important.

Moving forward, clinicians and academics must recognize that there are considerable challenges to the creation of therapies at each stage of the development pathway, and that traditional approaches have so far led to failure. As new agents become available for pre-clinical and clinical evaluation, consideration should be given to the following in order to increase the likelihood of successfully bringing a novel agent into clinical use:

- Consider exploring genetic studies for human target validation in the early phase of drug development.
- Explore the use of clinically relevant rodent models, including advanced models of infection, and the co-administration of conventional therapies as part of the pre-clinical development process.
- Explore the use of animals with comorbid illness or advanced age to more closely represent the clinical population that will be treated.
- Consider efficacy studies in non-rodent species prior to progression to human trials.
- Use biomarker/physiology-driven recruitment to select patient populations most likely to benefit from a specific novel intervention.
- Consider alternative patient-centered outcomes as a primary endpoint of treatment efficacy.
- Identify trials where novel adaptive designs may facilitate identification of target populations and exploration of the impact of combination therapies.

References

1. Shankar-Hari M, Bertolini G, Brunkhorst FM et al (2015) Judging quality of current septic shock definitions and criteria. Crit Care 19:1–5
2. The National Heart Lung Blood Institute Acute Respiratory Distress Syndrome Clinical Trials Network (2006) Comparison of two fluid-management strategies in acute lung injury. N Engl J Med 354:2564–2575
3. Gattinoni L, Quintel M (2016) How ARDS should be treated. Crit Care 20:1–3
4. Ziegler EJ, Fisher CJ Jr, Sprung CL et al (1991) Treatment of gram-negative bacteremia and septic shock with HA-1A human monoclonal antibody against endotoxin. A randomized, double-blind, placebo-controlled trial. The HA-1A Sepsis Study Group. N Engl J Med 324:429–436
5. Ranieri VM, Thompson BT, Barie PS et al (2012) Drotrecogin alfa (activated) in adults with septic shock. N Engl J Med 366:2055–2064
6. Fleischmann C, Scherag A, Adhikari NKJ et al (2015) Assessment of global incidence and mortality of hospital-treated sepsis. Current estimates and limitations. Am J Respir Crit Care Med 193:259–272
7. Lopez A, Lorente JA, Steingrub J et al (2004) Multiple-center, randomized, placebo-controlled, double-blind study of the nitric oxide synthase inhibitor 546C88: effect on survival in patients with septic shock. Crit Care Med 32:21–30
8. Bogdan C (2001) Nitric oxide and the immune response. Nat Immunol 2:907–916
9. Wang Z, Lambden S, Taylor V et al (2014) Pharmacological inhibition of DDAH1 improves survival, hemodynamics and organ function in experimental septic shock. Biochem J 460:309–316
10. Walley KR, Thain KR, Russell JA et al (2014) PCSK9 is a critical regulator of the innate immune response and septic shock outcome. Sci Transl Med 6:258ra143
11. Saia RS, Mestriner FL, Bertozi G, Cunha FQ, Carnio EC (2014) Cholecystokinin inhibits inducible nitric oxide synthase expression by lipopolysaccharide-stimulated peritoneal macrophages. Mediat Inflamm 2014:896029
12. Seok J, Warren HS, Cuenca AG et al (2013) Genomic responses in mouse models poorly mimic human inflammatory diseases. Proc Natl Acad Sci USA 110:3507–3512
13. Iskander KN, Osuchowski MF, Stearns-Kurosawa DJ et al (2013) Sepsis: multiple abnormalities, heterogeneous responses, and evolving understanding. Physiol Rev 93:1247–1288
14. Zolfaghari P, Pinto B, Dyson A, Singer M (2013) The metabolic phenotype of rodent sepsis: cause for concern? Intensive Care Med Exp 1:6
15. Correa TD, Jeger V, Pereira AJ, Takala J, Djafarzadeh S, Jakob SM (2014) Angiotensin II in septic shock: effects on tissue perfusion, organ function, and mitochondrial respiration in a porcine model of fecal peritonitis. Crit Care Med 42:e550–e559
16. Leong J, Zhou M, Jacob A, Wang P (2010) Aging-related hyperinflammation in endotoxemia is mediated by the α(2A)-adrenoceptor and CD14/TLR4 pathways. Life Sci 86:740–746
17. Holly MK, Dear JW, Hu X et al (2006) Biomarker and drug target discovery using proteomics in a new rat model of sepsis-induced acute renal failure. Kidney Int 70:496–506
18. Barochia A, Solomon S, Cui X, Natanson C, Eichacker PQ (2011) Eritoran tetrasodium (E5564) treatment for sepsis: review of preclinical and clinical studies. Expert Opin Drug Metab Toxicol 7:479–494
19. Opal SM, Laterre P, Francois B et al (2013) Effect of eritoran, an antagonist of md2-tlr4, on mortality in patients with severe sepsis: The access randomized trial. JAMA 309:1154–1162
20. Mullarkey M, Rose JR, Bristol J et al (2003) Inhibition of endotoxin response by e5564, a novel Toll-like receptor 4-directed endotoxin antagonist. J Pharmacol Exp Ther 304:1093–1102
21. Sha T, Sunamoto M, Kitazaki T, Sato J, Ii M, Iizawa Y (2007) Therapeutic effects of TAK-242, a novel selective Toll-like receptor 4 signal transduction inhibitor, in mouse endotoxin shock model. Eur J Pharmacol 571:231–239

22. Van Zee KJ, Moldawer LL, Oldenburg HS et al (1996) Protection against lethal Escherichia coli bacteremia in baboons (Papio anubis) by pretreatment with a 55-kDa TNF receptor (CD120a)-Ig fusion protein, Ro 45-2081. J Immunol 156:2221–2230
23. Brealey D, Karyampudi S, Jacques TS et al (2004) Mitochondrial dysfunction in a long-term rodent model of sepsis and organ failure. Am J Physiol Regul Integr Comp Physiol 286:R491–R497
24. Starr ME, Steele AM, Saito M, Hacker BJ, Evers BM, Saito H (2014) A new cecal slurry preparation protocol with improved long-term reproducibility for animal models of sepsis. PLoS One 9:e115705
25. Luna CM, Sibila O, Agusti C, Torres A (2009) Animal models of ventilator-associated pneumonia. Eur Respir J 33:182–188
26. Khatri M, Dwivedi V, Krakowka S et al (2010) Swine influenza H1N1 virus induces acute inflammatory immune responses in pig lungs: a potential animal model for human H1N1 influenza virus. J Virol 84:11210–11218
27. Tidswell M, Tillis W, Larosa SP et al (2010) Phase 2 trial of eritoran tetrasodium (E5564), a toll-like receptor 4 antagonist, in patients with severe sepsis. Crit Care Med 38:72–83
28. Solomon SB, Cui X, Gerstenberger E et al (2006) Effective dosing of lipid A analogue E5564 in rats depends on the timing of treatment and the route of Escherichia coli infection. J Infect Dis 193:634–644
29. Taylor FB Jr., Chang A, Esmon CT, D'Angelo A, Vigano-D'Angelo S, Blick KE (1987) Protein C prevents the coagulopathic and lethal effects of Escherichia coli infusion in the baboon. J Clin Invest 79:918–925
30. Rehberg S, Ertmer C, Vincent JL et al (2011) Role of selective V1a receptor agonism in ovine septic shock. Crit Care Med 39:119–125
31. Singer M, Deutschman CS, Seymour C et al (2016) The third international consensus definitions for sepsis and septic shock (sepsis-3). JAMA 315:801–810
32. Eichacker PQ, Parent C, Kalil A et al (2002) Risk and the efficacy of antiinflammatory agents: retrospective and confirmatory studies of sepsis. Am J Respir Crit Care Med 166:1197–1205
33. Bassi E, Park M, Azevedo LCP (2013) Therapeutic strategies for high-dose vasopressor-dependent shock. Crit Care Res Pract 2013:10
34. Huttunen R, Hurme M, Aittoniemi J et al (2011) High plasma level of long pentraxin 3 (PTX3) is associated with fatal disease in bacteremic patients: a prospective cohort study. PLoS One 6:e17653
35. Kim S, Mi L, Zhang L (2012) Specific elevation of DcR3 in sera of sepsis patients and its potential role as a clinically important biomarker of sepsis. Diagn Microbiol Infect Dis 73:312–317
36. Abraham E, Anzueto A, Gutierrez G et al (1998) Double-blind randomised controlled trial of monoclonal antibody to human tumour necrosis factor in treatment of septic shock. NORASEPT II Study Group. Lancet 351:929–933
37. Panacek EA, Marshall JC, Albertson TE et al (2004) Efficacy and safety of the monoclonal anti-tumor necrosis factor antibody F(ab')2 fragment afelimomab in patients with severe sepsis and elevated interleukin-6 levels. Crit Care Med 32:2173–2182
38. Bernard GR, Vincent JL, Laterre PF et al (2001) Efficacy and safety of recombinant human activated protein c for severe sepsis. N Engl J Med 344:699–709
39. Rubin EB, Buehler AE, Halpern SD (2016) States worse than death among hospitalized patients with serious illnesses. JAMA Intern Med 176:1557–1559
40. Iwashyna TJ, Deane AM (2016) Individualizing endpoints in randomized clinical trials to better inform individual patient care: the TARGET proposal. Crit Care 20:1–8
41. Gordon AC, Mason AJ, Thirunavukkarasu N et al (2016) Effect of early vasopressin vs norepinephrine on kidney failure in patients with septic shock: The vanish randomized clinical trial. JAMA 316:509–518
42. Rugo HS, Olopade OI, DeMichele A et al (2016) adaptive randomization of veliparib-carboplatin treatment in breast cancer. N Engl J Med 375:23–34

43. Lang T (2011) Adaptive trial design: could we use this approach to improve clinical trials in the field of global health? Am J Trop Med Hyg 85:967–970
44. Faisy C, Meziani F, Planquette B et al (2016) Effect of acetazolamide vs placebo on duration of invasive mechanical ventilation among patients with chronic obstructive pulmonary disease: A randomized clinical trial. JAMA 315:480–488
45. McCloskey RV, Straube RC, Sanders C, Smith SM, Smith CR (1994) Treatment of septic shock with human monoclonal antibody HA-1A. A randomized, double-blind, placebo-controlled trial. CHESS Trial Study Group. Ann Intern Med 121:1–5
46. Opal SM, Fisher CJ Jr., Dhainaut JF et al (1997) Confirmatory interleukin-1 receptor antagonist trial in severe sepsis: a phase III, randomized, double-blind, placebo-controlled, multicenter trial. The Interleukin-1 Receptor Antagonist Sepsis Investigator Group. Crit Care Med 25:1115–1124
47. Angus DC, Birmingham MC, Balk RA et al (2000) E5 murine monoclonal antiendotoxin antibody in gram-negative sepsis: a randomized controlled trial. E5 Study Investigators. JAMA 283:1723–1730
48. Abraham E, Reinhart K, Opal S et al (2003) Efficacy and safety of tifacogin (recombinant tissue factor pathway inhibitor) in severe sepsis: a randomized controlled trial. JAMA 290:238–247
49. Opal S, Laterre PF, Abraham E et al (2004) Recombinant human platelet-activating factor acetylhydrolase for treatment of severe sepsis: results of a phase III, multicenter, randomized, double-blind, placebo-controlled, clinical trial. Crit Care Med 32:332–341
50. Vincent JL, Marshall JC, Dellinger RP et al (2015) Talactoferrin in severe sepsis: results from the phase II/III Oral tAlactoferrin in Severe sepsIS Trial. Crit Care Med 43:1832–1838

Medicating Patients During Extracorporeal Membrane Oxygenation: The Evidence is Building

A. L. Dzierba, D. Abrams, and D. Brodie

Introduction

Extracorporeal membrane oxygenation (ECMO), which can support gas exchange or hemodynamics in patients with severe respiratory or cardiac failure, has demonstrated considerable evolution over the last decade [1], with a steady rise since 2009 in the number of ECMO-treated patients and number of centers providing ECMO support [2, 3]. With more adult patients being placed on ECMO support, there is an increased need to understand the complex changes in drug pharmacokinetics and pharmacodynamics that occur with the addition of an ECMO circuit to the management of a critically ill patient.

The relationship between the dose of a drug and the elicited response may be altered in critically ill patients as a result of pharmacokinetic and pharmacodynamic changes [4]. The use of extracorporeal mechanical support, such as ECMO, can further increase the variability of pharmacokinetic alterations [5]. Therefore, the combination of critical illness and ECMO presents considerable challenges to providing optimal pharmacotherapy. The ability to anticipate alterations in pharmacokinetics and pharmacodynamics in this patient population is essential for providing an individualized therapeutic plan that maximizes therapeutic benefit while minimizing potential toxicity.

Despite improvements in extracorporeal technology and resurgence in its use in respiratory and cardiac failure, there remains a paucity of data on pharmacotherapy in patients receiving ECMO. This chapter summarizes our current understanding

A. L. Dzierba
Department of Pharmacy, NewYork-Presbyterian Hospital, Columbia University Medical Center
New York, NY 10032, USA

D. Abrams · D. Brodie (✉)
Division of Pulmonary, Allergy and Critical Care, Columbia University College of Physicians and Surgeons
622 West 168th Street, New York, NY 10032, USA
e-mail: hdb5@cumc.columbia.edu

J.-L. Vincent (ed.), *Annual Update in Intensive Care and Emergency Medicine 2017*,
DOI 10.1007/978-3-319-51908-1_31

of the effects of ECMO on the pharmacokinetics and pharmacodynamics of several drug classes commonly used to manage these critically ill patients.

The Effect of Critical Illness and ECMO on Pharmacokinetics

Pharmacokinetics encompasses the absorption, distribution, metabolism and elimination of a drug, ultimately influencing the concentration at the targeted site of action. In contrast, pharmacodynamics denotes the relationship between the drug concentration and the physiologic and biochemical effects of the drug on the body, including the intensity of therapeutic and adverse effects. The relationship between pharmacokinetics and pharmacodynamics is influenced by the drug, the underlying disease process, and the presence of extracorporeal factors. The culmination of all of these factors can lead to considerable and unpredictable alterations in pharmacokinetics. Fig. 1 summarizes the effects of serum drug concentrations and the resultant pharmacokinetic changes influenced by critical illness and ECMO.

The elimination of drugs from the body is highly dependent on clearance of the drugs from the body and on volume of distribution. The patient's physiology and the specific physiochemical properties of drugs, such as protein binding, hydrophilicity, molecular weight, and degree of ionization at a given physiologic pH, may influence both clearance and volume of distribution. The presence of ECMO frequently leads to additional alterations, including an increased volume of distribution and either increased or decreased drug clearance [5].

The liver and the kidneys are the two major organ systems responsible for drug metabolism and elimination, with less significant elimination occurring through the biliary system, gastrointestinal tract and lungs. Critically ill patients often develop organ insufficiency or failure during the course of their illness thereby altering drug elimination rates. Decreased renal blood flow or function will lead to a decreased glomerular filtration rate, affecting drugs that are dependent on this route of elimination (mainly hydrophilic drugs), whereas decreases in hepatic perfusion or function may lead to toxicity through decreased enzymatic activity or decreases in extraction efficiency.

The distribution of drug throughout the body (volume of distribution) is largely dependent on the drug's hydrophilicity and its acid-ionization constant. Drugs that are hydrophilic will have a lower volume of distribution and their concentrations will primarily be influenced by fluid-shifts and large-volume fluid resuscitation. In contrast, lipophilic drugs penetrate into the tissues, leaving lower concentrations in the blood and increasing the apparent volume of distribution. The ECMO circuit may increase the volume of distribution through either hemodilution or sequestration of drugs [5, 6]. An initial increase in volume of distribution that occurs at the initiation of ECMO from the introduction of priming solutions (plasma, saline, or albumin), primarily affecting hydrophilic drugs, may result in decreased plasma concentrations and, potentially, therapeutic failure of a drug. This increased volume may also lead to the dilution of plasma proteins, notably albumin, affecting drugs that are highly protein-bound, leading to potential toxicities as a result of an increase in the proportion of the unbound fraction of a drug.

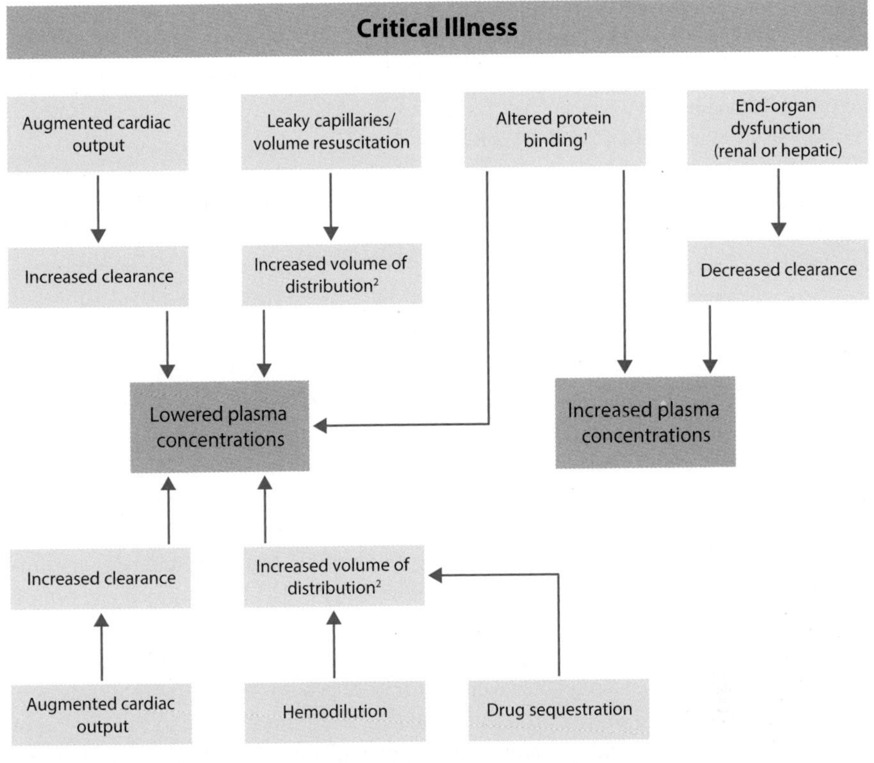

Fig. 1 Changes in pharmacokinetics with critical illness and extracorporeal membrane oxygenation. [1]increased α_1-acid glycoprotein and decreased albumin concentrations; [2]mostly affecting hydrophilic drugs

Modern extracorporeal circuits typically consist of cannulae, polyvinyl chloride (PVC) tubing, a centrifugal pump, and an artificial membrane for gas exchange (often termed a 'membrane oxygenator'). The membrane oxygenator and PVC tubing comprise a large surface area for potential drug sequestration, which may lead to drug loss over time, particularly for lipophilic drugs [5, 7, 8]. The composition of the tubing and membrane oxygenator may play a role in the amount of drug that is sequestered. Some studies have observed that both PVC tubing and the membrane oxygenators absorb drugs to a similar extent, whereas others have shown significant differences. This may be explained by both the age of the circuit and the type of pump used [8–12].

Albumin and α_1-acid glycoprotein, both synthesized in the liver, are the two major blood proteins that bind to drugs. In critical illness, albumin concentrations decrease in response to increased vascular permeability, decreased production and

Table 1 Effect of critical illness and extracorporeal membrane oxygenation (ECMO) on pharmacokinetics (PK) of drugs, based on degree of lipophilicity

	Hydrophilic drugs	Lipophilic drugs
Volume of distribution (Vd)	Low	High
Primary mode of clearance	Renal	Hepatic
Log *P*	Low	High
Potential effect of critical illness on PK	Increased Vd	No change in Vd
Effect of ECMO on PK	Increased Vd No change in clearance	Increased Vd Increased clearance

Log P: octanol-water partition coefficient (measure of drug's lipophilicity)

increased catabolism; whereas, α1-acid glycoprotein is an acute-phase reactant that may increase in response to physiologic stress. The changes in protein concentrations could affect both the amount of free drug available and the overall volume of distribution. Additionally the deposition of protein on the inner surface of the ECMO tubing may potentially increase the sequestration of drugs that have a high affinity for protein binding [13]. A recent *ex vivo* model tested the changes in concentrations over time of highly protein bound drugs [14]. Highly protein bound drugs in this experiment included ceftriaxone, caspofungin and thiopentone, all of which had significantly lower mean drug recoveries at 24 h (80, 56, and 12%, respectively) compared to drugs that were not highly protein bound [14].

Since lipophilic and highly protein bound drugs are more prone to sequestration in ECMO circuits, an understanding of the physicochemical properties of drugs can assist in determining the relationship between the dose administered and the anticipated blood concentration [5, 15]. The octanol-water partition coefficient or log *P*, is a common way to report the measure of a drug's lipophilicity [16]. Drugs with high log *P* values (around 2.0) will have a propensity to be very soluble in organic materials such as the PVC tubing used in the ECMO circuit. However, to date, there has been no characterization of the drug-circuit interaction beyond 24 h and, as such, little is known regarding the adsorptive capacity of the circuit over longer periods of ECMO support. Table 1 summarizes the effects of critical illness and ECMO on pharmacokinetics of drugs based on degree of lipophilicity of the drug.

Analgesia and Sedation

Patients receiving ECMO often require analgesia and sedation to reduce oxygen consumption, facilitate patient-ventilator synchrony, diminish patient stress and discomfort, and prevent patient-initiated device dislodgement or removal [1]. However, achieving the desired level of sedation and preventing delirium in the critically ill patient receiving ECMO remains a challenge in ICUs, owing to paradigm shifts in analgosedation regimens as well as pharmacokinetic alterations of commonly used analgesics and sedatives. Medication selection should be based on the patient's needs, with titration to a predetermined goal in accordance with recently published guidelines [17]. Limited data exist on the most appropriate opioid and sedative medication regimen to use in ECMO patients to achieve the desired level of sedation while minimizing excess sedative exposure. Commonly used intravenous opioids include fentanyl, hydromorphone and morphine, while sedatives often include propofol, dexmedetomidine and benzodiazepines. The choice of agent used is dependent on the desired physiological endpoint while balancing unwanted adverse effects of each individual agent.

Three *ex vivo* studies using adult ECMO circuits composed of PVC tubing and a hollow polymethylpentene fiber membrane oxygenator demonstrated significant losses of commonly used opioids and sedatives [6, 18, 19]. One investigation observed as much as a 93% loss in dexmedetomidine concentrations at 24 h [18]. Another study, measuring concentrations of morphine, fentanyl, and midazolam over a 24-hour period, demonstrated that the average drug recovery relative to baseline was lower with lipophilic drugs [6]. Only 3% of fentanyl and 13% of midazolam were detectable at 24 h; however, the ECMO circuit did not substantially alter morphine concentrations, with 103% recovery at 24 h. Of interest, in the first hour of ECMO support, up to 70% and 50% of fentanyl and midazolam, respectively, were lost in the circuit [6]. The most recent *ex vivo* study using adult ECMO circuits primed with human whole blood observed a recovery of only 30% of baseline propofol concentrations at 30 min and negligible concentrations at 24 h [19]. Additionally, midazolam concentrations were substantially reduced with 54% and 11% of baseline concentrations measured at 30 min and 24 h, respectively [19]. Similar findings have also been observed in neonatal circuits composed of PVC tubing and earlier generation silicone membrane oxygenators. These investigations observed up to a 68% loss of midazolam and a 98% loss of propofol within 40–120 min and up to a 30% reduction in lorazepam concentrations [11, 12].

Adult patients receiving ECMO for respiratory failure appear to have increased requirements of analgesia and sedation over time [20, 21]. The first case report demonstrating increased sedation requirements was in a 30-year-old man with severe respiratory failure requiring venovenous ECMO as a bridge to lung transplantation. Over 19 days of ECMO support, his requirements of morphine and propofol to maintain deep levels of sedation increased significantly [20]. A small, single-center, retrospective study observed an increase in opioid and sedative requirements over time in 29 consecutive patients requiring ECMO (13 venovenous, 16 venoarterial) where the sedation protocol was to keep patients heavily sedated during the first few days of ECMO followed by daily lightening of sedation when possible [21]. This study reported an increase in the average daily dose of midazolam and morphine of 18 mg ($p = 0.001$) and 29 mg ($p = 0.02$), respectively [21]. Interestingly, the authors did not find any significant increase in fentanyl requirements over time. Additionally, patients receiving venovenous ECMO had a significantly higher daily midazolam dose requirement than did patients receiving venoarterial ECMO ($p = 0.005$) [21]. A more recent single-center, prospective cohort study set out to determine the median daily dose of opioids and benzodiazepines in 32 patients receiving either venovenous or venoarterial ECMO [22]. In this mixed cohort the median daily dose of opioids and benzodiazepines, 3,875 micrograms and 24 mg respectively, was found to be lower than that reported from previous trials. Additionally, the authors did not find increasing requirements throughout the duration of ECMO support. The lower opioid and benzodiazepine requirements observed in this study could be a result of the study institution's analgosedation approach, lower goal sedation scores, and use of other non-benzodiazepine sedatives [22].

The only comparative trial to date is a recent retrospective cohort study that enrolled consecutive adult patients with severe respiratory failure with (n = 34) or without (n = 60) venovenous ECMO support requiring at least one sedative to maintain a level of wakefulness appropriate to maintain patient comfort and safety while optimizing oxygenation and ventilator support [23]. The authors found that the maximum median 6-hour sedative exposure was nearly twice as high in the ECMO group and was reached nearly 3 days later when compared to the group not receiving ECMO. However, there was no significant difference in 6-hour sedative exposure in adjusted analyses [23]. Therefore, this study challenges whether the increased requirements of opioids and sedatives are a result of circuit-related factors alone or whether other factors, such as tolerance, age or pharmacogenomics, play a central role.

Existing data are sparse to guide the appropriate dosing of opioids and sedatives in adult patients receiving ECMO in the context of modern extracorporeal technology. Many of the first-line agents used in the management of pain and sedation are lipophilic and therefore have a high propensity to be adsorbed or sequestered by the extracorporeal circuit [6, 11, 12]. One approach to achieving adequate sedation in patients receiving ECMO would be to start with continuous infusions of both an opioid and a sedative, anticipating requirements that exceed standard doses with the ultimate goal of minimizing the deleterious effects of sedative agents, especially benzodiazepines, with daily interruptions or down titrations. Additionally, clinicians should anticipate the need for significant dose reductions at the time of ECMO discontinuation given the likely rapid decrease in volume of distribution. Failure to do so could result in overuse of these medications. The reduction in dosing may be difficult to calibrate, so it is prudent to carefully monitor for signs of withdrawal and delirium. Consideration of adjunct agents, such as sub-anesthetic doses of ketamine, may help facilitate achieving sedation goals. Two uncontrolled studies demonstrated reductions in sedative rates with the addition of low-dose ketamine infusions [24, 25]. Most recently, a randomized trial did not show any differences in opioid or sedative requirements with the addition of low-dose ketamine to standard sedation practices as compared to standard sedation practices alone in patients receiving venovenous ECMO for severe respiratory failure [26]. Standard sedation practices consisted of infusions of fentanyl or hydromorphone and midazolam to achieve a Richmond Agitation Sedation Scale (RASS) of −5 at the initiation of ECMO. The median cumulative amount of fentanyl and midazolam equivalents in the low-dose ketamine group were almost twice and four times as high, respectively, when compared to the control group from ECMO initiation to the decision to achieve wakefulness [26]. However, patients receiving low-dose ketamine infusion had similar improvements in their RASS scores over the 72-hours after the decision to achieve wakefulness [26].

The incidence of delirium in patients receiving ECMO is not well characterized; however, given the high use of benzodiazepines in these patients, it may be reasonable to presume that the rates are as high as those reported in the critically ill patient population not receiving ECMO [27]. When appropriate, the use of a regimented analgosedation approach, daily interruption of sedation, and early mobilization may help minimize opioid and sedative exposure and thus reduce the incidence of delirium associated with these drugs, as appears to be the case in critically ill patients in general [17].

Antimicrobials

Infections are commonly encountered in critically ill patients and are associated with higher mortality [28]. In a critically ill patient, source control, in addition to timely and appropriate antimicrobial administration, remains the cornerstone of successful treatment of infection [29]. Selecting the appropriate dose of an antimicrobial can be challenging given the potential effects of critical illness and ECMO on drug concentrations, particularly considering that most antimicrobial dosing regimens have been established in healthy adults with normal physiology [5]. Changes in volume of distribution and clearance from critical illness and the ECMO circuit may affect pharmacodynamic parameters that ultimately determine the effectiveness of the antimicrobial agent. Inappropriate antimicrobial dosing may result in substantial drug losses, leading to therapeutic failure, development of resistance, and worse outcomes in patients with life-threating infections whereas an empiric increase in dose may potentially lead to accumulation and toxicity.

Vancomycin, a moderately protein bound, hydrophilic antimicrobial agent is commonly used to treat Gram-positive bacterial infections. Two *in vitro* ECMO studies observed steady vancomycin drug concentrations over 24 and 48-hour periods [6, 19]. In a matched cohort study of adult critically ill patients, those receiving ECMO had a similar volume of distribution and clearance of vancomycin compared to those not receiving ECMO in the first 24 h of therapy [30]. All patients received a 35 mg/kg loading dose over 4 h, followed by a continuous infusion targeting a serum concentration of 20–30 mg/l [30]. Linezolid, an alternative Gram-positive antimicrobial, was studied in three adult patients receiving ECMO, the results of which suggest that therapeutic targets may not be achieved with standard dosing when the minimum inhibitory concentration (MIC) is greater than 1 mg/l [31].

Aminoglycosides, including gentamicin and tobramycin, are hydrophilic drugs with low protein binding and with increased volume of distribution in the context of critical illness, resulting in decreased maximal concentrations. Additionally, in the context of a higher volume of distribution from the ECMO circuit, standard or higher initial doses may be needed with normal or extended intervals in order to provide sufficient peak concentrations. The study of aminoglycoside pharmacokinetic alterations during ECMO is largely limited to the neonatal population; however, one observational study in adult patients demonstrated comparable pharmacokinetics with amikacin in critically ill patients with or without ECMO support [32]. Therapeutic drug monitoring is readily available for this class of antimicrobial agents, making it feasible to target effective concentrations while limiting potential toxicity.

Extended-spectrum penicillins, cephalosporins and carbapenems are commonly used in the treatment of Gram-negative infections in the critically ill patient population. As a class, these antimicrobials are generally hydrophilic, largely dependent on renal elimination, and have moderate to low protein binding; however, variability exists with certain drugs such as ceftriaxone. Optimizing the time-dependent, bactericidal effect of this class will be achieved by maximizing the time concentrations above the MIC. The use of extended or continuous infusions seems to be a reasonable approach to optimize the pharmacodynamics in critically ill patients receiving ECMO [4].

Conflicting data have been reported on meropenem, a hydrophilic carbapenem with low protein binding. While some studies suggest a significant loss of meropenem within the ECMO circuit [6, 33, 34], other investigations have found no effect *in vivo* compared to other critically ill patients [35]. A recent retrospective, case-control study observed no differences in pharmacokinetic paramenters with either piperacillin/tazobactam or meropenem in patients receiving ECMO compared to those not receiving ECMO [35]. Of interest, nearly 30% of all drug levels measured for the two aformentioned drugs were subtherapeutic, which may be a consequence of other pathophysiological disturbances not controlled for in this critically ill population [35]. Mechanical circulatory support in general can induce a systemic inflammatory response, independent of the underlying critical illness, which, in turn, may augment renal clearance. Classes of antimicrobials in which direct correlations of augmented renal clearance and lower serum drug concentrations have been observed include beta-lactams, aminoglycocides and glycopeptides [36].

Regarding other antimicrobial drug classes, azithromycin pharmacokinetics appear to be similar between patients receiving ECMO and non-ECMO critically ill controls [37] and tigecycline levels in one patient were similar to expected levels based on population pharmacokinetics [38]. Concentrations of ciprofloxicin, a fluoroquinolone that is lipophilic with low to moderate protein binding, do not seem to be affected by ECMO [14]. To date there are no data on pharmacokinetic changes with polymyxin B or polymyxin E (colistin) that are used to treat multi-drug resistant Gram-negative infections. ECMO does not appear to affect oseltamivir pharmacokinetics directly; however, patients with renal dysfunction may experience impaired drug clearance [39–41].

Data on the pharmacokinetic changes of antifungal agents in adult patients receiving ECMO are limited to *in vitro* studies or case reports. While fluconazole does not seem to be affected by the ECMO circuit with a mean drug recovery of 91% at 24 h, voriconazole concentrations appear to be significantly affected, with up to a 71% loss at 24 h [14, 42]. Despite adequate serum concentrations of caspofungin at recommended doses, data suggest some sequestration by the ECMO circuit [43].

Lipophilic formulations of amphotericin B as well as posaconazole and isavuconazole, both highly protein bound, may result in significant sequestration within the ECMO circuit.

When designing an appropriate antimicrobial dosing regimen for patients receiving ECMO, the biochemical properties of each drug should be considered, generally favoring a high initial concentration while monitoring for potential toxicities. Whenever possible, monitoring of drug concentrations, including peaks and troughs as appropriate, will help inform an effective dose and interval. Individualized dosing strategies may be necessary, especially when targeting a specific microorganism. Further insight into pharmacokinetic changes of antimicrobials in adult ECMO patients will be provided with the ongoing Analgesia, Sedation, and Antibiotic Pharmacokinetics during Extracorporeal Membrane Oxygenation (ASAP ECMO) trial [44].

Limitations to Current Studies

Although there are known pharmacokinetic changes occurring as a consequence of ECMO support, there are very limited data addressing the clinical outcomes associated with these observations. For example, agents used for sedation or blood pressure control can be titrated to predetermined clinical endpoints, permitting the bedside clinician to use a dose for which the effects may be easily observed and measured. However, in the absence of therapeutic drug monitoring, attainment of adequate antimicrobial concentrations may not be so readily observed, instead requiring the clinician to rely on surrogate endpoints, such as white blood cell counts or temperature curves, to assess effectiveness. Much of the existing data is limited to simulated circuits that do not account for metabolism or elimination. Additionally studies have not addressed how changing blood flow rates or using different ECMO configurations could impact the amount of drug sequestered within the circuit. Finally, many of the studies do not have control subjects, have not addressed the effects of circuits over longer time intervals, and have not studied the impact of additional extracorporeal circuits, such as continuous renal replacement therapy, on pharmacokinetic parameters.

Future Directions

There is potential for novel strategies, such as altering the materials used in ECMO tubing or creating polymeric micelles for drug delivery, to minimize drug sequestration within the ECMO circuit. Absorption of lipophilic drugs to traditional medical grade PVC tubing containing di-ethylhexyl phthalate, a plasticizer, has been well established over the years. One *in vitro* study observed less adsorption capacity for lipophilic drugs when alternative materials, such as Teflon or silicone-caoutchouc mixture (SRT 460), were used [13]. Another method would be to encapsulate intravenous lipophilic drugs within micelles, a concept that has previously been demonstrated with gene therapy [45]. The idea is to solubilize appropriate portions of lipophilic drugs into the hydrophobic core, allowing attraction of the lipophilic tail to the surface of the ECMO tubing and drug release with minimal adherence to the surface of the tubing.

Conclusion

The pharmacokinetics and pharmacodynamics of drugs administered to critically ill patients are influenced by several factors, including the physiochemical properties of the drugs, the etiology and severity of the underlying illness, and the function of the organs responsible for drug metabolism. The presence of ECMO has an additional impact on drug distribution and metabolism, particularly due to increases in volume of distribution and sequestration by circuit components. Data are limited regarding the optimal regimen and dosing of sedatives and analgesics for critically ill patients receiving ECMO support, with the existing literature suggesting that, in many cases, higher amounts of analgosedation may be necessary to achieve therapeutic levels than would be expected for critically ill patients not receiving ECMO. Certain classes of antimicrobials may likewise be affected by ECMO, potentially leading to sub-therapeutic drug concentrations if usual dosing regimens are used. Emerging data from the ASAP ECMO trial should help inform the appropriate administration of many commonly used antimicrobials, sedatives and analgesics in patients receiving ECMO.

References

1. Brodie D, Bacchetta M (2011) Extracorporeal membrane oxygenation for ARDS in adults. N Engl J Med 365:1905–1914
2. Paden ML, Conrad SA, Rycus PT, Thiagarajan RR, ELSO Registry (2012) Extracorporeal Life Support Organization Registry Report 2012. Asaio J 59:202–210
3. Karagiannidis C, Brodie D, Strassmann S et al (2016) Extracorporeal membrane oxygenation: evolving epidemiology and mortality. Intensive Care Med 42:889–896
4. Roberts JA, Lipman J (2009) Pharmacokinetic issues for antibiotics in the critically ill patient. Crit Care Med 37:840–851
5. Shekar K, Fraser JF, Smith MT et al (2012) Pharmacokinetic changes in patients receiving extracorporeal membrane oxygenation. J Crit Care 27:741
6. Shekar K, Roberts JA, McDonald CI et al (2012) Sequestration of drugs in the circuit may lead to therapeutic failure during extracorporeal membrane oxygenation. Crit Care 16:R194
7. Preston TJ, Ratliff TM, Gomez D et al (2010) Modified surface coatings and their effect on drug adsorption within the extracorporeal life support circuit. J Extra Corpor Technol 42:199–202
8. Preston TJ, Hodge AB, Riley JB et al (2007) In vitro drug adsorption and plasma free hemoglobin levels associated with hollow fiber oxygenators in the extracorporeal life support (ECLS) circuit. J Extra Corpor Technol 39:234–237
9. Rosen DA, Rosen KR, Silvasi DL (1990) In vitro variability in fentanyl absorption by different membrane oxygenators. J Cardiothorac Anesth 4:332–335

10. Wildschut ED, Ahsman MJ, Allegaert K et al (2010) Determinants of drug absorption in different ECMO circuits. Intensive Care Med 36:2109–2116
11. Mulla H, Lawson G, von Anrep C et al (2000) In vitro evaluation of sedative drug losses during extracorporeal membrane oxygenation. Perfusion 15:21–26
12. Bhatt-Meht V, Annich G (2005) Sedative clearance during extracorporeal membrane oxygenation. Perfusion 20:309–315
13. Unger JK, Kuehlein G, Schroers A, Gerlach JC, Rossaint R (2001) Adsorption of xenobiotics to plastic tubing incorporated into dynamic in vitro systems used in pharmacological research – limits and progress. Biomaterials 22:2031–2037
14. Shekar K, Roberts JA, Mcdonald CI et al (2015) Protein-bound drugs are prone to sequestration in the extracorporeal membrane oxygenation circuit: results from an ex vivo study. Crit Care 19:164
15. Shekar K, Roberts JA, Barnett AG et al (2015) Can physicochemical properties of antimicrobials be used to predict their pharmacokinetics during extracorporeal membrane oxygenation? Illustrative data from ovine models. Crit Care 19:437
16. Poole SK, Poole CF (2003) Separation methods for estimating octanol-water partition coefficients. J Chromatogr B Analyt Technol Biomed Life Sci 797:3–19
17. Barr J, Fraser GL, Puntillo K et al (2013) Clinical practice guidelines for the management of pain, agitation, and delirium in adult patients in the ICU. Crit Care Med 41:263–306
18. Wagner D, Pasko D, Phillips K et al (2013) In vitro clearance of dexmedetomidine in extracorporeal membrane oxygenation. Perfusion 28:40–46
19. Lemaitre F, Hasni N, Leprince P et al (2015) Propofol, midazolam, vancomycin and cyclosporine therapeutic drug monitoring in extracorporeal membrane oxygenation circuits primed with whole human blood. Crit Care 19:40
20. Shekar K, Roberts JA, Ghassabian S et al (2012) Sedation during extracorporeal membrane oxygenation – why more is less. Anaesth Intensive Care 40:1067–1069
21. Shekar K, Roberts JA, Mullany DV et al (2012) Increased sedation requirements in patients receiving extracorporeal membrane oxygenation for respiratory and cardiorespiratory failure. Anaesth Intensive Care 40:648–655
22. DeGrado JR, Hohlfelder B, Ritchie BM, Anger KE, Reardon DP, Weinhouse GL (2016) Evaluation of sedatives, analgesics, and neuromuscular blocking agents in adults receiving extracorporeal membrane oxygenation. J Crit Care 37:1–6
23. Der Nigoghossian C, Dzierba AL, Etheridge J et al (2016) Effect of extracorporeal membrane oxygenation use on sedative requirements in patients with severe acute respiratory distress syndrome. Pharmacotherapy 36:607–616
24. Tellor B, Shin N, Graeta TJ, Avidan MS (2015) Ketamine infusion for patients receiving extracorporeal membrane oxygenation support: a case series. F1000Res 4:16
25. Floroff CK, Hassig TB, Cochran JB, Mazur JE (2016) High-dose sedation and analgesia during extracorporeal membrane oxygenation: A focus on the adjunctive use of ketamine. J Pain Palliat Care Pharmacother 30:36–40
26. Dzierba AL, Brodie D, Bacchetta M et al (2016) Ketamine use in sedation management in patients receiving extracorporeal membrane oxygenation. Intensive Care Med 42:1822–1823
27. Buscher H, Vaidiyanathan S, Al-Soufi S et al (2013) Sedation practice in veno-venous extracorporeal membrane oxygenation: an international survey. ASAIO J 59:636–641
28. Dellinger RP, Levy MM, Rhodes A et al (2013) Surviving Sepsis Campaign: international guidelines for management of severe sepsis and septic shock: 2012. Crit Care Med 41:580–637
29. Kumar A, Roberts D, Wood KE et al (2006) Duration of hypotension before initiation of effective antimicrobial therapy is the critical determinant of survival in human septic shock. Crit Care Med 34:1589–1596
30. Donadello K, Roberts JA, Cristallini S et al (2014) Vancomycin population pharmacokinetics during extracorporeal membrane oxygenation therapy: a matched cohort study. Crit Care 18:632

31. De Rosa FG, Corcione S, Baietto L et al (2013) Pharmacokinetics of linezolid during extracorporeal membrane oxygenation. Int J Antimicrob Agents 41:590–591
32. Gélisse E, Neuville M, de Montmollin E et al (2016) Extracoporeal membrane oxygenation (ECMO) does not impact on amikacin pharmacokinetics: a case-control study. Intensive Care Med 42:946–948
33. Shekar K, Roberts JA, Ghassabian S et al (2013) Altered antibiotic pharmacokinetics during extracorporeal membrane oxygenation: cause for concern? J Antimicrob Chemother 68:726–727
34. Shekar K, Fraser JF, Taccone FS et al (2014) The combined effects of extracorporeal membrane oxygenation and renal replacement therapy on meropenem pharmacokinetics: a matched cohort study. Crit Care 18:565
35. Donadello K, Antonucci E, Cristallini S et al (2015) Beta-lactam pharmacokinetics during extracorporeal membrane oxygenation therapy: A case-control study. Int J Antimicrob Agents 45:278–282
36. Udy AA, Roberts JA, Boots RJ, Paterson DL, Lipman J (2010) Augmented renal clearance: implications for antibacterial dosing in the critically ill. Clin Pharmacokinet 35:606–608
37. Turner RB, Rouse S, Elbarbry F et al (2016) Azithromycin pharmacokinetics in adults with acute respiratory distress syndrome undergoing treatment with extracorporeal-membrane oxygenation. Ann Pharmacother 50:72–73
38. Veinstein A, Debouverie O, Grégoire N et al (2012) Lack of effect of extracorporeal membrane oxygenation on tigecycline pharmacokinetics. J Antimicrob Chemother 67:1047–1048
39. Lemaitre F, Luyt CE, Roullet-Renoleau F et al (2012) Impact of extracorporeal membrane oxygenation and continuous venovenous hemodiafiltration on the pharmacokinetics of oseltamivir carboxylate in critically ill patients with pandemic (H1N1) influenza. Ther Drug Monit 34:171–175
40. Mulla H, Peek GJ, Harvey C et al (2013) Oseltamivir pharmacokinetics in critically ill adults receiving extracorporeal membrane oxygenation support. Anesth Intensive Care 41:66–73
41. Eyler RF, Heung M, Pleva M et al (2012) Pharmacokinetics of oseltamivir and oseltamivir carboxylate in critically ill patients receiving continuous venovenous hemodialysis and/or extracorporeal membrane oxygenation. Pharmacotherapy 32:1061–1069
42. Mehta NM, Halwick DR, Dodson BL et al (2007) Potential drug sequestration during extracorporeal membrane oxygenation: results from an ex vivo experiment. Intensive Care Med 33:1018–1024
43. Spriet I, Annaert P, Meersseman P et al (2009) Pharmacokinetics of caspofungin and voriconazole in critically ill patients during extracorporeal membrane oxygenation. J Antimicrob Chemother 63:767–770
44. Shekar K, Roberts JA, Welch S et al (2012) ASAP ECMO: Antibiotic, sedative and analgesic pharmacokinetics during extracorporeal membrane oxygenation: a multi-centre study to optimise drug therapy during ECMO. BMC Anesthesiol 12:29
45. Jones M, Leroux J (1999) Polymeric micelles – a new generation of colloidal drug carriers. Eur J Pharm Biopharm 48:101–111

Anti-Inflammatory Properties of Anesthetic Agents

F. F. Cruz, P. R. M. Rocco, and P. Pelosi

Introduction

For more than a century, experimental and clinical studies have reported that anesthetic agents have diverse effects on the immune system [1]. Despite rapid development in the fields of immunology and anesthesiology in recent decades, the specific mechanisms by which each anesthetic drug affects the immune system remain unclear. Here, we will define innate and adaptive immunity, present factors that can lead to immune dysregulation during the perioperative period, describe the effects of some of the most common anesthetic drugs on immune cells and cytokines, and discuss the possible clinical implications of the use of these drugs [2].

Innate and Adaptive Immunity

The immune system plays a vital role in survival by protecting us from the many potentially deadly infectious pathogens in our environment, as well as from cancer cells. The immune system is able to recognize pathogens and trigger their elimination through innate and then adaptive immune responses [3].

Innate immunity, also called natural or native immunity, is the first line of defense and refers to protective mechanisms that are present even before infection. Its principal components are the epithelial membranes (which block pathogen entry), phagocytic cells (neutrophils and macrophages), dendritic cells, natural killer (NK)

F. F. Cruz · P. R. M. Rocco
Laboratory of Pulmonary Investigation, Carlos Chagas Filho Institute of Biophysics, Federal University of Rio de Janeiro
Rio de Janeiro, 21941-902, Brazil

P. Pelosi (✉)
Department of Surgical Sciences and Integrated Diagnostics, IRCCS AOU San Martino IST, University of Genoa
16132 Genoa, Italy
e-mail: ppelosi@hotmail.com

J.-L. Vincent (ed.), *Annual Update in Intensive Care and Emergency Medicine 2017*,
DOI 10.1007/978-3-319-51908-1_32

cells and several plasma proteins, including the complement system. The most important cellular reaction of innate immunity is inflammation – the process, mediated by dendritic and NK cells, whereby phagocytic cells are recruited and activated to eliminate aggressor agents [2, 3].

Adaptive immunity, also called specific or acquired immunity, consists of mechanisms that are induced by the recognition of specific pathogen antigens. The adaptive immune system is mediated primarily by lymphocytes, and its function can be classified into two types: humoral immunity, mediated by B-lymphocytes and their secreted antibodies; and cell-mediated or cellular immunity, mediated mostly by T-lymphocytes and their cytokines, which play an important role in immune cell activation, regulation, and communication [2, 3].

Besides its role in host defense against infectious agents and tumor cells, the inflammatory response is essential for tissue reconstitution after injury caused by accidental or surgical insults. Dysregulation of this inflammatory process may increase susceptibility to infections, accelerate the growth and metastasis of residual cancer cells, and result in postoperative complications, such as wound healing disturbances and infections leading to sepsis followed by multiple organ failure and death [4].

Perioperative Immunosuppression

The perioperative immunosuppression observed in surgical patients is related to the neuroendocrine stress exerted through activation of the autonomic nervous system and the hypothalamic-pituitary-adrenal (HPA) axis. Surgical stress-induced release of hormones such as catecholamines (norepinephrine and epinephrine), adrenocorticotropic hormone and cortisol, via the autonomic nervous system and the HPA, mediates inhibitory effects on immune functions, as monocytes/macrophages and T-cells express both β2-adrenoreceptors and glucocorticoid receptors, which promote cellular signaling to inhibit the production of proinflammatory cytokines [5]. Moreover, cytokines such as interleukin (IL)-1, IL-6, and tumor necrosis factor (TNF)-α from monocytes/macrophages and lymphocytes activated by surgical stress may stimulate the HPA [6]. Therefore, the neuroendocrine system, as well as proinflammatory and anti-inflammatory cytokines, synergistically augments its suppressive effects on the immune system in the perioperative period.

In addition to the surgical stress response, intraoperative blood pressure management, blood transfusion, hyperglycemia, hypothermia, postoperative pain, and anesthesia, all of which are managed by anesthesiologists during surgical interventions, cause perioperative immunosuppression (Fig. 1; [4]). Anesthetic agents and anesthesia management are suspected of impairing several aspects of the inflammatory response process, either indirectly by modulating the stress response or directly by disturbing the functions of immune cells [1, 2, 4, 7].

Indeed, anesthetic drugs induce analgesia by affecting the transmission of nerve impulses and modulate surgical stress by acting on the HPA axis, thus affecting its immunomodulatory effects ([1, 2, 4]; Fig. 1). Recently, numerous studies have

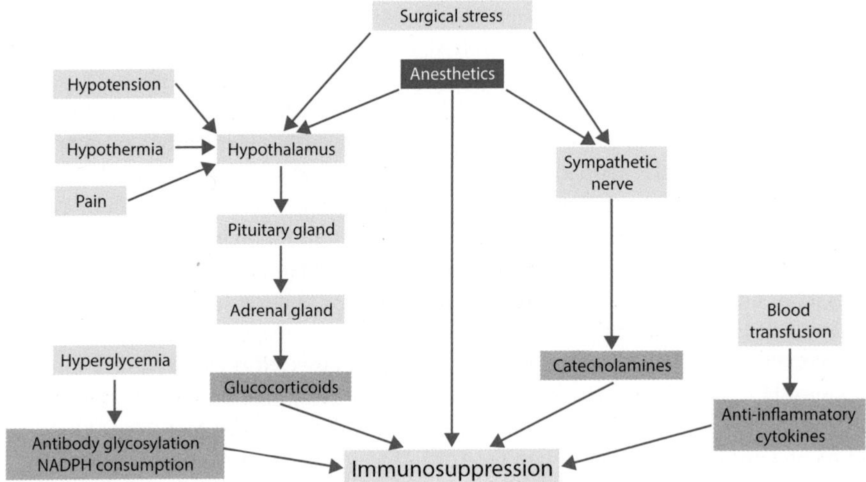

Fig. 1 Schematic diagram of possible modulators of immune competence during anesthesia and surgery. Anesthetics have direct effects on the immune system and indirect effects through neuro-immune-endocrine interactions during surgical stress

shown that, alongside the immunosuppression caused by surgical stress, anesthetics and analgesic agents commonly used in surgery and in intensive care may directly affect the functions of immunocompetent cells [4].

Diverse *in vitro* experiments with human immune cells *ex vivo* [2], *in vivo* tests [10] and animal models have demonstrated a wide range of effects of anesthetic drugs on the immune system, including changes in immune cell counts and their functionality and effects on the secretion patterns of diverse immune mediators, affecting the inflammatory response in the postoperative period [1–3].

Effects of General Anesthesia on Inflammation

The immune-modulating effects of anesthetics *in vitro* were first demonstrated more than 100 years ago [7]. The increasing knowledge of recent years is strongly related to developments in basic science and improvements in laboratory technique, e. g., cell separation and cell culture methods. It has been demonstrated that, at concentrations used clinically, different anesthetics depress the functions of the inflammatory response differentially.

Ketamine

Ketamine, an *N*-methyl-d-aspartate (NMDA)-receptor antagonist, acts at different levels of inflammation, interacting with inflammatory cell recruitment, cytokine production, and regulation of inflammatory mediators [11]. The immune-inhibitory effects of ketamine were recently found to be partly due to inhibition of transcription factor activator protein-1 and nuclear factor-kappa B (NF-κB), which regulate the production of several proinflammatory mediators [12]. The notion that ketamine interferes with immunity comes from the early observations of improved outcomes in critically ill patients and in experimental septic shock [13]. *In vivo*, a sub-anesthetic dose of ketamine produced a dose-dependent decrease in mortality with a significant reduction in production of TNF-α and IL-6 in septic rats [11, 14]. Intravenous administration of ketamine abolished albumin extravasation in a rat model of chemical peritonitis [14]. In other studies, anesthetic doses of ketamine attenuated lipopolysaccharide (LPS)-induced liver injury, with a reduction in cyclooxygenase (COX)-2, inducible nitric oxide synthase (iNOS), and NF-κB-binding activity [11, 14]. These data clearly indicate that ketamine may exert anti-inflammatory actions *in vivo*. These anti-inflammatory effects have also been found in clinical settings. Low-dose ketamine (0.25–0.5 mg/kg) significantly suppressed intraoperative and postoperative increases in serum IL-6 and C-reactive protein (CRP) in patients undergoing coronary artery bypass graft (CABG) surgery with cardiopulmonary bypass (CPB) [11, 14] and significantly decreased superoxide production. However, low-dose ketamine was not shown to have any anti-inflammatory effects in low-risk patients undergoing off-pump CABG. The link remains controversial [14].

Midazolam

Midazolam, a widely used benzodiazepine derivative, acts on GABA receptors by increasing neuronal permeability to chloride ions, leading to cell hyperpolarization. It is known to inhibit certain aspects of immune function [15]. Midazolam binds to peripheral receptors on macrophages and modulates their metabolic oxidative responsiveness *in vitro*. It has been suggested that clonazepam also binds to receptors on macrophages and inhibits their capacity to produce IL-1, IL-6, and TNF-α in a T-cell independent manner [16]; however, it was ineffective. These results demonstrate an *in vivo* immunosuppressive property of peripheral and mixed benzodiazepine receptor agonists (midazolam and diazepam) but not central-type receptor agonists (clonazepam), affecting characteristic phagocyte functions involved in host-defense mechanisms as well as in the inflammatory response [15]. Midazolam is also able to inhibit human neutrophil function and the activation of mast cells induced by TNF-α *in vitro,* and suppresses expression of IL-6 mRNA in human blood mononuclear cells [17]. When administered to LPS-stimulated macrophages, midazolam suppressed the respiratory burst of reactive oxygen species (ROS), inhibited NF-κB activation via suppression of IκB-α degradation, and inhibited p38 activation, which has been reported to play a critical role in LPS-mediated COX-2 and iNOS expression, pathways involved in the proinflammatory macrophage phenotype [18]. Nonetheless, midazolam infusion did not affect cytokine production in septic patients [15].

Propofol

Propofol, another GABA receptor agonist, has been shown to impair several monocyte and neutrophil functions of the innate immune system, including respiratory burst [19], chemotaxis [20], phagocytosis [21] and polarization [4]. While some authors have showed that the inhibitory properties on human neutrophils and complement activation of propofol are related to its lipid carrier vehicle [4, 22], others have suggested that propofol at least partly inhibits human neutrophil chemotaxis by suppressing the p44/42 mitogen-activated protein kinase (MAPK) pathway [4, 20]. In clinically relevant concentrations, propofol inhibits the production of a chemotactic agent in human neutrophils [4, 20]. The proliferative-suppressing effects of propofol were only observed in polymorphonuclear leukocytes (PMNs) obtained from critically ill patients who were primarily immunosuppressed [23]. Lymphocyte proliferation [4] and cytokine release in response to endotoxin were not found to be impaired in whole blood culture medium obtained from healthy volunteers [4, 24]. In an animal model of endotoxin-induced lung injury, propofol had anti-inflammatory effects. The underlying molecular mechanisms are still unclear; however, propofol is not known to inhibit activation of NF-κB [4]. Recent data suggest that propofol produces only cell-mediated immunomodulatory effects on innate immunity, and that these effects might be generated by its lipid solvent [4].

Opioids

The link between opioid use and alterations in host immune function is often mentioned in the literature, and has been formally documented since the early 19th century. The increased incidence of various local and systemic infections in intravenous drug abusers led to the conclusion that the causative link between drug use and infections could not be simply explained by the injection process, but that opiates themselves were acting to modulate immune function [25]. Different opioids affect immune function differently depending on drug factors, host factors, and the duration of exposure [26]. Morphine, fentanyl, remifentanil, methadone and codeine present strong immunomodulatory effects, while tramadol, hydrocodone, oxycodone, and buprenorphine present much weaker or no immune-modulating capacity [25]. This feature of opioids is often linked to central neuro-endocrine/neuro-paracrine and peripheral mechanisms and to peripheral actions mediated by mu-opioid receptors on immune cells [25].

The importance of centrally mediated mechanisms is supported further by the observation that opioids that cross the blood brain barrier (BBB) exert more immunomodulatory effects than opioids that do not cross the BBB [27]. Although opioid effects are largely attributed to decreased central sympathetic nervous system outflow, opioids can also cause direct sympathetic nervous activation, which may suppress the proliferation and function of some immune cell populations and primary and secondary lymphoid tissues [28]. The interaction of opioids with the HPA axis and its components (ACTH and cortisol production) is complex, species- and time-dependent, with different effects after acute and chronic administration. In humans, data are scarce; however, current evidence suggests that acute administration of opioids results in either a reduction or no change in ACTH or glucocorticoids. There is evidence that opioids attenuate the circadian rhythm of ACTH and cortisol, leading to consistent increments in circulating levels of these hormones, which might be sufficient to produce immune suppression [25].

Several studies have suggested that mu-opioid receptors are expressed on peripheral blood mononuclear cells [4, 29, 30]; however, in contrast to previous reports and despite using several validated methodologies, a recent investigation was unable to detect any opioid receptors or transcripts in mononuclear cells collected from venous blood [25].

There are well-documented, dose-dependent, immunosuppressive effects of morphine, which is known to impair monocyte and neutrophil function, NK cell-mediated cytotoxicity, lymphocyte and macrophage proliferation and cytokine release. Morphine promotes apoptosis by direct activation of the enzymes involved in cell apoptosis, inhibits leukocyte function by increasing intracellular concentrations of NO and cyclic AMP, and by inhibiting nuclear NF-κB via NO-dependent mechanisms [4]. Recent studies of the effects of synthetic opioids used in general anesthesia showed no more than transient immunomodulatory changes [1, 2, 4].

Fentanyl is known to enhance NK-cell cytotoxicity and increase NK and cytotoxic (CD8+) cell counts; however, the production of superoxide by PMNs and the number of circulating B- and T-lymphocytes remained unchanged in healthy volunteers [4, 31]. These effects of fentanyl on NK cells seem to be more centrally mediated, as fentanyl does not affect NK-cell activity directly. In two studies, sufentanil and alfentanil were observed to produce inhibitory effects on leukocyte migration, NK-cell activity, and mitogen-induced lymphocyte proliferation [1, 2, 4, 32].

Thiopental

When administered over prolonged periods, short- and intermediate-acting barbiturates, which act as GABA receptor agonists, may induce iatrogenic immunosuppression. A higher incidence of infections has been described in head-injured patients with increased intracranial pressure (ICP) who received prolonged infusions of thiopental [4, 33]. Thiopental is one of the most investigated anesthetic agents and is widely used for the induction of general anesthesia. Its inhibitory effects on the non-specific immune system have been well documented in several studies. In clinically used concentrations, thiopental has been shown to inhibit the bactericidal functions of leukocytes; neutrophil polarization, chemotaxis, adherence, phagocytosis, and respiratory burst; and monocyte chemotaxis [2]. In high concentrations, thiopental affects neutrophil and monocyte phagocytosis. In short, the described inhibitory effects of thiopental are indicative of direct cell-mediated inhibition of the immune response and a strong anti-inflammatory effect. In addition, thiopental is known to depress mitogen/antigen-induced lymphocyte proliferation in different culture mediums, and decreases the quantity of cytokines released in response to mitogens or endotoxins [34]. Recent studies have suggested that thiopental inhibits NF-κB activation [4]. Clinically, the immunosuppressive effects of thiopental are probably of minor clinical relevance, since it is often used only for induction of anesthesia [20].

Dexmedetomidine

Dexmedetomidine, an agonist of α_2-adrenergic receptors in certain regions of the brain, has been shown to reduce proinflammatory cytokine levels in experimental sepsis [35] as well as in critically ill [1, 4] and postoperative patients [36]. A significant decrease in leukocyte counts, CRP, IL-6, IL-8 and TNF-α levels in dexmedetomidine-treated patients is indicative of its anti-inflammatory potential when used as a perioperative adjunct [1, 2, 4]. A number of mechanisms of action have been postulated for dexmedetomidine, including: modulation of cytokine production by macrophages/monocytes during the stress response, which may also be stimulated via α2-adrenoceptors; inhibition of apoptosis; central sympatholytic effects, including stimulation of cholinergic anti-inflammatory pathways; and antinociceptive action involving interactions between pain and immune factors (proinflammatory cytokines) [1, 2, 4]. So far, however, these mechanisms remain unclear [37].

Volatile Anesthetics

Inhalational anesthetic agents have inhibitory effects on neutrophil function, decrease lymphocyte proliferation, and suppress cytokine release from peripheral blood mononuclear cells [1, 2, 38]. Halogenated anesthetics are known to suppress inflammatory cytokines in rat alveolar cells [4]. In contrast, exposure to volatile anesthetics and mechanical ventilation has been shown to induce increased gene expression of proinflammatory cytokines [38]. Volatile anesthetics affect the expression of iNOS by reversible inhibition of voltage-dependent calcium channels and decreased intracellular calcium concentrations. Thus, the *in vitro* effects of volatile anesthetics predominantly consist of inhibition of immune products, but these are generally transient, as well as dose- and time-dependent [1, 4, 38].

Sevoflurane

Anesthetic preconditioning to sevoflurane has been shown to promote protection from endotoxemia, ischemia–reperfusion injury, myocardial ischemia–reperfusion injury, among other disease models. Sevoflurane attenuated the activation of NF-κB and subsequent expression of NF-κB-dependent inflammatory mediators via Toll-like receptors (TLRs) [38]. Additionally, sevoflurane protects against vascular endothelium dysfunction induced by oxidative stress and inflammation through activation of the eNOS/NO pathway and inhibition of NF-κB. Endothelial dysfunction induced by oxidative stress and inflammation plays a critical role in the pathogenesis of cardiovascular diseases [37]. In particular, sevoflurane has been shown to induce a more pronounced suppression of cytokine release than isoflurane or enflurane.

Isoflurane

Isoflurane exposure leads to reduction in leukocyte counts and levels of systemic proinflammatory cytokines (TNF-α, IL-6 and IL-1β), as well as less macrophage activation and polarization toward the M2 phenotype. These effects were found to be protein kinase C-dependent and also due to systemic inhibition of NF-κB [38]. These findings suggest that pre-exposure to volatile anesthetics induces a systemic anti-inflammatory effect. On the other hand, exposure to isoflurane has been shown to lead to cognitive impairment and a small increase in IL-1β and activated caspase-3 levels in the hippocampi of both young adult and elderly rats. These results suggest that isoflurane induces neuroinflammation, which then leads to cognitive impairment.

Little is known regarding the mechanisms of volatile anesthetic-induced neuroinflammation, but isoflurane has been shown to open the BBB, increasing the permeation of intravascular substances into brain tissue. A recent study showed that exposure of H4 human neuroglioma cells to 2% isoflurane for 6 h activated NF-κB, increasing inflammatory cytokine production. Therefore, local activation of NF-κB is presumably a mechanism for isoflurane-induced neuroinflammation [39].

Effects of Regional and Local Anesthesia on Inflammation

With regard to their anti-inflammatory properties, local anesthetics have been shown to affect PMNs directly, as well as macrophage and monocyte function. Ropivacaine and lidocaine (100–300 mM) decreased TNF-α-induced upregulation of CD11b/CD18 surface expression on PMNs *in vitro* [40]. Thus, local anesthetics decrease PMN adherence, migration, and accumulation at the site of inflammation.

Since local anesthetics impair PMN presence and function, concerns have arisen that local anesthesia might increase susceptibility to infection, as local anesthetic-mediated depression of the PMN oxidative metabolic response may decrease the host's ability to control bacterial proliferation [41]. Antibacterial effects of local anesthetics have been reported *in vitro* and *in vivo*, but only at millimolar concentrations. Lidocaine (37 mM), for example, inhibits the growth of *Escherichia coli* and *Streptococcus pneumoniae*, but has no effect on *Staphylococcus aureus* or *Pseudomonas aeruginosa*. In contrast, other authors found that lidocaine reduced growth of all of the above-mentioned bacteria. Using a guinea pig wound model, lidocaine (74 mM) induced reduction of bacterial growth to approximately 30% in *S. aureus*-contaminated wounds. In summary, the anti-inflammatory properties of local anesthetics at systemic concentrations might, theoretically, increase the risk of infection, since antibacterial and antiviral effects are only attained with the use of high concentrations [1–3, 40, 41]. Nevertheless, this seems to be of minor importance in most studies, except for settings of severe bacterial contamination. Local anesthetics are known for their inhibition of excessive inflammatory responses without significant impairment of host immunity.

Clinical Implications of the Anti-inflammatory Properties of Anesthetics

Investigations of the immune effects of anesthetics have been derived mostly from *in vitro* studies, because human clinical studies are more complex, involving such variables as type and duration of surgery and patient complications. Although it is difficult to distinguish the relative contributions of surgical stress, anesthetics and analgesic agents to the patient's immune system, anesthesiologists must not ignore the immunosuppressive effects of anesthetic drugs on perioperative immunity [1].

In the Perioperative Period

Surgical trauma induces an endocrine, metabolic, hemodynamic and immune response that persists for at least a few days. It is generally accepted that the effect of anesthetics on the immune system is modest compared to the effects induced by major surgery or trauma; thus, anesthetics may not have any clinically significant effects on immune function in healthy patients anesthetized for short procedures, in whom the inflammatory response is usually balanced, well controlled and of limited duration [42]. An immunosuppressive effect of approximately 20% might not have great consequences for an immunocompetent patient. However, if the patient has a genetic predisposition to immune impairment or is already compromised, e. g., by aging, tumor burden, diabetes mellitus or malnutrition, the immunosuppressive effects of anesthetics might play a salient role in postoperative infectious complications, morbidity and mortality [43]. In addition, an increasing number of immunosuppressed elderly patients require anesthesia and intensive care treatment. Thus, the possible immunomodulatory effects of anesthetics must be widely comprehended and agents chosen wisely. Particularly in patients with cancer, immunosuppression after surgery accelerates the growth of residual malignant cells and promotes the establishment of new metastases [1, 42, 44]. On the other hand, the immunosuppressive effects of anesthetics that lead to anti-inflammatory responses may be therapeutically beneficial in distinct situations such as ischemia–reperfusion injury, the systemic inflammatory response syndrome, or acute respiratory distress syndrome (ARDS) [45]. Therefore, the effects of anesthetics on immunity may be not only adverse but also beneficial on the prognosis of specific patients. The immune effects of surgery and anesthetics affect the long-term outcomes of patients after surgery. Therefore, awareness of these immunological properties is helpful for daily anesthetic management.

In brief, the effect of anesthetics on the immune system has been less investigated *in vivo* than *in vitro*; current findings are contradictory and indicative of only minor clinical importance. At present, no one mode of anesthesia can be recommended in favor of another in terms of effect on the inflammatory response [1, 2, 4].

In addition to effects on non-specific cell-mediated immunity, some local anesthesia techniques can inhibit parts of the neuroendocrine response to surgery. Subarachnoid and epidural blockade blunts the increase in plasma levels of epinephrine, norepinephrine and cortisol induced by surgery. The reduction in the neuroendocrine stress response is most pronounced in connection with surgical procedures on the lower abdomen and lower extremities. In these cases, epidural anesthesia can provide complete blockade of all afferent neurogenic stimuli from the surgical field [40, 41], reducing the stress-related response, and can even reduce perioperative mortality and postoperative morbidity after some surgical procedures [1–4, 40, 41].

In the Intensive Care Unit

While a slight immunosuppressive effect of anesthesia during surgery is probably of minor importance because of the limited duration of exposure, critical care settings pose a different set of challenges. In the ICU, patients are often exposed to anesthetic agents for several days, and the side effects of immunosuppression have been shown to be clinically important in this population. In this context, as early as 1956, bone-marrow depression was described after prolonged ventilation with nitrous oxide [46].

Later, in 1983, increases in ICU mortality were reported after the introduction of etomidate for sedation [47]. Patients sedated with etomidate had a mortality of 77%, versus only 28% in patients not given this agent. It was later discovered that etomidate inhibits the synthesis of cortisol precursors and thus reduces levels of plasma cortisol. A high rate of infections has also been described in ICU patients receiving long-term thiopental infusions.

Propofol or benzodiazepines are most often used for long-term sedation in the ICU. Animal studies have shown reduced defense against infection following long-term infusion of propofol as well as benzodiazepines. A single study has shown increased plasma levels of proinflammatory cytokines (IL-1, IL-6, TNF-α) following long-term propofol infusion, while a reduction in proinflammatory cytokines was observed following benzodiazepine infusion. To avoid a potential detrimental effect of long-term sedation in critically ill patients, the duration and the doses of sedative agents should be kept as low as possible, not least because these patients are immunocompromised. Daily wake-up trials are recommended to reduce the risk of oversedation [1–4]

Conclusion

Anesthetics have long been suspected of impairing various aspects of immune system function, either indirectly by modulating the stress response or directly by affecting the functioning of immunocompetent cells. Although these effects are transient and may be of minor importance in subjects with normal immune systems, in patients with pre-existing immune dysfunction or multiple organ failure and in other high-risk groups, the influence of anesthetics and of the choice of anesthetic management technique on the perioperative inflammatory response may have clinical implications.

The effects of anesthetics on immunomodulation of inflammation are complex; immunosuppression can have positive as well as negative impact. Therefore, the choice and use of anesthetic agents are highly dependent on the immune status of each patient. Possible hazards associated with perioperative immunosuppression include increased risk of tumor metastasis and infection, whereas the anti-inflammatory effects of anesthetics may instead provide benefit in conditions associated with systemic and local inflammation [4].

References

1. Kurosawa S, Kato M (2008) Anesthetics, immune cells, and immune responses. J Anesth 22:263–277
2. Colucci DG, Puig NR, Hernandez PR (2013) Influence of anesthetic drugs on immune response: from inflammation to immunosuppression. OA Anesthetics 1:21–38
3. Friedman H, Newton C, Klein TW (2003) Microbial Infections, Immunomodulation, and Drugs of Abuse. Clin Microbiol Rev 16(2):209–219
4. Schneemilch CE, Schilling T, Bank U (2004) Effects of general anaesthesia on inflammation. Best Pract Res Clin Anaesthesiol 18:493–507
5. Elenkov IJ, Chrousos GP (2002) Stress hormones, proinflammtory and anti-inflammatory cytokines, and autoimmunity. Ann NY Acad Sci 966:290–303
6. Kennedy BC, Hall GM (1999) Neuroendocrine and inflammatory aspects of surgery: do they affect outcome? Acta Anaesthesiol Belg 50:205–209
7. Graham EA (1911) The influence of ether and ether anesthesia on bacteriolysis, agglutination and phagocytosis. J Infect Dis 8:147–175
8. Amin OAI, Salah HE (2011) The effect of general or spinal anaesthesia on pro- and anti-inflammatory intracellular cytokines in patients undergoing appendicectomy using flow cytometric method. Egypt J Anaesth 27:121–125
9. Colucci D, Harvey G, Gayol MC, Elena G, Puig N (2011) Halothane anesthesia in mice: effect on the phagocytic activity and respiratory burst of peritoneal macrophages. Neuroimmunomodulation 18:11–18
10. Simeonova GP, Slovov E, Usunov R, Halacheva K, Dinev DN (2008) Increased apoptosis of peripheral blood mononuclear cells (PBMC) during general and epidural anaesthesia in dogs. Vet Res Commun 32:619–626
11. Loix S, De Kock M, Henin P (2011) The anti-inflammatory effects of ketamine: state of the art. Acta Anaesthesiol Belg 62:47–58
12. Welters ID, Hafer G, Menzebach A et al (2010) Ketamine inhibits transcription factors activator protein 1 and nuclear factor-kappab, Interleukin-8 production, as well as CD11b and CD16 expression: studies in human leukocytes and leukocytic cell lines. Anesth Analg 110:934–941

13. Kock M, Loix S, Lavand'homme P (2013) Ketamine and peripheral inflammation. CNS Neurosci Ther 19:403–410
14. Hirota K, Lambert DG (2011) Ketamine: new uses for an old drug? Br J Anaesth 107:123–126
15. Memiş D, Hekimoğlu S, Vatan İ, Yandım T, Yüksel M (2007) Effects of midazolam and dexmedetomidine on inflammatory responses and gastric intramucosal pH to sepsis, in critically ill patients. Br J Anaesth 98:550–552
16. Zavala F, Haumont J, Lenfant M (1984) Interaction of benzodiazepines with mouse macrophages. Eur J Pharmacol 106:561–566
17. Nishina K, Akamatsu H, Mikawa K et al (1998) The inhibitory effects of thiopental, midazolam, and ketamine on human neutrophil functions. Anesth Analg 86:159–165
18. Kim SN, Son SC, Lee SM et al (2006) Midazolam inhibits proinflammatory mediators in the lipopolysaccharide-activated macrophage. Anesthesiology 105:105–110
19. Frohlich D, Rothe G, Schwall B et al (1996) Thiopentone and propofol, but not methohexitone nor midazolam, inhibit neutrophil oxidative responses to the bacterial peptide FMLP. Eur J Anaesthesiol 13:582–588
20. Jensen AG, Dahlgren C, Eintrei C (1993) Propofol decreases random and chemotactic stimulated locomotion of human neutrophils in vitro. Br J Anaesth 70:99–100
21. Mikawa K, Akamatsu H, Nishina K et al (1998) Propofol inhibits human neutrophil functions. Anesth Analg 87:695–700
22. Cleary TG, Pickering LK (1983) Mechanisms of intralipid effect on polymorphonuclear leukocytes. J Clin Lab Immunol 11:21–26
23. Pirttinkangas CO, Perttila J, Salo M (1993) Propofol emulsion reduces proliferative responses of lymphocytes from intensive care patients. Intensive Care Med 19:299–302
24. Hoff G, Bauer I, Larsen B, Bauer M (2001) Modulation of endotoxin-stimulated TNF-alpha gene expression by ketamine and propofol in cultured human whole blood. Anaesthesist 50:494–499
25. Al-Hashimi M, Scott WM, Thompson JP, Lambert DG (2013) Editor's choice: Opioids and immune modulation: more questions than answers. Br J Anaesth 111:80–88
26. Sacerdote P (2006) Opioids and the immune system. Palliat Med 20:s9–15
27. Hernandez M, Flores L, Bayer B (1993) Immunosuppression by morphine is mediated by central pathways. J Pharmacol Exp Ther 267:1336–1341
28. Hall DM, Suo JL, Weber RJ (1998) Opioid mediated effects on the immune system: sympathetic nervous system involvement. J Neuroimmunol 83:29–35
29. Bidlack JM (2000) Detection and function of opioid receptors on cells from the immune system. Clin Diagn Lab Immunol 7:719–723
30. Rittner HL, Brack A, Machelska H et al (2001) Opioid peptide-expressing leukocytes: identification, recruitment, and simultaneously increasing inhibition of inflammatory pain. Anesthesiology 95:500–508
31. Jacobs R, Karst M, Scheinichen D et al (1999) Effects of fentanyl on cellular immune functions in man. Int J Immunopharmacol 21:445–454
32. Sacerdote P, Gaspani L, Rossoni G et al (2001) Effect of the opioid remifentanil on cellular immune response in the rat. Int J Immunopharmacol 1:713–719
33. Eberhardt KE, Thimm BM, Spring A, Maskos WR (1992) Dose-dependent rate of nosocomial pulmonary infection in mechanically ventilated patients with brain oedema receiving barbiturates: a prospective case study. Infection 20:12–18
34. Chanimov M, Berman S, Weissgarten J et al (2000) Substances used for local and general anaesthesia in major surgery suppress proliferative responsiveness of normal rat peripheral blood mononuclear cells in culture. Eur J Anaesthes 17:248–255
35. Cavalcanti V, Santos CL, Samary CS et al (2014) Effects of short-term propofol and dexmedetomidine on pulmonary morphofunction and biological markers in experimental mild acute lung injury. Respir Physiol Neurobiol 203:45–50

36. Kang SH, Kim YS, Hong TH et al (2013) Effects of dexmedetomidine on inflammatory responses in patients undergoing laparoscopic cholecystectomy. Acta Anaesthesiol Scand 57:480–487
37. Li B, Li Y, Tian S et al (2015) Anti-inflammatory effects of perioperative dexmedetomidine administered as an adjunct to general anesthesia: a meta-analysis. Sci Rep 5:12342
38. Yoon-Mi L, Byeng CS, Kyung-Jin Y (2015) impact of volatile anesthetics on oxidative stress and inflammation. Biomed Res Int 2015:242709
39. Blum FE, Zuo Z (2013) Volatile anesthetics-induced neuroinflammatory and anti-inflammatory responses. Med Gas Res 3:16
40. Cassuto J, Sinclair R, Bonderovic M (2006) Anti-inflammatory properties of local anesthetics and their present and potential clinical implications. Acta Anaesthesiol Scand 50:265–282
41. Hahnenkamp K, Herroeder S, Hollmann MW (2004) Regional anaesthesia, local anaesthetics and the surgical stress response. Best Pract Res Clin Anaesthesiol 18:509–527
42. Toft P, Tønnesen E (2008) The systemic inflammatory response to anaesthesia and surgery. Curr Anaesth Crit Care 19:349–353
43. Homburger JA, Meiler SE (2006) Anesthesia drugs, immunity, and long-term outcome. Curr Opin Anaesthesiol 19:423–428
44. Vallejo R, Hord ED, Barna SA, Santiago-Palma J, Ahmed S (2003) Perioperative immunosuppression in cancer patients. J Environ Pathol Toxicol Oncol 22:139–146
45. Kelbel I, Weiss M (2001) Anesthetics and immune function. Curr Opin Anaesthesiol 14:685–691
46. Lassen HC, Henriksen E, Neukirch F, Kristensen HS (1956) Treatment of tetanus; severe bone-marrow depression after prolonged nitrous-oxide anaesthesia. Lancet 270:527–530
47. Fellows IW, Byrne AJ, Allison SP (1983) Adrenocortical suppression with etomidate. Lancet 2:54–55

Part XII
The Extremes of Age

Facing the Ongoing Challenge of the Febrile Young Infant

A. DePorre, P. L. Aronson, and R. McCulloh

Introduction

Fever in young infants (i. e., infants ≤ 90 days of life) is a frequent complaint encountered by health care providers, and medical decision-making regarding testing, disposition, and treatment of the febrile infant can be challenging. In the developed world, these otherwise well-appearing young infants are commonly evaluated by clinicians in the ambulatory and emergency department (ED) setting, and they pose a significant conundrum to clinicians for a variety of reasons.

Fever is often the only sign of illness in young infants, making it clinically difficult to differentiate infants with a benign self-limiting illness from those with a more serious illness that could progress to sepsis, permanent disability or death if left untreated. Because of this clinical uncertainty, many febrile young infants undergo invasive testing, are administered empiric antibiotics and are admitted to

A. DePorre
Department of Pediatrics, Division of Hospital Medicine, Children's Mercy Hospital
2401 Gillham Rd, Kansas City, MO 64108, USA
Department of Pediatrics, University of Missouri—Kansas City, University of Kansas Medical Center
Kansas City, MO 64108, USA

P. L. Aronson
Departments of Pediatrics and Emergency Medicine, Section of Pediatric Emergency Medicine, Yale School of Medicine
New Haven, CT 06511, USA

R. McCulloh (✉)
Department of Pediatrics, Division of Hospital Medicine, Children's Mercy Hospital
2401 Gillham Rd, Kansas City, MO 64108, USA
Department of Pediatrics, University of Missouri—Kansas City, University of Kansas Medical Center
Kansas City, MO 64108, USA
Division of Infectious Disease, Children's Mercy Hospital
Kansas City, MO 64108, USA
e-mail: rmcculloh@cmh.edu

J.-L. Vincent (ed.), *Annual Update in Intensive Care and Emergency Medicine 2017*,
DOI 10.1007/978-3-319-51908-1_33

the hospital. Currently there is no consensus regarding the optimal management and treatment strategy for the febrile young infant. While multiple criteria have been developed to stratify infants based on their risk for serious bacterial infections, the most commonly-used of these criteria are over 25 years old, and these criteria do not account for the changing incidence and epidemiology of invasive infections in young infants or for advances in medical technology for identifying bacteria and viruses responsible for severe infections. Finally, current treatment recommendations largely ignore the potential negative consequences of over-testing, including false-positive test results, excessive antibiotic use and the psychological and financial hardships to which patients' families may be subjected in the course of evaluating these at-risk infants.

In this chapter, we will highlight the historical context of febrile infant management, review important definitions and terminology, discuss the most clinically relevant viral and bacterial causes of fever in the young infant, describe current risk stratification tools guiding medical-decision making, and outline research and clinical practice improvement priorities for improving the management of the febrile young infant.

Historical Context

Since the mid-1970s, there have been numerous published recommendations for the suggested work-up and treatment of nontoxic young febrile infants. These recommendations have changed through the years as medical technology, antibiotic agents and maternal and neonatal healthcare have advanced, and as emerging information is shared. Many of the first recommendations were based on prior reports of occult bacteremia in children, which most often were caused by *Streptococcus pneumoniae*, *Hamophilus influenzae type b*, and *Neisseria meningitidis*, leading to invasive meningitis [1, 2]. Early reports focusing on infants in the first 1–3 months of life identified *Streptococcus agalactiae* (hereafter referred to as Group B Streptococci [GBS]) and enterobacteraceae, especially *Escherichia coli* and *Salmonella spp.*, as common causes of bacteremia and meningitis [3–5]. Due in part to these risks, in the 1970s and early 1980s it was generally recommended that all febrile infants have blood, urine and cerebrospinal fluid (CSF) cultures drawn, receive empiric antibiotics, and be admitted to the hospital pending culture results, though the exact age limit for when this strategy should generally be employed varied widely.

In the mid-1980s, reflecting healthcare overutilization and risks associated with previous recommendations, risk-stratification algorithms based on clinical and laboratory features were created that identified infants at lower risk for serious bacterial infection who could safely be monitored outside of the hospital and often without antibiotics [6]. The most commonly used criteria in the US that were developed during this time include the Boston, Milwaukee, Philadelphia, and Rochester criteria. These criteria, developed largely on single-site experiences with evaluating febrile infants at tertiary medical centers, were effective in identifying infants at relatively low risk for bacterial meningitis and bacteremia (negative predictive value

[NPV] 93–100%) [7–10]. These criteria form the basis for many local and professional society recommendations and clinical practice guidelines currently in use by healthcare providers [6, 11].

However, while these criteria demonstrate reasonably high reliability for identifying infants at low risk for serious bacterial infection, there are increasing limitations. First, these criteria were not designed to identify febrile young infants at high-risk for bacterial infection. Second, none of the risk-stratification systems reliably identified low-risk infants younger than 1 month of age. Additionally, none of the algorithms could account for subsequent technological advances for rapidly and reliably diagnosing viral infection in young infants, which can greatly affect the likelihood of an infant having a bacterial infection [12]. Given these limitations, it is unsurprising that contemporary practices in evaluating and managing young febrile infants vary widely in both the inpatient and outpatient settings [11, 13].

Definitions

Fever in young infants is defined as a rectally-obtained temperature ≥ 38 °C (100.4 F). Temperature taken by touch, in the axilla or the ear is less accurate, although studies have also shown that caregiver reports of fever correlated with rectal thermometer measurement in up to 79% of patients [14, 15]. Thus, it is recommended that infants solely with caregiver report of fever be taken as seriously as those with findings of fever at the clinical visit.

Common terms used in discussions focused on febrile young infants that warrant further definition include 'serious bacterial infection' and 'invasive bacterial infection'. The term serious bacterial infection classically includes bacterial urinary tract infection (UTI), bacteremia and bacterial meningitis. Occasionally, in cases where a known bacterial pathogen is identified as the cause, bacterial pneumonia, enteritis, skin and soft tissue infections and bone infections are included under the term serious bacterial infection [16].

More recently, the phrase invasive bacterial infection has been used to describe infants with bacterial meningitis or bacteremia, reflecting the generally good outcomes of infants diagnosed with UTI [17]. Some experts recommend the sole use of infection source (e.g., meningitis, bacteremia, UTI, etc.) to promote clarity in nomenclature.

Epidemiology of Infections in Febrile Infants

Viruses are thought to cause the majority of febrile illnesses in young infants, and identifying a viral infection is often associated with a lower risk of bacterial infection in these infants (Table 1). A comprehensive description of the exact epidemiology and incidence of bacterial causes of fever in the young infant is difficult. To date, no large-scale, multi-site estimates of bacterial infection prevalence have been conducted, with available reports relying on data obtained primarily from sin-

Table 1 Common viral illnesses presenting as fever in young infants and association with bacterial illness. Data from references [21, 24, 25, 45–48]

Virus	Recommended diagnostic test	Association with bacterial illness
Enterovirus (EV)	CSF EV PCR; EV serum PCR if EV sepsis is suspected	Low risk for concomitant bacterial meningitis and bacteremia. Decreased risk for UTI
Human parechovirus (HPeV)	CSF HPeV PCR	Insufficient data, but likely decreased risk of bacterial meningitis, bacteremia, and UTI
Respiratory syncytial virus (RSV)	Nasopharyngeal RSV Ag detection or RSV RT-PCR	Low risk for concomitant bacterial meningitis or bacteremia. Decreased risk for UTI
Influenza A/B	Nasopharyngeal Influenza A/B Ag detection or Influenza A/B RT-PCR	Low risk for concomitant bacterial infection
Human rhinovirus (hRV)	Nasopharyngeal rhinovirus PCR	Unknown. Due to prolonged viral shedding, unable to solely attribute febrile illness to rhinovirus
Adenovirus (ADV)	Nasopharyngeal adenovirus RT-PCR	Unknown. Due to prolonged viral shedding, unable to solely attribute febrile illness to adenovirus
Human parainfluenza virus (HPIV) 1,2,3,4	Nasopharyngeal HPIV 1,2,3,4 RT-PCR	Insufficient data, but likely low risk of concomitant bacterial infection
Rotavirus (ROTA)	Stool rotavirus Ag detection, stool rotavirus enzyme immunoassay or rotavirus PCR	Insufficient data, but likely low risk of concomitant bacterial infection
Herpes simplex virus (HSV) Types 1 and 2	CSF HSV PCR, viral culture or PCR of vesicles Surface cultures in neonates (mouth, nasopharynx, conjunctivae, perianal) Serum HSV PCR (if available)	Insufficient data, but likely low risk of concomitant bacterial infection
Human herpes virus-6 (HHV-6)	Plasma HHV-6 RT-PCR; HHV-6 serologic antibody titers	Insufficient data, but likely low risk of concomitant bacterial infection

PCR: polymerase chain reaction; *RT-PCR*: reverse-transcriptase polymerase chain reaction; *CSF*: cerebrospinal fluid; *UTI*: urinary tract infection

gle-site surveys over varying time periods. High-quality data on the prevalence of bacterial infections in different age groups is also lacking [1]. Overall, bacterial infections are identified in roughly 8–10% of febrile infants.

Viral Infections

Herpes simplex virus (HSV) is a rare but significant cause of morbidity and mortality among febrile infants, being identified in <0.3% of febrile infants, but with an associated mortality of >15%, a risk that is increased with delay in initiation of antiviral therapy [18, 19]. The majority of neonatal HSV disease is transmitted to the newborn by active maternal shedding of the virus during the peripartum period.

Infection most commonly occurs in the first month of life, and it is exceedingly rare in children older than 6–8 weeks of age. HSV infection can be categorized as limited to skin, eye, mouth (SEM disease); disseminated disease/sepsis; or meningoencephalitis (which can complicate both sepsis and SEM disease), and can be caused by either HSV-1 or HSV-2. Fever can be the only feature of HSV infection, although it may be lacking in up to 50% of infants ultimately diagnosed with HSV disease, and other clinical symptoms, including vesicular rash, seizures, ill or toxic appearance, irritability, lethargy, conjunctivitis, bulging fontanel and temperature instability, can aid in the diagnosis [20]. These clinical symptoms, along with laboratory findings, such as elevated liver function tests and CSF pleocytosis, are more commonly found in infants with HSV than without, and the presence of any of these signs and symptoms should prompt the consideration of HSV testing and empiric treatment with acyclovir.

Enterovirus is one of the most common causes of febrile illness in young infants and its incidence varies seasonally, with rates being highest in the summer and fall. During these times, enterovirus infection is found in 40–50% of admitted febrile infants [21]. Because enterovirus-positive infants have a low rate of concomitant bacterial infections, management of enterovirus-positive infants often consists of supportive care alone. A rare manifestation of enterovirus infection in neonates includes severe viral sepsis, which is generally associated with maternal acute infection with enterovirus near the time of delivery. Treatment for enterovirus sepsis is also limited to supportive care with the possible addition of intravenous immune globulin, as no FDA-approved or compassionate-use antiviral therapy is currently available. Testing for enterovirus is encouraged, especially during summer and fall seasons, as a confirmed diagnosis allows clinicians to safely decrease hospital length of stay and antibiotic exposure for otherwise well-appearing febrile infants [22].

Human Parechovirus (HPeV) is a relatively recently described cause of viral meningitis and encephalitis among febrile infants. Similar to enterovirus, HPeV is a picornavirus with seasonal variation, and treatment consists largely of supportive care. Compared to enterovirus-positive infants, HPeV-positive infants typically appear more acutely ill and more often require ICU care [23]. While the rates of concomitant bacterial infections are thought to be low (similar to those of enterovirus), suggesting that HPeV-infants could be monitored off antibiotics, further data are needed to confirm this [23].

Respiratory viruses, particularly respiratory syncytial virus (RSV), influenza viruses A and B, rotavirus, and rhinovirus are also commonly identified in the febrile infant (Table 1). With the exception of rotavirus, these viruses often cause respiratory symptoms, most commonly manifested as bronchiolitis. Because well-appearing febrile RSV-positive infants are at low risk for bacterial meningitis and bacteremia, but still have a notable risk for bacterial UTI [24], management and testing of these infants should include urinalysis and urine culture, and in most well-appearing infants without evidence of UTI, antibiotics and routine lumbar punctures can be safely delayed or avoided. Similarly, the risk of bacterial infection among infants with influenza or rotavirus is low [25]. The detection of rhinovirus in the otherwise well-appearing febrile infant does not necessarily decrease an infant's risk for concomitant bacterial infection because, due to its long shedding period, detection of the virus may not correlate with acute viral illness [26].

Other viruses and their potential association with the risk of bacterial infection in febrile young infants are detailed in Table 1.

Bacterial Infections

A description of the exact epidemiology and incidence of bacterial causes of fever in the young infant is difficult, as recent large datasets are lacking. However, meta-analyses and data from single-center or regional data in the United States suggest that while the majority of bacterial infections used to be due to GBS, and *Listeria* was of relatively greater concern, *E. coli* and other Gram-negative bacteria now account for the majority of infections, and *Listeria monocytogenes* is a rarely encountered pathogen [27, 28].

In addition to *E. coli*, other Gram-negative infections of importance include *Klebsiella pneumoniae, Citrobacter spp., Enterobacter spp., Salmonella spp.* and *Serratia marcescens*. About 20% of serious bacterial infections are thought to be due to Gram-positive bacteria [15]. The most commonly-isolated Gram-positive organisms include GBS, *Staphylococcus aureus* and *Enterococcus spp. L. monocytogenes* is now considered an extremely rare cause of serious bacterial infection in the United States [27–29].

UTIs are the most common cause of serious bacterial infection, with *E. coli* causing the majority of infections. It is thought that UTIs occur in roughly 9% of all febrile infants who undergo medical evaluation, making up roughly 85% of all serious bacterial infection in this population [16, 24]. Despite the relatively high incidence of UTI among febrile infants, consensus regarding the disposition and treatment duration of febrile young infants with UTI is lacking. The perceived risk of developing concomitant bacteremia or meningitis and/or long-standing renal injury drives common practice, which frequently includes hospital admission, invasive CSF testing, and often a 2-week course of parenteral antibiotics.

It is now questioned whether these infants should be treated less conservatively, as the risk of bacterial meningitis, shock, or death is thought to be extremely low in otherwise well-appearing infants [17]. While the risk of bacteremia secondary to UTI remains substantial, it is unlikely to be associated with adverse effects, and recent studies on well-appearing infants with bacteremia secondary to UTI show similar clinical outcomes between those treated with a prolonged course of parenteral antibiotics vs. those treated with shorter courses of parenteral antibiotics [17, 30, 31].

Bacteremia and bacterial meningitis in febrile infants are thought to occur at an incidence of roughly 1.8–2% and 0.5–0.7%, respectively [13, 24]. Unlike UTI, bacterial meningitis is associated with a 5% mortality risk and long-term sequelae, such as hearing loss, seizures, motor problems, hydrocephalus, and cognitive and behavioral problems, underscoring the need for early detection and treatment of bacteremia (which may lead to bacterial meningitis) and bacterial meningitis [32].

Tools for Risk Stratification

A combination of age, clinical appearance and laboratory values is commonly used to identify young febrile infants at risk for a serious bacterial or viral infection.

The Rochester, Philadelphia, Milwaukee and Boston criteria all use the above combination to identify infants at low risk for serious bacterial infection. While the laboratory tests used, interpretation of test results, empirical antibiotic use, and age at which criteria should be applied, vary across these tools, there are many similarities among them (Table 2). Regardless of laboratory values, febrile infants who are ill-appearing or <28 days old are identified as at higher risk for serious bacterial infection. It is generally recommended that young febrile infants be evaluated with a complete blood count with differential, urinalysis, blood, and urine culture. Blood and urine tests are often obtained simultaneously, and obtaining CSF depends on which strategy is used. Chest radiographs are not routinely recommended.

Although useful in predicting illness severity in older infants and children, the Yale Observational Score, a scoring system that uses clinical signs and symptoms to determine the risk of serious bacterial or viral illness, is not an accurate risk-stratification tool among young febrile infants <8 weeks of age [33].

A sequential approach for identifying febrile young infants at low risk for invasive bacterial infection has been proposed. Highlighting UTI as the most common bacterial infection in young febrile infants, this approach recommends evaluating age, clinical appearance and urinalysis results prior to obtaining blood samples [34]. This step-by-step approach has been prospectively validated and has a high sensitivity (92%) and NPV (99.3%) [36].

There has been much debate about the utility of certain biomechanical markers as part of a febrile infant evaluation. While an abnormal white blood cell (WBC) count in a febrile young infant is associated with serious bacterial infection, it is not a specific marker for serious bacterial infection (positive predictive value of 30–43.8% for WBC <5,000 or >15,000/mm^3) [12].

Compared to an abnormal WBC, elevated C-reactive protein (CRP) and procalcitonin (PCT) values are associated with serious bacterial infection with a greater sensitivity and specificity, with PCT being more sensitive than CRP for diagnosis of invasive bacterial infection [34, 36]. CRP can often be elevated in viral infections and does not rise as acutely as PCT levels do, which can cause both false positive and negative results, respectively. While PCT use has been widely investigated in the adult sepsis literature, its use in febrile young infants has been mostly limited to European studies. Using PCT is limited in many non-European countries, as it is not widely available, is not rapidly performed and is associated with high laboratory costs [34, 36]. Combining PCT, CRP and presence of leukocyte esterase or nitrites on urinalysis into a single "lab score" has better specificity to predict the presence of serious bacterial infection than do WBC, CRP or PCT alone, but has a low sen-

Table 2 Clinical and laboratory findings of common low-risk criteria. Adapted from [12]

	Boston	Milwaukee	Philadelphia	Rochester
Age range	28–89 days	28–56 days	29–60 days	$\leq$ 60 days
History	No immunizations or antimicrobials in prior 48 h	Not defined	Not defined	Term infant; no prior antibiotics; no underlying disease; no hospitalization longer than mother
Physical exam	Well appearing; no signs of focal infection	Well appearing; no signs of focal infection	Well appearing; no signs of focal infection	Well appearing; no signs of focal infection
Laboratory parameters	CSF < 10 WBC/mm^3 WBC < 20,000 mm^3 UA < 10 WBC/hpf CXR without infiltrate (if obtained)	CSF < 10/mm^3 WBC < 15,000/mm^3 UA < 5–10 WBC/hpf; UA no bacteria, negative leukocyte esterase, negative nitrites CXR without infiltrate	CSF < 8 WBC/mm^3 WBC < 15,000/mm^3 UA < 10 WBC/hpf CXR without infiltrate (if obtained)	WBC > 5,000 and < 15,000/mm^3 ABC < 1,500/mm^3 UA $\leq$ 10 WBC/hpf CXR without infiltrate (if obtained) Stool: WBC $\leq$ 5/hpf smear (if indicated)
Management strategies for high risk	Hospitalize, empiric antibiotics	Not defined	Hospitalize, empiric antibiotics	Hospitalize, empiric antibiotics
Management strategy for low risk	Home/outpatient ok Empiric antibiotics, outpatient follow up required	Home/outpatient ok i.m. ceftriaxone 50 mg/kg followed by outpatient follow up within 24 h Must have reliable caretaker	Home/outpatient ok No antibiotics, but outpatient follow up is required	Home/outpatient ok No antibiotics, but outpatient follow up is required

CXR: chest X-ray; *UA*: urinalysis; *CSF*: cerebrospinal fluid; *WBC*: white blood cells; *ABC*: absolute band count; *hpf*: high power field; *i.m.*: intramuscular sitivity [37]. New research has also identified that an infant produces a unique host response, called an RNA-biosignature, secondary to bacterial infection, which can be detected by microarray analysis. Data on the role of RNA-biosignatures in the management of the febrile young infant are emerging and future studies are needed to evaluate their utility in the clinical setting [38].

Emerging evidence on 1) the changing epidemiology and incidence of bacterial infections; 2) patient outcomes with certain bacterial infections, such as UTIs; 3) the low risk of concomitant bacterial infections among infants with viral illnesses; 4) risk of serious illness with viral illnesses such as enterovirus and HSV; and 5) the need for judicious testing that limits the negative consequences of febrile infant evaluations is reshaping how infants are risk-stratified.

Many health care centers and institutions have created site-specific practice guidelines for the management of the febrile young infant, some of which advocate for more judicious testing and risk-stratify febrile infants based on viral status. These guidelines have been associated with good outcomes, including decreased hospital costs, hospital lengths of stay, and antibiotic exposure without any increase in adverse events [39]. However, guidelines vary widely across institutions, and not all guidelines advocate for more judicious testing and antibiotic use, which can affect health care costs and contributes to the observed variation in practice [11].

Therapeutic Options

For those infants at low risk of serious infection, outpatient management with close monitoring and primary care follow-up is recommended. Antibiotic administration is dependent on which strategy is used, but, in general, antimicrobials should not be given to well-appearing febrile infants until after blood, urine and CSF cultures are obtained.

High-risk infants require hospitalization for empiric intravenous antimicrobials pending bacterial and viral testing results. Hospital length of stay depends on culture and viral testing results. While many clinicians observe infants on empiric antibiotics until all bacterial cultures are negative for 36–48 h, this practice varies widely and is rapidly changing. New evidence has suggested that, due to advances in automated culture detection, an observation period pending negative bacterial culture results at 24–36 h is often appropriate and can reduce antibiotic exposure, hospital length of stay, and healthcare costs without an increase in missed bacterial infections [39, 40]. In addition, due to the low risk of concomitant bacterial infections, in otherwise well-appearing enterovirus-positive infants, short observation periods of no more than 24 h are generally recommended [39]. Other potential adjustments to management based on virological test results and PCT results are detailed in Table 3.

Hospital admission can often come at a time when infant-family bonding is just beginning, and therefore should focus on maximizing family bonding by encouraging breast feeding, skin-to-skin contact, and maintaining previous routines, while minimizing unnecessary tests and interventions.

Table 3 Diagnostic tests and their utility in the well-appearing febrile young infant. Data from references [22, 25, 49, 50]

Test	Indications	Potential role in management
RSV testing	Infants with respiratory symptoms	If positive, may safely avoid LPs, antibiotic exposure, and hospitalizations
EV testing	Infants undergoing LP and CSF studies	If positive, may consider discontinuing antibiotics, discharge home if bacterial cultures negative at 24–36 h
Influenza testing	Infants with respiratory symptoms, especially during high regional prevalence	If positive, may consider discontinuing antibiotics, discharge home if bacterial cultures negative at 24–36 h
Procalcitonin	Otherwise low-risk infants with negative virological testing	If normal/minimal elevation: may consider initial inpatient observation off antibiotics, avoidance of LP, or outpatient management

LP: lumbar puncture; *CSF*: cerebrospinal fluid; *RSV*: respiratory syncytial virus; *EV*: enterovirus

Empiric antibiotic choices should cross the blood brain barrier and target the most common pathogens, such as *E. coli* and GBS. In a large regional study, almost 80% of infants with meningitis were infected with ampicillin-resistant organisms, highlighting the need for identification of and treatment according to regional and institution-specific antibiotic resistance patterns [16]. Medication side-effects are also a factor when determining appropriate antibiotic choices. For example, in infants <28 days old who are already at increased risk for kernicterus, ceftriaxone is generally avoided as it can cause further increases in serum bilirubin levels.

Commonly-used antibiotic regimens for infants <28 days old include ampicillin and either an aminoglycoside, such as gentamicin, or a third-generation cephalosporin, such as cefotaxime. For infants >28 days of age, a third-generation cephalosporin, such as ceftriaxone, is often used as monotherapy. For those infants at risk of HSV infection, acyclovir should be empirically administered pending HSV test results.

Unintended Consequences of Testing/Treatment

The risk of delayed care of a febrile young infant with a serious infection drives invasive testing, hospitalization and antibiotic use, but in some cases these interventions are unnecessary and can often have unintended negative consequences, such as vulnerable child syndrome, family stress, prolonged hospital stay, increased hospital costs, and iatrogenic complications.

Vulnerable child syndrome is a well-described syndrome in which a caregiver's perception of their child as being vulnerable leads to a dysfunctional parent-child relationship. Clinical features of vulnerable child syndrome in the caregiver include excessive separation anxiety, over-protective behavior, difficulties with discipline, and excessive use of the medical system; children can display impaired sleeping habits, difficulties in school, exaggerated separation anxiety, and hypochondria [41, 42]. Children hospitalized early in life, such as those born premature, those with congenital malformations, or those with a suspected serious illness (which one could argue includes suspected meningitis) have been shown to be more prone to vulnerable child syndrome [42].

Parents of hospitalized infants who were interviewed in an effort to better characterize the stress and difficulties families of febrile infants face have previously described believing that their infant had a weak immune system and could rapidly deteriorate or die. Parents have also reported feeling an overwhelming sense of responsibility, a lack of control, experiencing disruption of breast-feeding and increased financial stress [43].

Potentially unnecessary or avoidable testing of febrile infants can cause negative consequences by prolonging hospitalizations and increasing healthcare-related costs. Due to the development of a reliable rapid HSV polymerase chain reaction (PCR) test, many infants at low risk of HSV infection (i. e., well-appearing infants without any historical risks, signs, or symptoms of HSV) are tested and given empiric acyclovir pending PCR results. This testing and empiric treatment of all febrile infants may increase hospital length of stay, and healthcare costs without conferring any additional benefits [44].

Iatrogenic harm caused by the management and treatment of febrile infants has not been well studied. Common sources of iatrogenic harm likely include antimicrobial pre-treated CSF cultures and traumatic lumbar punctures [45], which may cause unnecessary antibiotic exposure; radiation exposure from x-rays or other imaging; and phlebitis or venous injury during blood draws or infusions. Due to the relatively low incidence of bacterial infections among febrile infants, bacterial cultures have a low positive predictive value, and can often result in false-positive culture results. False-positive test results likely lead to even further caregiver stress, invasive testing, antibiotic exposure, hospital days and healthcare costs.

Conclusion/Future Priorities

Caring for the febrile young infant is often challenging, as the fear of not properly treating a serious illness can often lead to unnecessary testing, antibiotics and hospitalization. To better guide management descisions, future research priorities should focus on using large multi-regional data to identify the incidence and epidemiology of bacterial infections, and further attempts should be made to identify infants at high-risk of invasive bacterial and HSV infection. Viral testing should be incorporated into febrile infant evaluations, as identification of a virus may decrease antibiotic exposure, invasive testing and hospitalization. Continued efforts should be made towards the study of novel diagnostic tools such as RNA biosignatures. Finally, there is a large gap in our understanding of the consquences of current febrile infant managment methods, and future efforts should focus on better delineating the risks and unintended consequences of testing, antibiotic administration and hospilization of young febrile infants.

References

1. Teele DW, Pelton SI, Grant MJA et al (1975) Bacteremia in febrile children under 2 years of age: Results of cultures of 600 consecutive febrile children seen in a walk-in clinic. J Pediatr 87:227–230
2. Long SS (1984) Approach to the febrile patient with no obvious focus of infection. Pediatr Rev 5:305–315
3. Crain EF, Shelov SP (1982) Febrile infants: Predictors of bacteremia. J Pediatr 101:686–689
4. Crain EF, Gershel JC (1988) Which febrile infants younger than two weeks of age are likely to have sepsis? A pilot study. Infect Dis J 7:561–564
5. Roberts KB, Borzy MS (1977) Fever in the first eight weeks of life. Johns Hopkins Med J 141:9–13
6. Baraff LJ (2000) Management of fever without source in infants and children. Ann Emerg Med 36:602–614
7. Baker DM, Bell LM, Avner JR (1993) Outpatient management without antibiotics of fever in selected infants. N Engl J Med 329:1437–1441
8. Bonadio WA, Hagen E, Rucka J, Shallow K, Stommel P, Smith D (1993) Efficacy of a protocol to distinguish risk of serious bacterial infection in the outpatient evaluation of febrile young infants. Clin Pediatr 32:401–404
9. McCarthy PL, Sharpe MR, Spiesel SZ et al (1982) Observation scales to identify serious illness in febrile children. Pediatrics 70:802–809
10. Dagan R, Powell KR, Hall CB, Menegus MA (1985) Identification of infants unlikely to have serious bacterial infection although hospitalized for suspected sepsis. J Pediatr 107:855–860
11. Aronson PL, Thurm C, Williams DJ et al (2015) Association of clinical practice guidelines with emergency department management of febrile infants ≤56 days of age. J Hosp Med 10:358–365
12. Hui C, Neto G, Tsertsvadze A et al (2012) Diagnosis and Management of Febrile Infants (0–3 Months). Evidence Report/Technology Assessments, No. 205. AHRQ Publication No. 12-E004-EF. http://www.ahrq.gov/research/findings/evidence-based-reports/er205-abstract.html#Report. Accessed Nov 20, 2016
13. Pantell RH, Newman TB, Bernzweig J et al (2004) Management and outcomes of care of fever in early infancy. JAMA 291:1203–1212
14. Callanan D (2003) Detecting fever in young infants: reliability of perceived, pacifier, and temporal artery temperatures in infants younger than 3 months of age. Pediatr Emerg Care 19:240–243
15. Hooker EA, Smith SW, Miles T, King L (1996) Subjective assessment of fever by parents: comparison with measurement by noncontact tympanic thermometer and calibrated rectal glass mercury thermometer. Ann Emerg Med 28:313–317
16. Byington CL, Rittichier KK, Bassett KE et al (2003) Serious bacterial infections in febrile infants younger than 90 days of age: the importance of ampicillin-resistant pathogens. Pediatrics 111:964–968
17. Schnadower D, Kuppermann N, Macias CG et al (2010) Febrile infants with urinary tract infections at very low risk for adverse events and bacteremia. Pediatrics 126:1074–1083
18. Caviness AC, Demmler GJ, Almendarez Y, Selwyn BJ (2008) The prevalence of neonatal herpes simplex virus infection compared with serious bacterial illness in hospitalized neonates. J Pediatr 153:164–169
19. Shah SS, Aronson PL, Mohamad Z, Lorch SA (2011) Delayed acyclovir therapy and death among neonates with herpes simplex virus infection. Pediatrics 128:1153–1160

20. Kimberlin DW (2004) Neonatal herpes simplex infection. Clin Microbiol Rev 17:1–13
21. Rittichier KR, Bryan PA, Bassett KE et al (2005) Diagnosis and outcomes of enterovirus infections in young infants. Pediatr Infect Dis J 24:546–550
22. King RL, Lorch SA, Cohen DM, Hodinka RL, Cohn KA, Shah SS (2007) Routine cerebrospinal fluid enterovirus polymerase chain reaction testing reduces hospitalization and antibiotic use for infants 90 days of age or younger. Pediatrics 120:489–496
23. Sharp J, Harrison CJ, Puckett K et al (2013) Characteristics of young infants in whom human parechovirus, enterovirus or neither were detected in cerebrospinal fluid during sepsis evaluations. Pediatr Infect Dis J 32:213–216
24. Levine DA, Platt SL, Dayan PS et al (2004) Risk of serious bacterial infection in young febrile infants with respiratory syncytial virus infections. Pediatrics 113:1728–1734
25. Bender JM, Ampofo K, Gesteland P et al (2010) Influenza virus infection in infants less than three months of age. Pediatr Infect Dis J 29:6–9
26. Loeffelholz MJ, Trujillo R, Pyles RB et al (2014) Duration of rhinovirus shedding in the upper respiratory tract in the first year of life. Pediatrics 134:1144–1150
27. Biondi EA, Evans R, Mischler R et al (2013) Epidemiology of bacteremia in febrile infants in the United States. Pediatrics 132:990–996
28. Leazer R, Perkins AM, Shomaker K, Fine B (2016) A meta-analysis of the rates of Listeria monocytogenes and Enterococcus in febrile infants. Hosp Pediatr 6(4):187–195
29. Greenhow TL, Hung YY, Herz A, Losada E, Pantell RH (2014) The changing epidemiology of serious bacterial infections in young infants. Pediatr Infect Dis J 33:595–599
30. Schroeder AR, Shen MW, Biondi EA et al (2016) Bacteraemic urinary tract infection: management and outcomes in young infants. Arch Dis Child 101:125–130
31. Roman HK, Chang PW, Schroeder AR (2015) Diagnosis and management of bacteremic urinary tract infection in infants. Hosp Pediatr 5:1–8
32. de Jonge RC, van Furth AM, Wassenaar M, Gemke RJ, Terwee CB (2010) Predicting sequelae and death after bacterial meningitis in childhood: a systematic review of prognostic studies. BMC Infect Dis 10:232
33. Baker MD, Avner JR, Bell LM (1990) Failure of infant observation scales in detecting serious illness in febrile, 4- to 8-week-old infants. Pediatrics 85:1040–1043
34. Mintegi S, Bressan S, Gomez B et al (2014) Accuracy of a sequential approach to identify young febrile infants at low risk for invasive bacterial infection. Emerg Med J 31:e19–24
35. Gomez B, Mintegi S, Bressan S et al (2016) Validation of the step-by-step approach in the management of young febrile infants. Pediatrics 138:e20154381
36. Jhaveri R, Byington CL, Klein JO, Shapiro ED (2011) Management of the non-toxic-appearing acutely febrile child: a 21st century approach. J Pediatr 159:181–185
37. Bressan S, Gomez B, Minteg S et al (2012) Diagnostic performance of the lab-score in predicting severe and invasive bacterial infections in well-appearing young febrile infants. Pediatr Infect Dis J 31:1239–1244
38. Mahajan P, Kuppermann N, Mejias A et al (2016) Association of RNA biosignatures with bacterial infections in febrile infants aged 60 days or younger. JAMA 316:846–857
39. Byington CL, Reynolds CC, Korgenski K et al (2012) Costs and infant outcomes after implementation of a care process model for febrile infants. Pediatrics 130:e16–24
40. Vamsi SR, Bhat RY, Lewis LE, Vandana KE (2014) Time to positivity of blood cultures in neonates. Pediatr Infect Dis J 33:212–214
41. Kokotos F (2009) The vulnerable child syndrome. Pediatr Rev 30:193–194
42. Rautaya P, Lehtonen L, Helenius H, Sillanpää M (2003) Effect of newborn hospitalization on family and child behavior a 12-year follow-up study. Pediatrics 111:277–283
43. De S, Tong A, Isaacs D, Craig JC (2014) Parental perspectives on evaluation and management of fever in young infants: an interview study. Arch Dis Child 99:717–723
44. Shah SS, Volk J, Mohamad Z, Hodinka RL, Zorc JJ (2010) Herpes simplex virus testing and hospital length of stay in neonates and young infants. J Pediatr 156:738–743

45. Pingree EW, Kimia AA, Nigrovic LE (2015) The effect of traumatic lumbar puncture on hospitalization rate for febrile infants 28 to 60 days of age. Acad Emerg Med 22:240–243
46. Byington CL, Enriquez FR, Hoff C et al (2004) Serious bacterial infections in febrile infants 1 to 90 days old with and without viral infections. Pediatrics 113:1662–1666
47. Mintegi S, Garcia-Garcia JJ, Benito J et al (2009) Rapid influenza test in young febrile infants for the identification of low-risk patients. Pediatr Infect Dis J 28:1026–1028
48. Messacar K, Breazeale G, Wei Q, Robinson CC, Dominguez SR (2015) Epidemiology and clinical characteristics of infants with human parechovirus or human herpes virus-6 detected in cerebrospinal fluid tested for enterovirus or herpes simplex virus. J Med Virol 87:829–835
49. Byington CL, Castillo H, Gerber K et al (2002) The effect of rapid respiratory viral diagnostic testing on antibiotic use in a children's hospital. Arch Pediatr Adolesc Med 156:1230–1234
50. Milcent K, Faesch S, Gras-Le Guen C et al (2016) Use of procalcitonin assays to predict serious bacterial infection in young febrile infants. JAMA Pediatr 170:62–69

Post-Discharge Morbidity and Mortality in Children with Sepsis

O. C. Nwankwor, M. O. Wiens, and N. Kissoon

Introduction

Pediatric sepsis is a major contributor to childhood morbidity and mortality, accounting for about 23% of deaths in pediatric intensive care units (PICUs) [1] and about 30% of in-hospital morbidity. In addition, one in every five survivors exhibits a new functional disability. The Global Burden of Disease puts deaths from infectious diseases, and hence mostly sepsis, as the number one killer in children under 5 years of age. Although there are no systematic data from low and middle income countries, this high burden of mortality disproportionality plagues these countries. However, deaths are not only due to in-hospital demise because many children succumb without access to medical care or after hospital discharge.

For example, a systematic review of 13 studies done in low and middle income countries showed a consistent trend of post-discharge mortality similar to, and in some cases exceeding, in-hospital mortality [2]. Post-discharge mortality was most common in the first weeks to months following discharge and in children who were young, malnourished, had been previously admitted, were infected with human immunodeficiency virus (HIV) or had pneumonia. These observations suggest opportunities for early and inexpensive interventions to decrease the burden of morbidity and mortality in these contexts. In resource-rich settings, such as the United States, post-discharge mortality and morbidity pose similar, although less

O. C. Nwankwor
Division of Pediatric Critical Care Medicine, Department of Pediatrics, Regional Children's Hospital at Cooper University Hospital
Camden, NJ, USA
Division of Critical Care Medicine, Department of Pediatrics, Alfred 1. DuPont Hospital for Children
Wilmington, DE, USA

M. O. Wiens · N. Kissoon (✉)
Child and Family Research Institute, BC Children's Hospital & University of British Columbia
4480 Oak Street, Vancouver, BC V6H 3V4, Canada
e-mail: nkissoon@cw.bc.ca

J.-L. Vincent (ed.), *Annual Update in Intensive Care and Emergency Medicine 2017*,
DOI 10.1007/978-3-319-51908-1_34

burdensome concerns, because in most cases follow-up of children can be assured. In the US, the long-term post-discharge mortality rate approximates the mortality rate during in-patient admission among children with severe sepsis, and almost half of the survivors are readmitted within a median of 3 months [3]. Most children in the US are less than one year of age, have neurologic or hematologic organ dysfunction, blood stream or cardiovascular infections and comorbidities. Thus, there are opportunities for improving outcomes, even in resource-rich areas.

Aside from the concerns of mortality, morbidity is also of significant concern. Globally, as many as 39% of children who survived severe sepsis experienced some degree of deterioration of function at 28 days [4]. In low and middle income countries, because of the high burden of mortality, and the social and economic context of these settings, morbidity has taken a back seat and its burden has been largely ignored although it is likely to be higher and include a significant contribution from malnutrition. These observations present unique opportunities for the development and validation of outcome measures, such as health-related quality of life and functional status measures to better understand and develop interventions for post-discharge morbidity in these complex settings [2, 5].

Decreasing sepsis-associated morbidity and mortality relies on early recognition, aggressive treatment and context specific guidelines and protocols for follow-up care beyond hospital admission. Early recognition of sepsis relies on a useful definition to identify at-risk children.

Early Recognition

The systemic inflammatory response syndrome (SIRS) criteria, used to define sepsis by the International Consensus Conference [6], were intended to be used for research purposes and have not been very useful to clinicians in the early recognition of sepsis globally. In resource-rich areas, SIRS has not proven practical primarily because of its high sensitivity and low specificity. In low and middle income countries, the SIRS-based sepsis definition is not only poorly specific, it is also difficult to apply since it relies on laboratory parameters such as leukocyte count, not routinely available in all settings (Table 1). A recent study from Uganda found that nearly all children who were admitted with an infection were captured by the SIRS criteria, suggesting that its measure does little to further identify at-risk children [7].

Early Aggressive Treatment

Once recognized, aggressive treatment has been shown to improve outcomes in all settings. In resource rich settings, adherence to international guidelines has made great inroads in decreasing mortality [8–10]. However, a myriad of reports has shown that guidelines need to be context specific and the international guidelines cannot be adopted in many areas of the world due to lack of resources. This has

Table 1 Definition of sepsis based on context. Adapted from references [7] and [11]

	Sepsis definition by International Consensus (SIRS criteria)	Suggested sepsis definition in resource-limited settings
	Confirmed or highly suspected presence of infection caused by a pathogen plus any 2 of the following, one of which must be abnormal temperature or leukocyte count	Confirmed or highly suspected presence of infection caused by a pathogen plus any 2 of the following, one of which must be abnormal temperature
Temperature	< 36 °C or > 38.5 °C (core temp)	< 36 °C or > 38.5 °C (axillary or oral)
Heart rate (beats/min) – bradycardia or tachycardia	0–1 yr: < 90 – > 180 2–5 yrs: > 140	0–1 yr: < 90 – > 180 2–5 yrs: > 140
Respiratory rate (breaths/min) – tachypnea	0–1 yr: > 34 2–5 yrs: > 22	0–1 yr: > 34 2–5 yrs: > 22
White cell count (counts × 10^3/mm^3) – leukocytosis or leukopenia	0–1 yr: < 5 – > 17.5 2–5 yrs: < 6 – > 15.5	– Not included – Not readily available – Presence of malaise/ill-looking

SIRS: systemic inflammatory response syndrome

prompted the development of guidelines for a variety of international settings to improve the treatment of pediatric sepsis [11].

Follow-up Care Post Discharge

Common to all guidelines from resource rich to resource-poor settings is the fact that none has a robust approach to post-discharge care. For example, the ubiquitous Integrated Management of Childhood Illness (IMCI) guidelines, which form the foundation of the treatment of severe infections in many low and middle income countries, do not address the vulnerable post-discharge period. The same can be said for the Surviving Sepsis Campaign in North America and Europe. A lack of recognition that post-discharge morbidity and mortality represent a high burden in all settings, and a paucity of research to identify interventions to reduce this burden, has precluded any incorporation of post-discharge interventions in current guidelines.

The newly adapted sustainable development goals of the United Nations has set specific targets to reduce preventable neonatal and under-5 deaths [12]; targets that will be beyond the reach of most regions of the world unless the issues of post-discharge mortality can be addressed. Improvement in post-discharge outcomes will rely on research in the epidemiology of post-discharge morbidity and mortality as well as efforts to improve outcomes through a variety of means, including risk prediction, improved discharge planning, education, pharmacotherapeutic interventions, and addressing a variety of related issues, such as poverty and infrastructure challenges.

The aim of this chapter is to draw the attention of policy makers and care providers to this neglected but very important preventable contributor to child morbidity and mortality. In doing so we embrace a holistic approach that builds on the protocols, guidelines and bundles in sepsis management so as to direct appropriate and adequate resources towards care during the vulnerable period after a child is discharged from the hospital.

Issues Relating to Post-discharge Mortality

Infectious diseases including pneumonia, diarrhea and malaria remain a leading cause of under-5 mortality [13]. The final common pathway leading to death for most infectious diseases, including these, is sepsis [14]. While issues surrounding the epidemiology of post-discharge mortality are complex, there are several potential factors that may be causally related to its high burden.

Limited Resources in Poorly Resilient Health Systems

The IMCI, an initiative of the World Health Organization (WHO), has been widely adopted in low and middle income countries settings, and has made inroads in reducing in-patient mortality. However, this approach leaves no direct measure to reduce post-discharge mortality. To further improve outcomes from sepsis, all children should be afforded post-discharge follow-up, but this is often not practical because of the inordinate demand on limited resources. The identification of high-risk children can facilitate follow-up of the most vulnerable children while at the same time ensuring the responsible use of resources [15, 16]. However, there are limited data on post-discharge mortality in most resource limited settings [17, 18]. This is because of several factors, including that many children die in the community and the limited resources reduce the ability to ensure follow-up of all children with sepsis post-discharge. This was highlighted during the Ebola outbreak in western Africa with collapse of the most basic health systems [19], where mortality was high in low and middle income countries, but non-existent in those afflicted who had access to contemporary care. In non-resilient systems, decreasing morbidity and mortality will rely on innovative approaches to identify children who are at high risk and develop interventions that are sustainable in the clinical context.

Poor Illness Recognition and Care Seeking Behavior

To reduce child morbidity and mortality in the under-5 age group, caregivers should be able to easily recognize the symptoms of the commonest infectious diseases, and be able to seek care promptly. Recent evidence suggests that in low and middle income countries, the ability of caregivers to recognize diseases such as diarrhea, malaria or pneumonia, to recognize danger signs, and to seek appropriate health care, is very low [20]. These issues appear to be more prominent in rural areas, where the use of traditional care practices is also high. Other factors influencing appropriate care-seeking include severity of illness, socioeconomic status, cost of care and in some regions the sex of the child with boys more likely to receive care.

Poverty, Lack of Money and Transport

Of the 19.2 million episodes of severe acute lower respiratory infections in the under-5 age group, 38% of the cases did not reach the hospital [21]. Furthermore, 81% of the cases that did not get to the hospital died compared to 19% of those that were admitted to the hospital. Even when access and low health-seeking behavior are not present, there exists a high referral burden on hospitals, stretching their personnel, medication and facility supplies. In resource-limited settings, the WHO recommendation of home treatment for severe pneumonia with oral antibiotics has been shown to be effective in Asia [22]. To reduce poverty and all its associated health inequities, education of girls has been shown to be a strong predictor for improved health among infants and children [23]. Government and policy makers of low and middle incomes countries should ensure that every girl receives some level of formal education.

Difficulty in Accessing Timely Care

In many parts of the world, health systems for critically ill children are fragmented, with children often subject to many delays prior to definitive care. In addition, suboptimal care and iatrogenic-induced adverse events are often commonplace in such settings. For example, in South Africa, caregivers experience significant difficulty in accessing healthcare for their critically ill children. EMS delays result in parents either driving their own vehicles or using public transport to bring their children to the hospital, regardless of severity of illness [24]. At many hospitals, there are no clear directions to locate the trauma or emergency area. In many cases, long waiting times and the use of non-medical staff to make determinations on how sick the children are limits timely access to care. Caregivers can also experience difficulties due to language barriers.

Lack of Faith in Health Systems

In Uganda, some caregivers refused to go back to the hospital when their children became sick again after they had been discharged because they thought that there was no improvement from their earlier visits and no need to go back. To address this issue, caregiver education given by community health workers who are drawn from within the community should be encouraged. Trusted community health workers

(CHWs) contribute to improving health outcomes among mothers and their newborn babies through education [25].

Addressing Post-discharge Morbidity and Mortality in Resource-rich Areas

Improving the functional outcomes of children who survive sepsis is a priority [26, 27]. The Sepsis Prevalence, Outcomes and Therapy (SPROUT) study showed that 25% of children with sepsis died while 17% of the survivors had new moderate or worse disability at discharge [28]. In this study, 21% of patients with sepsis had severe acute kidney injury (AKI), and half of these patients either died or developed moderate functional disability. Similarly, data from the Researching Severe Sepsis and Organ Dysfunction in Children (RESOLVE) trial showed that of the 298 children who were 28-day survivors of severe sepsis, 18% showed poor functional outcomes, and 34% had deterioration of their functional status compared to their baseline [4].

In the United Kingdom and Ireland, school-aged children who were admitted to the PICU with central nervous system (CNS) infection and septicemia underperformed on neuropsychological function measures and some performed academically worse 3–6 months after discharge from the ICU [29]. These studies clearly show the significant burden of post-discharge morbidity, justifying an increased focus on this vulnerable period. Interventions that include physical and occupational therapy should be instituted early. Child life specialists and hospital schooling should be encouraged.

Addressing Post-discharge Morbidity and Mortality in Low and Middle Income Countries

In resource-limited areas, our understanding of post-discharge mortality is increasing, but morbidity is largely ignored. The fact that morbidity ranges from subtle to severe, that measurement is rarely straight forward and that resources are limited are key barriers in addressing this issue. However, efforts to understand and implement simple measures to decrease or avert post-discharge morbidity are important. These may include discharge follow-up of kidney function for children with AKI; neurological follow-up for those with CNS infections, and expansion of services in school to include individualized learning plans for children who have residual functional disability.

Addressing morbidity may also influence and avert mortality and improve quality of life and productivity. For reasons outlined earlier, a key step in addressing post-discharge mortality begins with the identification of patient groups who are at high risk of death during the post-discharge period [15].

Disease-specific Risk Groups

Severe malnutrition and pneumonia are common among children who die during the post-discharge period in Bangladesh [18] as well as Kenya, and undernourished children have an eight-fold increase in post-discharge mortality compared to their community peers [17, 30]. In Gambia, post-discharge mortality was high among children with pneumonia, meningitis and sepsis and severe malnutrition [31]. Among Malawian children, post-discharge mortality was common among HIV positive children, children under 12 months, and those with severe malnutrition at admission or disability [32].

Bacterial meningitis is a leading cause of morbidity and mortality in African children, and up to 18% of children die after discharge [33]. CNS infections (including meningoencephalitis), even in developed countries, are associated with poor functional outcomes, more severe educational difficulties and deficits in neuropsychological performance [4, 29].

Children who were admitted with gastroenteritis were also at a significantly higher risk of death within the first three months after been being discharged alive [34]. In Bangladesh, most deaths in the first 3 months after discharge from the hospital were associated with either a new respiratory infection or gastrointestinal symptoms [18].

Other Risk Groups

In children with severe malaria, post-discharge mortality was associated with severe anemia, jaundice, less parasitemia, elevated lactate dehydrogenase (LDH), increased transfusions and elevated levels of angiopoietin-2 (Ang-2) biomarker [35]. Furthermore, levels of Ang-2 in the highest quartile were associated with a 1.2-fold increase in post-discharge mortality.

In Bangladesh, young age has been shown to be significantly associated with post-discharge mortality [18]. Many of these young children are severely malnourished at the time of discharge, and are vulnerable to community-acquired infections when they return home. Most die at home within one month of discharge, often without any contact with the hospital.

A higher risk of post-discharge mortality has also been observed in children who were discharged against medical advice [36]. In Cote d'Ivoire, the proportion of children who were taken away prematurely from the hospital was closely related to the cost of medication, the availability of essential drugs at the hospital and the families' inability to pay for the cost of hospitalization [37].

Use of Risk Data for Risk Classification

A recent study, with the objective of developing a robust post-discharge prediction model, used the disease and context factors outlined above, and incorporated them

Table 2 Prediction of post-discharge mortality. Model characteristics at probability cut-offs ensuring model sensitivity of >80%. Adapted from [16]

Model	AUC (95% CI)	Probability Cut-Off	Sensitivity (95% CI)	Specificity (95% CI)	PPV	NPV
1	0.82 (0.75 to 0.87)	0.035	82.0 (72.3 to 91.6)	66.2 (63.5 to 68.9)	11.1	98.6
2	0.81 (0.75 to 0.87)	0.040	80.3 (70.4 to 90.3)	67.5 (64.8 to 70.2)	11.3	98.5
3	0.80 (0.74 to 0.86)	0.031	80.3 (70.4 to 90.3)	63.4 (60.7 to 66.2)	10.2	98.4
4	0.80 (0.73 to 0.86)	0.035	82.0 (72.3 to 91.6)	61.4 (58.6 to 64.2)	9.9	98.5

30% of children would be flagged as high risk (positive predictive value [PPV]: 0.11) and require further follow-up and 80% of those children who eventually died would have been correctly identified and singled out for more intensive follow-up management. 70% of the children could be safely discharged, with a low risk of mortality during the post-discharge period (negative predictive value [NPV]: 0.99). *AUC*: area under the curve

via a Delphi process into a set of candidate predictors [38]. In stratifying post-discharge mortality risk, Wiens et al. then developed a predictive model that included mid-upper arm circumference (mm), oxygen saturation (SpO_2, %) at admission, time since previous hospitalization, the presence of an abnormal Blantyre coma scale (BCS) at admission and HIV status (Table 2). This model had a sensitivity of 82% and specificity of 66% [16] in identifying children with post-discharge mortality. This model uses variables that are easily and reliably collected when a patient is being admitted to the hospital in a low and middle income country setting. Such prediction models can help with early and focused discharge planning in high-risk children.

Post-Discharge Interventions to Ensure Follow-up and Return to Care

Risk Classification

The PAediatric Risk Assessment (PARA) Mobile App was designed to predict inpatient and post-discharge mortality among children under 5 years old who are admitted with a proven or suspected infection. This application uses a previously derived regression model for the prediction of mortality both during and following hospitalization, using demographic, anthropometric and clinical indicators collected on admission [39] (Fig. 1). Using this app, high-risk patients can be identified and thus targeted for appropriate post-discharge care.

Education and Follow-up

Community-based health interventions that are culturally sensitive and economically soft improve health outcomes. In Nepal, infant mortality rate was improved in

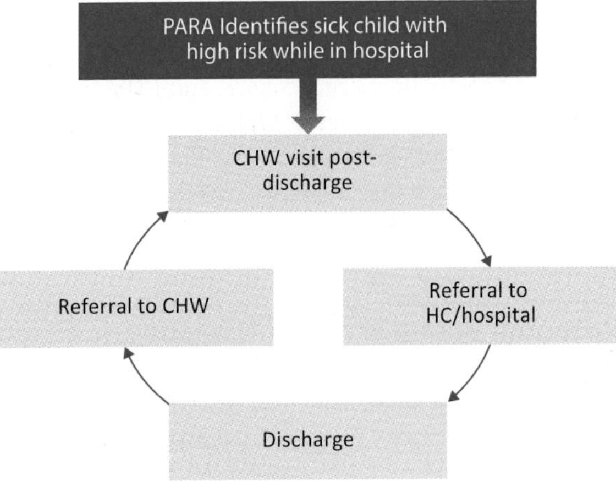

PARA App

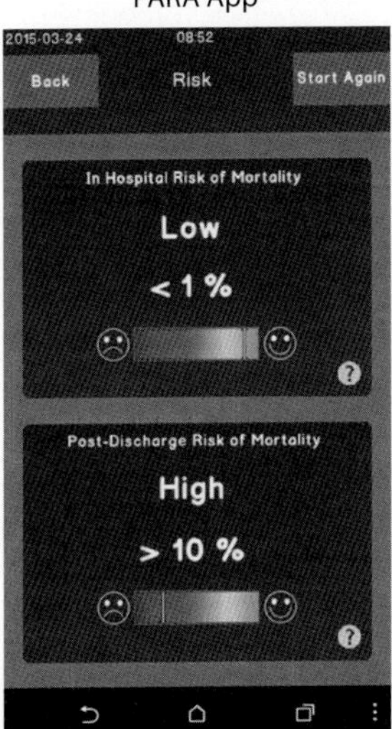

- Education for mother
  - Post-discharge vulnerability
  - Health behavior
  - Early recognition
  - Early health seeking
- Incentives for mother
  - New bed net
  - Oral rehydration solution
  - Soap

Fig. 1 Home referral and discharge kit. *CHW*: community health worker; *HC*: health clinic; *PARA*: PAediatric Risk Assessment Mobile app

a program where local female health facilitators held group meetings every month with groups of women [40]. In a similar study, CHWs were quite effective in treating severe neonatal sepsis [41].

Recently, a study in Uganda demonstrated the effectiveness and feasibility of a discharge bundle of care among children admitted with a proven or suspected infection [42]. This bundle consisted of a post-discharge referral for follow-up and a Discharge Kit. The referral for post-discharge care, provided by a discharge nurse, encouraged follow-up during the first few days following discharge, by either a CHW or at a local health center. The Discharge Kit consisted of brief educational counseling paired with simple household incentives to reinforce education. The educational counseling consisted of an explanation of the child's vulnerability during the discharge period and discussed three main themes of action: (1) prevention through hygiene and other health behaviors (e. g., mosquito net use); (2) recognition of signs of early illness recurrence; and (3) prompt healthcare seeking. This intervention improved healthcare seeking following discharge three-fold, from about 30 to 90%. Further, it increased post-discharge re-admissions by 50%, an important achievement given that most post-discharge deaths occurred at home and that half of the re-admissions were directly attributed to the scheduled post-discharge.

Potential Post-discharge Therapeutic Interventions

Since nutritional status is key in determining risk of infection, trajectory of acute disease and outcomes in post-discharge period, modifiable risk factors associated with malnutrition should be potential treatment targets for ill children [16, 30]. These should include, in the immediate acute illness period, anthropometric measures to determine nutritional state and addressing nutrient composition of both therapeutic/supplementary feeds. Critically ill children who are severely malnourished should be started on a nutritional regime for severe acute malnutrition, while still treating the child's primary disease or reason for admission.

Other potential target points for addressing malnutrition include addressing suboptimal infant nutrition practices at the community level, addressing issues of food insecurity, understanding the roles of unhealthy microbiomes in the gut that might be responsible for a tropical sprue type of picture and malabsorption and recurrence of infection. Community Management of Acute Malnutrition (CMAM) programs (an initiative of the WHO, World Food Program, and UNICEF), would be helpful in addressing severe acute malnutrition in the setting of sepsis. As part of the program, children with severe acute malnutrition are treated at home with ready-to-use food therapy [RUTF]. In Malawi, under-5 mortality rates have decreased since the initial trial of these RUFT packages [43].

Zinc supplementation has been shown to reduce treatment failure in infants less than 4 months of age with serious bacterial infection, and reduce diarrheal and pneumonia-related morbidity and mortality [44, 45]. It is therefore possible that zinc could also play a role as an adjunctive medication for children continuing antibiotic treatment during the post-discharge period. In children with malaria and severe anemia, intermittent preventive therapy for malaria with monthly artemether-lumefantrine during the post-discharge period showed an absolution reduction in primary events of re-admittance or death [46]. Although interventions such as oral home amoxicillin have shown some efficacy in the treatment of pneumonia, increasing antimicrobial resistance and access to antibiotics are significant concerns to such approaches [47].

While it is known that daily cotrimoxazole prophylaxis prevents mortality and re-admissions in children who are HIV-positive, disappointingly, in children with severe acute malnutrition who were HIV-negative, daily cotrimoxazole did not reduce mortality.

Remaining Gaps and the Way Forward

Strengthening Community Health Worker Systems

Since poverty is pervasive in most low and middle income countries among segments of the populace, cost of hospital care, transport issues, healthcare seeking behaviors and mistrust of healthcare systems continue to plague health outcomes in terms of post-discharge mortality and morbidity, especially in resource-limited settings. CHWs are locals who in most cases are trusted, could provide tailored low-cost preventive, curative and other actionable follow-up care.

Education of Girls

Maternal education has been associated with positive health outcomes for infants and children. Every nation-state in low and middle income countries should provide some level of formal education to all girls in their society. This in the long-term would be cost-effective, as it would reflect on reduced mortality and morbidity for children.

Long Follow-up Period

An extended follow-up period after hospital discharge will, in the short-term, ensure that at the period children are most vulnerable, they hopefully would be seen for scheduled visits for any organ dysfunction management to mitigate any potential associated morbidity. In the long-term, it also provides an opportunity to watch for outcomes in children who had decreased functional status immediately after discharge. It also provides the space to follow these children and accurately time any potential mortality or morbidity event.

Conclusions

Since the number of children with sepsis dying during the post-discharge period approximates the number dying during hospitalization, models that assist in the identification of vulnerable children could be incorporated into clinical care. Furthermore, sepsis guidelines, including the IMCI guidelines, should take into consideration the neglected issue of post-discharge mortality further strengthening the premise that sepsis and its management are a continuum that stretches beyond the acute phase of illness [16]. Although limited data currently exist on interventions to improve post-discharge outcomes, discharge planning for all children with sepsis should start at the initial patient intake for hospital admission. An approach that engages community partners, such as local health centers and CHWs, should be encouraged. The prominence of malnutrition in post-discharge mortality, suggests that nutritional interventions may play a key role in further reducing this burden. Finally, addressing post-discharge morbidity in both research and practice will be imperative to ensure that survivors can lead productive and healthy lives, and that adequate resources can be made available to those experiencing lasting impact from sepsis.

References

1. Weiss SL, Fitzgerald JC, Pappachan J et al (2015) Global epidemiology of pediatric severe sepsis: the sepsis prevalence, outcomes, and therapies study. Am J Respir Crit Care Med 191:1147–1157
2. Wiens MO, Pawluk S, Kissoon N et al (2013) Pediatric post-discharge mortality in resource poor countries: a systematic review. PLoS One 8:e66698
3. Czaja AS, Zimmerman JJ, Nathens AB (2009) Readmission and late mortality after pediatric severe sepsis. Pediatrics 123:849–857
4. Farris RW, Weiss NS, Zimmerman JJ (2013) Functional outcomes in pediatric severe sepsis: further analysis of the researching severe sepsis and organ dysfunction in children: a global perspective trial. Pediatr Crit Care Med 14:835–842
5. Aspesberro F, Riley C, Kitagawa M, Zimmerman J (2015) Improving long-term outcomes for pediatric patients. http://www.sccm.org/Communications/Critical-Connections/Archives/Pages/Improving-Long-Term-Outcomes-for-Pediatric-Patients.aspx. Accessed Nov 10, 2016
6. Goldstein B, Giroir B, Randolph A, International Consensus Conference on Pediatric Sepsis (2005) International pediatric sepsis consensus conference: definitions for sepsis and organ dysfunction in pediatrics. Pediatr Crit Care Med 6:2–8
7. Wiens MO, Larson CP, Kumbakumba E et al (2016) Application of sepsis definitions to pediatric patients admitted with suspected infections in Uganda. Pediatr Crit Care Med 17:400–405
8. Han YY, Carcillo JA, Dragotta MA et al (2003) Early reversal of pediatric-neonatal septic shock by community physicians is associated with improved outcome. Pediatrics 112:793–799
9. de Oliveira CF, de Oliveira DS, Gottschald AF et al (2008) ACCM/PALS haemodynamic support guidelines for paediatric septic shock: an outcomes comparison with and without monitoring central venous oxygen saturation. Intensive Care Med 34:1065–1075
10. Larsen GY, Mecham N, Greenberg R (2011) An emergency department septic shock protocol and care guideline for children initiated at triage. Pediatrics 127:e1585–1592
11. Dunser MW, Festic E, Dondorp A et al (2012) Recommendations for sepsis management in resource-limited settings. Intensive Care Med 38:557–574
12. You D, Hug L, Ejdemyr S et al (2015) Global, regional, and national levels and trends in under-5 mortality between 1990 and 2015, with scenario-based projections to 2030: a systematic analysis by the UN Inter-agency Group for Child Mortality Estimation. Lancet 386:2275–2286
13. Liu L, Oza S, Hogan D et al (2015) Global, regional, and national causes of child mortality in 2000–13, with projections to inform post-2015 priorities: an updated systematic analysis. Lancet 385:430–440
14. Kissoon N, Daniels R, van der Poll T, Finfer S, Reinhart K (2016) Sepsis-the final common pathway to death from multiple organ failure in infection. Crit Care Med 44:e446
15. Wiens MO, Kumbakumba E, Kissoon N, Ansermino JM, Ndamira A, Larson CP (2012) Pediatric sepsis in the developing world: challenges in defining sepsis and issues in post-discharge mortality. Clin Epidemiol 4:319–325
16. Wiens MO, Kumbakumba E, Larson CP et al (2015) Postdischarge mortality in children with acute infectious diseases: derivation of postdischarge mortality prediction models. BMJ Open 5:e009449

17. Moisi JC, Gatakaa H, Berkley JA et al (2011) Excess child mortality after discharge from hospital in Kilifi, Kenya: a retrospective cohort analysis. Bull World Health Organ 89:725–732
18. Chisti MJ, Graham SM, Duke T et al (2014) Post-discharge mortality in children with severe malnutrition and pneumonia in Bangladesh. PLoS One 9:e107663
19. Kruk ME, Myers M, Varpilah ST, Dahn BT (2015) What is a resilient health system? Lessons from Ebola. Lancet 385:1910–1912
20. Geldsetzer P, Williams TC, Kirolos A et al (2014) The recognition of and care seeking behaviour for childhood illness in developing countries: a systematic review. PLoS One 9:e93427
21. Nair H, Simoes EA, Rudan I et al (2013) Global and regional burden of hospital admissions for severe acute lower respiratory infections in young children in 2010: a systematic analysis. Lancet 381:1380–1390
22. World Health Organization (2014) Revised WHO classification and treatment of childhood pneumonia at health facilities. World Health Organization, Geneva, pp 6–14
23. Wamani H, Tylleskar T, Astrom AN, Tumwine JK, Peterson S (2004) Mothers' education but not fathers' education, household assets or land ownership is the best predictor of child health inequalities in rural Uganda. Int J Equity Health 3:9
24. Jones CH, Ward A, Hodkinson PW et al (2016) Caregivers' Experiences of pathways to care for seriously ill children in cape town, south africa: a qualitative investigation. PLoS One 11:e0151606
25. Singh D, Cumming R, Negin J (2015) Acceptability and trust of community health workers offering maternal and newborn health education in rural Uganda. Health Educ Res 30:947–958
26. Pollack MM, Holubkov R, Funai T et al (2014) Pediatric intensive care outcomes: development of new morbidities during pediatric critical care. Pediatr Crit Care Med 15:821–827
27. Rennick JE, Childerhose JE (2015) Redefining success in the PICU: new patient populations shift targets of care. Pediatrics 135:e289–291
28. Fitzgerald JC, Basu RK, Akcan-Arikan A et al (2016) Acute kidney injury in pediatric severe sepsis: an independent risk factor for death and new disability. Crit Care Med 44:2241–2250
29. Als LC, Nadel S, Cooper M, Pierce CM, Sahakian BJ, Garralda ME (2013) Neuropsychologic function three to six months following admission to the PICU with meningoencephalitis, sepsis, and other disorders: a prospective study of school-aged children. Crit Care Med 41:1094–1103
30. Ginsburg AS, Izadnegahdar R, Berkley JA, Walson JL, Rollins N, Klugman KP (2015) Undernutrition and pneumonia mortality. Lancet Glob Health 3:e735–736
31. Chhibber AV, Hill PC, Jafali J et al (2015) Child mortality after discharge from a health facility following suspected pneumonia, meningitis or septicaemia in rural Gambia: a cohort study. PLoS One 10:e0137095
32. Kerac M, Bunn J, Chagaluka G et al (2014) Follow-up of post-discharge growth and mortality after treatment for severe acute malnutrition (FuSAM study): a prospective cohort study. PLoS One 9:e96030
33. Ramakrishnan M, Ulland AJ, Steinhardt LC, Moisi JC, Were F, Levine OS (2009) Sequelae due to bacterial meningitis among African children: a systematic literature review. BMC Med 7:47
34. Snow RW, Howard SC, Mung'Ala-Odera V et al (2000) Paediatric survival and re-admission risks following hospitalization on the Kenyan coast. Trop Med Int Health 5:377–383
35. Conroy A, Hawkes M, McDonald C et al (2016) Host biomakers are associated with response to therapy and long-term mortality in pediatric severe malaria. Open Forum Infect Dis 3:ofw134
36. Veirum JE, Sodeman M, Biai S, Hedegård K, Aaby P (2007) Increased mortality in the year following discharge from a paediatric ward in Bissau, Guinea-Bissau. Acta Paediatr 96:1832–1838
37. Gloyd S, Kone A, Victor AE (1995) Pediatric discharge against medical advice in Bouake Cote d'Ivoire, 1980–1992. Health Policy Plan 10:89–93

38. Wiens MO, Kissoon N, Kumbakumba E et al (2016) Selecting candidate predictor variables for the modelling of post-discharge mortality from sepsis: a protocol development project. Afr Health Sci 16:162–169
39. English LL, Dunsmuir D, Kumbakumba E et al (2016) The PAediatric Risk Assessment (PARA) Mobile app to reduce postdischarge child mortality: design, usability, and feasibility for health care workers in Uganda. JMIR Mhealth Uhealth 4:e16
40. Manandhar DS, Osrin D, Shrestha BP et al (2004) Effect of a participatory intervention with women's groups on birth outcomes in Nepal: cluster-randomised controlled trial. Lancet 364:970–979
41. Baqui AH, Arifeen SE, Williams EK et al (2009) Effectiveness of home-based management of newborn infections by community health workers in rural Bangladesh. Pediatr Infect Dis J 28:304–310
42. Wiens MO, Kumbakumba E, Larson CP et al (2016) Scheduled follow-up referrals and simple prevention kits including counseling to improve post-discharge outcomes among children in Uganda: A proof-of-concept study. Glob Health Sci Pract 4:422–423
43. Murray E, Manary M (2014) Home-based therapy for severe acute malnutrition with ready-to-use food. Paediatr Int Child Health 34:266–270
44. Bhatnagar S, Wadhwa N, Aneja S et al (2012) Zinc as adjunct treatment in infants aged between 7 and 120 days with probable serious bacterial infection: a randomised, double-blind, placebo-controlled trial. Lancet 379:2072–2078
45. Yakoob MY, Theodoratou E, Jabeen A et al (2011) Preventive zinc supplementation in developing countries: impact on mortality and morbidity due to diarrhea, pneumonia and malaria. BMC Public Health 11(Suppl 3):S23
46. Phiri K, Esan M, van Hensbroek MB, Khairallah C, Faragher B, ter Kuile FO (2012) Intermittent preventive therapy for malaria with monthly artemether-lumefantrine for the post-discharge management of severe anaemia in children aged 4–59 months in southern Malawi: a multicentre, randomised, placebo-controlled trial. Lancet Infect Dis 12:191–200
47. Laxminarayan R, Matsoso P, Pant S et al (2016) Access to effective antimicrobials: a worldwide challenge. Lancet 387:168–175

Emergency Abdominal Surgery in the Elderly: How Can We Reduce the Risk in a Challenging Population?

X. Watson and M. Cecconi

Introduction

Emergency laparotomy is a common surgical intervention with an estimated 1 in 1,100 patients in the UK undergoing the procedure annually [1]. Both substandard care and poor outcomes have been demonstrated by the National Confidential Enquiry into Patient Outcome and Death (NCEPOD), and morbidity and mortality have consistently been higher in patients undergoing emergency versus elective surgery [2]. In 2010, data collected by the Emergency Laparotomy Network (ELN) demonstrated a crude 30-day mortality of 14.9% [3].

Emergency general surgery constitutes approximately 8–26% of all hospital admissions and is associated with substantial cost across the entire care pathway. The morbidity and mortality associated with emergency laparotomy is well known to increase with age and emergency procedures carry a much higher age-adjusted incidence for each decade above 60 years of age [4]. Perioperative mortality in the elderly is estimated to be between 15–20% and has been shown to reach between 40–50% in patients aged 80 or above [5]. Elderly patients may survive the surgical procedure but not the complications that ensue, with perioperative complications having been demonstrated to be strong predictors of outcome and mortality increasing up to threefold in their presence [5]. In addition, of those patients who survive the surgical insult, many will have increased dependency requiring additional care which adds further burden to an increasingly stretched healthcare system from a resource and financial aspect.

X. Watson (✉)
Department of Anaesthesia and Intensive Care, Kingston Hospital
Galsworthy Road, Kingston, KT2 7QB, UK
e-mail: ugm2xw@doctors.org.uk

M. Cecconi
Department of Anaesthesia and Intensive Care, St George's University Hospitals NHS Trust
London, SW17 0QT, UK

J.-L. Vincent (ed.), *Annual Update in Intensive Care and Emergency Medicine 2017*,
DOI 10.1007/978-3-319-51908-1_35

At present, approximately 17% of the population is aged 65 years or above and it is estimated that this number will increase by two thirds to reach 15.8 million by 2031 with 5% aged over 90 years [6]. The elderly population pose a significant challenge to clinicians in the perioperative period owing to both high comorbidity and low functional reserve. In the elective setting, there may be time to optimize these patients preoperatively but patients presenting with an acute abdomen are often septic with fluid and electrolyte imbalances superimposed on a poor pre-morbid state. These patients therefore require careful perioperative management with a multidisciplinary team approach. Although over recent years there have been significant improvements in the care of the acute surgical patient, improvements in surgical holistic care have been slow to emerge and further research is warranted on how best to manage this high-risk cohort in the perioperative period.

In this chapter, we provide an overview of the challenges associated with emergency surgery in an ageing population and describe what we can do as clinicians to reduce the risk of morbidity and mortality in the perioperative period.

Preoperative Care

As stated, the elderly cohort represents a complex population with contributing factors such as frailty, pre-existing comorbidity, cognitive dysfunction and polypharmacy. The care patients receive in the preoperative period will notably have an influence on their surgical outcome and it is of critical importance that these patients undergo rapid diagnosis and appropriate resuscitation. In the elderly patient presenting with an acute abdomen, diagnosis is not always straightforward and can be challenging. Patients may not always present with typical features of an 'acute abdomen' and signs of abdominal sepsis may not be as obvious as in the younger cohort; therefore a high of index of suspicion is required. The NECEPOD report from 2010 found that a delay in diagnosis and subsequently treatment had a significant impact on the perioperative outcome of these patients, with a significant delay from admission to surgery occurring in over 1 in five elderly patients [7]. The use of early computed tomography (CT) imaging has been shown to improve the management of the elderly with an acute abdomen and its liberal use has been recommended, as the long term adverse effects of radiation are considered less of an issue in the elderly [6, 8]. As part of a comprehensive geriatric preoperative assessment, accurate risk assessment and screening for frailty should be undertaken in a timely manner. Frailty can be described as a "state of vulnerability to poor resolution of homeostasis" and is a consequence of cumulative decline in many physiological systems [9]. There are five main indicators of frailty, namely weight loss, low energy, exhaustion, slow gait speed and poor grip strength, and although these can be measured in the elective setting, time often does not permit its accurate identification in the acute setting and the results may be confounded by the surgical insult.

A recent study that evaluated the ability of six frailty screening instruments to predict outcome after emergency abdominal surgery found that four out of the six were able to accurately and independently predict postoperative mortality with the

Vulnerable Elderly Survey (VES-13) being the most accurate [10]. In addition to identification of frailty, the "Higher Risk General Surgical Patient" report advocates that an accurate perioperative risk assessment should be undertaken with the patient [11]. Although numerous risk prediction models currently exist, such as the American Society of Anesthesiologists (ASA), Acute Physiology and Chronic Health Evaluation (APACHE)-11 and Portsmouth Physiological and Operative Severity Score for the Enumeration of Mortality and Morbidity (P-POSSUM) systems, they can be cumbersome, requiring multiple inputs and do not always take into account the complexity of the disease process or the underlying frailty of the patient. The American College of Surgeons has recently developed an online risk prediction tool for use in both elective and emergency surgery and this has been widely validated [12]. A thorough risk assessment is not only important for the clinician to help plan perioperative management but also allows for an honest discussion with the patient and family about the patient's best interests. A recent study showed that, without the use of a risk prediction tool, the likelihood of survival in patients aged 90 or above with high ASA grade, septic shock and dependent living was less than 10% and therefore these factors alone could be used to guide whether surgical treatment is in the patient's best interests [13].

As highlighted in the recent Association of Anaesthetists of Great Britain and Ireland (AAGBI), patients with capacity have the right to make decisions about their treatment and respecting their wishes is of paramount importance. Not all patients with operative pathology should undergo surgery and avoiding futile surgery, although a difficult task, may be the right decision for an individual patient. In patients in whom the decision has been made to take to the operating room, preoperative optimization should be undertaken although the risks of optimizing vs delaying surgery need to be taken into account. Evidence has shown that operative delay before emergency laparotomy is associated with poorer outcome and therefore optimization and surgery should occur simultaneously rather than separately [14]. Although it is well-recognized that opportunities for optimization in the emergency setting may be limited, every effort should be made to ensure that these patients are cared for in an appropriate setting with early involvement of senior clinicians. It is well-known that elderly patients are unable to tolerate hypovolemia as well as the younger population and, therefore, there should be a low threshold for the diagnosis or suspicion of shock in these patients. Studies from elderly trauma patients have suggested that a systolic blood pressure of 110 mmHg may be indicative of shock and compounded with a reduced cardiac reserve may necessitate optimization of preload and contractility with the use of vasopressors and inotropes in a critical care environment [15].

Additionally, these patients may be at risk of pulmonary complications due to an obstructed gastrointestinal tract on a background of pulmonary disease and reduced immunity. Early placement of a nasogastric tube is therefore recommended. The development of acute kidney injury (AKI) may also be seen in the preoperative period due to cumulative factors such as hypovolemia, polypharmacy and pre-existing renal insufficiency and diabetes. Ensuring careful and adequate fluid resuscitation is therefore imperative and may be guided by the use of hemodynamic monitoring to target dynamic indices. The use of goal-directed therapy is discussed in more detail later but should be considered early in the preoperative period. In addition to early resuscitation, prompt administration of antibiotics if there is any evidence of sepsis is of paramount importance and should be seen as a priority. In 2015, Huddart et al. on behalf of the ELPQuiC Collaborator group demonstrated that the use of a pathway quality improvement bundle was associated with a significant reduction in mortality after emergency laparotomy surgery [3]. The bundle was based upon key recommendations made in the Royal College of Surgeons of England and Department of Health publications and was implemented in four UK hospitals. The bundle consists of five elements which are:

1) all emergency admissions have an early warning score assessed on presentation, with graded escalation policies for senior clinical and intensive care unit (ICU) referral;
2) broad-spectrum antibiotics to be given to all patients with suspicion of peritoneal soiling or with a diagnosis of sepsis;
3) once the decision has been made to carry out laparotomy, the patient takes the next available place in the emergency operating room (or within 6 h of decision being made);
4) start resuscitation using goal-directed techniques as soon as possible, or within 6 h of admission;
5) admit all patients to the ICU after emergency laparotomy.

Although this bundle is applicable to all patients undergoing emergency abdominal surgery, it is apparent that since the elderly population constitute a significant proportion of these high-risk patients, that this bundle should be implemented as part of a comprehensive geriatric protocol-driven pathway. In addition, a multidisciplinary approach should be employed in the preoperative period to ensure that optimum care is delivered and that the pathway is adhered to at all times.

Intraoperative Care

There are numerous variables that can be optimized intraoperatively with the aim of improving outcome and reducing postoperative complications. The importance of delivering expert operative care with senior involvement cannot be underestimated and evidence has demonstrated that lack of consultant involvement is associated with higher rates of complications and mortality [16]. Surgical intervention in this high-risk cohort should be delivered by a surgeon of consultant grade with similar expectations for the provision of anesthesia [6]. The implementation of the ELPQuiP bundle as described in the study by Huddart et al. demonstrated that its use led to a significant improvement in patient care at one hospital by the direct involvement of senior surgeons and anesthetists [3]. A guideline published in 2014 by the AAGBI on the 'Perioperative care of the elderly patient' describes standards of care that should be adhered to both in the elective and emergency setting

[17]. The AAGBI guideline highlights the importance of temperature control in the elderly as it is well known that perioperative hypothermia is common and associated with increased complications, such as delirium, cardiac dysfunction, increased length of stay and poor wound healing [17]. Frail elderly patients are increasingly prone to the adverse effects of hypothermia and, therefore, regular assessment of temperature and active measures to avoid hypothermia should be taken promptly. Such measures include fluid warming and forced air warming and these should be employed throughout the perioperative period. All patients undergoing emergency surgery should also be monitored as per AAGBI guidelines and it is recommended that invasive monitoring be considered in elderly patients undergoing emergency surgery. As previously stated, these patients are likely to be hypovolemic and in shock and, therefore, an invasive arterial catheter inserted prior to induction is advocated. The NCEPOD report in 2007 concluded that intraoperative hypotension is common with a reported incidence of 47% and it is likely that this is a contributing factor to the poor outcomes observed. A recent study conducted by Wickham et al., which examined the incidence of hypotension in the elderly, found that hypotension (defined as >20% reduction in systolic blood pressure) occurred in up to 83% of elderly patients undergoing anesthesia, with invasive arterial monitoring being used in 1 in five patients [18]. They also showed that up to 39% of patients experienced a drop of >40% from their baseline, a degree of hypotension that has been linked to stroke, myocardial ischemia and AKI. The use of central venous pressure (CVP) monitoring is contentious as it is well documented that there is a poor correlation between CVP and blood volume, and changes in CVP are not predictive of fluid status, particularly in the elderly with poorly compliant ventricles [19]. However, the insertion of a CVP line may facilitate the administration of vasopressors and inotropes in the intra- and postoperative periods.

Fluid management is challenging in the elderly patient as there is a reduced homeostatic compensation for fluid loss, coupled with the fact these patients are likely to be septic and hypovolemic by the time they receive surgical intervention. Careful administration of fluid boluses individualized to the patient is therefore advocated and the use of early goal-directed fluid therapy was recommended in the ELPQuiP bundle, to be commenced as soon as possible or within 6 h of admission. The intraoperative goal of the anesthetist is to achieve hemodynamic stability and ensure adequate oxygen delivery and this can be facilitated by the use of hemodynamic monitoring. There has been increased interest in the use of goal-directed fluid therapy recently and the significant advancements in less-invasive hemodynamic monitoring over the years has led to the concept of goal-directed fluid therapy becoming further embedded in clinical practice. Goal-directed fluid therapy using hemodynamic monitoring allows the 'real-time' measurement of cardiovascular variables and dynamic parameters of fluid responsiveness to guide administration of intravenous fluids, vasopressors and inotropic therapy [21]. Fluid responsiveness can be defined as an increase in stroke volume (SV) or cardiac output by 10–15% in response to a fluid challenge, although the rate and volume of fluid is variable.

Various monitors currently exist in clinical practice and due to the large body of evidence supporting the use of the esophageal Doppler monitor, The National

Institute for Health and Care Excellence (NICE) recommend that it "should be considered in patients undergoing major or high-risk surgery" [22]. However, at present there is little evidence for its use in the elderly or in emergency surgery and it may be less accurate in the elderly due to a poorly compliant aorta resulting in overestimation of cardiac output and inadequate fluid administration [17]

Recent evidence for the use of goal-directed fluid therapy has been conflicting. Despite high quality evidence from a meta-analysis demonstrating that the use of hemodynamic monitoring coupled with therapy reduces morbidity and mortality in high-risk surgical patients [22], recent studies have cast doubt on its benefits with a large randomized controlled trial demonstrating no reduction in mortality, but a significant reduction in postoperative complications when a planned sub-analysis was performed [23]. At present the use of early goal-directed fluid therapy is recommended as per the ELPQuiP bundle and we await further studies.

Elderly patients are also at risk of developing postoperative pulmonary complications and the method by which these patients are ventilated intraoperatively may influence their perioperative outcome. Postoperative pulmonary complications are common after abdominal surgery and are a significant cause of increased hospital stay and mortality. The reported incidence is variable but postoperative pulmonary complications have been reported to occur in up to 28% of patients undergoing emergency surgery [24]. Although there are numerous risk factors for their development, evidence has highlighted that increasing age remains a significant risk factor after adjustment for the presence of co-morbidities and there is a threefold increase in the likelihood of their development in patients aged 70–79 years [25]. There has been recent interest in the implementation of protective lung ventilation in patients undergoing abdominal surgery. Protective lung ventilation, defined as the use of low tidal volumes (6–8 ml/kg/ideal body weight [IBW]), application of positive end-expiratory pressure (PEEP) and use of recruitment maneuvers is a well-established practice in the management of patients with acute respiratory distress syndrome (ARDS). A meta-analysis conducted by Tao et al., published in 2014, concluded that the use of PLV could reduce the incidence of pulmonary complications [26]. In addition, a recent double-blind randomized controlled trial conducted by Futier et al. found a statistically significant reduction in complications in patients receiving protective lung ventilation compared to the control group ($p = 0.001$) [27]. However, this study looked at a relatively small number of patients ($n = 400$) and only included patients undergoing elective surgery. There is currently no standardized guidance on how patients undergoing emergency surgery should be ventilated and whether there is in fact any correlation between mode of ventilation and development of postoperative pulmonary complications. We eagerly await the results of a Pan-London study "Adoption of Lung Protective ventilation in patients undergoing Emergency laparotomy surgery" which aims to answer this question. At present, it is recommended that anesthetists give careful consideration to how these patients are ventilated with particular emphasis on preventing both barotrauma and atelectasis, both of which can lead to adverse outcomes.

Other considerations that need to be taken into account in the intraoperative period include blood transfusion and patient positioning. Anemia is common in the elderly patient for a multitude of reasons and is associated with myocardial ischemia, falls, failure to wean and poor wound healing [7]. Data from observational studies suggest that patients aged over 65 years have a higher mortality when there is significant intraoperative blood loss compared to younger patients and a reduced mortality when the preoperative hematocrit is 30–36% and surgical blood loss is <500 ml [28]. The NICE guidelines published in 2015 relating to blood transfusion advocate a restrictive transfusion regime with a transfusion threshold of 7 g/dl in patients who do not have active hemorrhage or acute coronary syndrome [29]. Regarding patient positioning, the elderly patient is prone to the development of preventable peripheral neve injuries including the ulnar nerve when in the supine position. The AAGBI therefore recommend that likely areas of potential nerve injury should be thoroughly padded prior to the start of surgery and assessed every 30 min for the duration of the procedure.

Postoperative Care

The quality of care that elderly patients receive in the postoperative period is of crucial importance and is likely to significantly affect their perioperative outcome. The ELPQuiC bundle recommends that all patients post-emergency laparotomy surgery be admitted to the ICU and there is currently an ongoing need for provision of high dependency or intensive care support for elderly patients after major surgery [3]. At present, not all postoperative patients are managed in the ICU and studies have highlighted that patients who develop complications and are not admitted to the ICU have a higher mortality compared to those who are admitted immediately postoperatively [30]. Provision of good quality of care is also essential to avoid the concept of 'failure to rescue' whereby a potentially treatable or avoidable postoperative complication arises and results in death.

This concept is believed to be occur more frequently in the elderly and can result from either failure to recognize that a complication has ensued or failure to adequately treat the complication [6]. It should be noted, however, that although this concept is important to remember, not all patients die from potentially remediable complications. Early involvement of the multidisciplinary team as part of a comprehensive geriatric assessment has been shown to reduce hospital stay, ICU admissions and costs [31].

However, despite compelling evidence from the orthopedic community, which has welcomed the involvement of orthogeriatricians, the collaborative multidisciplinary team approach is yet to gain full acceptance in the wider surgical community. A recent survey undertaken in the UK found that <30% of hospitals regularly included geriatric medicine input into the care of their surgical patients and that funding was the main barrier. Further research into this promising area is, therefore, definitely warranted. In addition to early medical input, early involvement of a nutritionist and dietician is imperative as up to 80% of elderly patients have been found to be either malnourished or at risk of malnourishment [4]. Regular input from physiotherapists is also advocated to help mobilization and reduce complica-

Table 1 Risk factors for delirium in elderly patients. Adapted from [34]

Predisposing	Critical illness	Iatrogenic
Increasing age	Acidosis	Immobilization
Dementia	Anemia	Over sedation
Depression	Electrolyte disturbance	Uncontrolled pain
Stroke	Sepsis	Sleep disturbances
Visual and hearing impairment	Pyrexia	Medication (opioids, benzodiazepines, anticholinergic)
Functional dependence		
Immobility		

tions such as deep vein thrombosis and pneumonia. Finally, early recognition of delirium is necessary and the process of recognizing and reducing the development of cognitive dysfunction should continue into the postoperative period. The occurrence of postoperative delirium is common and often underdiagnosed with reported incidences in the elderly population of up to 50% in patients undergoing emergency surgery [32]. Both older age and emergency surgery are two out of eleven risk factors for the development of delirium in the ICU [33]. A table describing the risk factors for delirium (adapted from NICE guidance) can be seen in Table 1 [34]. In 2015, the American Geriatrics Society's Geriatrics for Specialists Initiative published recommendations on the treatment of delirium which included the use of interdisciplinary teams, early mobility and walking, avoiding restraints, sleep hygiene, and adequate nutrition, fluids and oxygen. Ensuring adequate analgesia and avoiding the use of opioids was also recommended. The incidence of perioperative pain in the elderly with cognitive impairment is often underestimated and the adverse effects of pain are well documented in the literature [33]. NICE recommend that the DSM-IV (Diagnostic and Statistical Manual of Mental Disorders) criteria or short-CAM (confusion assessment method) should be used regularly to identify delirium early and that drugs believed to precipitate delirium, including benzodiazepines, opioids, antihistamines (including cyclizine), atropine and sedative hypnotics, be avoided if at all possible [35].

Trainee and surgeon education is another area that warrants further exploration. It is not surprising to discover that the majority of surgical trainees have not received any formal training in geriatric medicine. A recent study found that implementation of a formal geriatric teaching program to surgical trainees led to improved recognition and treatment of medical geriatric issues, such as delirium and acute renal impairment [36]. Conversely, increasing the understanding of surgical management in geriatric trainees may be of use and lead to an improved collaborative approach. Although this article has highlighted various areas that are thought to influence outcome in the emergency surgical setting, further research on the elderly population undergoing high-risk surgery is essential. It is appreciated however that undertaking research in emergency surgery can be challenging due to issues such as consent and urgency of intervention. Data analysis of studies have shown that elderly patients are often underrepresented in surgical trials and geriatric patients are less likely to be enrolled in acute research compared to the middle-aged population [37]. Future studies should therefore focus on this area to allow the same standards of care to be achieved in emergency surgery as they are for elective surgery.

Conclusion

In summary, the elderly population is rapidly growing and the number of older patients undergoing emergency laparotomy surgery continues to increase. The associated morbidity and mortality in such a complex and challenging cohort remains high, although implementation of quality improvement pathways, such as the ELPQuiP model, has been associated with promising results with reductions in mortality. Anesthetists play a key role in the patient's perioperative journey and by highlighting awareness of poor outcomes and implementing strategies to identify and reduce complications early, we can hope to improve perioperative outcomes. Improvement and change cannot be achieved alone and a collaborative multidisciplinary approach is advocated. It is clear at present that further research into the care of the elderly surgical patient is warranted and increased participation in national audit initiatives and quality improvement projects are required to drive further improvement.

References

1. Shapter SL, Paul MJ, White SM (2012) Incidence and annual cost of emergency laparotomy in England: is there a major funding shortfall? Anaesthesia 67:474–478
2. Shah AA, Haider AH, Zogg CK et al (2015) National estimates of predictors of outcomes for emergency general surgery. J Trauma Acute Care Surg 78:482–490
3. Huddart S, Peden C, Swart M et al (2015) Use of a pathway quality improvement care bundle to reduce mortality after emergency laparotomy surgery. Br J Surg 102:57–66
4. Desserud K, Veen T (2016) Emergency general surgery in the geriatric patient. Br J Surg 103:e52–61
5. Svenningsen P, Manoharan T, Foss NB, Lauritsen ML, Bay-Nielsen M (2014) Increased mortality in the elderly after emergency abdominal surgery. Dan Med J 61:A4876
6. Torrance A, Powell S, Griffiths E (2015) Emergency surgery in the elderly: challenges and solutions. Op Acc Em Med 7:55–68
7. Richards T (2007) An age old problem. BMJ 335:698
8. Esses D, Birnbaum A, Bijur P, Shah S, Gleyzer A, Gallagher EJ (2002) Ability of CT to alter decision making in elderly patients with acute abdominal pain. Am J Emerg Med 22:270–272
9. Clegg A, Young J, Iliffe S, Rikke MO, Rockwood K (2013) Frailty in elderly people. Lancet 381:752–762
10. Kenig J, Zychiewicz B, Olszewska U, Barczynski M, Nowak W (2015) Six screening instruments for frailty in older patients qualified for emergency abdominal surgery. Arch Gerontol Geriatr 61:437–442
11. Anderson I, Eddleston J, Grocott M et al (2011) The Higher Risk General Surgical Patient: Towards Improved Care For A Forgotten Group. The Royal College of Surgeons, London.
12. Bilimoira K, Liu Y, Paruch J et al (2013) Development and evaluation of the ACS NSQIP surgical risk calculator: A decision aid and informed consent tool. J Am Coll Surg 217:833–842

13. Al-Temimi MH, Griffee M, Enniss TM, Preston R, Vargo D, Overton S (2012) When is death inevitable after emergency laparotomy? Analysis of the American College of Surgeons National Surgical Quality Improvement Program database. J Am Coll Surg 215:503–511
14. Stoneham M, Murray D, Foss N (2014) Emergency surgery: the big three – abdominal aortic aneurysm, laparotomy and hip fracture. Anaesthesia 69:70–80
15. Brown JB, Gestring ML, Forsythe RM, Stassen NA, Billiar TR, Peitzmann AB (2015) Systolic blood pressure criteria in the National Trauma Triage Protocol for geriatric trauma: 110 is the new 90. J Trauma Acute Care Surg 78:352–359
16. Saunders DI, Murray D, Pichel AC, Varley S, Peden CJ (2012) Variations in mortality after emergency laparotomy: the first report of the UK Emergency Laparotomy Network. Br J Anaesth 109:368–375
17. Griffiths R, Beech F, Brown A (2014) Perioperative care of the elderly. Anaesthesia 69:81–98
18. Wickham A, Highton D, Martin D (2016) Care of elderly patients: a prospective audit of the prevalence of hypotension and the use of BIS intraoperatively in 25 London hospitals. Perioper Med 5:12
19. Marik PE, Cavallazzi R (2013) Does the central venous pressure predict fluid responsiveness? An updated meta-analysis and a plea for some common sense. Crit Care Med 41:1774–1781
20. Hamilton M, Cecconi M, Rhodes A (2011) A systematic review on the use of pre-emptive haemodynamic intervention to improve perioperative outcomes in moderate and high risk surgical patients. Anaesth Analg 112:1392–1402
21. Cove ME, Pinsky MR (2012) Perioperative haemodynamic monitoring. Best Pract Res Clin Anaesthesiol 26:453–462
22. National Institute of Health and Care Excellence (2011) MTG 3. CardioQ-ODM oesophageal Doppler monitor. http://www.nice.org.uk/nicemedia/live/13312/52624/52624.pdf. Accessed August 2016
23. Pearse RM, Harrison DA, MacDonald N et al (2014) Effect of a perioperative, cardiac output-guided hemodynamic therapy algorithm on outcomes following major gastrointestinal surgery: a randomized clinical trial and systematic review. JAMA 311:2181–2190
24. Serejo LG, Pereira de Silvia-Junior F, Bastos JP (2007) Risk factors for pulmonary complications after emergency abdominal surgery. Respir Med 10:808–813
25. Sieber FE, Barnett SR (2011) Preventing postoperative complications in the elderly. Anesthesiol Clin 29:83–97
26. Tao T, Bo L, Chen et al (2014) Effect of protective ventilation on postoperative pulmonary complications in patients undergoing general anesthesia: a meta-analysis of randomized controlled trials. BMJ 4:e005208
27. Futier E, Constantin JM, Paugam-Burtz C et al (2013) IMPROVE Study Group. A trial of intraoperative low-tidal volume ventilation in abdominal surgery. N Engl J Med 369:428–437
28. Wu WC, Smith TS, Henderson WG (2010) Operative blood loss, blood transfusion, and 30-day mortality in older patients after major non cardiac surgery. Ann Surg 252:11–17
29. National Institute of Clinical health and Excellence (2015) Blood transfusion. www.nice.org.uk/guidance/NG24. Accessed September 2016
30. Symons NR, Moorthy K, Almoudaris AM et al (2013) Mortality in high-risk emergency general surgical admissions. Br J Surg 100:1318–1325
31. Partridge JS, Harari D, Martin FC, Dhesi JK (2014) The impact of pre-operative comprehensive geriatric assessment on postoperative outcomes in older patients undergoing scheduled surgery: a systematic review. Anaesthesia 69:8–16
32. National Institute of Clinical health and Excellence (2010) Delirium: Diagnosis, Prevention and Management. https://www.nice.org.uk/guidance/cg103. Accessed August 2016
33. Harsoor SS (2011) Emerging concepts in postoperative pain management. Indian J Anaesth 55:101–103
34. Lloyd DG, Ma D, Vizcaychipi MP (2012) Cognitive decline after anaesthesia and critical care. Continuing Educ Anaesth Crit Care Pain 12:105–109

35. Clegg A, Young JB (2011) Which medications to avoid in people at risk of delirium: a systematic review. Age Ageing 40:23–29
36. Barbas AS, Haney JC, Henry BV, Heflin MT, Lagoo SA (2014) Development and implementation of a formalized geriatric surgery curriculum for general surgery residents. Gerontol Geriatr Educ 35:380–394
37. Hempenius L, Slaets JP, Boelens MA, Van Asselt DZ, de Bock GH, Wiggers T (2013) Inclusion of frail elderly patients in clinical trials: solutions to the problems. J Geriatr Oncol 4:26–31

Part XIII
Simulation

Patient-Specific Real-Time Cardiovascular Simulation as Clinical Decision Support in Intensive Care Medicine

M. Broomé and D. W. Donker

Introduction

Decision making in intensive care medicine is based on combining knowledge about pathophysiology and pharmacology, incorporating available scientific results from multiple sources ideally including the whole spectrum ranging from case studies to randomized controlled trials. It is clear to everyone involved in caring for patients with life-threatening disease that almost infinite variations exist in combinations of underlying diseases and in the presenting pathophysiology. Some reaction patterns and symptoms are encountered on a regular basis, such as an inflammatory state accompanied by capillary fluid leakage and hypotension caused by vasodilatation. This clinical picture is often associated with renal insufficiency and progressive pulmonary failure. Occasionally, it may also be combined with right or left heart failure due to changes in loading conditions, or underlying (non-)ischemic or toxic inflammatory cardiomyopathy. The complexity of this multitude of changes in multiorgan physiology on top of underlying acute and chronic diseases creates diagnostic and therapeutic challenges. It seems as if even the most experienced doctors experience significant problems to correctly understand the relative importance of each contributing factor when many variables change in parallel.

Simulation models offer a realistic alternative to analyze single and multiple factors changing in a complex system, such as the cardiovascular system. During the last few decades, simulation of circulatory physiology has evolved along several different conceptual lines. Early models describing the left ventricle as a time-vary-

M. Broomé (✉)
School of Technology and Health, KTH Royal Institute of Technology
Alfred Nobels Allé 10, 141 52 Huddinge, Sweden
ECMO Centre, Astrid Lindgren Children's Hospital, Karolinska University Hospital
171 76 Stockholm, Sweden
e-mail: michael.broome@karolinska.se

D. W. Donker
Department of Intensive Care Medicine, University Medical Centre Utrecht
3584 CX Utrecht, Netherlands

J.-L. Vincent (ed.), *Annual Update in Intensive Care and Emergency Medicine 2017*,
DOI 10.1007/978-3-319-51908-1_36

ing elastance [1] and the arterial system as a two-element Windkessel [2] have been replaced by closed-loop models with all cardiac chambers and a better representation of the vascular tree including many 0D segments or 1D arterial vessels with propagation of flow and pressure waves [3]. A lot of emphasis has been put on simulating the arterial side of the circulation, while the venous side has been less well described, despite the fact that both a healthy and a failing heart are extremely dependent on filling. This is probably related to the fact that arterial pressure rather than flow and filling pressures are usually measured in clinical practice. Cardiac filling and preload is largely determined by pressures and compliance in the low pressure part of the circulatory system, that is veins and capillaries, where physiology is less well studied. To simulate clinically meaningful pathophysiology in the intensive care setting, a model does not only need to include left ventricular and arterial physiology, but implicitly the interaction between intrathoracic pressures and filling conditions as well as the interdependency between the right and left sides of the heart. This, in turn, requires the design of more complex models including many parameters, which also renders the clinical validation process much more difficult. Moreover, the massive contemporary increase in computational power has made it possible to simulate parts of the system with 3D finite element modeling enabling high spatial and temporal resolution analysis of stresses, strain and flow patterns in, for example, the aorta [4] or the left ventricle [5].

These models create beautiful multicolored animations, but their physiologic relevance is hampered by artificial boundary conditions dictated by both lack of complete understanding of tissue properties and also computational issues. Examples of these boundary conditions are constant pressure or flow profiles as inlet and outlet, rigid walls of arteries, lack of cardiac AV-valves and atria, the absence of a pericardium, predefined ventricular movement patterns, which do not account for longitudinal pumping. It is therefore doubtful if physiological output from 3D models adds any hemodynamic benefits compared to 0D and 1D models. In addition, 3D modeling often requires many hours of computation time in order to simulate just a single heart-beat even when using extremely powerful computers. This scenario limits the clinical availability of data and renders its practical use unrealistic for the intensive care setting. Renewed interest has, therefore, been focusing on the computationally simpler models, with which simulations can be run in real-time within a clinical environment [6]. However, even for these models, more validation work is needed before realistic modeling can be a regular clinical tool and serve decision making in complex situations. In this chapter, we highlight a few possible future directions of cardiovascular modeling embedded in clinical decision-making scenarios.

Model Development

Model development and validation are ongoing processes. Creating a perfect model of a complex system, such as the cardiovascular system, is in fact impossible. Every part of the model has built-in limitations and assumptions that can be violated.

From a strict traditional scientific point-of-view, validation can only be performed in a specified group of patients within the (patho-)physiological range studied. However, the real benefits of a simulation model are particularly appreciated when it can be used as a prediction tool outside the already established and well-known physiology. This way of using a model means that uncertainties are introduced, but it can still generate useful hypotheses about relationships between disease entities and new treatment strategies, which is superior to justifying important decisions purely on 'clinical experience' and subjective beliefs.

The current model is built with cardiac and vascular building blocks as published previously [7–10]. The basic version of the model is a generic physiology of a healthy 30-year-old. The parameters of this generic model can be scaled according to a set of rules to create healthy models of the circulatory system in differently sized persons, based on age, weight and length (Table 1). Furthermore, deliberate modification of parameters enables creation of a full range of pathologies including left and/or right systolic and diastolic heart failure as well as valvular regurgitation and stenosis. Atrial and ventricular septal shunts and a persistent duct can be combined with valve and chamber properties to create complex and realistic individualized cardiac pathology. In this context, it should be realized that a patient with a specific type of structural heart disease inevitably develops inherent secondary changes in physiology. For example, short-term adaptations of autonomic tone and changes in blood-volume will modify the physiology considerably within minutes to hours. Thus, cardiogenic shock due to systolic left heart failure will be accompanied by an increase in sympathetic tone causing vasoconstriction and tachycardia as well as an increase in blood volume to preserve blood pressure and cardiac output. Within days and weeks, significant structural vascular and cardiac remodeling will occur, spanning from the subcellular to the organ level, which clinically manifests itself, e. g., as hypertrophy and dilatation. In clinical reality, all these processes are intermingled and constantly ongoing, which makes it impossible to differentiate with certainty between primary and secondary changes. To simulate all these processes in detail and in parallel is practically not only difficult, but sometimes also unnecessary or even unwanted. It is, in our experience, often better to change only one parameter at a time and build a specific disease state in a stepwise manner. This strategy enables better control of the physiological contributions of both primary and secondary changes and improves pathophysiological understanding.

Generic Model

The current closed-loop real-time model consists of 27 vascular segments, six in the pulmonary circulation and 21 in the systemic circulation, the four cardiac chambers with corresponding valves, atrial and ventricular septal interactions, the pericardium and intrathoracic pressure (Fig. 1). The cardiovascular simulation model has been published elsewhere [7–10]. Briefly, the cardiac chambers are represented as time-varying elastances (Fig. 2) and the closed-loop vascular system segments are characterized by non-linear resistances, compliances, inertias and viscoelastances. Each

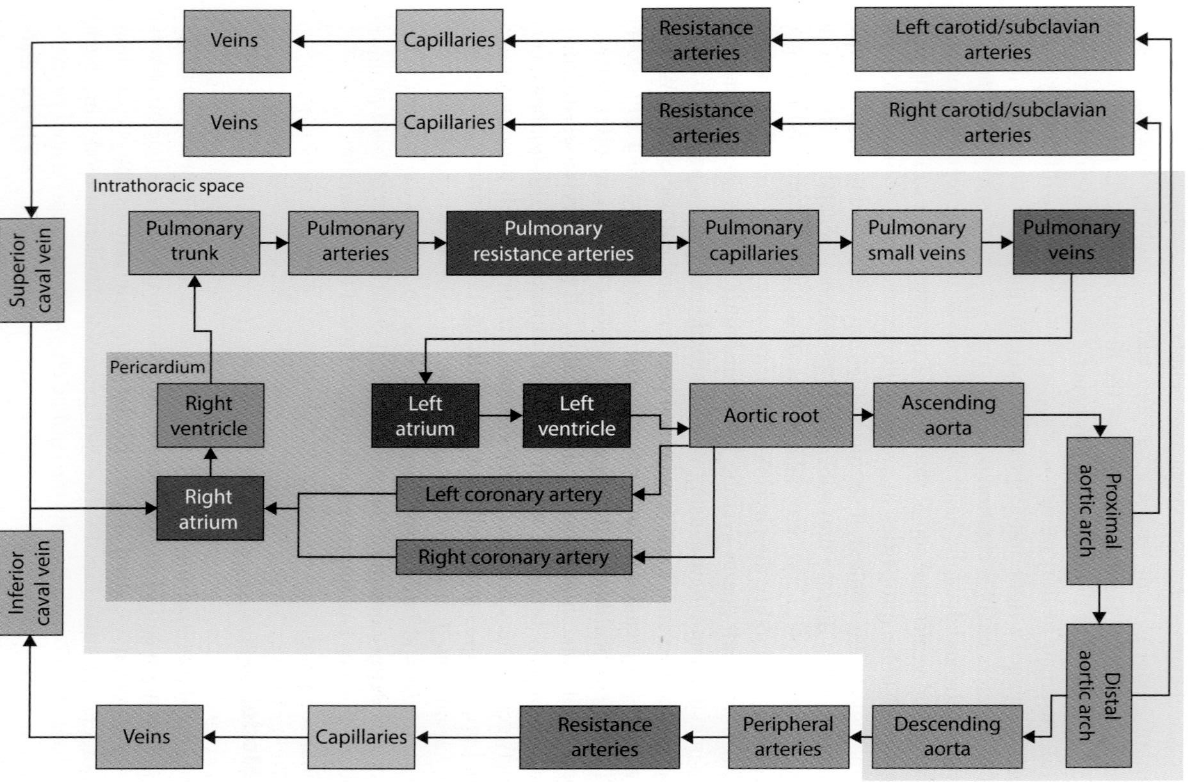

Fig. 1 Block diagram showing an overview of the simulation model. Cardiac chambers are contained within the pericardium (*dark yellow*). The aortic arch and pulmonary circulation are located inside the intrathoracic space (*light yellow*). Peripheral arteries in the lower part of the figure represent vessels supplying the lower body, whereas the head and the upper extremities are supplied by the combined carotid/subclavian arteries shown in the upper part of the diagram

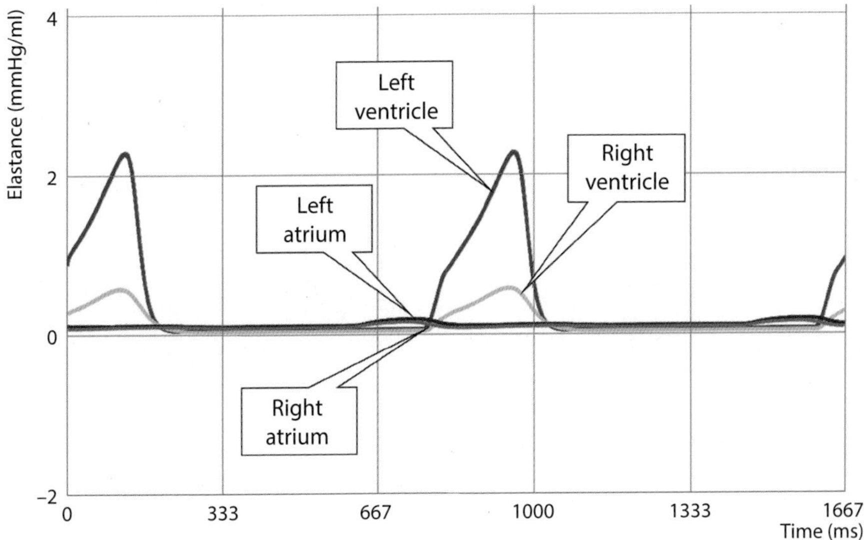

Fig. 2 Cardiac elastance. The amplitude of the function represents contractility and the basal level passive stiffness. The steepness of rise and fall represents synchronicity of contraction and relaxation

compartment is characterized by pressure, volume, flow and oxygen saturation being updated with 4,000 Hz (every 0.25 ms) in real-time. No cardiovascular autonomic reflexes or autoregulatory features are included in the simulations presented, but can be activated in the model to analyze and better understand possible secondary effects of the interventions in question. Valves are simulated as dynamically opening and closing elements depending on pressure gradients and flow (Fig. 3). Atrial and ventricular septal defects as well as a persistent congenital duct connecting the pulmonary artery and aorta can all be simulated.

Vascular Compartments

Each vascular compartment is characterized by length, radius, wall thickness, tissue stiffness (Young's modulus) and the number of parallel vessels. The radius changes dynamically based on intravascular pressure and wall properties, but the other features are assumed constant. Resistance, stiffness, inertance and viscoelastance are calculated and updated dynamically based on these physical properties. Despite the fact that most of these properties are impossible to measure clinically in individual patients, a combination of physics and basic physiological and medical knowledge makes it possible to estimate parameter values [10].

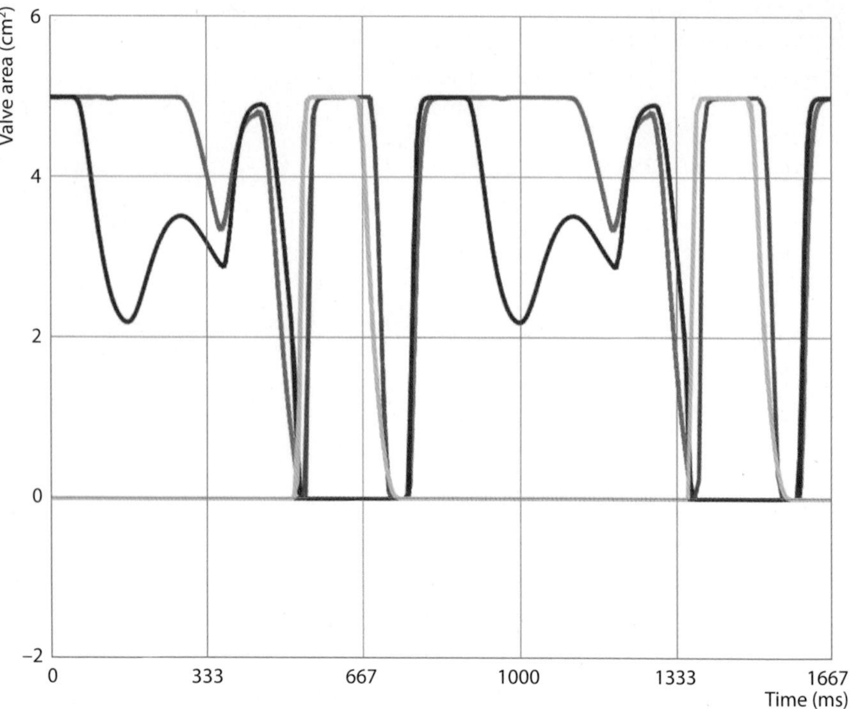

Fig. 3 Valve areas. The aortic valve area (*red*), pulmonary valve area (*yellow*), tricuspid valve area (*blue*) and mitral valve area (*brown*) are indicated in the figure. Please note that the tricuspid and mitral valves partly close during diastasis

Cardiac Chambers

Contractile properties and basal compliance of cardiac chambers are determined by time-varying elastance functions (Fig. 2), which are independent of loading conditions at any given clinical state. Parameter values can be adapted to clinically measured variables, such as ejection fraction, cardiac dimensions and 'invasive' pressure measurements, similar to cardiac catheterization, in a semi-autonomic way.

Valves

The most important valvular properties are the open and closed areas. Flow resistance and inertia are calculated based on these values. In addition, opening and closure behavior are characterized based on separate time constants ([3]; Fig. 3). Validation and fine-tuning of these parameters are done by comparison of valvular flow profiles and transvalvular pressure gradients as available from Doppler echocardiography and cardiac catheterization.

Table 1 Scaling of physiological parameters. Representative examples illustrating the importance of scaling model parameters to the size and age of the patient

Parameter	Scaling principle	1-year old 80 cm, 10 kg	30 years old 170 cm, 70 kg	70 years old 170 cm, 85 kg
Heart rate	$BSA^{-1/3}$	112	72	70
Ascending aortic radius	$BSA^{1/2}$	0.748 cm	1.47 cm	1.68 cm
Ascending aortic length	Body length	1.88 cm	4.00 cm	4.00 cm
Systemic capillary number	BSA	$4.16 \cdot 10^9$	$16.0 \cdot 10^9$	$17.6 \cdot 10^9$
Aortic stiffness Youngs' modulus	$1{,}000 + 1{,}000 \cdot \text{age}$	1,033 mmHg	2,000 mmHg	3,333 mmHg
Left ventricular-contractility	BSA^{-1}	10.8 mmHg/ml	2.80 mmHg/ml	2.54 mmHg/ml

BSA: Body surface area

Model Scaling

It is common sense to index vascular resistance and cardiac output to body surface area (BSA) in clinical practice, which enables a straightforward comparison to generally accepted reference values in all patients. Similar principles apply to scaling of vascular dimensional parameters. The cross sectional area of major vessels scales against BSA, while the length of, e. g., the aorta, scales against the length of the patient only. Small vessels, such as resistance arterioles, capillaries and venules, have the same size in all ages and sizes of patients, but the number of parallel vessels scales against BSA. Somewhat less obvious scaling principles apply to contractile properties of the heart, but these algorithms are based on creating realistic stroke volumes and mean arterial and venous pressures in different age groups. The same is true for blood volume changes during ageing and growth. In general, tissue stiffness increases with increasing age as evident when measuring pulse wave velocity and diastolic cardiac properties. Passive stiffness values change with age in vessels and cardiac chambers. Precise values and mechanisms are unknown, but a combination of published data and intellectual reasoning provides realistic results, although more validation would be advantageous. Some examples of scaling principles are shown in Table 1.

Autoregulatory Features

Local vascular autoregulation has two important components, metabolic and myogenic, both serving to keep blood flow in the tissues adequate. Metabolic autoregulation dilates local resistance arterioles when metabolism increases to adapt flow to the needs of the tissue. In the model, this is controlled by local venous oxygen saturation, although more complex control is found in reality [11]. The myogenic control mechanism is a local stretch reflex, reacting with vascular constriction, when the arterial vessel wall is stretched to keep flow constant despite blood pressure changes [12]. This is in the model controlled by vascular wall tension. The baroreceptor reflex acts through the sympathetic branch of the autonomic nervous system and will react within seconds when pressure in the great arteries changes [13]. A decrease in blood pressure will result in tachycardia, an increase in cardiac contractility, systemic arteriolar vasoconstriction and venous capacitance increasing venous return. All of the above-mentioned autoregulatory reflexes can be activated in the model, but are deactivated as default to allow the user to control the physiology manually, since changing parameters one-by-one likely improves understanding by deciphering complexity step-by-step. Nevertheless, it should be kept in mind that these reflexes are constantly acting in our patients and all potentially have a profound importance for clinical hemodynamics.

Long-term Remodeling

In general, every different entity of cardiovascular disease results in structural remodeling processes within the human cardiovascular system and beyond, and thereby creates characteristic organ manifestations. For example, a specific increase in cardiac chamber or vascular wall tension within the cardiac cycle will result in a distinct hypertrophic phenotype, as seen, for example, in the left ventricle of patients with aortic valve stenosis or arterial hypertension. In a similar way, an increase in flow, which manifests itself as an increase in wall shear stress, will result in dilatation, as seen in for example regurgitant valvular disease or pulmonary shunts. Remodeling can be both beneficial and detrimental. After interventions, some degree of reverse remodeling can almost always be expected within months depending on individual characteristics [14]. When predicting results of hemodynamic interventions, it is important to distinguish between acute and secondary changes due to (reverse) remodeling. Algorithms in the model are being developed for cardiac, pericardial and vascular remodeling and all of these model features require separate validation.

Patient-specific Adaptation

A key feature in the prediction of individual treatment responses is the reliability of the simulation of an individual hemodynamic state before an intended intervention. The precision needed differs for different scenarios. When contemplating qualitatively gross left ventricular unloading effects of a ventricular assist device in systolic left heart failure, it might even suffice to use a generic patient; but in a child with pulmonary hypertension, right ventricular hypertrophy and combined pulmonary valvular stenosis after multiple previous corrections, a more detailed approach is needed. A major challenge in patient-specific adaptation is to translate clinically available information, such as continuous monitoring of vital parameters, data from a cardiac catheterization and echocardiographic study, to model parameters. In general, clinical data are not sufficient to determine the large number of model parameters in a rigorous way, but a strategy of combining physiological knowledge with mathematical fitting algorithms is needed to achieve reasonable results in a semi-automatic way. Obviously, post-intervention physiology will be affected not only by the intervention itself, but also by short-term autoregulatory effects and long-term structural remodeling.

Simulation of Treatment Options

The model and its user interface software contain treatment options like the intra-aortic balloon pump, an ascending aortic axial pump (Impella™), venovenous and venoarterial extracorporeal membrane oxygenation (ECMO), left and right ventricular assist devices and positive pressure mechanical ventilation, incorporating resultant cardiovascular effects.

Future Implications of Patient-specific Adaptation

To illustrate how simulation could advance current daily practice, three different clinical scenarios have been constructed and will be discussed further below:

1. a 65-year old female with severe cardiogenic shock due to systolic left heart failure caused by an acute myocardial infarction and supported with venoarterial ECMO;
2. a 44-year old male with right heart failure due to progressive pulmonary hypertension in need of a palliative atrial septostomy;
3. a 5-year old boy with an uncorrected Tetralogy of Fallot with a ventricular septal defect (VSD), right heart hypertrophy and dilatation due to a residual pulmonary stenosis despite earlier catheter-based valvular interventions.

Extracorporeal Membrane Oxygenation in Cardiogenic Shock

The cardiac unloading effect of venoarterial ECMO in cardiogenic shock caused by left heart systolic failure is often disappointing [7, 15]. A progressive increase in left heart loading and oxygen consumption with increasing ECMO flow has been suggested [7, 16]. A virtual case representing a 65-year old woman with left heart systolic failure due to an acute myocardial infarction was simulated by decreasing left ventricular contractility from 2.8 to 0.8 mmHg/ml resulting in left atrial pressure (LAP) of 14 mmHg, a decrease in cardiac output from 5.8 to 3.2 l/min and a systemic arterial pressure of 80/55 mmHg (Fig. 4a).

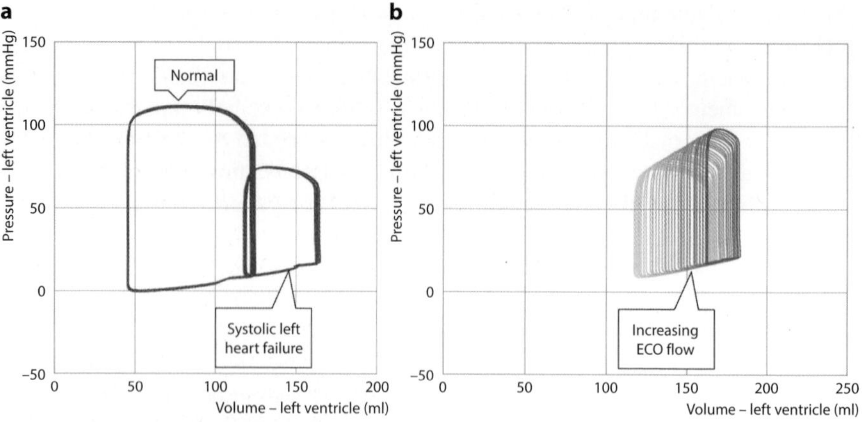

Fig. 4 Simulated pressure-volume loops in systolic left heart failure and venoarterial ECMO. Pressure-volume loops in left panel represent the left ventricle in a 65-year old female with normal function and systolic left heart failure (**a** left panel) and left heart dilatation with increasing venoarterial ECMO flow 0–4 l/min (**b** right panel). Pressure and volume variations arise from ongoing spontaneous breathing with inherent variation of intrathoracic pressures and related hemodynamic effects

A further increase in LAP to 20 mmHg was seen when increasing ECMO flow from 0 to 4 l/min (Fig. 4b). Some LV unloading was accomplished in the model by systemic arterial vasodilatation aiming for a mean arterial pressure (MAP) of 60 mmHg, but unloading was still considered unsatisfactory and other adjunct therapies were explored. For example, the addition of an intra-aortic balloon pump to ECMO decreased LAP from 20 to 18 mmHg and end-systolic left ventricular volume from 164 to 151 ml (Fig. 5). Alternatively, an axial pump placed through the aortic valve reaching a flow 2.5 l/min and an adjustment of the systemic vascular resistance to a MAP of 70 mmHg decreased LAP from 20 to 10 mmHg and end-systolic left ventricular volume from 164 to 109 ml (Fig. 5). Another therapeutic option would be to create an atrial septostomy with a diameter of 10 mm, which enables LAP to be decreased from 20 to 9 mmHg and left ventricular end-systolic volume from 164 to 119 ml.

Palliative Atrial Septostomy in Pulmonary Hypertension

Progressive right heart failure is seen in end-stage idiopathic pulmonary hypertension in adults. Symptoms are mainly related to venous congestion, but also due to the lack of ability to increase cardiac output in response to changes in workload [17]. Right atrial pressure (RAP) is usually much higher than LAP as indicated by an atrial septum bulging from the right to left side of the atrium as visualized on echocardiograms. It has long been known that performing a balloon atrial septostomy in these patients can result in palliative symptomatic relief [17]. This

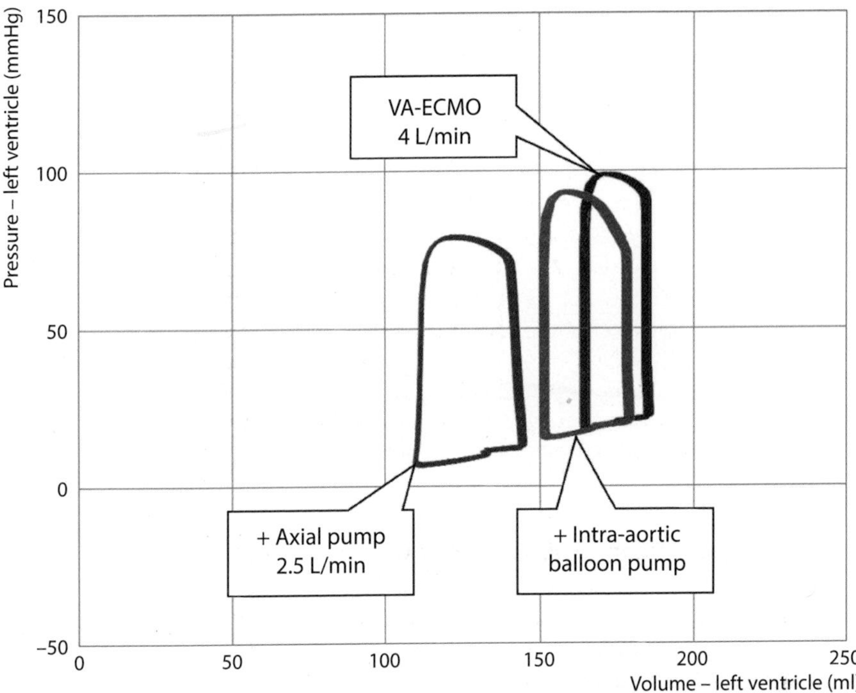

Fig. 5 Simulated pressure-volume loops during venoarterial ECMO with adjunct therapies. Pressure-volume in *gray* represents the left ventricle in a 65-year old female with systolic left heart dilatation supported by venoarterial ECMO with a flow of 4 l/min. Left ventricle pressure-volume loops in *red* illustrate the unloading effect of an intra-aortic balloon pump, whereas loops in *purple* show the unloading effect of a transaortic axial pump flow of 2.5 l/min with an adjusted systemic vascular resistance aiming for a mean arterial pressure of 70 mmHg. Pressure and volume variations due to ongoing breathing with inherent variation of intrathoracic pressures and related hemodynamic effects

intervention reduces venous congestion and increases left heart filling and cardiac output, although a 'price is paid' as right-left shunting of deoxygenated blood occurs.

A correctly sized atrial septal defect will result in an arterial saturation of about 85% and an increase in oxygen transport. By simulating the effects of different sizes of 'implantable' atrial flow regulator devices in a fictive 44-year old male with right heart failure due to progressive pulmonary hypertension, possible benefits and pitfalls of this treatment can be analyzed in detail (Fig. 6; Table 2).

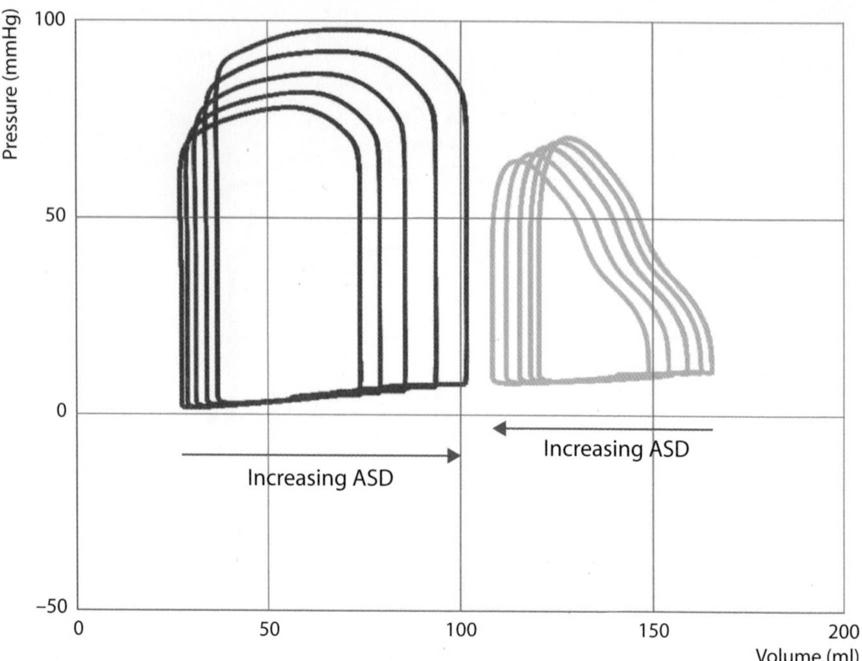

Fig. 6 Simulated pressure-volume loops representing effects of atrial septal shunting in pulmonary hypertension. Increasing atrial septal defect (ASD) size results in a less dilated right ventricle (*yellow*) and improved left ventricular (*red*) filling

Table 2 Simulated hemodynamic effects of atrial septal shunting in pulmonary hypertension. Arterial oxygen saturation decreases due to right-left shunting with increasing size of the atrial septal defect, but systemic oxygen delivery increases due to an increase in right-left shunting and cardiac output

		No device	Ø 4 mm	Ø 6 mm	Ø 8 mm	Ø 10 mm
RAP	mmHg	10	10	10	10	9
LAP	mmHg	4	4	5	6	6
Cardiac output	l/min	3.36	3.62	3.94	4.31	4.67
Arterial oxygen saturation	%	92	87	82	76	72
Qp/Qs	–	1:1	0.89:1	0.81:1	0.70:1	0.63:1
Oxygen delivery	ml/min	577	590	604	619	634

RAP: right atrial pressure; *LAP*: left atrial pressure; *Qp/Qs*: pulmonary-systemic flow ratio

Pulmonary Valve Dilatation in Corrected Tetralogy of Fallot

Tetralogy of Fallot is an important group of congenital heart defects with a pulmonary outflow restriction either in the right ventricular outflow tract or in the

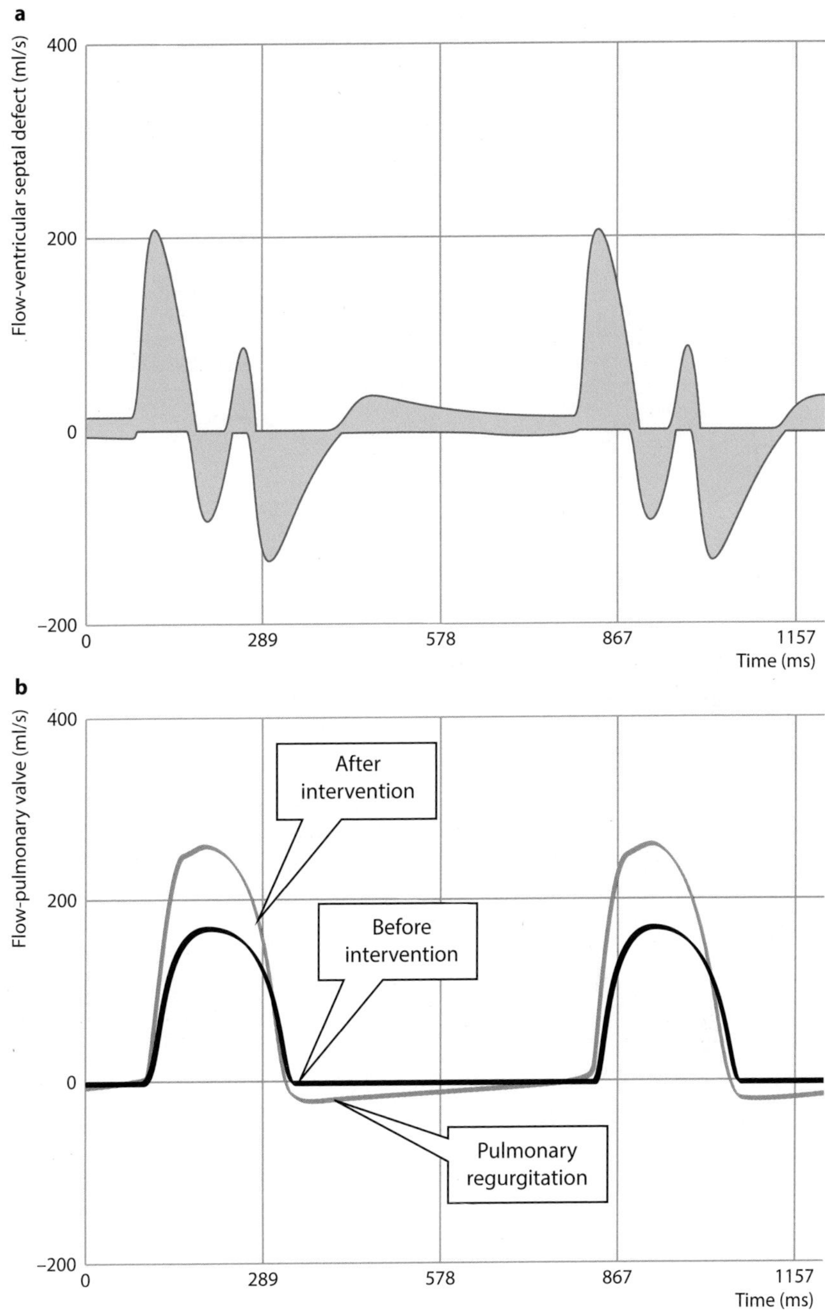

Fig. 7 Simulated VSD and pulmonary valve flows in 5-year old boy with uncorrected Tetralogy of Fallot. A bi-directional left-right VSD flow with a non-restrictive VSD Ø 10 mm and pulmonary stenosis Ø 8 mm (**a**) is seen prior to the intervention. Pulmonary valve flow (**b**) increases after intervention (*orange*) compared to before intervention (*black*), although a diastolic pulmonary regurgitant flow is also seen post-intervention

pulmonary valve itself combined with a VSD, an overriding aorta and secondary right ventricular hypertrophy.

Tetralogy of Fallot is the most common cyanotic congenital heart defect in the western world [18]. The pulmonary valve may exhibit anything ranging from only slight narrowing to total absence. In a severe case with pulmonary valve atresia, blood shunts from right to left through the VSD (Fig. 7a), and pulmonary blood flow is provided solely by an open ductus arteriosus in the early neonatal period.

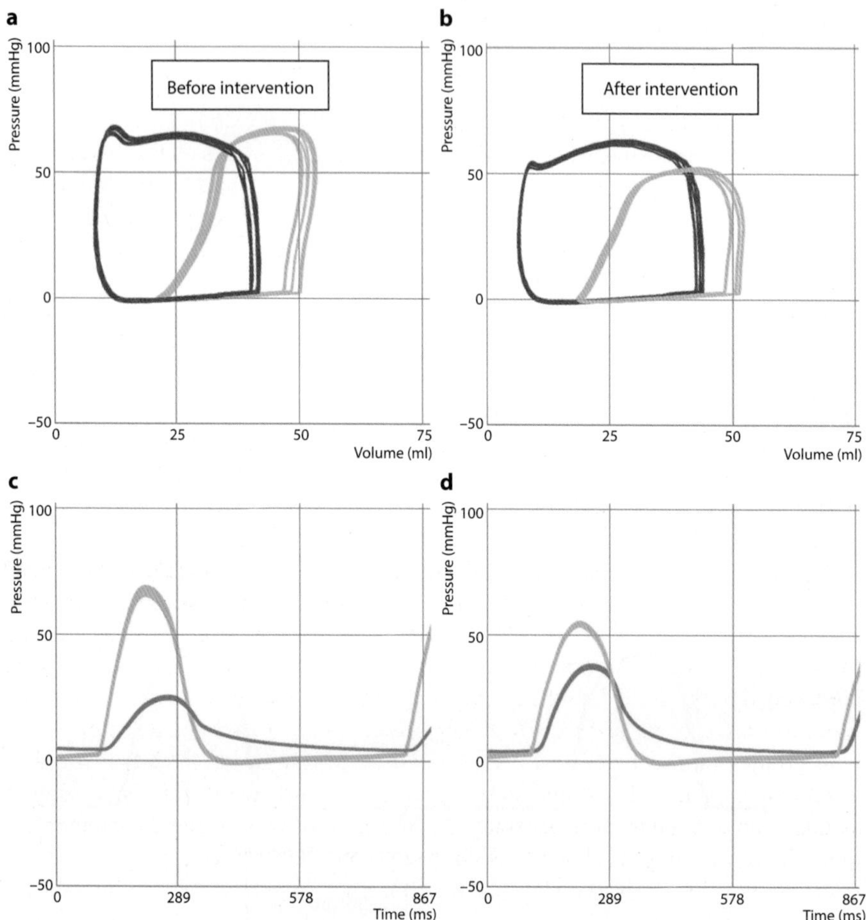

Fig. 8 Simulated pressure-volume (PV) loops and pressures in 5-year old boy with an uncorrected Tetralogy of Fallot. The upper panel shows PV-loops from the left (*red*) and right (*yellow*) ventricle with a non-restrictive VSD Ø 10 mm and pulmonary stenosis Ø 8 mm (**a**) and after pulmonary valve dilatation to Ø 12 mm with some residual pulmonary regurgitation (**b**). The lower panel shows right ventricular (*yellow*) and pulmonary artery (*orange*) pressures before (**c**) and after (**d**) intervention. Peak-to-peak gradient decreases from almost 50 mmHg to less than 20 mmHg. Pressure and volume variations due to ongoing spontaneous breathing

With repeated catheter-based dilatations of the pulmonary valve increasing flow through the pulmonary circulation can be achieved, although some degree of pulmonary valve regurgitation often results after the interventions. Combinations of valvular stenosis and regurgitation can be explored in a simulation of a fictive 5-year old boy with a previously uncorrected tetralogy of Fallot. Results of a successful percutaneous valve dilatation are shown in Fig. 7b and 8, with an open valve diameter increasing from 8 to 12 mm.

Future Perspective

A large variety of complex hemodynamic scenarios can realistically be simulated in adult and pediatric patients in real-time. This enables possible effects of planned interventions to be explored and analyzed and greatly improves pathophysiological understanding. Moreover, it enables quantitative estimates of all relevant parameters to be generated, which, in turn, enables clinicians to create an 'educated guess' on the relative importance of contributing factors. Model validation and development of dedicated algorithms for patient-specific simulation including appropriate parameter settings remain challenging endeavors. Moreover, the complexity increases when indirect hemodynamic effects mediated by neuro-humoral influences, autoregulatory reflexes and structural remodeling are taken into account, which is possible in current models. However, it is not realistic to build a perfect model, since understanding of cardiovascular physiology is far from complete. In addition, individual variation, due to genetic and environmental factors, induces important sources of errors in acute hemodynamics and in secondary effects related to autoregulation and remodeling.

Current decisions based on clinical experience and the knowledge of individual doctors are, however, not foolproof. Thus, the key question remains when patient-specific modeling reaches the state of maturation that enables decision making to be improved beyond current clinical practice. This question can potentially be approached with clinical studies comparing different modes of decision making. From a formal scientific perspective this needs to be done separately in every patient group. It may, therefore, be more realistic to introduce simulation software as an educational tool first and slowly progress towards clinical decision support as this approach gains more acceptance and can be used as a true complementary tool adding meaningful clinical insight to current methods. Grouping of patients with complex disease is also difficult, since disease presentations by definition vary among individuals.

0D-models can be run in real-time and interventions thus tested within minutes. This increases usability and optimizes understanding, since fast feed-back is a key to efficient learning.

3D-models often require hours to simulate one heart-beat on supercomputers and are therefore not readily available as clinical tools. Furthermore, these complex models often suffer from severe restrictions due to artificial boundary conditions violating fundamental physiological rules. There are specific clinical problems, where detailed 3D-simulations are needed for full understanding, such as in regional left ventricular hypokinesia/dyskinesia in ischemic heart disease and left ventricular dyssynchrony due to electrophysiological disturbances. These problems may be approached by combining detailed 3D-modeling of the left ventricle with 0D- or 1D-models of the remaining circulatory system. In these circumstances it is crucial to include both the right side of the heart, atria, the pericardium, the venous, pulmonary and arterial vasculature, since symptoms in heart failure and other cardiovascular disorders are usually related to the interaction between the heart, the vasculature and surrounding structures.

The advantages with real-time simulation and fast feed-back are so large that low order models with 0D-components should be preferred whenever possible. It is our experience that this is possible in the majority of hemodynamic challenges encountered in intensive care medicine.

Model validation is an ongoing process. Some clinically relevant conclusions can be drawn from models already at the current stage of development [3, 7–9, 19–21]. In other areas, more development and validation is needed. It is suggested that interested clinicians start to become acquainted with these tools already now, because a lot of creativity and deep understanding can be found in the process of comparing clinical experience with simulation models with open, but also critical eyes.

Conclusion

Real-time computer simulation of patient-specific complex cardiovascular disease is readily available. Automatic algorithms featuring scaling and adaptation to specific disease states and individual patient characteristics are key elements of clinical decision-support simulation software. Using this method, realistic predictions can be accomplished in individual case scenarios, which may support planned interventions and device-related treatment modalities. Clinical validation is ongoing and considered of utmost importance in order to allow reliable clinical decision making and for simulation to enter the often complex clinical arena.

References

1. Suga H, Sagawa K, Shoukas AA (1973) Load independence of the instantaneous pressure-volume ratio of the canine left ventricle and effects of epinephrine and heart rate on the ratio. Circ Res 32:314–322
2. Stergiopulos N, Westerhof BE, Westerhof N (1999) Total arterial inertance as the fourth element of the windkessel model. Am J Physiol 276:H81–H88
3. Mynard JP, Davidson MR, Penny DJ, Smolich JJ (2011) A simple versatile model of valve dynamics for use in lumped parameter and one-dimensional cardiovascular models. Int J Numer Meth Biomed Engng 28:626–641
4. Prahl Wittberg L, van Wyk S, Fuchs L, Gutmark E, Backeljauw P, Gutmark-Little I (2016) Effects of aortic irregularities on blood flow. Biomech Model Mechanobiol 15:345–360

5. Cheng Y, Oertel H, Schenkel T (2005) Fluid-structure coupled CFD simulation of the left ventricular flow during filling phase. Ann Biomed Eng 33:567–576
6. Shi Y, Lawford P, Hose R (2011) Review of zero-D and 1-D models of blood flow in the cardiovascular system. Biomed Eng Online 10:33
7. Broome M, Donker DW (2016) Individualized real-time clinical decision support to monitor cardiac loading during venoarterial ECMO. J Transl Med 14:4
8. Lindfors M, Frenckner B, Sartipy U, Bjallmark A, Broome M (2016) Venous cannula positioning in arterial deoxygenation during veno-arterial extracorporeal membrane oxygenation – a simulation study and case report. Artif Organs April 18, Epub ahead of print
9. Broman M, Frenckner B, Bjallmark A, Broome M (2015) Recirculation during veno-venous extra-corporeal membrane oxygenation – a simulation study. Int J Artif Organs 38:23–30
10. Broome M, Maksuti E, Bjallmark A, Frenckner B, Janerot-Sjoberg B (2013) Closed-loop real-time simulation model of hemodynamics and oxygen transport in the cardiovascular system. Biomed Eng Online 12:69
11. Goodman AH, Einstein R, Granger HJ (1978) Effect of changing metabolic rate on local blood flow control in the canine hindlimb. Circ Res 43:769–776
12. Folkow B (1989) Myogenic mechanisms in the control of systemic resistance. Introduction and historical background. J Hypertens Suppl 7:S1–S4
13. Pilowsky PM, Goodchild AK (2002) Baroreceptor reflex pathways and neurotransmitters: 10 years on. J Hypertens 20:1675–1688
14. Kehat I, Molkentin JD (2010) Molecular pathways underlying cardiac remodeling during pathophysiological stimulation. Circulation 122:2727–2735
15. Boulate D, Luyt CE, Pozzi M et al (2013) Acute lung injury after mechanical circulatory support implantation in patients on extracorporeal life support: an unrecognized problem. Eur J Cardiothorac Surg 44:544–549
16. Ostadal P, Mlcek M, Kruger A et al (2015) Increasing venoarterial extracorporeal membrane oxygenation flow negatively affects left ventricular performance in a porcine model of cardiogenic shock. J Transl Med 13:266
17. McLaughlin VV, Shah SJ, Souza R, Humbert M (2015) Management of pulmonary arterial hypertension. J Am Coll Cardiol 65:1976–1997
18. Villafane J, Feinstein JA, Jenkins KJ et al (2013) Hot topics in tetralogy of Fallot. J Am Coll Cardiol 62:2155–2166
19. Lumens J, Arts T, Broers B et al (2009) Right ventricular free wall pacing improves cardiac pump function in severe pulmonary arterial hypertension: a computer simulation analysis. Am J Physiol Heart Circ Physiol 297:H2196–H2205
20. Kerckhoffs RC, Lumens J, Vernooy K (2008) Cardiac resynchronization: insight from experimental and computational models. Prog Biophys Mol Biol 97:543–561
21. Arts T, Delhaas T, Bovendeerd P, Verbeek X, Prinzen FW (2005) Adaptation to mechanical load determines shape and properties of heart and circulation: the CircAdapt model. Am J Physiol Heart Circ Physiol 288:H1943–H1954

Making the Best Use of Simulation Training in Critical Care Medicine

A. Mahoney, J. Vassiliadis, and M. C. Reade

Introduction

Oscar Wilde once quipped that "*experience is the one thing you can't get for nothing*". While this may once have been true, simulation-based education in critical care aims to achieve just that, by exposing participants to complex situations in a realistic but safe environment, in which their performance becomes a powerful vehicle for learning, through non-judgmental debriefing and participant reflection. The aim is to decrease adverse events for patients and at the same time improve the quality and efficiency of healthcare professional training.

In this chapter, we outline the history of simulation-based education in critical care before considering the theoretical underpinnings, advantages, and limitations of the various forms of simulation. The influence of stress on learning and performance will be discussed and the chapter will conclude by outlining core principles for best-practice use of simulation-based education within critical care.

A. Mahoney
2nd General Health Battalion, Australian Regular Army
Brisbane, QLD, Australia

J. Vassiliadis
Sydney Clinical Skills and Simulation Centre, Royal North Shore Hospital
Sydney, NSW, Australia
Discipline of Emergency Medicine, Sydney Medical School
Sydney, NSW, Australia
Royal Australian Naval Reserve
Sydney, NSW, Australia

M. C. Reade (✉)
2nd General Health Battalion, Australian Regular Army
Brisbane, QLD, Australia
Military Medicine and Surgery, University of Queensland
Brisbane, QLD, Australia
Australian Defense Force Joint Health Command
Canberra, ACT 2610, Australia
e-mail: m.reade@uq.edu.au

J.-L. Vincent (ed.), *Annual Update in Intensive Care and Emergency Medicine 2017*,
DOI 10.1007/978-3-319-51908-1_37

History of Simulation in Critical Care

Simulation may be defined as a teaching method that evokes and replicates substantial aspects of the real world in a fully interactive manner [1]. Like many industries that involve 'routine but risky' activities, the critical care disciplines of anesthesia, intensive care and emergency medicine were early proponents of simulation [2]. The first cardiopulmonary resuscitation (CPR) trainer, 'Resusci-Anne', was developed by Laerdal in the 1960s and shortly thereafter the first patient simulator was produced by Gordon [3]. Together with the development of 'standardized patients' by Barrows in the 1980s, these innovations marked the beginning of the modern era of medical simulation [1, 4]. Subsequently, Gaba and colleagues built upon this foundation by integrating technology-based simulators with standardized patients and confederates within a replicated work environment, the Comprehensive Anesthesia Simulation Environment (CASE), which would be familiar to contemporary users of purpose-designed simulation centers [2].

The rapid evolution of simulation technology in the second half of the 20th century coincided with exposition of new educational theories, which recognized concrete experiences relevant to the workplace as the foundation of adult learning. From the 1990s onward, curriculum designers have increasingly integrated simulation within undergraduate and postgraduate medical education, often bridging the transition between theoretical instruction and application of knowledge in clinical environments [5].

In the 21st century, simulation-based education has become almost 'infinitely scalable'. Simulator complexity ranges from improvised models fashioned in the workplace, through isolated limb part-task trainers, to highly sophisticated hybrid devices used in conjunction with standardized patients. Similarly, the context in which simulation-based education is practiced ranges from purpose built centers to individualized 'just-in-time' training at the bedside. The technology, theory and application of contemporary simulation-based education will be explored in greater detail in subsequent sections.

Modes of Simulation

Simulated clinical environments can be achieved using standardized patients, full body mannequins, part-task trainers, computer-generated simulators or hybrid simulators.

Standardized patients are either actors given a script or patients trained to present their condition in a reproducible way. Part-task trainers are models used for deliberate practice of procedural skills, such as model arms for venepuncture [6]. Full body mannequins are familiar to all who have completed CPR training. Computer-generated simulators are virtual environments, often used to familiarize learners with the operation of a piece of equipment that would otherwise be unavailable to them; virtual bronchoscopy is a notable example [7].

Hybrid simulators combine simulated patients with part-task trainers, allowing contextualization of learning; examples include the model developed by the Swedish military to teach control of catastrophic hemorrhage [8], or damage control surgery simulators employed by the Australian Defense Force (Fig. 1).

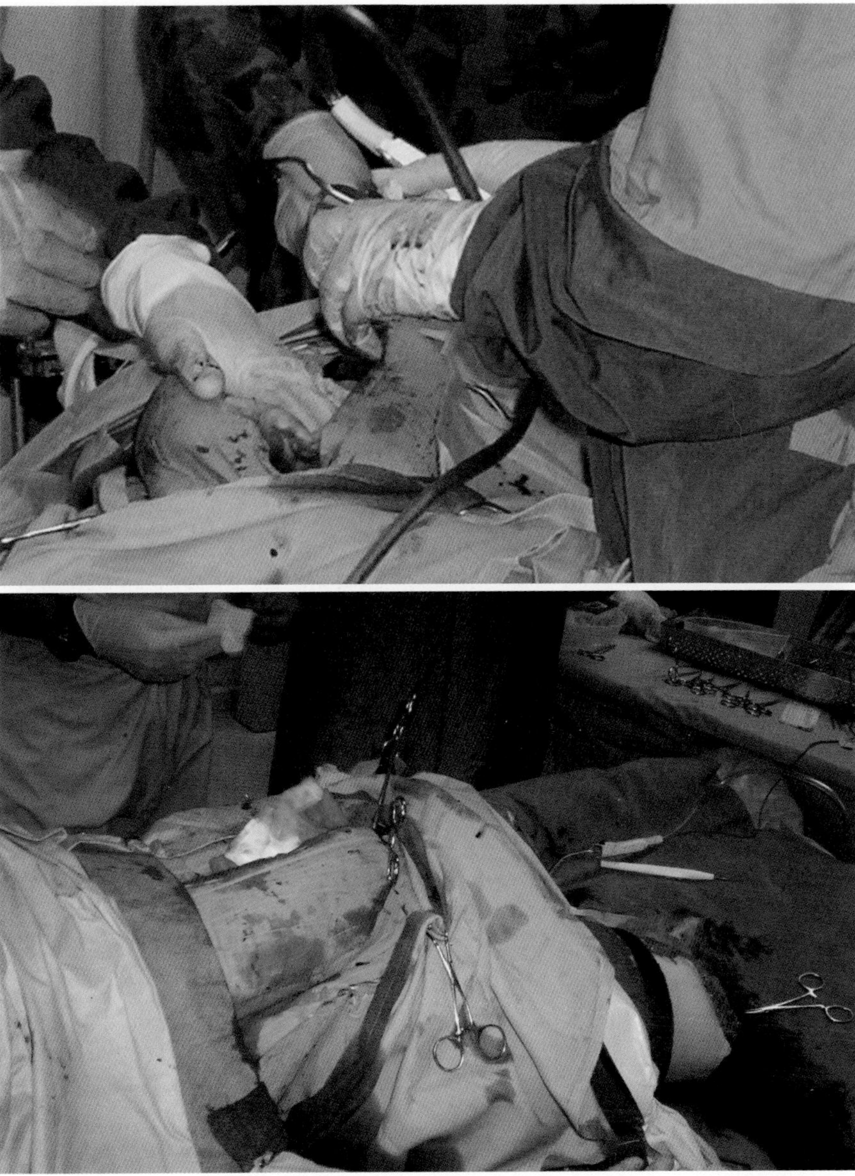

Fig. 1 Australian Defense Force damage control surgery simulations. Figures reproduced with Courtesy of the Sydney Clinical Skills and Simulation Centre

Justification for the Use of Simulation

Theoretical, practical and ethical imperatives, together with published evidence of efficacy, justify the use of simulation in critical care education.

Theoretical Imperative

The use of simulation-based education in critical care medicine is supported by several theories of adult learning. Knowles' constructivist theory of adult learning, 'androgogy', assumes that adult learners possess a reservoir of experience that forms a resource for learning and that they are internally motivated to apply knowledge in a manner purposeful to their workplace [9]. The associated experiential learning model proposed by Kolb also emphasizes concrete experience as the catalyst for reflection and consolidation of understanding [10]. Indeed, Kolb argues that it is only when learners test the implications of their learning in new situations that their understanding is consolidated; hence some authors have argued that repeated simulation following debriefing represents an ideal learning encounter [11]. Similarly, transformative learning theorists, such as Mezirow, suggest that learners encountering a disorienting dilemma are triggered to engage in critical reflection on their existing cognitive schema, thereby transforming their perspective [12].

These theories establish concrete experience, critical reflection and application of lessons to the workplace as the *sine qua non* of adult learning. Consequently, with the exception of direct clinical experience, simulation has greater face validity than any other teaching technique for promoting adult learning in critical care.

Practical Imperative

Simulation allows learners to be exposed to high-risk situations that they would rarely encounter in the workplace [1]. This may be particularly beneficial for medical practitioners who are 'transitioning' to a role that will require them to exercise a greater degree of clinical responsibility; for example junior doctor to specialist trainee, or specialist trainee to junior consultant [13].

Ethical Imperative

Learning through contact with patients has long been considered the foundation of medical education. Unfortunately, 'hands-on' teaching may have ethical implications when learning objectives relate to complex or critically ill patients. Traditionally, learning through supervised practice on patients has been justified by the utilitarian judgement that society needs a well-trained medical workforce. However, the principle of non-maleficence dictates that learners should not harm patients. Therefore iatrogenic injuries caused by clinicians in the course of their learning can only be justified when all reasonable efforts have been taken to minimize harm to patients, including the use of alternative educational approaches such as simulation [14].

Efficacy of Simulation-based Education

A commonly employed means of evaluating the efficacy of educational interventions is through use of Kirkpatrick's hierarchy, the four levels of which are reaction, learning, behavior and results [15]. This section will precis the evidence in support of simulation-based education for each of the four Kirkpatrick levels.

Reaction

Several meta-analyses and systematic reviews have established that simulation is viewed positively by almost all learners [16, 17]. Unfortunately, perceived value does not reliably predict post-simulation performance [18].

Learning

Both self-reported and objectively measured knowledge transfer has been demonstrated after simulation-based education. Notable examples include improved skills acquisition for advanced cardiac life support, central venous catheter insertion, thoracocentesis and fiberoptic intubation [19]

Behavior

Behavioral changes have been demonstrated after simulation-based education programs, both in repeat simulation and in the workplace. Examples include improved bedside skills among intensive care residents [20], improved adherence to trauma treatment protocols [21], and improved management of simulated malignant hyperthermia cases [22]. However, the duration of behavioral change has varied significantly between studies [16].

Results

Within the Kirkpatrick levels of evaluation, 'results' refers to the impact of the intervention on organizationally meaningful endpoints, such as patient outcomes. Historically, while there has been an abundance of evidence supporting simulation driven improvements in knowledge and certain behaviors, there has been a paucity of data pointing to patient-centered gains [6].

Recently however, a number of studies has established causal links between simulation-based education and key clinical goals. Improved central line insertion success and reduced infection rates have been reported in several Canadian studies of simulation-based mastery learning [23]. With regard to more complex learning outcomes, for pediatric medical emergency teams at one hospital in Edinburgh, implementation of regular simulation training resulted in earlier recognition of deteriorating patients, more patients transferred from the ward to intensive care and a lower hospital mortality [24]. Similarly, a Hawaiian trauma center improved the timeliness and completeness of treatment through an *in situ* simulation program [21].

Fidelity in Simulation

A 'perfect' simulation would be indistinguishable from the clinical environment in which learners work. Often it is said that a simulation that closely replicates the clinical environment has 'high fidelity'. However, for a number of reasons the unitary conception of fidelity is unhelpful and arguably the term should be eschewed in favor of more tightly defined concepts.

Fidelity is multifaceted. 'Reality' in the setting of simulation has several dimensions. One model makes reference to physical reality, conceptual (semantical) reality and emotional (phenomenal) reality [25, 26]. Each of these concepts is outlined below.

Physical Reality

Physical reality includes those aspects of the simulation environment that can be measured or directly observed, for example the physical characteristics of a resuscitation mannequin or of the monitoring equipment.

Conceptual Reality

Conceptual reality includes those aspects of the simulated environment that are 'facts only by human agreement', such as concepts and the relationship between them. An example of conceptual reality is the observation that when the mannequin loses blood, the blood pressure falls. Importantly with regard to conceptual reality, the manner in which this information is communicated to the participant is not relevant; simulated monitoring, a verbal description or signs exhibited by the mannequin would function equally well. Hence, conceptual realism may be achieved independently of physical realism [25].

Emotional Reality

Emotional reality refers to the emotional states and beliefs that learners experience during simulation. Simulation is a social construct that is experienced in two ways: firstly, as a complex real-time situation and secondly as a learning encounter intended to replicate a particular clinical context [25]. Successful simulation results in learners experiencing the clinical scenario envisaged by the teacher, which relates to the intended goals of the session. Learners are then able to make conceptual sense of the scenario despite shortcomings in physical reality.

Practical Implications

The most salient question arising from the multidimensional model of simulated reality outlined above is – which aspect of reality matters most? The answer depends upon the intended learning objectives.

Traditional conceptions of fidelity were often conflated with physical reality. Simulation centers and mannequins were regularly modified to more closely replicate real life patients and artefacts. Unfortunately, increasing physical reality does not reliably increase learner engagement [25]. Rather, learners need to be willing to enter into a 'fiction contract' and their willingness may be more heavily determined by the conceptual and emotional reality of the scenario than its tangible trappings.

Manual dexterity tasks may require a greater focus on the physical properties of the requisite movements. This does not imply that the simulator must be an exact replication of the tissues or equipment, but rather there needs to be sufficient similarity to allow the learner to engage. The threshold for engagement will vary from task to task and from learner to learner. Indeed, it has been demonstrated that a simulator found to have characteristics suitable for learning of one procedural skill, such as fiberoptic intubation, may be unsuitable for the teaching of an ostensibly similar skill, such as videolaryngoscopy [27].

On the other hand, conceptual fidelity is paramount for scenarios designed to develop learners' clinical reasoning. Further, emotional fidelity leading to high engagement synergistically enhances the physical and conceptual realism of simulation [26]; this observation is explored in a later section on the role of stress in simulation training.

Cognitive Frames

'Frames' are a construct proposed by Goffman to explain how learners make sense of situations [28]. Frames are cognitive structures incorporating attitudes, beliefs, information and prior experiences; one example would be the 'difficult airway frame' of the anesthetist or the 'penetrating thoracic trauma' frame of the emergency physician. The frame is used consciously or unconsciously and determines the elements of a situation that occupy a person's attention and those which influence their behavior. When a situation exceeds the boundaries of a learner's primary frame, they will experience difficulty in making sense of the situation [25].

Simulation has a role in affording learners a safe environment, where they may refine their primary frames through personal reflection and as a result of feedback from expert tutors. However, in order to ensure that learners are accessing a primary frame that will later be useful to them in the workplace, it is important that the simulation possesses sufficient conceptual and emotional reality to allow them to experience the scenario intended by the teacher.

Simulation Center Training

Designated simulation centers developed as a result of efforts to provide an immersive learning environment that faithfully replicated the clinical workplace. Simulation centers are well suited to simulation-based education that involves large numbers of participants; requires extended periods of deliberate practice with part-task trainers; employs equipment that is too bulky or fragile to be easily transported to the clinical setting; or involves extensive use of video recording and playback [29]. Simulation center-based training also benefits from the presence of an experienced faculty, ample space for private debriefing and physical isolation from the workplace, which minimizes interruptions.

Numerous simulation center-based courses have been developed in critical care disciplines. Notable among these is the Effective Management of Anaesthetic Crises course developed by the Australian and New Zealand College of Anaesthetists, which has been successfully exported to several other regions. This course reinforces didactic teaching through immersive simulation, with a focus on crisis resource management and anesthesia non-technical skills [30].

Early, intensive simulation center 'boot camps' have also been developed to aid transition of clinicians from one phase of their career to the next. Wayne and colleagues reported significantly improved performance procedural skills, recognition of the deteriorating patient and communication skills after a two day workshop [31].

Notwithstanding the success of programs based in dedicated facilities, simulation centers also have shortcomings. They are expensive to establish and maintain, require clinicians to obtain leave from clinical duties to attend and only infrequently involve interdisciplinary teams when running scenarios.

In situ Training

In the early 2000s, an alternative mode of simulation-based education emerged in which simulation occurred in the workplace. Termed '*in situ*', 'mobile' or even 'guerilla' simulation, this method typically employs a blended approach, with patient simulators embedded within actual clinical environments [32]. *In situ* simulation has several advantages, as outlined below.

First, *in situ* simulation uses "real teams", who are simultaneously responsible for the care of real patients [33]. This enhances the conceptual and emotional reality of simulation and affords team members the opportunity to get to know one another. Further, *in situ* simulation can facilitate orientation to a new operating environment, as demonstrated in Fig. 2, which shows a Royal Australian Navy treatment team rehearsing patient handling and evacuation procedures while deployed at sea on a disaster relief mission to Fiji. From an experiential learning perspective, the concrete experience provided by *in situ* simulation, being more functionally aligned with the actual work of the learner, would be expected to lead to improved learning outcomes.

Second, unlike the controlled environment of a simulation center, *in situ* simulation involves actual components of the health delivery system. *In situ* simulation may therefore identify 'accidents waiting to happen' within the clinical environment, contributing to enhanced organizational safety. One example of this effect is reported by Walker and colleagues, who identified a number of such 'latent conditions' through a program of unannounced *in situ* cardiac arrest simulations at various locations throughout their hospital [34]. It should be noted that in tightly

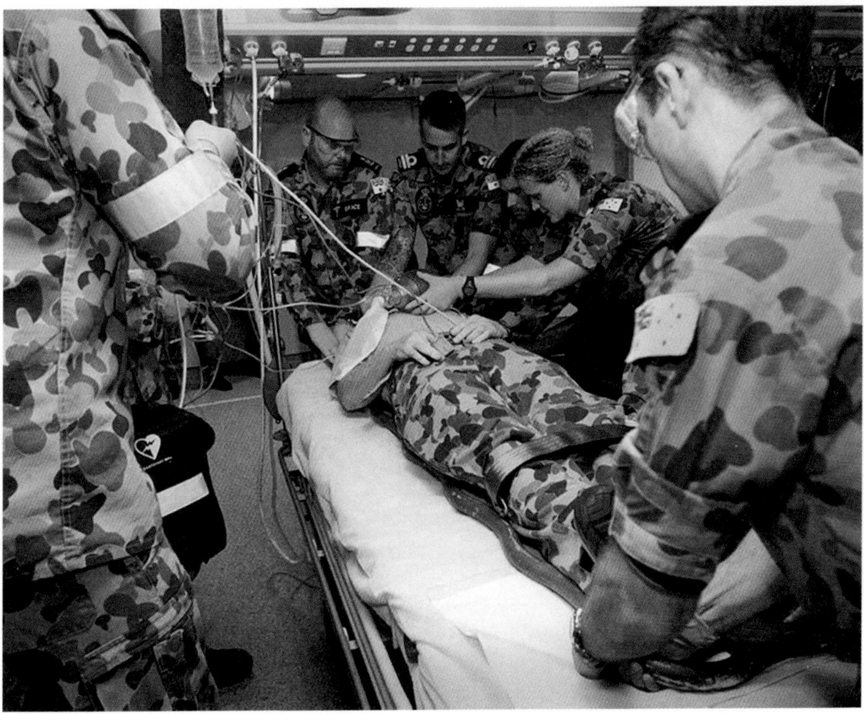

Fig. 2 Royal Australian Navy treatment team rehearsing resuscitation at sea. © Commonwealth of Australia 2015, reproduced with permission

coupled environments such as intensive care, identification of these hazards during real arrests could have catastrophic consequences for patients.

Third, *in situ* simulation offers the opportunity to deliver 'just in time' training in order to better prepare clinicians for the performance of complex procedural skills. Successful implementation of this approach has recently been reported for fiberoptic bronchoscopy [35] and for transthoracic echocardiography [36].

Fourth, *in situ* training allows teams to frequently practice infrequent events. The durability of behavioral changes produced by sporadic simulation center sessions has been questioned; brief *in situ* reinforcement training may offer one answer to this problem.

Finally, *in situ* training is more efficient, as simulation can be accommodated in quieter phases of a department's operational rhythm, meaning that there is no requirement to relieve staff to attend off-site simulation center activities.

It should be noted that *in situ* simulation is not a replacement for training in simulation centers. The two approaches are complementary and often have different objectives. Simulation center learning often forms part of a broader course of instruction that has both technical and non-technical learning objectives. In contrast, *in situ* training is uniquely suited to improving the function of actual clinical teams through enhanced communication, problem solving and reflection.

Stress, Learning and Performance: Implications for Simulation-based Education

Stress is a complex psychological and neurohormonal response triggered when an environmental threat exceeds the capacity of an individual's coping mechanisms. Learner stress is an important consideration when planning simulation-based education in critical care. Simulation itself may be stressful [37] and it is important to consider how stress influences the learning and performance of simulation participants. Having recognized that simulation can engender stress, educators are invited to consider whether manipulation of learner stressors during simulation sessions might facilitate the development of effective coping strategies for stress in the workplace.

Stress and Performance

Stress can be beneficial. It has been suggested that when confronted with an obstacle, learners appraise the situation in two stages: first they determine the demands of overcoming the obstacle; then they assess the personal and environmental resources available. When the resources are sufficient to meet the demands, the learner encounters a 'challenge'; when resources are insufficient, the learner encounters a 'threat' and manifests a stress response [38].

Stress can also impair performance in the simulation environment. Several studies, including that by Krage and colleagues, have demonstrated that the quality of

CPR declines in the presence of experimentally introduced distractors, such as noise and scripted interruptions by confederates [39]. Interestingly, the stress-induced degradation in performance in this study was found to be no less for experienced than for junior practitioners.

Stress and Learning

Stress affects learners' ability to store, retain and retrieve information. The link between stress and memory seems intuitive; nearly all critical care practitioners can recall a stressful clinical encounter that has indelibly etched a lesson in their mind. However, not all stressful experiences are so readily recalled and this may be due to the differing impact of stress on working memory, memory consolidation and memory retrieval [38].

Working memory, the ability to manipulate stored information for short periods, is impaired by stress. A recent study by Prottengeier and colleagues demonstrated this in a group of medical students, paramedics and anesthetists who were asked to complete simple mental arithmetic whilst performing endotracheal intubation and other airway maneuvers. As cognitive load increased, procedural errors increased and speed of performance decreased [40]. In contrast, at least one study has noted that learners who exhibit a 'challenge response', marked by sympathetic nervous system activation without the other neurohormonal sequelae of the stress response such as elevated cortisol, retain normal working memory [38].

Stress, while degrading working memory, appears to enhance memory consolidation. Events leading to hypophyseal-pituitary-adrenal (HPA) axis activation and raised serum cortisol tend to be recalled in greater detail and for longer than events that do not trigger the stress response. This reinforces the maxim about enhanced learning 'under the gun'. However, it should be noted that it is the aspect of the event that triggered the stress response that is consolidated in the learner's mind. This is pertinent for simulation-based education facilitators because simulation sessions can expose learners to fear of judgement by their peers; if this 'socioevaluative' aspect of simulation is the main source of stress, then the intended learning outcomes and key points from debriefing may not be consolidated [38].

Hence, it would seem preferable for learner stress to arise from features of the case itself, or from realistic distractors such as those offered by competing workplace demands during *in situ* simulation.

Despite potential to enhance memory consolidation, stress also impairs memory retrieval. As in the case of working memory, this negative effect manifests at the point at which learners move from being challenged by a scenario to being overwhelmed.

Simulation and Manipulation of the Stress Response

Stress imprints memories; but learners do not always remember what simulation-based education facilitators hope they might. Sources of stress should be selected carefully such that they are conceptually linked to the information to be retained. Indiscriminate stress created by noise, abstract distractors or intimidating facilitators is likely to consolidate the impression that simulation is not worthwhile.

Stress Modulation and Stress Inoculation Training

Unfortunately, no matter how effectively participants may assimilate the intended learning outcomes of simulation-based education, the effect of the stress response on memory retrieval all but guarantees that these lessons will not initially be translated into clinical practice. This line of inquiry has led several authors to wonder whether simulation-based education might not also allow learners to become 'inoculated' against stress and thus inured to its consequences.

A form of cognitive-behavioral therapy, stress inoculation training was developed in the 1970s by Meichenbaum. As originally described it had three phases: conceptualization; skills acquisition and consolidation; and application and follow through. Conceptualization teaches the learner about the nature of stress and encourages them to evaluate the efficacy of their existing coping strategies. Learners are then trained in problem solving, cognitive restructuring, relaxation techniques, self-monitoring and de-arousal techniques. Cognitive restructuring aims to regulate negative emotions; relaxation and de-arousal techniques aim to ameliorate the physiological response to stress [38]. Finally, learners are exposed to stressors analogous to those likely to be encountered in the workplace. When applied to reduce 'performance' anxiety, that which is associated with a particular role or task, mental rehearsal and graduated exposure likely render real life events less novel and thereby increase the sense of predictability and control [41]. Simultaneously, stress inoculation training enhances self-efficacy beliefs, favorably influencing the balance between perceived threat and perceived cognitive and emotional resources, thus reducing the likelihood of stress response activation [42].

Simulation-based stress inoculation training has been extensively adopted by military forces around the world [42]. Several techniques successfully applied in military contexts would readily translate to critical care simulation-based education.

Cognitive Control Strategies

A variety of techniques can be employed to assist learners in focusing their attention on task-relevant information, whilst excluding distractions. Attentional training is one such approach. Participants use simulation to identify distractors likely to be present in their workplace, such as bystanders, family or environmental influences, and then develop strategies to manage these distractors. During simulation, participants can be encouraged to affirm their ability to perform through 'positive self-talk' while simultaneously 'parking' distracting or negative thoughts for later consideration. These strategies are also commonly taught to athletes by performance psychologists, who may be enlisted to participate in simulation sessions focusing on stress modulation.

Physiological Control Strategies

Controlled breathing, muscle relaxation and biofeedback techniques all aim to allow learners to ameliorate the physical sequelae of stress.

Overlearning

Overlearning refers to repeatedly practicing a task to a point beyond proficiency in order to increase automaticity and thereby reduce the impact of stress-induced failure of memory retrieval [41]. This technique has been criticized because of its potential to reduce learners' flexibility when encountering novel situations. However, overlearning has particular merit where learners must consolidate skills that are always done exactly the same way; preparation of emergency drugs or checking of intubation and ventilation apparatus are notable examples.

Mental Practice

Like the cognitive control strategies mentioned above, mental practice is extensively employed in the military and by elite athletes [41]. Mental rehearsal is particularly helpful in preparing learners to execute complex or daunting tasks. Mental rehearsal, by anticipating and mentally overcoming obstacles to success, can both reduce the impact of encountered stressors during simulation and improve self-efficacy beliefs.

Hyper-realistic Team-centered Training

Once learners have developed skills that allow them to exclude distractors, control negative thoughts, affirm their competence and regulate the physiological response to stress, they are ready to practice under 'operational conditions'. Simulation should be used to present learners with the full range of conceivable workplace stressors, including unexpected equipment failure, unhelpful colleagues, concurrent emergencies, uncertain diagnosis and unexpected patient death.

Introduction of stressors should be progressive. Critical care simulation often has two goals: teaching new skills and consolidating existing competences. Given that generalized stress may detract from knowledge retention, it has been recommended that the intensity of stressors should only be increased after successful demonstration of task proficiency [41].

Directions for Future Research

Extant simulation-based education research has demonstrated that simulation is well accepted by learners, that it results in knowledge transfer and that it can change clinical behaviors. Future research is likely to seek further evidence of the organizational benefits of different simulation-based education strategies. In particular, it is necessary to explore further the differing effects of *in situ* and simulation center based training on stress, performance, knowledge transfer and retention so that critical care educators may select an appropriate range of simulation activities to meet the needs of their organization. Consideration should also be given to the challenge of determining how learning acquired through simulation translates into practice. Learning can be content- and context-specific; therefore, strong performance in one skill domain and setting does not predict performance in another. There is still a paucity of research in which learning acquired through simulation-based education has been rigorously evaluated in the workplace using measures other than repeated simulation. Further research should aim to clarify the transferability and durability of particular knowledge, skills and attitudes developed through differing simulation-based education approaches.

The role of stress in simulation also remains incompletely elucidated. Research should seek to identify ways of reducing the intrinsic socioevaluative stressors of simulation through evidence-based improvements in simulation conduct and debriefing practice. Simultaneously, it is important to determine whether deliberate introduction of conceptually and emotionally realistic stressors into simulation activities can lead to improved memory consolidation, as well as potentially 'inoculating' learners against the effects of stressors in the workplace.

Conclusion

We conclude by offering some principles for making best use of simulation-based education in critical care:

- Approach simulation with an understanding of adult learning principles. Design sessions to maximize efficacy of reflection, consolidation and experimentation.
- Choose a form of simulation appropriate to the intended learning outcomes and the experience of the learner. For individual procedural skill teaching, consider part-task trainers with high physical realism. For individual clinical skills teaching in large learner cohorts, consider simulation integrated within a broader curriculum conducted at a purpose built center. When assisting experienced practitioners to refine their performance, consider highly contextualized *in situ* simulation, carefully designed to maximize conceptual and emotional realism.
- Be mindful of the effects of stress on performance. Exclude stressors that are not related to the intended learning objectives, but consider introducing clinical stressors in a graduated, purposeful manner that has potential to enhance the psychological resilience of the learners. Consider inclusion of stress-inoculation strategies within the simulation-based education program.
- Use simulation-based education to build effective teams and create a safer workplace. The evolving practice of *in situ* simulation has great potential to strengthen the performance of clinical teams as well as enhancing organizational safety through identification of latent threats to patient safety.

References

1. Jones F, Passos-Neto C, Braghiroli O (2015) Simulation in medical education: Brief history and methodology. Princ Pract Clin Res 1:56–63
2. Gaba D, DeAnda A (1988) A comprehensive anesthesia simulation environment: Re-creating the operating room for research and training. Anesthesiology 69:387–394
3. Cooper J, Taqueti V (2008) A brief history of the development of mannequin simulators for clinical education and training. Postgrad Med J 84:563–570
4. Barrows H (1993) An overview of the uses of standardized patients for teaching and evaluating clinical skills. Acad Med 68:443–451
5. Rosen M (2008) The history of medical simulation. J Crit Care 23:157–166
6. Weller J, Nestel D, Marshall S, Brooks P, Conn J (2012) Simulation in clinical teaching and learning. Med J Aust 196:1–5
7. Kennedy CC, Maldonado F, Cook DA (2013) Simulation-based bronchoscopy training: Systematic review and meta-analysis. Chest 144:183–192
8. Silverplats K, Jonnson A, Lundberg L (2016) A hybrid simulator model for the control of catastrophic external junctional haemorrhage in the military environment. Adv Simul 1:1–5
9. Knowles M (1984) Androgogy in Action. Josey-Bass, San Francisco
10. Kolb D (1984) Experiential Learning. Prentice-Hall, New Jersey
11. Stocker M, Burmester M, Allen M (2014) Optimisation of simulated team training through the application of learning theories: A debate for a conceptual framework. BMC Med Educ 14:1–9
12. Mezirow J (2000) Learning as Transformation: Critical Perspectives on a Theory in Progress. Josey-Bass, San Francisco
13. Cleland J, Patey R, Thomas I, Walker K, O'Connor P, Russ S (2016) Supporting transitions in medical career pathways: The role of simulation-based education. Adv Simul 1:1–9
14. Ziv A, Wolpe P, Small S, Glick S (2006) Simulation-based medical education: An ethical imperative. Simul Healthc 1:252–256
15. Kirkpatrick D (1994) Evaluating Training Programs: The Four Levels. Berret-Koekler, San Francisco
16. Lorello G, Cook D, Johnson R, Brydges R (2014) Simulation-based training in anaesthesiology: A systematic review and meta-analysis. Br J Anaesth 112:231–245
17. Cook D, Hatala R, Brydges R et al (2011) Technology-enhanced simulation for health professions education: A systematic review and meta-analysis. JAMA 306:978–988
18. Le Blanc V (2012) Simulation in anaesthesia: State of the science and looking forward. Can J Anaesth 59:193–202
19. McGaghie W, Issenberg B, Cohen E, Barsuk J, Wayne D (2011) Does simulation-based medical education with deliberate practice yield better results than traditional clinical education? A meta-analytic comparative review of the evidence. Acad Med 86:706–711
20. Schroedel C, Corbridge T, Cohen E et al (2012) Use of simulation-based education to improve resident learning and patient care in the medical intensive care unit: A randomized trial. J Crit Care 27:e7–e13
21. Steinemann S, Berg B, Skinner A et al (2011) In situ, multidisciplinary, simulation-based teamwork training improves early trauma care. J Surg Educ 68:472–476
22. Chopra V, Gesink B, De Jong J, Bovill J, Spierdijk J, Brand R (1994) Does training on an anaesthesia simulator lead to improvement in performance? Br J Anaesth 73:293–297
23. Barsuk J, Cohen E, Potts S et al (2014) Dissemination of a simulation-based mastery learning intervention reduces central-line associated bloodstream infections. Bmc Qual Saf 23:749–756
24. Theilen U, Leonard P, Jones P et al (2013) Regular in situ simulation training of paediatric medical emergency team improves hospital response to deteriorating patients. Resuscitation 84:218–222
25. Diekmann P, Gaba D, Rall M (2007) Deepening the theoretical foundations of patient simulation as social practice. Simul Healthc 2:183–193

26. Rudolph J, Simon R, Raemer D (2007) Which reality matters? Questions on the path to high engagement in healthcare simulation. Simul Healthc 2:161–163
27. Murray D (2014) Progress in simulation education: Developing an anesthesia curriculum. Curr Opin Anesthesiol 27:610–615
28. Goffman E (1974) Frame Analysis: An Essay on the Organization of Experience. Northeastern University Press, Boston
29. Gaba D (2004) The future of simulation in health care. Qual Saf Health Care 13:e2–e10
30. Weller J, Morris R, Watterson L et al (2006) Effective management of anaesthetic crises: Development and evaluation of a college-accredited simulation-based course for anaesthesia education in Australia and New Zealand. Simul Healthc 1:209–214
31. Wayne D, Cohen E, Singer B et al (2014) Progress towards improving medical school graduates' skills via a "boot camp" curriculum. Simul Healthc 9:33–39
32. Rosen M, Hunt E, Pronovost P, Federowicz M, Weaver S (2012) In situ simulation in continuing education for the health care professions: A systematic review. J Contin Educ Health Prof 32:243–254
33. Patterson M, Blike G, Nadkarni V (2008) In situ simulation: Challenges and results. In: Henriksen K, Battles J, Keyes M (eds) Advances in Patient Safety: New Directions and Alternative Approaches. Agency for Healthcare Research and Quality, Rockville
34. Walker S, Sevdalis N, McKay A et al (2013) Unannounced in situ simulations: Integrating training and clinical practice. BMJ Qual Saf 22:453–458
35. De Oliviera G, Glassenberg R, Chang R, Fitzgerald P, McCarthy R (2013) Virtual airway simulation to improve dexterity among novices performing fibreoptic intubation. Anaesthesia 68:1053–1058
36. Neelankavil J, Howard-Quijano K, Hsieh T et al (2012) Transthoracic echocardiography simulation in an efficient method to train anesthesiologists in basic transthoracic echocardiography skills. Anesth Analg 115:1042–1051
37. Piquette D, Tarshis J, Sinuff T, Fowler R, Pinto R, Le Blanc V (2014) Impact of acute stress on resident performance during simulated resuscitation episodes: A prospective randomized cross-over study. Teach Learn Med 26:9–16
38. Le Blanc V (2009) The effect of acute stress on performance: Implications for health professions education. Acad Med 84:S25–S33
39. Krage R, Tjon Soei Len L, Schober P et al (2014) Does individual experience affect performance during cardiopulmonary resuscitation with additional external distractors? Anaesthesia 69:983–989
40. Prottengeier J, Petzoldt M, Jess N et al (2016) The effect of a standardised source of divided attention in airway management. Eur J Anaesthesiol 33:195–203
41. Robson S, Manacapilli T (2014) Enhancing Performance under Stress: Stress Inoculation Training in Battlefield Airmen. Rand Corporation, Santa Monica
42. Wiederhold M, Wiederhold B (2010) Using Advanced Prosthetics for Stress Inoculation Training and to Teach Life Saving Skills. NATO, Brussels

Part XIV
Organization and Quality of Care

We Have Good Enough Data to Support Sepsis Performance Measurement

H. C. Prescott and V. X. Liu

Introduction

The past couple of years have witnessed many changes in sepsis. In 2016, the European Society of Intensive Care Medicine and the Society of Critical Care Medicine definitions task force released an updated sepsis definition (Sepsis-3) based on sequential organ failure assessment (SOFA) scores, and also released a new tool (qSOFA) to screen for highest-risk sepsis at the bedside [1]. What was once a clear and stable set of definitions and guidelines has now become uncertain for some. These changes correspond to a growing sense of unrest among the sepsis community, including researchers, clinicians and healthcare systems. Improved sepsis survival, it is argued, may simply have resulted from nothing more than diluting the sample of the 'truly sick' sepsis patients. Three long-awaited, multicenter randomized clinical trials (RCTs) found no benefit to protocol-based care over "usual care" [2–4].

These developments have led many clinicians to feel that the rules of the game for sepsis have not only changed, but that we lack RCT data to guide our care. When asked to integrate what decades of hard work have taught us about defining and treating sepsis, the world's leading experts repeat a common refrain: "early identification and treatment". When asked how we tell if a patient is adequately resuscitated – if there are objective goals we can use – they tell us "use your best clinical judgment." And, as we debate the merits of qSOFA versus systemic inflam-

H. C. Prescott (✉)
Division of Pulmonary and Critical Care Medicine, University of Michigan
Ann Arbor, MI 48104, USA
VA Center for Clinical Management Research, Health Services Research & Development Center of Innovation, Ann Arbor Veteran's Affairs Hospital
Ann Arbor, MI, USA
e-mail: hprescot@med.umich.edu

V. X. Liu
Kaiser Permanente Division of Research
Oakland, CA, USA

J.-L. Vincent (ed.), *Annual Update in Intensive Care and Emergency Medicine 2017*,
DOI 10.1007/978-3-319-51908-1_38

matory response syndrome (SIRS), Sepsis-3 versus prior sepsis definitions, and the veracity of sepsis epidemiology, front-line clinicians and quality leaders are feeling increasingly bewildered.

The uncertainty regarding sepsis definitions and treatment comes at a challenging time. The US Centers for Medicare & Medicaid Services (CMS) has recently recognized the need to standardize care in sepsis – a goal many have been working on for decades. The CMS initiative, known as SEP-1, went into effect October 1, 2015 and calls for all US hospitals to submit data on adherence to 3-hour and 6-hour early management bundles for septic Medicare beneficiaries (Table 1) – specifically, for patients with suspected infection, two or more SIRS criteria, and evidence of sepsis-induced organ dysfunction (Table 2).

Critics have warned that the CMS measure has many flaws and is liable to worsen care for patients ([5]; Table 3). Concerns focus on both the uncertainty of sepsis treatment (e. g., limited evidence for early antibiotics in septic patients without shock) and the SEP-1 performance measure itself (e. g., the "all-or-nothing" approach to scoring bundle compliance; the need to document volume status and tissue perfusion assessment in patients with persistent hypotension following initial fluid resuscitation) [6]. However, while there is no simple way to tell if quality care is being provided to patients with sepsis, we believe that there is sufficient evidence and consensus about sepsis care to support performance measurement.

Table 1 Overview of Center for Medicare & Medicaid Services' early management bundle for severe sepsis and septic shock

Target Population		Process Measures	Time Frame	
Severe sepsis	Septic shock		3 h	6 h
X	X	Obtain blood cultures (prior to antibiotics)	X	
X	X	Measure lactate	X	
X	X	Administer broad-spectrum antibiotics	X	
	X	Resuscitate with 30 ml/kg crystalloid fluid if hypotensive or lactate > 4 mmol/l	X	
	X	Administer vasopressors if hypotension persists despite fluid resuscitation (e. g., systolic blood pressure < 90 mmHg or mean arterial pressure < 65 mmHg)		X
X	X	Repeat lactate measurement if initial value is elevated (> 2.0 mmol/l)		X
	X	Document responsiveness to fluid resuscitation in patients with septic shock if there is persistent hypotension after initial fluid resuscitation (e. g., through (a) focused physical exam [vital signs, cardiopulmonary examination, peripheral pulse examination, and skin examination] or (b) 2 of the following: central venous pressure measurement, straight leg raise, bedside cardiac ultrasound, or central venous oxygen saturation measurement)		X

Table 2 Centers for Medicare & Medicaid Services operational definitions of severe sepsis and septic shock for SEP-1 performance measure

Severe Sepsis Definition	Suspected infection
	Two or more SIRS criteria (temperature > 38 or < 36 C, heart rate > 90, respiratory rate > 20, white blood cell count > 12,000 or 4,000 or containing > 10% bandemia)
	One of more signs of sepsis-induced organ dysfunction (systolic blood pressure < 90 mmHg or decrease > 40 mmHg from baseline, lactate > 2.0 mmol/l, urine output < 0.5 ml/kg/h for > 2 h, bilirubin > 2.0 mg/dl, platelets < 100,000 μl, international normalized ratio > 1.5, altered mental status)
Septic Shock Definition	Severe sepsis, plus hypoperfusion despite fluid resuscitation or lactate > 4.0 mmol/L

SIRS: systemic inflammatory response syndrome

Table 3 Select arguments against implementing the Centers for Medicare & Medicaid Services' SEP-1 performance measure

Concerns about mandating early antibiotics	"*there are worrisome parallels between SEP-1 and the former CMS rule requiring clinicians to administer antibiotics for pneumonia within 4 h of presentation*" [5]
	"*the SEP-1 mandate has the potential to magnify the flaws of the 4-hour pneumonia rule. It sets too rigid rules for managing an uncertain condition*" [5]
	"*the only real evidence [in favor of early antibiotics] (albeit not great evidence) is for patients who have septic SHOCK*" [6]
Concerns about "All-or-nothing" bundle compliance	"*SEP-1 is an "all-or-nothing" measure, meaning that unless a hospital can demonstrate perfect compliance and perfect documentation for all components of the bundle, it will not receive any credit*" [5]
	"*hospitals will not be acknowledged for some cases in which they provided excellent care and their patients had favorable outcomes*" [5]
	"*This "all-or-nothing" bundle approach paradoxically treats a failure to administer timely antibiotics identically to failure to document resuscitation endpoints in the clinical notes*" [29]
Concerns about documentation	"*the rule's uncertainty's are amplified by the considerable administrative burden*" [5]
	"*the measure's specifications are complex, and many of the required data elements require manual chart abstraction. Hospitals are already struggling under the crushing weight of onerous quality reporting requirements, and this measure only increases the burden*" [29]
Concerns about the definition of severe sepsis and septic shock	"*we have a reimagining of septic shock. Somehow, septic shock now includes a lactate > 4*" [6] "*SEP-1 requires abstractors to document systemic inflammatory response syndrome and to differentiate between sepsis and severe sepsis. These concepts are at odds with the latest sepsis definitions*" [5]

Standardizing Sepsis Care Today

As clinicians, we work in a world of imperfect approximations. While some experts argue that national programs to address sepsis should be put on hold until we have better data and methods [7], we disagree. The best approach for health systems in the face of imperfect measurement and information is not to put sepsis performance measurement on hold – but rather to focus on incentivizing the undeniable features of good sepsis care.

Sepsis Is an Urgent Problem

We know that sepsis is a costly and deadly. By conservative estimates, the condition kills more than 150,000 Americans (and 5 million people around the world) each year [8, 9]. It contributes to at least one third of all US hospital deaths [10], costs over $US 23 billion in US acute hospitalizations alone [8], and exacts a massive and persistent toll on patients and families long after they leave the hospital [11, 12]. Yet, public awareness of sepsis remains poor. In contrast to cardiovascular emergencies like myocardial infarction and stroke – where lay person knowledge of presenting symptoms is common – just over half of Americans are aware of the term 'sepsis', and only a quarter can identify the key symptoms [13].

Treatment Works

We also know that, even with our imperfect understanding of sepsis and paucity of positive RCT data to guide care, sepsis mortality has improved over time – so something has worked. Some of the mortality reduction is due to greater detection of less sick sepsis cases – the so-called 'Will Rogers' phenomenon – but not all of it. Several studies with careful adjustments for temporal changes in case-mix detect true mortality improvements [14, 15], and the available data argues that sepsis quality improvement programs can and do work [16–19].

There Is Consensus About the Key Elements of Good Sepsis Treatment

The core requirements of the SEP-1 early sepsis resuscitation bundle are lactate measurement, blood cultures, broad-spectrum antibiotics, and repeat lactate measurement if the initial level is elevated [20]. Patients with hypotension must also receive 30 ml/kg crystalloid followed by vasopressors if hypotension persists despite fluid resuscitation. And, if patients remain hypotensive despite initial fluid resuscitation, then vasopressors must be administered, and an assessment of volume status and tissue perfusion must be documented.

Table 4 Mandated Multicenter Sepsis Quality Improvement Studies

Setting	Intervention Resuscitation Bundle	Target Population	Outcome
Intermountain Health, 2004–2010	Serum lactate measured within 3 h of ED admission Blood cultures prior to antibiotics Broad-spectrum antibiotics within 3 h of ED admission If hypotensive (SBP < 90 mm Hg or MAP ≤ 65 mm Hg) or lactate ≥ 4 mmol/l, then resuscitate with 20–40 ml/kg (predicted body weight) crystalloid If hypotensive despite fluid resuscitation, administer vasopressor If septic shock or lactate ≥ 4 mmol/l, CVP and $ScvO_2$ measures obtained through central catheter with tip in SVC. If CVP ≥ 8 cm H_2O and $ScvO_2$ < 70%, administer ionotropes and/or packed rec cells if hematocrit < 30%	Severe sepsis: infection, SIRS, plus evidence of end-organ dysfunction including lactate ≥ 2 mmol/l Septic Shock: hypotension despite adequate fluid administration or lactate ≥ 4 mmol/l	Reduced in-hospital mortality
Kaiser Permanente Northern California, 2011–2014	(Initial lactate measurement in all patients with SIRS and/or blood cultures was already standard practice) Antibiotics within 3 h Repeat lactate measurement within 1–4 h of initial lactate 30 ml/kg (or at least 2 l) intravenous fluid within 3 h	Intermediate lactate: infection, SIRS, lactate ≥ 2 and ≤ 4 mmol/without hypotension	Reduced in-hospital mortality; association strongest for patients with heart failure or kidney disease history

CVP: central venous pressure; *ED*: emergency department; *MAP*: mean arterial pressure; *$ScvO_2$*: systemic venous oxygen saturation; *SBP*: systolic blood pressure; *SVC*: superior vena cava; *SIRS*: systemic inflammatory response syndrome

Aside from reassessing and documenting volume status and tissue perfusion, these treatment elements are consistently included in sepsis treatment bundles across a variety of organizations [21], and are also required components of mandated sepsis protocols in all New York state hospitals under 2013 legislation known as Rory's Regulations. And, the data is clear about these initial elements of treatment: health system-wide implementation of lactate measurement, blood cultures, early antibiotics, and crystalloid fluid bolus for hypotension and/or elevated lactate in clinically suspected sepsis patients result in a net mortality reduction ([18]; Table 4). There is also data to support crystalloid resuscitation in patients with intermediate lactate [19] who are included in the SEP-1 definition of septic shock.

Certainly, some patients with clinically suspected sepsis turn out to have some other condition. But, even under imperfect, real-world conditions, treating all patients with clinically suspected sepsis results in a net survival benefit [18, 19]. (When it comes to documenting volume status and tissue perfusion, however, we agree with critics that the substantial effort associated with auditing this exam documentation is not warranted).

The recent negative trials of early goal-directed therapy should not change our thinking about the key elements of good sepsis care. While protocolized early sepsis resuscitation was no better than usual care among the 31 high volume academic centers in the ProCESS trial [2] (or for centers participating in PRoMISe [4] and ARISE [3]), patients in both arms consistently received early antibiotics, lactate measurement, and fluid resuscitation. Rather, the take-home lessons from these trials are: (1) "usual care" has evolved over the past 15 years such that patients are now getting antibiotics and fluid earlier – the average patient in ProCESS received >2 l intravenous fluid prior to enrollment; (2) patients in all arms of these trials overwhelmingly received the key elements of good sepsis care – 76% of ProCESS patients had received antibiotics prior to enrollment [2]; and (3) if one cannot provide expert 'usual care', then he/she can just follow the protocol-based standard therapy arm of the ProCESS trial and know that he/she is providing care every bit as good as that delivered at some of the best centers in the US by highly experienced resuscitationists.

Outcomes Measures Cannot Replace Process Measures

Quality improvement in healthcare is built on measuring structure, processes, and outcomes. Since our ultimate goal is to reduce sepsis mortality, some have argued that we should mandate hospitals to report sepsis-related mortality alone. A life may be saved, after all, but the hospital is nonetheless penalized because an element of recommended care was missed. Should not the saved life count more than the missed element of care?

There are several reasons why measuring sepsis-related mortality alone is not a straight-forward solution. First, we cannot simply count the number of patients who survive or die during sepsis hospitalization. We have to account for the differences in the patients between hospitals. Consider the challenges of comparing outcomes between two hypothetical hospitals (Fig. 1). Given the sheer number of factors that influence death (age, sex, race, number and severity of chronic co-morbidities, access to health care, illness severity on presentation, etiology of sepsis, etc. and the non-linear interactions between these various factors), adjusting for differences in patient population to generate a fair risk-adjusted assessment of sepsis-related mortality by hospital is not easy, and is likely to require hospitals to report just as much information as SEP-1.

Second, in-hospital mortality is biased by discharge practices – some hospitals are more likely to discharge patients immediately before their death, lowering in-hospital mortality but not 30-day mortality [22]. Even worse, when it is clear that a patient is not getting better quickly, and the best course of action may be to transition the focus to comfort only, there is a tension between doing what is in the best interest of the patient (allowing the patient to die peacefully) and what is in the best interest of hospital performance measurement (keeping the patient alive just long enough to transfer to another facility). And, while we hope that a physician would always act in the interest of the patient, we should not intentionally design

Which hospital is better at treating sepsis?

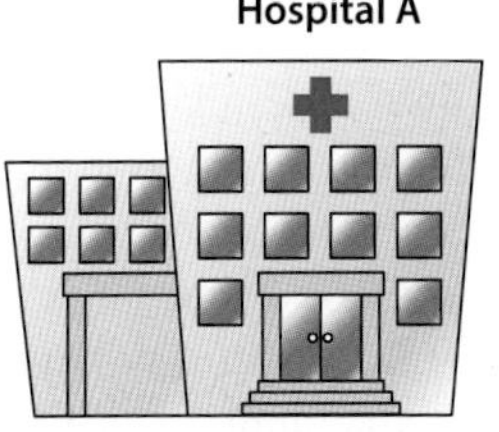

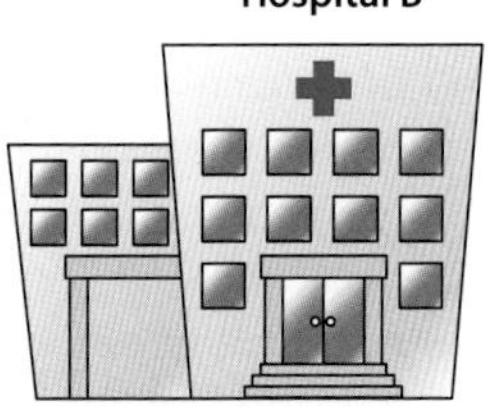

Fig. 1 The challenge of comparing sepsis outcomes between hospitals

systems that push against the patients' best interests. For now, the optimal approach for integrating code status into mortality metrics remains unclear [23, 24].

Third, the discordance between process and outcome measures cuts both ways. A hospital may provide the best possible sepsis care, but the patient may still die. Should not the excellent care provided (for which the hospital has complete control) count more than the death, for which the hospital ultimately does not have complete control?

Fourth, we do not know the 'optimal' rate of sepsis-related mortality. Sepsis contributes to one out of every two to three deaths in US hospitals [10]. It is a common cause of death among people with a variety of chronic conditions, such as malignancies and neurodegenerative disease. It is unrealistic to believe that we can prevent all sepsis-related deaths. But the optimal, or achievable, rate of sepsis-related mortality is not clear – that is, the rate at which sepsis is part of the dying process of those fated to die soon, but does not kill those who ought to survive. By contrast, all patients who present to the hospital without care limitations should receive optimal early treatment of sepsis.

We Are Not Just Repeating Prior Failures

Drawing parallels to process measures for early antibiotics in pneumonia, some experts have cautioned that SEP-1 will likely drive over-use of antibiotics, aggressive fluid resuscitation, and precipitate complications such as *Clostridium difficile* infection [5]. But, this comparison inherently discounts the higher stakes for patients who are potentially septic.

Unlike patients with simple infection, patients with possible sepsis (i. e., patients with organ dysfunction or shock that may be due to infection) are likely to be dead the next morning without antibiotics. Moreover, the sicker patients for whom we may worry most about over-resuscitation (those with heart failure or end-stage renal disease) are the exact patients who derive the bulk of the benefit from sepsis treatment bundles [19] – suggesting that our tendency to limit fluid volume in these patients is detrimental, and that incentivizing resuscitation may save lives.

Sepsis performance measures may indeed increase the initiation of antibiotics, with the potential for negative antibiotic-related sequelae (development of multidrug-resistant organisms, *C. difficile* infection). While we await better tools to rapidly rule in/out infection, as well as better evidence on which patients must get early antibiotics, we can reduce the risk for negative antibiotic-associated sequelae by stopping antibiotics promptly if infection remains unconfirmed after a couple days and also by limiting treatment duration in those with confirmed infection. Shortening antibiotic duration may be a safer approach to antibiotic stewardship than limiting antibiotic initiation in patients with organ failure or shock that is potentially due to sepsis [25].

The Infrastructure to Measure Quality Now Will Get Us Better Care Faster

The mandate to report sepsis-related outcomes is spurring hospitals to build the infrastructure necessary to promote high-quality sepsis care [5], which is an important outcome in and of itself. Declines in acute myocardial infarction mortality began with the American Heart Association's "Get with the Guidelines" quality improvement initiative [26], before widespread availability of troponin measurements, when our tests for acute myocardial infarction were deeply imperfect. Moreover, much of the acute myocardial infarction mortality improvement results from early percutaneous intervention, which happens before definitive testing necessarily occurs. Sepsis mandates could also catalyze quality improvement collaboratives, which may themselves advance the science of sepsis diagnosis and treatment [27].

We Should Not Sit on Our Hands Waiting for a Better Definition

Waiting for a perfect (or even a better) sepsis definition will not work. We have struggled to define the condition since the dawn of medicine and are unlikely to solve the problem soon. We know that "sepsis is not a specific illness but rather a syndrome encompassing a still-uncertain pathobiology", and "no gold standard diagnostic test exists" [1]. Because of this, all proposed definitions of sepsis are necessarily incomplete, imperfect, conceptual, and aspirational. In fact, we do not yet have a gold standard for determining whether or not a patient is infected. Tracking culture and antibiotic orders in the electronic medical record will also reflect only clinician-recognized cases, and cannot distinguish between sepsis-related and non-sepsis-related organ dysfunction.

We are, perhaps, at the dawn of a new era of molecular characterization, but the pay-off remains distant and uncertain. Meanwhile, patients are dying of sepsis today, and the best available evidence indicates that lactate measurement, blood cultures, early broad-spectrum antibiotics, and fluid resuscitation saves lives. The new definition is the best one available based on the state of the science, and one that will support effective use of the sepsis bundle. We believe that all hospitals should track these core process measures in patients with clinically suspected sepsis.

Now, to be clear, we fully agree that big financial penalties, all-or-nothing bundle compliance, and overly onerous measures are unlikely to be the right approach to incentivizing productive change. But, the core ingredients of SEP-1 (lactate measurement, blood cultures, broad-spectrum antibiotics, and fluid resuscitation) are right, and the best approach for health systems in the face of imperfect measurement is not to walk away from sepsis altogether – but rather to focus on incentivizing the key features of good sepsis care.

For sepsis mandates to be successful at improving care, clinicians must work within the spirit of the mandate, rather than attempting to game the system [28]. Clinicians not operating under a mandate must still hold themselves to a high standard, measure things and behave as if they were operating under a mandate – or create one.

Conclusion

Sepsis is a major cause of death. While we debate nuances of sepsis and septic shock definitions and treatment, the core ingredients of good sepsis care are clear, and real world implementation of sepsis treatment bundles reduces mortality. Thus, we believe the best approach for health systems is not to walk away from sepsis altogether – but rather to incentivize the key features of good sepsis care in all patients with clinically suspected sepsis.

References

1. Singer M, Deutschman CS, Seymour CW et al (2016) The Third International Consensus Definitions for Sepsis and Septic Shock (Sepsis-3). JAMA 315:801–810
2. Yealy DM, Kellum JA et al (2014) A randomized trial of protocol-based care for early septic shock. N Engl J Med 370:1683–1693
3. Peake SL, Delaney A, Bailey M et al (2014) Goal-directed resuscitation for patients with early septic shock. N Engl J Med 371:1496–1506
4. Mouncey PR, Osborn TM, Power GS et al (2015) Trial of early, goal-directed resuscitation for septic shock. N Engl J Med 372:1301–1311
5. Klompas M, Rhee C (2016) The CMS Sepsis Mandate: Right disease, wrong measure. Ann Intern Med 165:517–518
6. Weingart S (2015) We are Complicit – A glimpse into the current state of severe sepsis/septic shock quality measures. http://emcrit.org/blogpost/current-state-of-severe-sepsis-quality-measures. Accessed Nov 10, 2016
7. Rhee C, Gohil S, Klompas M (2014) Regulatory mandates for sepsis care – reasons for caution. N Engl J Med 370:1673–1166
8. Aguency for Healthcare Research and Quality (2016) HCUPnet, Healthcare Cost and Utilization Project. http://hcupnet.ahrq.gov/. Accessed October 23, 2016
9. Fleischmann C, Scherag A, Adhikari NKJ et al (2016) Assessment of global incidence and mortality of hospital-treated sepsis. Current estimates and limitations. Am J Respir Crit Care Med 193:259–272

10. Liu V, Escobar GJ, Greene JD et al (2014) Hospital deaths in patients with sepsis from 2 independent cohorts. JAMA 312:90–92
11. Cameron JI, Chu LM, Matte A et al (2016) One-year outcomes in caregivers of critically ill patients. N Engl J Med 374:1831–1841
12. Iwashyna TJ, Ely EW, Smith DM, Langa KM (2016) Long-term cognitive impairment and functional disability among survivors of severe sepsis. JAMA 304:1787–1794
13. Sepsis Alliance. Sepsis Awareness Research 2016. http://sepsis.org/files/sasepsisawareness2016.pdf Accessed November 10, 2016
14. Kaukonen KM, Bailey M, Suzuki S, Pilcher D, Bellomo R (2014) Mortality related to severe sepsis and septic shock among critically ill patients in Australia and New Zealand, 2000–2012. JAMA 311:1308–1316
15. Prescott HC, Kepreos KM, Wiitala WL, Iwashyna TJ (2015) Temporal changes in the influence of hospitals and regional healthcare networks on severe sepsis mortality. Crit Care Med 43:1368–1374
16. Ferrer R, Artigas A, Levy MM et al (2008) Improvement in process of care and outcome after a multicenter severe sepsis educational program in Spain. JAMA 299:2294–2303
17. Levy MM, Dellinger RP, Townsend SR et al (2010) The Surviving Sepsis Campaign: results of an international guideline-based performance improvement program targeting severe sepsis. Intensive Care Med 36:222–231
18. Miller RR 3rd, Dong L, Nelson NC et al (2013) Multicenter implementation of a severe sepsis and septic shock treatment bundle. Am J Respir Crit Care Med 188:77–82
19. Liu VX, Morehouse JW, Marelich GP et al (2016) Multicenter implementation of a treatment bundle for patients with sepsis and intermediate lactate values. Am J Respir Crit Care Med 193:1264–1270
20. Centers for Medicare & Medicaid Services & The Joint Commission (2016) NQF-endorsed voluntary consensus standards for hospital care. In: Specifications Manual for National Hospital Inpatient Quality Measures Discharges 10-01-15 (4Q15) through 06-30-16 (2Q16), Version 5.0a. http://www.nhfca.org/psf/resources/Updates1/SEP-1%23Measure%23Information%23Form%23(MIF).pdf. Accessed Nov 10, 2016
21. Kramer RD, Cooke CR, Liu V, Miller RR, Iwashyna TJ (2015) Variation in the contents of sepsis bundles and quality measures. a systematic review. Ann Am Thorac Soc 12:1676–1684
22. Hall WB, Willis LE, Medvedev S, Carson SS (2012) The implications of long-term acute care hospital transfer practices for measures of in-hospital mortality and length of stay. Am J Respir Crit Care Med 185:53–57
23. Walkey AJ, Weinberg J, Wiener RS, Cooke CR, Lindenauer PK (2016) Association of do-not-resuscitate orders and hospital mortality rate among patients with pneumonia. JAMA Intern Med 176:97–104
24. Kim YS, Escobar GJ, Halpern SD, Greene JD, Kipnis P, Liu V (2016) The natural history of changes in preferences for life-sustaining treatments and implications for inpatient mortality in younger and older hospitalized adults. J Am Geriatr Soc 64:981–989
25. Spellberg B (2016) The New Antibiotic Mantra – "Shorter Is Better". JAMA Intern Med 176:1254
26. Lewis WR, Peterson ED, Cannon CP et al (2008) An organized approach to improvement in guideline adherence for acute myocardial infarction: results with the Get With The Guidelines quality improvement program. Arch Intern Med 168:1813–1819
27. Cooke CR, Iwashyna TJ (2014) Sepsis mandates: improving inpatient care while advancing quality improvement. JAMA 312:1397–1398
28. Sjoding MW, Iwashyna TJ, Dimick JB, Cooke CR (2015) Gaming hospital-level pneumonia 30-day mortality and readmission measures by legitimate changes to diagnostic coding. Crit Care Med 43:989–995
29. Barbash IJ, Kahn JM, Thompson BT (2016) Opening the debate on the new sepsis definition. medicare's sepsis reporting program: two steps forward, One Step Back. Am J Respir Crit Care Med 194:139–141

The Use of Health Information Technology to Improve Sepsis Care

J. L. Darby and J. M. Kahn

Introduction

Sepsis is a critical illness syndrome defined by a dysregulated immune response to infection leading to life threatening organ dysfunction [1]. Sepsis is the most common cause of death among hospitalized patients in the United States, and its incidence is only expected to rise as the population ages and greater numbers of people live with chronic medical conditions that put them at risk [2, 3]. Because of the large clinical and economic burden associated with sepsis, it is increasingly the focus of local, national, and global quality improvement efforts. Yet despite these efforts, many patients with sepsis do not receive evidence-based care process consistent with published international clinical practice guidelines. For example, one recent national quality improvement initiative showed that only 25% of patients received all recommended care practices, even after a program of intensive guideline dissemination and education [4].

To address these gaps, critical care providers and health care quality improvement specialists are increasingly turning to health information technology (IT) to improve sepsis care. Health IT can be broadly defined as the use of electronic systems for creating, storing, retrieving, and processing data in the health care arena [5]. At a minimum, health IT typically takes the form of electronic medical records (EMRs), which are quickly becoming the norm, with nearly 60% of hospitals now reporting some degree of EMR use [6]. As computing power increases and artificial intelligence systems become more sophisticated, health IT is now being extended to include real-time decision support and advanced predictive analytics. For these

J. L. Darby
University of Pittsburgh School of Medicine
Pittsburgh, PA, USA

J. M. Kahn (✉)
Dept of Critical Care Medicine and Dept of Medicine and Health Policy & Management,
University of Pittsburgh School of Medicine
602B Scaife Hall, 3550 Terrace Street, Pittsburgh, PA 15261, USA
e-mail: kahnjm@upmc.edu

J.-L. Vincent (ed.), *Annual Update in Intensive Care and Emergency Medicine 2017*,
DOI 10.1007/978-3-319-51908-1_39

reasons, it is natural to apply health IT to the problem of the quality gap, particularly in the case of sepsis for which timely recognition and treatment is paramount for survival [7].

In this chapter, we discuss the role of health IT in the effort to improve quality of sepsis care. We focus on three major areas in which health IT may be particularly salient: increasing sepsis recognition, improving adherence to evidence-based sepsis care, and facilitating population-based sepsis quality improvement. We conclude by discussing some of the limitations of health IT approaches and outlining key areas for future research and development. Overall, we discuss how health IT, used critically and judiciously, holds the potential to further the mission of quality at the level of the patient, the hospital, and the health system.

IT Strategies to Increase Sepsis Recognition

Early recognition is a cornerstone of effective sepsis care. Robust observational data indicate that timely administrative of appropriate antimicrobial agents are associated with increased survival in sepsis [8]. And although clinical trials suggest that fully protocolized early goal-directed therapy is not associated with survival, all patients in these trials were rapidly diagnosed with sepsis and were given antibiotics and fluids prior to enrollment [9], strengthening the value of early recognition as a means to improve survival.

Unfortunately, sepsis remains difficult to identify, particularly in its early stages before organ failure develops. The central challenge in recognizing sepsis is undoubtedly related to the enigmatic nature of sepsis itself, a syndrome for which no gold standard diagnostic test exists and that is without pathognomonic features even on autopsy. The Sepsis-3 definition, a recent attempt to both simplify and codify the process of identifying sepsis, addressed this problem by linking sepsis identification to the presence of organ dysfunction [1], moving away from the indicators of the systemic inflammatory response which are nearly ubiquitous in hospitalized patients [10].

Although the Sepsis-3 definition is not without controversy, it does create a useful framework for using the EMR to screen emergency department and hospitalized patients for sepsis, and in turn provide real-time alerts for bedside providers about the potential presence of sepsis. Sepsis alerts work by integrating data in the EMR and applying algorithms to determine the likely presence of sepsis. Given the uncertainties of the syndrome itself and the difficulty of accurately identifying sepsis under the best of circumstances, it is unrealistic to think about sepsis alerts as a means of completely superseding clinical intuition. However, using EMRs to stratify risk and prompt further evaluation for high-risk patients is a reasonable and potentially high-value way to incorporate information technology into a sepsis screening protocol.

Several examples of real-time sepsis alerts have been published (Table 1; [11–20]). These examples predate the Sepsis-3 definition and therefore generally use the older criteria for sepsis based on some combination of organ failure and the systemic

Table 1 Selected studies evaluating electronic sepsis alerts

Author, year [ref]	Setting	N	Sensitivity [%]	Specificity [%]	Notes
Thiel, 2010 [11]	General floor	13,937	55	93	Multiple cohorts were described. Here performance is reported for the validation set
Sawyer, 2011 [12]	General floor	89	NR	NR	Implementation of a prior real-time alert [11] led to escalation of therapy in alerted patients but did not change clinical outcomes
Nelson, 2011 [13]	ED	33,460	64	99	Applying the alert in practice led to increased use of blood cultures before antibiotics
Hooper, 2012 [14]	ICU	442	99	82	Applying the alert in practice did not influence care patterns or clinical outcomes
Alsolamy, 2014 [15]	ED	49,838	93	98	For patients referred to the ICU, the alert preceded ICU referral by a median of 4 h
Umscheid, 2015 [16]	General floor	4,575	16*	97*	In a separate implementation phase, applying the alert led to increased sepsis recognition but not change in clinical outcomes
Harrison, 2015 [17]	ICU	587	80	96	68% of patients receiving an alert were observed to have experienced treatment delays that might have been otherwise mitigated
Brandt, 2015 [18]	General floor	164	100	62	Timing of alert was generally similar to the time of sepsis onset as determined by clinical adjudication
Amland, 2016 [19]	General floor	6,200	83	92	51% of patients with the alert already had infection suspected, although 25% of patients with alert had no antibiotics ordered at the time
Idrees, 2016 [20]	ED	55	NR	NR	Implementation of a real-time alert led to inconsistent changes in processes and no improvements in clinical outcomes

NR: not reported; *ED*: emergency department; *ICU*: intensive care unit. *The reference standard was not sepsis but a composite outcome of ICU transfer, rapid response team call, or death

inflammatory response. For this reason, as well as reasons related to the vagaries of the EMR, the alerts are of widely varying sensitivity and specificity such that they are of generally low positive and negative predictive value. Moreover, most alerts have not been compared to the generally accepted reference standard of in-person clinical screening, and most have not been evaluated for use in clinical practice to determine if they actually change provider behavior or influence clinical outcomes.

These limitations highlight several challenges that remain before sepsis alerts can be broadly applied in practice. First, the accuracy of current alerts remains unacceptably low. An ideal alert would detect sepsis with a high sensitivity (to maximize the potential for early intervention) while maintaining a high specificity (to minimize alert fatigue due to unhelpful over-firing of alerts). However, most sepsis sniffers, particularly those that rely on markers of the systemic inflammatory response or organ failure criteria, lack sufficient specificity, increasing the number of false positives and increasing the likelihood of over treatment and alarm fatigue. Alternatively they are very specific but lack sensitivity, increasing the number of false negatives and thus precluding early intervention in those who need it most. Indeed, at least one published study of provider perceptions of these alerts found that most providers did not feel they were very useful for precisely these reasons [21].

Second, sepsis sniffers must address the limitations inherent in existing EMRs, which contain data from multiple sources and of widely varying quality. This problem reflects the difference between EMR 'knowledge' and provider knowledge. The EMR is only as good as the data in it. To the degree that important data elements are either entered inaccurately or entered in free text fields that are difficult to process in a standardized fashion (e. g., altered mentation, a key component of the new sepsis definition), sepsis alerts may miss key cases, reducing sensitivity and overall utility.

Third, sepsis alerts are not useful if the provider has already diagnosed the patient with sepsis and is taking appropriate action. In order to trigger a useful alert, the EMR must know not only what the provider knows but also what the provider may not yet have discovered. An ideal alert would selectively fire for patients where the algorithm has detected a failure of recognition on the part of the clinician and not for patients that have been identified as septic by both the EMR and provider. This issue also reflects a key limitation with the Sepsis-3 framework itself. Sepsis-3 uses organ failures as a marker for the dysregulated immune response, and indeed organ failures are for the most part easy to recognize in the EMR. However, an ideal sepsis alert would identify sepsis *before* organ failures occur, providing time for clinicians to act quickly to prevent organ failure in the first place.

Potential strategies to improve sepsis alerts and make them more useful at the bedside include natural language processing to better use the unstructured data in the EMR and machine learning techniques to increase the accuracy.

Natural language processing uses the qualitative written word to make quantitative inference [22]. In lieu of capturing and analyzing discrete data, searching written notes for words and phrases that reflect the way clinicians think about sepsis could help both improve sepsis detection and reduce redundant alerting. For example, if the clinician recently wrote a note that includes the phrase "sepsis – giving broad spectrum antibiotics and actively fluid resuscitating", an alert is unlikely to be useful. That said, an important limitation of using natural language processing in alerts is that, at present, clinical notes are not always written in real time. Indeed, EMRs are paradoxically perceived as slowing down the process of writing notes [23]. As EMR functionality improves, it is possible that note writing will be streamlined enough for them to be written in real-time and act as a feasible reservoir for early detection information, increasing the value of natural language processing.

Machine learning uses advanced computational processes to identify latent patterns in data [24]. Most current sepsis alerts are not based on machine learning but instead are based on outdated Boolean algorithms in which sepsis is either present or absent based on a series of 'if-then' logic statements (e. g., 'if X and Y then Z'). Machine learning may provide more robust algorithms that can flexibly make use of time-varying data, narrow time windows, and the uncertainty inherent in the EMR. Combined with advances in computing, machine learning algorithms can also hand handle more variables, different types of variables (e. g., free text and numerical), and more complex interactions between variables simultaneously. In this way, machine learning may provide an avenue to identify complex syndromes in the EMR.

IT Strategies to Improve Adherence to Evidence-based Care

A second potential use of health IT is in spurring clinicians to use evidence-based practice in patients already diagnosed with sepsis. Sepsis-specific treatments include early appropriate antibiotics, early fluid resuscitation, avoidance of starch-based resuscitation fluids, and regular hemodynamic assessments to ensure response to treatment [7]. In addition, there are a number of supportive treatments that apply to the broader critically ill population including those with sepsis, such as lung-protective ventilation in acute lung injury, daily assessment for readiness to wean from mechanical ventilation, avoidance of deep-sedation, and use of a restrictive red blood cell transfusion threshold, among others [25].

One way in which the EMR could be leveraged to improve adherence to these treatments is through real-time decision support and prompts [26]. Prompts are a ubiquitous tool for behavior change that can be as low-tech as a hand washing sign in a public restroom. Human-based prompting for evidence-based practice is associated with improved use of guideline-recommended treatments and improved clinical outcomes, both with in-person prompts [27] and remote prompts via telemedicine [28]. In theory, the EMR could be used to screen patients for whether or not they are receiving an evidence-based practice and then, when quality deficits are suspected, alerting the clinician about the opportunity to improve care. Prompts could also be used as a disincentive to unwanted care, such as a real-time alert that the patient does not have a sufficiently low hemoglobin value to justify a red blood cell transfusion [29].

Another more innovative approach to prompting would rely not on static algorithms to determine evidence-based practice but instead on the 'wisdom of crowds' to help guide clinicians toward more evidence-based choices. This approach might be particularly useful when the evidence behind a certain therapy is unproven, or if multiple valid clinical decisions might be correct. At the hospital level, the EMR might be able to recognize the ordering practices of physicians and draw off the collective body of clinical knowledge to make suggestions to physicians about what orders they might want to place – similar to Google's autocomplete functionality. For example, in selecting an antibiotic in patients with sepsis, the EMR could integrate data from the hospital antibiogram and all the past prescribing patterns for similar patients to suggest the antibiotic that is most likely to be appropriate. In this way, local, regional and national practice patterns could iteratively shape the prescribing behavior of individual physicians.

A third approach would be to use the EMR to leverage the principles of behavioral economics to improve decision making. Behavioral economics is the science of how economic principles related to heuristics and biases impact our decisions. One example is the use of 'nudge' principles to guide clinicians toward evidence-based practices [30]. When given a list of items to choose from, otherwise unbiased respondents are more likely to select the first option on the list compared to later items [31]. The EMR could be used to prioritize lists of treatment options such that the highest value option is listed first. For example, instead of typing the antibiotic name into a computerized physician order entry (CPOE) system, a user could type 'antibiotics' and be offered a list, with the EMR identifying and placing first the best antibiotic from the patient's current cultures, past history, and the institution's antibiogram. In this way, health IT could still preserve physician autonomy while at the same time nudging physicians to choose the best treatment based on available data.

All of these options can serve to make sepsis therapy more patient-specific, furthering the mission of the 'personalized medicine' movement. In sepsis studies to date, the heterogeneity of the patient population has largely been accepted rather than parsed through to select more homogenous subgroups. The generalized grouping of similar presentations in vastly different patients under the heading of 'sepsis' may have contributed to the field's difficulty in identifying sepsis-specific pharmacological treatment. Recent advances in detecting immunologic biomarkers may hold the key to stratifying sepsis patients into subgroups to be studied and treated in a more specialized fashion [32]. Rather than ignore this variation, the EMR could ultimately be used to not only identify but also make intelligent use of this variation, quantifying sepsis phenotypes and suggesting the treatments that are thought to reflect each phenotype's underlying pathophysiology.

There is still much research to be done, but is it not hard to imagine the EMR being able to recommend crystalloid versus colloid fluids for volume resuscitation, a vasopressor choice based on venous access and drug costs, or an antibiotic based on culture results; all while incorporating information about the patient's specific sepsis phenotype. Given that sepsis still lacks specific pharmacologic targets, the next wave of innovation may well be embracing the empiric nature of treatment while refining the characteristics that we consider as part of an empiric approach.

IT Strategies to Facilitate Population-based Sepsis Quality Improvement

A third strategy for health IT-based sepsis quality improvement involves the potential for IT to enable larger, population-based approaches to measuring and improving sepsis quality. Population-based strategies for sepsis quality improvement can take several forms, including regional quality improvement collaboratives in which hospitals band together to pool resources and share strategies for quality improvement, as well as government-led efforts to incentivize quality improvement through health policy, such as pay-for-performance and public reporting of quality data. Each of these could be facilitated and made more effective by the innovative use of health IT.

Regional Quality Improvement Collaboratives

Regional quality improvement collaboratives provide a forum for hospitals to share strategies for quality improvement, including protocols, care bundles, and educational platforms [33]. Central to these collaboratives is the notion of sharing data. Data sharing is essential for creating clinical registries to measure quality and compare quality across providers, a process known as 'benchmarking'. At present most quality improvement collaboratives share data manually, through web-based data entry for relevant patients. This process is cumbersome and expensive, limiting participation in large sepsis collaboratives, such as the Surviving Sepsis Campaign [34]. The rise of EMRs means, in theory, that data could be transmitted and analyzed by these collaboratives electronically, increasing the efficiency of data sharing and lowering the costs required to participate. Automated electronic data sharing can also increase the number of data elements that can be shared, expanding the scope and scale of these registries.

Health Policy Approaches

Health policy is a critical tool for incentivizing sepsis quality improvement on a large scale. These approaches include the public reporting of quality data, by which risk-adjusted outcome data are made available to patients to enable consumer choice and motivate poor performing hospitals to improve [35], and pay-for-performance, by which health care purchasers provide greater reimbursement to higher performing providers as a way of rewarding high performers and incentivizing quality improvement among poor performers [36]. Although sepsis-focused policy initiatives are still in their infancy, they are gaining steam. For example, the United States government now requires all US hospitals to report data on adherence to selected sepsis care processes, and New York State will soon publically report risk-adjusted sepsis outcomes for all hospitals in the state as part of its nascent sepsis-regulations [37].

Similar to regional quality improvement collaboratives, central to these activities is the availability of multicenter data. In the past, most policy-oriented quality improvement programs used administrative claims data. Although useful, these data lack both reliable process data and sufficiently granular clinical data for meaningful risk-adjustment models. As a result, health systems are typically required to perform manual data collection and data entry, a process which is onerous and expensive. The claims data are a stopgap, but improving the accuracy of sepsis outcomes measures requires access to more accurate and comprehensive patient data that can only be provided by the EMR.

Despite this need, there are several major barriers to the use of EMR-data for population-based quality improvement. These include limited interoperability across different EMRs, including differing variable names and differing data structures, as well as a lack of secure transmission capabilities precluding large-scale sharing of data while still respecting the need for patient privacy. Recent advances in health IT can help solve both of these problems. One key advance is the advent of so-called 'distributed data networks' which facilitate data sharing across organizations while accounting for differing data structures and maintaining the privacy and confidentiality of medical records [38].

Under a distributed data network model, all original patient-level data including personal identifiers remains at the host institution, while group level data (e. g., summary statistics on the characteristics of patients with sepsis) and de-identified patient-level data (e. g., key clinical variables and outcomes for specific patients) are sent to a central repository for pooling across hospitals (Fig. 1). Differences in variable names and data structures are handled by specially designed software that can 'translate' the different languages spoken by different hospitals and different EMRs. These models are currently being used in the US, where software such as I2B2 and Shrine are used to facilitate large-scale Clinical Data Research Networks as part of the US Patient Centered Outcomes Research Institute [39–41]. These networks satisfy each hospital's need for independence and data security while still allowing for robust data sharing and data integrity.

Limitations and Pitfalls

Despite the promise of health IT as a tool for sepsis quality improvement, there are a number of potential limitations and pitfalls that still must be addressed. First is the general perception that the use of technology itself is equivalent to quality improvement and the notion that technology is often allowed to create its own demand, a concept known as 'technological determinism'. Technological determinism is particularly prevalent among intensive care unit (ICU) providers, which have long been enamored with new technologies for monitoring that later are shown to have minimal impact on patient outcomes, such as pulmonary artery catheters. It is essential that we do not let information technology fall into this trap. IT itself is not quality improvement, it is merely a tool for quality improvement. Simply introducing a sepsis alert into an EMR will not ensure that providers will better recognize sepsis –

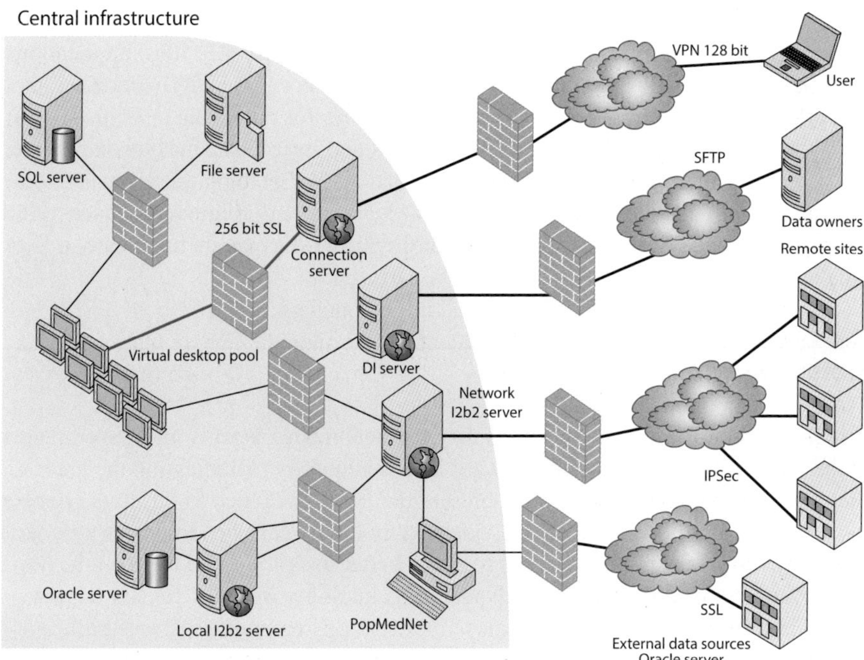

Fig. 1 Schematic for a distributed data network for regional sepsis quality improvement. Data from remote sites is sent to a central source via an I2b2 server which de-identifies and standardizes the data, which are then made accessible to remote users for benchmarking, quality improvement or research

such alerts must be rigorously evaluated and refined to ensure that they are meeting their goals, and abandoned if it is determined that the unintended consequences outweigh the benefits.

Second, there are reasonable concerns about the 'over-protocolization' of care that can occur when we remove physicians from the decision-making process. Such efforts can lead to physician burnout and restrict physician decision making in a way that could paradoxically reduce the quality of care. In one sense, addressing this problem means acknowledging that the practice of medicine has changed over the last few decades, and efforts to standardize care are not in contradiction to the art of medicine but are now part of the art of medicine. At the same time, it is essential that we ensure that electronic decision support is designed in a way to encourage thoughtful decision-making at the periphery and allow clinicians to refine treatment plans based on their clinical expertise. In this way, well-designed electronic interfaces have the potential to actually increase intellectual engagement by streamlining decision trees and eliminating pointless distractions.

Third, it is important to pay attention to how technology affects organization and workflow. In part because medicine existed for thousands of years without IT, and in part because most health IT interfaces are poorly designed without proper attention to the needs of the end users, adoption of health IT can be quite traumatic both to individual users and to the organization as a whole [42]. Ideal applications of health IT will enhance health workflows or disrupt unhealthy workflows, not disrupt already healthy workflows, making it easier for clinicians to do their jobs. The best health IT ultimately 'disappears', such that its use becomes second nature. At present, health IT has failed in that respect. As we develop these applications, it is essential that we prioritize the user experience and continue to place value on organizational dynamics, ensuring that the technology exists in service to high quality care, not in parallel to high quality care.

Conclusions

Improving quality in sepsis is a priority for healthcare systems and governments alike. One of the clearest paths forward in sepsis quality is harnessing the growing field of information technology. At present the EMR has failed to fulfill its promise as a tool for quality improvement, not only in sepsis care but in health care writ large; however, several approaches to make better use of health IT are on the horizon. As we devote resources to advancing technology, we must remain cognizant of the pitfalls of these new capabilities, implementing technological capabilities not simply because they exist but rather because they truly move the needle on sepsis quality for patients and providers alike.

Acknowledgement

The authors gratefully acknowledge the assistance of Daniel Ricketts in preparing the figure.

References

1. Singer M, Deutschman CS, Seymour CW et al (2016) The Third International Consensus Definitions for Sepsis and Septic Shock (Sepsis-3). JAMA 315:801–810
2. Liu V, Escobar GJ, Greene JD et al (2014) Hospital deaths in patients with sepsis from 2 independent cohorts. JAMA 312:90–92
3. Gaieski DF, Edwards JM, Kallan MJ, Carr BG (2013) Benchmarking the incidence and mortality of severe sepsis in the United States. Crit Care Med 41:1167–1174
4. Rhodes A, Phillips G, Beale R et al (2015) The Surviving Sepsis Campaign bundles and outcome: results from the International Multicentre Prevalence Study on Sepsis (the IMPreSS study). Intensive Care Med 41:1620–1628
5. Jones SS, Rudin RS, Perry T, Shekelle PG (2014) Health information technology: an updated systematic review with a focus on meaningful use. Ann Intern Med 160:48–54
6. Adler-Milstein J, DesRoches CM, Furukawa MF et al (2014) More than half of US hospitals have at least a basic EHR, but stage 2 criteria remain challenging for most. Health Aff 33:1664–1671

7. Dellinger RP, Levy MM, Rhodes A et al (2013) Surviving Sepsis Campaign: International guidelines for management of severe sepsis and septic shock: 2012. 41:580–637
8. Kumar A, Roberts D, Wood KE et al (2006) Duration of hypotension before initiation of effective antimicrobial therapy is the critical determinant of survival in human septic shock. Crit Care Med 34:1589–1596
9. Angus DC, Barnato AE, Bell D et al (2015) A systematic review and meta-analysis of early goal-directed therapy for septic shock: the ARISE, ProCESS and ProMISe Investigators. Intensive Care Med 41:1549–1560
10. Churpek MM, Zadravecz FJ, Winslow C et al (2015) Incidence and prognostic value of the systemic inflammatory response syndrome and organ dysfunctions in ward patients. Am J Respir Crit Care Med 192:958–964
11. Thiel SW, Rosini JM, Shannon W et al (2010) Early prediction of septic shock in hospitalized patients. J Hosp Med 5:19–25
12. Sawyer AM, Deal EN, Labelle AJ et al (2011) Implementation of a real-time computerized sepsis alert in nonintensive care unit patients. Crit Care Med 39:469–473
13. Nelson JL, Smith BL, Jared JD, Younger JG (2011) Prospective trial of real-time electronic surveillance to expedite early care of severe sepsis. Ann Emerg Med 57:500–504
14. Hooper MH, Weavind L, Wheeler AP et al (2012) Randomized trial of automated, electronic monitoring to facilitate early detection of sepsis in the intensive care unit. Crit Care Med 40:2096–2101
15. Alsolamy S, Al Salamah M, Al Thagafi M et al (2014) Diagnostic accuracy of a screening electronic alert tool for severe sepsis and septic shock in the emergency department. BMC Med Inform Decis Mak 14:105
16. Umscheid CA, Betesh J, VanZandbergen C et al (2015) Development, implementation, and impact of an automated early warning and response system for sepsis. J Hosp Med 10:26–31
17. Harrison AM, Thongprayoon C, Kashyap R et al (2015) Developing the surveillance algorithm for detection of failure to recognize and treat severe sepsis. Mayo Clin Proc 90:166–175
18. Brandt BN, Gartner AB, Moncure M et al (2015) Identifying severe sepsis via electronic surveillance. Am J Med Qual 30:559–565
19. Amland RC, Hahn-Cover KE (2016) Clinical decision support for early recognition of sepsis. Am J Med Qual 31:103–110
20. Idrees M, Macdonald SP, Kodali K (2016) Sepsis Early Alert Tool: Early recognition and timely management in the emergency department. Emerg Med Australas 28:399–403
21. Guidi JL, Clark K, Upton MT et al (2015) Clinician perception of the effectiveness of an automated early warning and response system for sepsis in an academic medical center. Ann Am Thorac Soc 12:1514–1519
22. Hripcsak G, Friedman C, Alderson PO et al (1995) Unlocking clinical data from narrative reports: a study of natural language processing. Ann Intern Med 122:681–688
23. Payne TH, Corley S, Cullen TA et al (2015) Report of the AMIA EHR-2020 Task Force on the status and future direction of EHRs. J Am Med Inform Assoc 22:1102–1110
24. Pinsky MR, Dubrawski A (2014) Gleaning knowledge from data in the intensive care unit. Am J Respir Crit Care Med 190:606–610
25. Halpern SD, Becker D, Curtis JR et al (2014) An official American Thoracic Society/American Association of Critical-Care Nurses/American College of Chest Physicians/Society of Critical Care Medicine policy statement: the Choosing Wisely® Top 5 list in Critical Care Medicine. Am J Respir Crit Care Med 190:818–826
26. Balas EA, Weingarten S, Garb CT et al (2000) Improving preventive care by prompting physicians. Arch Intern Med 160:301–308
27. Weiss CH, Moazed F, McEvoy CA et al (2011) Prompting physicians to address a daily checklist and process of care and clinical outcomes: a single-site study. Am J Respir Crit Care Med 184:680–686
28. Kahn JM, Gunn SR, Lorenz HL et al (2014) Impact of nurse-led remote screening and prompting for evidence-based practices in the ICU. Crit Care Med 42:896–904

29. Rana R, Afessa B, Keegan MT et al (2006) Evidence-based red cell transfusion in the critically ill: quality improvement using computerized physician order entry. Crit Care Med 34:1892–1897
30. Bourdeaux CP, Davies KJ, Thomas MJC et al (2014) Using "nudge" principles for order set design: a before and after evaluation of an electronic prescribing template in critical care. BMJ Qual Saf 23:382–388
31. Emanuel EJ, Ubel PA, Kessler JB et al (2016) Using behavioral economics to design physician incentives that deliver high-value care. Ann Intern Med 164:114–119
32. Calfee CS (2016) Precision medicine: an opportunity to improve outcomes of patients with sepsis. Am J Respir Crit Care Med 194:137–139
33. Nadeem E, Olin SS, Hill LC et al (2013) Understanding the components of quality improvement collaboratives: a systematic literature review. Milbank Q 91:354–394
34. Levy MM, Dellinger RP, Townsend SR et al (2010) The Surviving Sepsis Campaign: Results of an international guideline-based performance improvement program targeting severe sepsis. Crit Care Med 38:367–374
35. Reineck LA, Le TQ, Seymour CW et al (2015) Effect of public reporting on intensive care unit discharge destination and outcomes. Ann Am Thorac Soc 12:57–63
36. Kahn JM, Scales DC, Au DH et al (2010) An official American Thoracic Society policy statement: pay-for-performance in pulmonary, critical care, and sleep medicine. Am J Respir Crit Care Med 181:752–761
37. Cooke CR, Iwashyna TJ (2014) Sepsis mandates: improving inpatient care while advancing quality improvement. JAMA 312:1397–1398
38. Brown JS, Holmes JH, Shah K et al (2010) Distributed health data networks: a practical and preferred approach to multi-institutional evaluations of comparative effectiveness, safety, and quality of care. Med Care 48:45–51
39. Murphy SN, Weber G, Mendis M et al (2010) Serving the enterprise and beyond with informatics for integrating biology and the bedside (i2b2). J Am Med Inform Assoc 17:124–130
40. Weber GM, Murphy SN, McMurry AJ et al (2009) The Shared Health Research Information Network (SHRINE): a prototype federated query tool for clinical data repositories. J Am Med Inform Assoc 16:624–630
41. Amin W, Tsui FR, Borromeo C et al (2014) PaTH: towards a learning health system in the Mid-Atlantic region. J Am Med Inform Assoc 21:633–636
42. Edmondson AC, Bohmer RM, Pisano GP (2001) Disrupted routines: team learning and new technology implementation in hospitals. Adm Sci Q 46:685

Beyond Semantics: 'Disproportionate Use of Intensive Care Resources' or 'Medical Futility'?

E. J. O. Kompanje and J. Bakker

Introduction

Patients suffering from acute and life-threatening dysfunction of one or more vital organs are commonly treated in an intensive care unit (ICU) using advanced resources. The use of these resources is usually highly valued by most stakeholders as appropriate and timely (Fig. 1). However, the goal of intensive care is not the use of advanced resources but to use these if needed to achieve complete restoration of prior physical and mental health status, or an acceptable quality of life. However, significant comorbid conditions are already present on admission in more than half of ICU patients [1], resulting in a prolonged ICU stay, significant morbidity and mortality and increased associated costs. Surviving patients are frequently faced with decreased quality of life and debilitating morbidity. Over the past two decades, the use of life-sustaining measures has increased significantly in ICU patients including those with chronic and irreversible organ dysfunctions, debilitating comorbid conditions and/or altered quality of life [2–4]. In trying to reverse the acute organ dysfunction on top of already present morbidity we increasingly use costly and scarce resources with questionable benefice. This can, in contrast to the appropriate use of resources, be judged as inappropriate. Although it seems logical and desirable to avoid this, intensivists are often reluctant to withhold or withdraw

E. J. O. Kompanje
Department of Intensive Care Medicine, Erasmus MC University Medical Center
3000 CA Rotterdam, Netherlands

J. Bakker (✉)
Department of Intensive Care Medicine, Erasmus MC University Medical Center
3000 CA Rotterdam, Netherlands
Division of Pulmonary, Allergy, and Critical Care Medicine, Columbia University Medical Center
622 West 168th St, New York, NY 10032, USA
Division of Pulmonary, Critical Care and Sleep Medicine, Bellevue Hospital, New York University
New York, NY, USA
e-mail: jb3387@cumc.columbia.edu

J.-L. Vincent (ed.), *Annual Update in Intensive Care and Emergency Medicine 2017*,
DOI 10.1007/978-3-319-51908-1_40

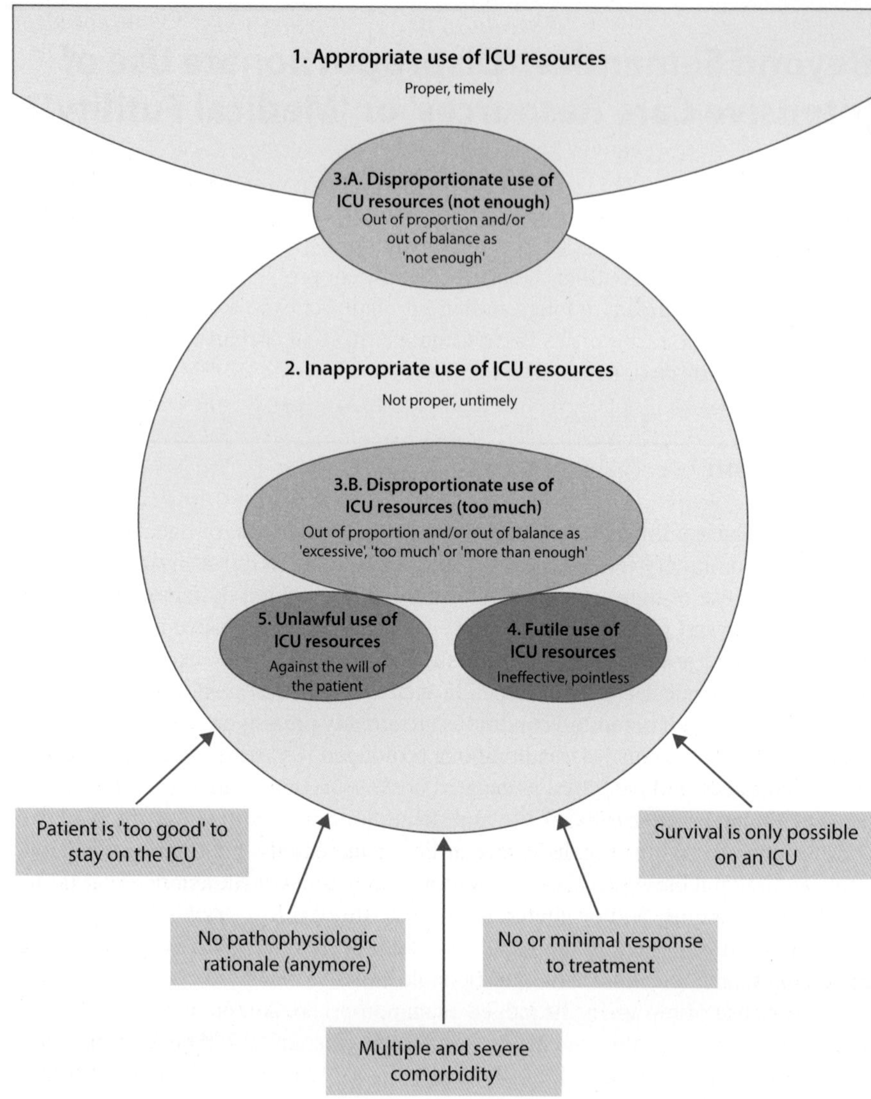

Fig. 1 Inappropriate use of ICU resources

life-sustaining measures. Most frequently this is related to the uncertainty of the prognosis, doubt whether the provided care is beneficial or not, or because patients or family members urge them to start and continue even the most aggressive treatment. However, the clinical situation of the patient and/or the emotional condition of the relatives may limit the ability of clinicians to adequately identify patients' preferences and values, before or shortly after ICU admission. In addition, one third of the relatives cannot correctly reflect the wishes of their loved-ones [5] and underestimate the quality of life of their loved one [6].

Frequently it takes several days after starting invasive care treatment before ICU clinicians learn from the relatives that this may be at odds with patient's values, should she/he have been able to express her/his own wishes. Clearly, none of the stakeholders benefit from this growing and worrying situation as inappropriate care compromises patient dignity and, in addition, represents harm. Moreover, the relatives may be exposed to guilt and complicated grief [7].

Although the above outlines a current and urgent problem, delivering non-beneficial ICU care is already a longstanding problem. Already a decade ago, 73% of European ICU physicians and 87% of Canadian ICU physicians declared that they frequently admitted patients with unrealistic perspectives [8, 9]. In a prevalence study, 27% (445/1,651) of the physicians and nurses stated that they had cared for at least one patient receiving disproportionate care [10], and 60% indicated that similar situations were rather common. Due to the increased use of technical life-sustaining measures, spontaneous death has become rare in the ICU, and a decision to withhold/withdraw life-sustaining measures is frequently made in the anticipation of death [11, 12]. Different cultural, ethical, financial, and legal frameworks that prevail in various countries, often lead to delayed end-of-life decision-making [13, 14]. In-depth psychological factors in each individual decision-maker (physicians, nurses and surrogates) worsen the actual picture [15]. This results in unnecessary patient suffering and relatives' burden given rise to loss of dignity in the dying process [16, 17]. In addition, conflicts between staff and family and within the ICU-staff, moral distress, compassion fatigue and burnout among physicians and nurses, lead to huge staff turnover [10, 18, 19]. These elements as well as many others plead for avoiding inappropriate care.

Resources on the ICU include several care components. First, they include the unit (building, including heating and air conditioning/filtering), and material facilities (beds, equipment [e. g., monitoring, mechanical ventilator, dialysis, extracorporeal membrane oxygenation (ECMO), and medication pumps], invasive tools [e. g., catheters], medications, infusion fluids and the use of other services [e. g. laboratories, administration, and radiology]). Second, they contain the costs of the care-providers (physicians, nurses, physiotherapists, etc.). The sum of these resources is essentially to decrease the risk of death of patients admitted to the ICU with life-threatening conditions [20].

To improve decision-making, stimulate constructive deliberation and facilitate the ICU experience for all parties involved, we propose to change terminology and define different categories of use of ICU resources.

'Inappropriate' Use of ICU Resources

Appropriate use of these ICU resources is adequate, timely and proper following moral standards and codes of the professions. Inappropriate use of ICU resources therefore can be defined as 'not proper' or 'untimely'. Inappropriate use of ICU resources includes disproportionate use of ICU resources as 'excessive, too much, or more than enough, but also as 'not enough', and 'futile use of ICU resources', and even 'unlawful use of ICU resources' (Fig. 1).

'Disproportionate' Use of ICU Resources

Proportionate use of ICU resources could be defined as care that reduces a patient's risk of death in acute and life-threatening conditions. Improving or restoring quality of life by avoiding long-term physical or mental sequels is also 'proportionate'. However, disproportionate use of ICU resources is perceived by most health care providers, patients and their relatives, and/or society as disproportionate and/or out of balance, in relation to the condition of the patient or the expected outcome or reduction in risk of death of the patient.

Patients can be 'too good' or 'not sick enough' to be admitted to the ICU [21] or the use of ICU resources can be 'not enough' in terms of inadequate treatment (Fig. 1). Inadequate treatment can take place due to incompetence of the physician, due to financial reasons or at the explicit request of the patient. On the other hand, in extreme situations some interventions can be proportionate while others are disproportionate in the same patient (e. g., an artificial heart may be disproportionate, but ECMO proportionate), whereas in others both may be disproportionate. More prevalent, disproportionate use of ICU resources is judged as 'too much' or 'more than enough'. In only a small proportion of the cases can the inappropriate use of ICU resources be judged as futile, in the sense of ineffective or pointless. Another small part of inappropriate use of ICU resources can be judged as unlawful (e. g., when used against the will of the patient, Fig. 1).

So, in contrast to earlier publications on end-of-life issues where futility of care/use of resources has been introduced, the use of the terms inappropriate and disproportionate use of ICU resources would be a better reflection of current ICU practice.

Medical Futility

Medical futility as a concept and the use of the term 'futile care' is controversial and troublesome. In the ICU, futile care can be defined as the initiation or prolongation of 'ineffective, pointless or hopeless' use of ICU resources. Therefore, medical futility is by definition inappropriate. However the inappropriate or disproportionate use of ICU resources does not need to be futile (Fig. 1). An example of medical futility would be the use of mechanical ventilation in a brain dead patient who is not an organ donor. Medical futility in this definition is rather rare in the ICU.

'Non-beneficial Treatment'

Another frequently used term is non-beneficial treatment, which is defined as treatment that is not expected to cure or ameliorate the disease state and not expected to improve or restore patient's quality of life to a satisfactory level [22]. It is a synonym of futile.

Disproportionate Use of ICU Resources in the Sense of 'More Than Enough'

Others than the patient and/or her/his relatives can judge the use of ICU resources to be 'more than enough' if the prolonged use is not in the patient's best interest. Physicians involved in the care of patients with severe organ-failure should question themselves if there are medical interventions used in these patients that they can label as disproportionate because they, the nurses, or relatives of the patients are sufficiently confident that the interventions will not be beneficial. Excessive resources are sometimes used to provide life-sustaining medical care at the end of life frequently associated with a poor quality of death [21]. Especially in older patients and in patients with multiple comorbidities, this could be labeled as 'too much' or 'more than enough'.

Because we have the possibility and the resources to postpone and orchestrate death for a, sometimes, indefinite time, we have the moral responsibility to deliberate whether the continued use is still in the best interest of the patient. Alternatively, we should question ourselves whether admission to the ICU is primarily in the patient's interest.

Disproportionate Use of ICU-resources in the Sense of 'Too Much'

The initiation or prolongation of the use of ICU resources is 'too much' and thus disproportionate care if (Fig. 1):

1. The condition of the patient is known to be reversible, however,
   a. patient is 'too good', 'not sick enough' to legitimate ICU admission;
   b. it is certain or nearly certain that the treatment will not achieve the goals that the patient has specified or is against the will of the patient (e. g., advanced directives);
   c. further treatment and rehabilitation after ICU discharge will require a social network that is not present or cannot be organized;
   d. severe or multiple underlying comorbidities are highly likely to compromise recovery (see bullets 2a and 3).
2. The condition of the patient is irreversible or has become irreversible (according to current knowledge) during the ICU stay (i. e., cannot be solved by advanced ICU support even after a prolonged attempt):

   a. No effective treatment is available or the prolonged treatment has no real pathophysiologic rationale (anymore). Patients can be admitted for an intervention, but the use of resources is restricted (e. g., patients with advanced chronic obstructive pulmonary disease [COPD] can be admitted to receive non-invasive ventilation, however, neither resuscitation nor mechanical ventilation will be offered in case of further deterioration); we can even imagine giving in-ICU non-ICU care just to help prevent the patient becoming critically ill.
   b. Effective treatment is available, however, the patient is not responding to therapy, even when treatment is at its maximal level and it is not plausible anymore to assume that cure will occur (e. g., in a patient with acute respiratory distress syndrome [ARDS] with refractory hypoxemia despite a trial of corticosteroids).
   c. Effective treatment has already been given to the patient with no or only minimal response (marginally effective interventions).
3. The condition for which reason the patient was admitted is resolved; however prolonged life-sustaining treatment can only be delivered in an ICU (e. g., in cases of failure to wean from mechanical ventilation in an otherwise stable situation with no indication or possibility of ventilation outside the ICU).
4. It is certain or nearly certain that the treatment will not achieve the goals that the patient has specified or is against the patient's will (e. g., in patients with advanced directives).

Why Not Use the Concept 'Medical Futility' or the Term 'Futile Care'?

1. Contrary to the term 'futile care', 'disproportionate use of ICU resources' entails a potential bidirectional discrepancy between the administered care and the prognosis: this may be 'not enough' or 'too much'/'more than enough'. Although 'disproportionate' as 'not enough' is rare on the ICU [10], it is necessary to consider this aspect as well, as both situations may arise for different health care providers caring for the same patient (e. g., nurses may judge the situation as 'more than enough', whereas the physicians still sees opportunities for the patient) [23].
2. Disproportionate use of ICU resources is determined by the patient's wishes, a surrogate's report of the patient's preferences and values, severity of illness, comorbidity, response to (previous) treatment, life expectancy, quality of life, costs of use of ICU resources and cost of long-term follow-up for society, in which the burdens outweigh the benefits.
   Futile interventions are determined by only one factor, which is the patient's (estimated by the doctor) expected prognosis or course of the condition [24].
3. 'Futile care' presupposes a high degree of certainty regarding the final fatal prognosis, as the term implies that the patient will die, despite this care. However, this term does not take real life situations into account, such as the difficulty

to predict an individual patient's survival. This is a common situation in the ICU, where the use of life-sustaining technology (e. g., mechanical ventilation, vasoactive medication, ECMO, continuous veno-venous hemofiltration [CVVH]) virtually excludes a patient's spontaneous death [11, 12]. On the other hand, withdrawal of life-sustaining measures in a patient who is dependent on these measures can lead to the self-fulfilling prophecy that the treatment *was* futile, judged from the fact that the patient died after withdrawal [25–29].

4. 'Futile care' does not take into account that physicians and nurses have an evolving opinion concerning a patient's prognosis and burden during the course of treatment. Frequently, nurses consider care as futile much earlier than does the physician [30] depending on the patient's evolution, among other things. They are also sometimes more pessimistic [23]. In this respect, the proposed terminology recognizes another phase than futile care: these are situations during which the physician or nurse starts to doubt whether the level of care they are administering is still proportionate. An open and honest communication within the team is necessary to acknowledge the situation of disproportionate care as perceived by one of the healthcare providers. This is the first step to reach a consensus between all parties involved.
5. Every physician's or nurse's view of a specific situation is influenced by his/her reflection of his/her emotional past, cultural background, sex, clinical context, family requests and moral consciousness, formed by education, socialization and conscious moral consent [31, 32]. In practice, the term 'futile' care applies only as an absolute term when different expert health care providers agree that care is provided in a pointless, hopeless situation.
6. Futility does not recognize all the palliative care and comfort measures that should be maintained when life-sustaining measures are withheld or withdrawn (e. g., care after death of the patient, family conferences, as well as informal compassionate care).
7. Futility can be a source of family guilt during bereavement [34].

When the use of ICU resources is deemed inappropriate, two possible scenarios are possible:

1. It should be withheld or withdrawn. The most important reason to do this is because it prolongs unnecessary suffering by the patient and his/her relatives and loss of dignity. Furthermore, prolonging scarce and costly medical care without prospect is unjust. Third, prolongation of inappropriate use of ICU resources can lead to compassion fatigue, burnout and high staff turnover in health care providers. Fourth, prolongation of inappropriate use of ICU resources can be seen as a violation of ethical principles, such as nonmaleficence, beneficence and justice.
2. Inappropriate use of ICU resources can be prolonged in some cases, but only for a short period of time, in accordance with the patient and her/his relatives. This period should be used as time to help the patient and relatives accept that prolongation of the use of ICU-measures is out of proportion and thus inappropriate.

Conclusion

We propose the use of 'disproportionate use of ICU resources' instead of 'futile use of ICU resources'. This is beyond semantics. Contrary to the term 'futile care', 'disproportionate use of ICU resources' entails a potential bidirectional discrepancy between the administered care and the prognosis: this may be 'not enough' or 'too much'/'more than enough'. Disproportionate use of ICU resources is determined by a patient's wishes, a surrogate report of patient's preferences and values, severity of illness, comorbidity, response to (previous) treatment, life expectancy, quality of life, costs of use of ICU resources and cost of long-term follow-up for society, in which the burdens outweigh the benefits. Futile interventions are determined by only one factor, which is the patient's (estimated by the doctor) expected prognosis or course of the condition.

References

1. Vincent JL, Moreni R, Takala J et al (1996) The SOFA (Sepsis-related Organ Failure Assessment) score to describe organ dysfunction/failure. Intensive Care Med 22:707–710
2. Angus DC, Barnato AE, Linde-Zwirble WT et al (2004) ICU End-of Life peer group. Use of intensive care at the end of life in the united states: an epidemiologic study. Crit Care Med 32:638–643
3. Wunsch H, Linde-Zwirbe WT, Harrison DA, Barnato AE, Rowan KM, Angus DC (2009) Use of intensive care services during terminal hospitalizations in England and the united states. Am J Respir Crit Care Med 180:875–880
4. Quill CM, Ratcliffe SJ, Harhay MO et al (2014) Variation in decisions to forgo life-sustaining therapies in US ICUs. Chest 146:573–582
5. Shalowitz DI, Garrett-Mayer E, Wendler D (2006) The accuracy of surrogate decision makers. Arch Intern Med 166:493–497
6. Hofhuis J, Hautvast JL, Schrijvers AJ et al (2003) Quality of life on admission to the intensive care: can we query the relatives? Intensive Care Med 29:974–979
7. Rodriguez Villar S, Sanchez Casado M, Prigerson HG et al (2012) Incidence of prolonged grief disorder in relatives of patients who die during or after admission in intensive care unit. Rev Esp Anesthesiol Reanim 59:535–541
8. Palda VA, Bowman KW, Mclean RF, Chapman MG (2005) "Futile" care: Do we provide it? Why? A semistructured, Canada-wide survey of intensive care unit doctors and nurses. J Crit Care 20:207–213
9. Giannini A, Consonni D (2006) Physicians' perceptions and attitudes regarding inappropriate admissions and resource allocation in the intensive care setting. Br J Anaesth 96:57–62
10. Piers R, Azoulay E, Ricou B et al (2011) APPROPRICUS study group of the ESICM. Perception of appropriateness of care among European and Israeli Intensive care unit nurses and doctors. JAMA 306:2694–2703
11. Prendergast TJ, Luce JM (1997) Increasing incidence of witholding and withdrawal of life support from the critically ill. Am J Respir Crit Care Med 155:15–20
12. Sprung CL, Cohen SL, Sjokvist P et al (2003) Ethicus study group. End-of-life practices in European intensive care units: the ETHICUS Study. JAMA 290:790–797
13. Lind R, Lorem GF, Nortvedt P, Hevroy O (2011) Family members' experiences of "wait and see" as communication strategy in end-of-life decisions. Intensive Care Med 37:1143–1150

14. Jensen HI, Ammentorp J, Erlandsen M, Ording H (2011) Withholding or withdrawing therapy in intensive care units: an analysis of collaboration among healthcare professionals. Intensive Care Med 37:1696–1705
15. Kets de Vries MFR (2009) The denial of death. In: Sex, Money, Happiness and Death. The Quest for Authenticity. Palgrave Macmillan, Basingstoke, pp 168–175
16. Wright AA, Zhang B, Ray A et al (2008) Associations between end-of-life discussions, patient mental health, medical care near death, and caregiver bereavement adjustment. JAMA 300:1665–1673
17. Kross EK, Engelberg RA, Gries CJ, Nielsen EL, Zatzick D, Curtis JR (2011) ICU care associated with symptoms of depression and posttraumatic stress disorder among family members of patients who die in the ICU. Chest 139:795–801
18. Azoulay E, Timsit JF, Sprung C et al (2009) Prevalence and determinants of intensive care unit conflicts. Am J Respir Crit Care Med 180:853–860
19. Embriaco N, Azoulay E, Barrau K et al (2007) High level of burnout in intensivists: prevalence and associated factors. Am J Respir Crit Care Med 175:686–692
20. Tan SS, Hakkaart-van Rooijen L, Al MJ et al (2008) A microcosting study of intensive care unit stay in the Netherlands. J Intensive Care Med 23:250–257
21. Zhang B, Wright AA, Haiden A et al (2009) Heath care cost in the last week of life : associations with end of life conversations. Arch Intern Med 169:480–488
22. Andereck WS, McGaughey JW, Schneiderman LJ et al (2014) Seeking to reduce nonbeneficial treatment in the ICU: an exploratory trial of proactive ethics intervention. Crit Care Med 42:824–830
23. Frick S, Uehlinger DE, Zuercher Zenklusen RM (2003) Medical futility: predicting outcome of intensive care unit patients by nurses and doctors – a prospective comparative study. Crit Care Med 31:456–461
24. Sprung CL, Baras M, Lapichino G et al (2012) The Eldicus prospective, observational study of triage decision making in European intensive care units: part I – European Intensive Care Admission Triage Scores. Crit Care Med 40:125–131
25. Poncet MC, Toullic P, Papazian L et al (2007) Burnout syndrome in critical nursing staff. Am J Respir Crit Care Med 175:698–704
26. Murphy DJ (1997) The economics of futile interventions. In: Zucker MB, Zucker HD (eds) Medical Futility. Cambridge University Press, Cambridge, pp 123–135
27. Angus DC, Truog RD (2016) Toward better ICU use at the end of life. JAMA 315:255–256
28. Wilkinson D (2009) The self-fulfilling prophecy in intensive care. Theor Med Bioeth 30:401–410
29. Azoulay E, Pochard F, Garrouste-Orgeas M et al (2003) Decisions to forgo life-sustaining therapy in ICU patients independently hospital death. Intensive Care Med 29:1895–1901
30. Azoulay E, Garrouste M, Goldgran-Toledano D et al (2012) Increased nonbeneficial care in patients spending their birthday in the ICU. Intensive Care Med 38:1169–1176
31. Becker KJ, Baxter AB, Cohen WA et al (2001) Withdrawal of support in intracerebral hemorrhage may lead to self-fulfilling prophecies. Neurology 56:766–772
32. Rushton CH (2006) Defining and addressing moral distress: tools for critical care nursing leaders. AACN Adv Crit Care 17:161–168
33. Weiner JS, Cole SA (2004) Three principles to improve clinician communication for advance care planning: overcoming emotional, cognitive, and skill barriers. J Palliat Med 7:817–829
34. Stroebe M, Schut H, Stroebe W (2007) Health outcome of bereavement. Lancet 370:1960–1973

Reflections on Work-Related Stress Among Intensive Care Professionals: An Historical Impression

M. M. C. van Mol, E. J. O. Kompanje, and J. Bakker

Introduction

Medical doctors have experienced significant changes in the delivery of healthcare over time. Long and tense working hours, increased administrative burden, impaired work-life balance, and frequent burden of liability and lawsuits have changed daily practice [1]. In addition, increased expectations from patients and families and a complex process of shared decision-making, lead to severe stress in health care providers [2]. This work-related stress can have a negative impact on an individual's joy in work, increase the chances of medical errors, and jeopardize quality of care [3, 4]. It might even result in long-term absenteeism or a threatening brain and skill drain if the professionals leave their jobs prematurely to preserve their own health, ultimately leading to economic burdens [5]. Reports have indicated that this increased work-related stress may cause suicide among doctors [6].

Physicians appear to be more likely to die by suicide than other health care professionals and twice as likely compared to the general population, although, it is still quite a rare occurrence. Each year, approximately 400 physicians in the USA die by suicide, which is more than by motor vehicle, drowning, homicide, and plane crashes together [7]. Historically, various health care professionals have been acknowledged as particularly vulnerable to work-related stress, with a number of

M. M. C. van Mol (✉) · E. J. O. Kompanje
Department of Intensive Care Medicine, Erasmus MC University Medical Center
3000 CA Rotterdam, Netherlands
e-mail: m.vanmol@erasmusmc.nl

J. Bakker
Department of Intensive Care Medicine, Erasmus MC University Medical Center
3000 CA Rotterdam, Netherlands
Division of Pulmonary, Allergy, and Critical Care Medicine, Columbia University Medical Center
New York, NY, USA
Division of Pulmonary, Critical Care, Sleep Medicine, Bellevue Hospital, New York University
New York, NY, USA

J.-L. Vincent (ed.), *Annual Update in Intensive Care and Emergency Medicine 2017*,
DOI 10.1007/978-3-319-51908-1_41

Table 1 Types of stress responses experienced by healthcare professionals

Anxiety	Moral distress
Burnout	Post-traumatic stress
Compassion fatigue	Secondary traumatic stress
Countertransference	Secondary victimization
Depression	Substance abuse
Empathic distress/strain/fatigue/overload	Suicide
Emotional distress	Vicarious trauma/stress
Exhaustion	Wounded healer

prevalent stress responses such as burnout, compassion fatigue, and traumatic stress (see Table 1 for an overview).

A 2014 study on the prevalence of burnout among physicians in the USA found that more than 54% reported at least one symptom of burnout, measured using the Maslach Burnout Inventory (MBI) [8]. Among all domains, the field of critical care scored highest in the prevalence of burnout (55%) [9]. However, during the same period, a nationwide study on burnout among Dutch intensivists found a very low burnout rate with a prevalence of only 4.4% [10]. In a recent systematic literature review on emotional distress among intensive care professionals, we suggested that the true magnitude of work-related stress remains unclear due to a lack of unity in concepts, related measuring instruments, and cut-off points [11]. In this chapter, we provide a historical impression and trends in work-related stress responses among intensive care professionals.

The Origin of Stress

Stress describes a person's response to a threat or some other change in the environment, which goes beyond one's resources for coping with the obstacle (events, people, and situations). Similarly, in a psychological definition, stress is, "the condition in which person – environment transactions lead to a perceived discrepancy between the physical or psychological demands of a situation and the resources of the individual's biological, psychological, or social systems" [12].

Stress increases immediately if a defiant change or threat occurs. A certain amount of stress is necessary and important to perform activities and work tasks [13], also called eustress. The pathogenic role of stress was identified by physiologist Walter B. Cannon (1871–1945) in the 'fight-or-flight' response, as this mobilizes an individual to combat the threat or to flee in face of the stressful event [14]. This process could have negative consequences if the burden exceeds the individual's capacity or when it becomes a chronic stress. A little later, this theory was expanded to the General Adaption Syndrome by Hans Selye (1907–1982), a medical doctor at Johns Hopkins University. He showed that environmental stressors activate the HPA axis (hypothalamus, pituitary gland, and adrenal cortex) and consequently increase cortisol levels associated with an immediate increase in blood pressure and heart rate. In a chronic phase, these cortisol levels can lead to cell damage and depletion of the body's energy reserves [15]. Finally, the psychologist Richard Lazarus (1922–2002) found that cognitive appraisal processes can influence both the stress and the emotional experience [16]. The appraisal of a situation causes an emotional, or affective, response that is going to be based on that appraisal. An important aspect of this appraisal theory is that it accounts for individual variances in emotional reactions to the same event. Therefore, work-related stress might have different effects in individual healthcare professionals even in situations of equal stress.

Both physical warning signs (headaches, sleeping disturbances, low back pain and stomach problems) and mental responses (irritability or hostility, loss of concentration, low self-confidence and emotional instability) can indicate individual stress reactions [12]. However, these are non-specific symptoms that do not depict the origin of stress and subsequently constrain effective coping mechanisms and the development of preventive strategies.

Exhaustion and Burnout

The Roman physician Galen (129–c216) wrote one of the earliest discussions on exhaustion, which he believed was an imbalance of the four humors – blood, yellow bile, black bile and phlegm. An increase in black bile "slowed the body's circulation and clogged up the brain's pathways, bringing about lethargy, torpor, weariness, sluggishness and melancholy" [17]. Although this idea found no scientific basis, even today many people with exhaustion, and subsequent foggy thinking, experience their brains filled with a tar-like liquid causing an extreme mental tiredness. Many people throughout history have felt overtired, suggesting that fatigue and exhaustion could be part of the human condition.

Burnout was first described by Herbert J. Freudenberger (1926–1999). He borrowed the term from the drug scene where it originally referred to the catastrophic influence of chronic drug abuse, and applied this concept to volunteers at the St Mark's Free Clinic in New York's East Village who felt a gradual emotional depletion, loss of motivation, and reduced commitment [18]. At the same time, burnout was used by Maslach in a description of social workers who felt emotionally exhausted and developed negative perceptions about their clients. Since 1970, a considerable body of knowledge about the nature of burnout, its causes and consequences, and its prevalence in specific domains has emerged [19].

Burnout is currently seen as the most prevalent career crisis of the twenty-first century. It is now characterized by a combination of three factors: emotional exhaustion, depersonalization and diminished personal accomplishment [18, 19]. An official Critical Care Societies Collaborative statement provides an extensive summary of the symptoms, the causative factors and consequences of burnout in the intensive care unit (ICU) [20]. Some of the risk factors for burnout include individual characteristics, such as perfectionism, a compromised work-life balance and a neurotic personality. However, organizational aspects, such as an increased workload and too many work hours, are related to high rates of burnout as well. Although some contradictions exist, younger professionals are at higher risk of burnout compared to older and more experienced professionals [11]. Some studies have reported that female ICU professionals are at higher risk [4, 21], whereas others found no difference between men and women [22, 23].

The Maslach Burnout Inventory (MBI) is seen as the standard tool for measuring the severity of burnout [21, 24, 25]. The MBI is a highly reliable and validated 22-item self-report questionnaire that evaluates the three domains of burnout in independent subscales [26]. However, since its development, the operationalization and measurement of burnout have differed across studies [11, 20]. Measuring only exhaustion, as an equivalent to burnout, is not sufficient and induces erroneously high prevalence rates. The high burnout rates as currently reported in public discussions are also confounded by the limited methodologic quality of the majority of the studies [27]. Cross-sectional studies may suffer from reverse causation, thus mixing cause and effect of work-related stress to burnout and emotional exhaustion. In addition, the low response rates, seen in some studies to be as low as 19% [8], could result in selection bias. Therefore, this cost of caring is overestimated. The concept of burnout might be misused to indicate an overall exhaustion with life; fatigue and tiredness may be a part of the human condition. It is highly recommended that burnout is investigated using longitudinal international studies in a valid and comparative manner, with clear cut-off points in all three domains, to indicate the significance of the problem among intensive care professionals.

Post-traumatic Stress During War

Crocq and Crocq provide an all-encompassing historical overview on the diseases that are currently labeled as post-traumatic stress disorder (PTSD) [28]. The authors stated that the first reported phenomenon of psychological consequences after witnessing terrifying situations emerged during early battles: "The first case of chronic mental symptoms caused by sudden fright in the battlefield is reported in the account of the battle of Marathon by Herodotus, written in 440 BC". Hippocrates (c460–377 BC) also mentioned frightening battle dreams, and centuries later, Shakespeare wrote a line of poetry in his 'Romeo and Juliet' on the awakening of soldiers by re-experiencing past battles in their dreams. In 1678, a Swiss physician used "nostalgia", which was followed by the "traumatic neurosis" of the German physician, Oppenheim, in 1884, to label similar psychological signs. In 1871, the physician Jacob Mendes Da Costa (1833–1900) described psychological war symptoms as the so-called "irritable heart". He studied over 300 servicemen during the American Civil War (1861–1865) with complaints of chest pain, fatigue, dyspnea, palpitations, headaches and dizziness. He assumed a somatic cause from excessive marching [29]. However, later on, the irritable heart was also observed in civilians, especially young women who performed strenuous work and who were highly emotional. The term 'neurasthenia' or 'nervous exhaustion' was introduced in 1880 by the neurologist George Beard (1839–1883) [30] who assumed for the first time that there was a certain predisposition in soldiers, which could be recognized before they were sent to battle.

After the First World War (1914–1918), the cardiologist Thomas Lewis (1881–1945) described 'the soldier's heart' and the 'effort syndrome' [31]. Complaints were again shortness of breath, dizziness, headache, sighing, palpitations, chest pain, fatigue, confusion, forgetfulness and lack of concentration. The condition was explained as being somatically caused, such as from lack of sleep in the trenches and the effects of poisonous gas. Another term used during this war was, 'shell shock' (also named 'trench neurosis', 'gas neurosis' and 'buried-alive neurosis'), which differed from the above mentioned syndromes by also giving rise to symptoms such as irritation, speech disorders, forgetfulness and other cognitive complains. Soldiers with a history of a 'weak' personality, family psychiatric disorders and a fragile physical constitution were predisposed to develop this condition. In the Second World War (1939–1945), once again soldiers suffered from the previously described symptoms. The terms 'combat neurosis', 'battle fatigue', 'operational fatigue' and 'combat exhaustion' were introduced to name this complex of symptoms. Obviously, these conditions were more a psychological or a psychiatric condition than related to somatic stresses. The symptoms were supposed to disappear after the war, but the phrase "You can take the man out the war, but you can never take the war out of the man" proved to be more truthful than expected. Even the term 'the old sergeant syndrome' was introduced when it became evident that veterans might suffer chronically from their war experiences. During the Vietnam War (1955–1975), the incidence was much lower than in the previous wars, but still soldiers suffered from 'combat stress' and 'battle stress reactions'.

Post-traumatic Stress in Healthcare

In 1952, the first edition of the Diagnostic and Statistical Manual of Mental Disorders (DSM-1) was developed by the American Psychiatric Association (APA). This manual included 'gross stress reaction' to mention a stress syndrome that is a response to an exceptional physical or mental stress, such as a natural catastrophe or battle. In DSM-II (1968), this category disappeared, perhaps because of the peaceful era in which the manual was revised, only to be re-entered in DSM-III (1980), after the Vietnam War, as 'post-traumatic stress disorder'. The PTSD diagnostic criteria were again revised in DSM-5, and are presented in Table 2, including the persistent effortful avoidance of distressing trauma-related stimuli among others (category 309.81 F43.10) [32]. A structured interview, such as the Clinician-Administered PTSD Scale for DSM-5 or the PTSD Symptom Scale-Interview, establishes the PTSD diagnosis. Disadvantages of these interviews are the prolonged administration time and the special training to guarantee the validity of the diagnosis. Although a number of self-report measurement instruments, such as the Davidson Trauma Scale or the Impact of Event Scale-Revised, assess the symptoms of PTSD, these measures do not accomplish a diagnosis of PTSD because of too many biased responses [33]. The estimated lifetime prevalence of PTSD in the National Comorbidity Survey Replication among adult Americans was 6.8% with a twelve-month prevalence of 3.5% [34].

Some researchers have suggested that intensive care professionals experience a traumatic work environment; these studies have found that 21–29% of respondents tested positive for symptoms of PTSD [35, 36]. Most of the traumatic events

Table 2 Criteria of post-traumatic stress disorder, adopted from DSM-5 manual

Criterion A: stressor	
The person was exposed to: death, threatened death, actual or threatened serious injury, or actual or threatened sexual violence, as follows: (one required)	
1	Direct exposure
2	Witnessing, in person
3	Indirectly, by learning that a close relative or close friend was exposed to trauma. If the event involved actual or threatened death, it must have been violent or accidental
4	Repeated or extreme indirect exposure to aversive details of the event(s), usually in the course of professional duties (e. g., first responders, collecting body parts; professionals repeatedly exposed to details of child abuse). This does not include indirect non-professional exposure through electronic media, television, movies or pictures
Criterion B: intrusion symptoms	
The traumatic event is persistently re-experienced in the following way(s): (one required)	
1	Recurrent, involuntary, and intrusive memories. Note: Children older than six may express this symptom in repetitive play
2	Traumatic nightmares. Note: Children may have frightening dreams without content related to the trauma(s)
3	Dissociative reactions (e. g., flashbacks) which may occur on a continuum from brief episodes to complete loss of consciousness. Note: Children may reenact the event in play
4	Intense or prolonged distress after exposure to traumatic reminders
5	Marked physiologic reactivity after exposure to trauma-related stimuli
Criterion C: avoidance	
Persistent effortful avoidance of distressing trauma-related stimuli after the event:(one required)	
1	Trauma-related thoughts or feelings
2	Trauma-related external reminders (e. g., people, places, conversations, activities, objects or situations)
Criterion D: negative alterations in cognition and mood	
Negative alterations in cognition and mood that began or worsened after the traumatic event: (two required)	
1	Inability to recall key features of the traumatic event (usually dissociative amnesia; not due to head injury, alcohol, or drugs)
2	Persistent (and often distorted) negative beliefs and expectations about oneself or the world (e. g., "I am bad," "The world is completely dangerous")
3	Persistent distorted blame of self or others for causing the traumatic event or for resulting consequences
4	Persistent negative trauma-related emotions (e. g., fear, horror, anger, guilt or shame)
5	Markedly diminished interest in (pre-traumatic) significant activities
6	Feeling alienated from others (e. g., detachment or estrangement)
7	Constricted affect: persistent inability to experience positive emotions

Table 2 (Continued)

Criterion E: alterations in arousal and reactivity	
Trauma-related alterations in arousal and reactivity that began or worsened after the traumatic event: (two required)	
1	Irritable or aggressive behavior
2	Self-destructive or reckless behavior
3	Hypervigilance
4	Exaggerated startle response
5	Problems in concentration
6	Sleep disturbance
Criterion F: duration	
Persistence of symptoms (in Criteria B, C, D, and E) for more than one month	
Criterion G: functional significance	
Significant symptom-related distress or functional impairment (e. g., social, occupational)	
Criterion H: exclusion	
Disturbance is not due to medication, substance use, or other illness	
Specify if: with dissociative symptoms In addition to meeting criteria for diagnosis, an individual experiences high levels of either of the following in reaction to trauma-related stimuli:	
1	Depersonalization: experience of being an outside observer of or detached from oneself (e. g., feeling as if "this is not happening to me" or one were in a dream)
2	Derealization: experience of unreality, distance, or distortion (e. g., "things are not real")
Specify if: with delayed expression. Full diagnosis is not met until at least six months after the trauma(s), although onset of symptoms may occur immediately	

presented in these studies on PTSD, such as verbal abuse, massive bleeding in the patient, or stress related to feeling overextended due to an inadequate professional to patient ratio, do not meet the DSM-5 criteria for PTSD. Although these situations may be stressful and may result in negative personal effects, this should not lead to the medicalization of normal human emotional responses or turn to overdiagnosis with potential overtreatment [37]. Witnessing a person's death, which is stated as a potential risk for PTSD, and providing palliative care might raise feelings of grief and pain in intensive care professionals, in particular if the patient is of a younger age or in a comparable situation to the professional's own surroundings. These feelings should be considered as normal human reactions and part of the normal process of dealing with one's emotions. The majority of individuals recover spontaneously after a traumatic situation [38]. Many people are exposed to loss or potentially traumatic events throughout their life span. However, most of them successfully endure the temporary emotional disturbance, with no apparent interference in functioning at work or in close relationships [39]. This process typically occurs because many individuals show resilience, which is the capacity to stay mentally healthy and to positively adapt after experiencing profound events. Intensive care professionals may have adapted their individual coping strategies to the demanding work environment to find emotional balance.

Thus, apart from some exceptional cases, such as being involved in a medical error, a natural disaster, or a war situation, it is very unlikely that intensive care professionals are traumatized by their emotionally demanding work. PTSD, and its related symptoms stemming from war veterans, is completely different from work-related stress in ICU professionals.

The Foundation of Compassion Fatigue

In the early 1980s, the term 'compassion fatigue' was used in American policy documents in reference to immigration and in the early 1990s to describe the lack of interest in homeless people by the general public. In 1992, Carol Joinson, a nurse educator in Texas, described compassion fatigue as the loss of compassion due to repeated exposure to suffering during work [40]. Slightly later, the psychologist Charles Figley defined this phenomenon as secondary traumatic stress resulting from a deep involvement with a primarily traumatized person because of the "more friendly framing" [41]. Figley proposed in 1995 that compassion fatigue is an excessive empathic reaction after witnessing another's suffering, resulting in symptoms such as anxiety, irritability, intrusive thoughts, hypervigilance or startle reactions, and avoidance of patient care. Although conceptually different, since then compassion fatigue and secondary traumatic stress have been used interchangeably, with suggested similarities between vicarious traumatization and burnout [11]. While compassion fatigue has been studied predominantly in the nursing field [42, 43], high risks were also found in physicians, ranging from 9 to 20% [44, 45].

Some scientists posed critical notes on the empirical understanding of compassion as a fundamental element of compassion fatigue, which is not equivalent to empathy, as used by Figley [46, 47]. His model identifies empathic ability as the capacity of health care providers to notice pain in others, and as a response, to project themselves into this emotional energy, thus feeling the pain, grief, desperation, or anger. However, a fundamental and profound theory on the concept of compassion is lacking. Thus, being empathic all of the time is perhaps too much of a good thing, with distancing or dehumanization as the result. Additionally, The Professional Quality of Life Scale, the newest modified measuring instrument on compassion fatigue, evaluates items responding to secondary stress [48]. This seems to be insufficient to meet the concept of compassion in the first place. In the last two decades, compassion fatigue has become a fashionable hype that should be critically reexamined or erased in favor of a new debate on work-related stress among intensive care professionals.

The Positive Approach of Work Engagement

In 1990, Robert Louis Kahn, an American psychologist, first described "personal engagement". He stressed the psychological conditions of personal engagement and disengagement at work. In optimal engagement, the individual's values co-

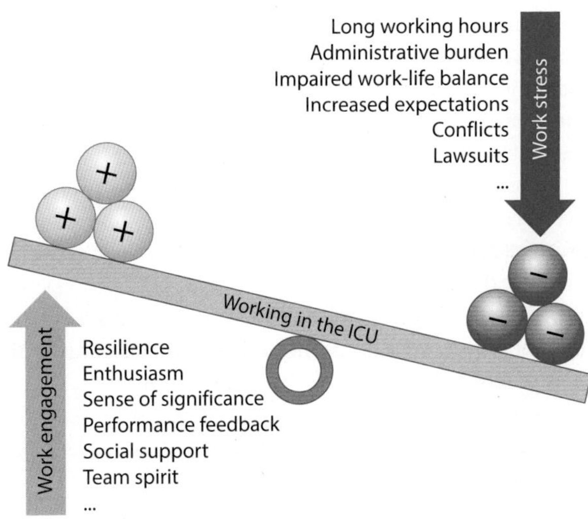

Fig. 1 Work engagement as a counterbalance to work-related stress

incide with the role of performance in all aspects (physical, cognitive, and emotional) while working [49]. In a further development, work engagement has been defined as a positive, fulfilling, work-related state of mind, which is characterized by vigor, dedication, and absorption [26]. Wilmar Schaufeli et al. stated that, "Vigor is characterized by high levels of energy and mental resilience while working, the willingness to invest effort in one's work, and persistence even in the face of difficulties; dedication by being strongly involved in one's work, and experiencing a sense of significance, enthusiasm, inspiration, pride, and challenge; and absorption by being fully concentrated and happily engrossed in one's work, whereby time passes quickly and one has difficulties with detaching oneself from work" [26]. Engaged employees believe in themselves, generate their own positive feedback, set higher goals, have values that match with the organization, and show a sustained healthy state. As illustrated in Fig. 1, work engagement with its positive labeled elements is the counterbalance to work-related stress. In general, work engagement is influenced by job autonomy, social support, performance feedback, and personal resources such as self-efficacy, flexibility and adaptability. Work engagement is firmly grounded in the Job-Demands-Resources Model [26].

From Historical Facts to Future Direction

Health care organizations should think of improvements and provide support in daily practice, in addition to individual activities to promote well-being, such as self-care in nutrition, sleep, exercise, and spending time with family or friends [4, 8]. The urge of a call for action has been heard and endorsed by all healthcare providers now. Evidence-based interventions are needed to address the most effective contributing factors; however, persuasive randomized controlled trials in this domain have not yet been performed [20]. Probably, there is not one simple solution that will fit all. Stimulating a healthy work environment is a multidimensional challenge, a traffic map with multiple roads leading to the same point of interest. Some promising suggestions are to regulate the environment and workload, have adequate administrative support systems, and find meaning in work [4].

Education and early recognition of the stress-related consequences among intensive care professionals could provide some answers as well. Furthermore, personal development of resilience may provide the basic adaptability to flourish in the hectic and ever demanding ICU environment. ICU professionals have learned to respond to these emotionally difficult situations. Indeed, we must take care of ourselves [50]; however, we should not forget that working in the ICU can be exciting and pleasurable too.

References

1. Sprung CL, Cohen R, Marini JJ (2016) Excellence in intensive care medicine. Crit Care Med 44:202–206
2. Curtis JR, Ciechanowski PS, Downey L et al (2012) Development and evaluation of an interprofessional communication intervention to improve family outcomes in the ICU. Contemp Clin Trials 33:1245–1254
3. West CP, Huschka MM, Novotny PJ et al (2006) Association of perceived medical errors with resident distress and empathy – A prospective longitudinal study. JAMA 296:1071–1078
4. Spickard A Jr, Gabbe SG, Christensen JF (2002) Mid-career burnout in generalist and specialist physicians. JAMA 288:1447–1450
5. Böckerman P, Ilmakunnas P (2008) Interaction of working conditions, job satisfaction, and sickness absences: evidence from a representative sample of employees. Soc Sci Med 67:520–528
6. Legha RK (2012) A history of physician suicide in America. J Med Humanit 33:219–244
7. Gunter TD (2016) Physician Death by Suicide: Problems Seeking Stakeholder Solutions. http://www.peertechz.com/Depression-Anxiety/pdf/ADA-2-110.pdf. Accessed November 10, 2016
8. Shanafelt TD, Hasan O, Dyrbye LN et al (2015) Changes in burnout and satisfaction with work-life balance in physicians and the general US working population between 2011 and 2014. Mayo Clin Proc 90:1600–1613
9. Peckham C (2016) Medscape Lifestyle Report 2016: Bias and Burnout. http://www.medscape.com/features/slideshow/lifestyle/2016/public/overview#page=2. Accessed 18 August 2016
10. Meynaar IA, van Saase JLCM, Feberwee T, Aerts TM, Bakker J, Thijsse W (2015) Burnout among dutch intensivists. Neth J Crit Care 24:12–17
11. van Mol MMC, Kompanje EJO, Benoit DD, Bakker J, Nijkamp MD (2015) The prevalence of compassion fatigue and burnout among healthcare professionals in intensive care units: a systematic review. PLoS One 10:e0136955
12. Sarafino EP (2002) Health Psychology. Biopsychosocial Interactions, 4th edn. John Wiley & Sons, New York, p 613
13. Piquette D, Reeves S, Leblanc VR (2009) Stressful intensive care unit medical crises: How individual responses impact on team performance. Crit Care Med 37:1251–1255
14. Cannon WB (1929) Bodily Changes In Pain, Hunger, Fear And Rage. Appleton, New York
15. Selye H (1983) The stress concepts. Past, present and future. In: Cooper CL (ed) Stress Research Issues for the Eighties. John Wiley, Chichester, pp 1–20

16. Lazarus RS (1993) From psychological stress to the emotions: A history of changing outlooks. Ann Rev Psychol 44:1–22
17. Schaffner AK (2016) Exhaustion: A History. Columbia University Press, New York
18. Schaufeli WB, Leiter MP, Maslach C (2009) Burnout: 35 years of research and practice. Career Dev Int 14:204–220
19. Leiter MP, Bakker AB, Maslach C (2014) Burnout at Work: A Psychological Perspective. Psychology Press, London
20. Moss M, Good VS, Gozal D, Kleinpell R, Sessler CN (2016) An official critical care societies collaborative statement – burnout syndrome in critical care health-care professionals: a call for action. Chest 150:17–26
21. Embriaco N, Azoulay E, Barrau K et al (2007) High level of burnout in intensivists: prevalence and associated factors. Am J Respir Crit Care Med 175:686–692
22. Bellieni CV, Righetti P, Ciampa R, Iacoponi F, Coviello C, Buonocor G (2012) Assessing burnout among neonatologists. J Matern Fetal Neonatal Med 25:2130–2134
23. Guntupalli KK, Fromm RE Jr (1996) Burnout in the internist-intensivist. Intensive Care Med 22:625–630
24. Barbosa FT, Leão BA, Sales Tavares GM, Peixoto dos Santos JGR (2012) Burnout syndrome and weekly workload of on-call physicians: Cross-sectional study. Sao Paulo Med J 130:282–288
25. Galvan ME, Vassallo JC, Rodríguez SP et al (2012) Physician's burnout in pediatric intensive care units from Argentina. Arch Argent Pediatr 110:466–473
26. Schaufeli WB, Salanova M, Gonz'alez-rom'a V, Bakker AB (2002) The measurement of engagement and burnout: A two sample confirmatory factor analytic approach. J Happiness Stud 3:71–92
27. Seidler A, Thinschmidt M, Deckert S et al (2014) The role of psychosocial working conditions on burnout and its core component emotional exhaustion – a systematic review. J Occup Med Toxicol 9:10
28. Crocq MA, Crocq L (2000) From shell shock and war neurosis to posttraumatic stress disorder: a history of psychotraumatology. Dialogues Clin Neurosci 2:47–55
29. Da Costa JM (1951) On irritable heart: a clinical study of a form of functional cardiac disorder and its consequences. Am J Med 11:559–567
30. Beard GM (1880) A Practical Treatise On Nervous Exhaustion (Neurasthenia); Its Symptoms, Nature, Sequences, Treatment. W Wood and Company, New York
31. Lewis T (1918) Soldier's heart and effort syndrome. Shaw and Sons, London
32. American Psychiatric Association (2013) Diagnostic and Statistical Manual Of Mental Disorders (DSM-5®). American Psychiatric Publishing, Washington
33. National Center for Post Traumatic Stress Disorder (2014) PTSD Overview and Assessment. http://www.ptsd.va.gov/professional/index.asp. Accessed 02 September 2016
34. Kessler RC, Berglund P, Demler O, Jin R, Merikangas KR, Walters EE (2005) Lifetime prevalence and age-of-onset distributions of DSM-IV disorders in the national Comorbidity Survey Replication. Arch Gen Psychiatry 62:593–627
35. Czaja AS, Moss M, Mealer M (2012) Symptoms of posttraumatic stress disorder among pediatric acute care nurses. J Pediatr Nurs 27:357–365
36. Mealer M, Jones J (2013) Posttraumatic stress disorder in the nursing population: a concept analysis. Nurs Forum 48:279–288
37. Nimmo A, Huggard P (2013) A systematic review of the measurement of compassion fatigue, vicarious trauma, and secondary traumatic stress in physicians. Australas J Disaster Trauma Stud 2013:37–44
38. Sijbrandij MA, Olff M, Reitsma JB, Carlier IVE, de Vries MH, Gersons BPR (2007) Treatment of acute posttraumatic stress disorder with brief cognitive behavioral therapy: a randomized controlled trial. Am J Psychiatry 164:82–90
39. Bonanno GA (2004) Loss, trauma, and human resilience: have we underestimated the human capacity to thrive after extremely aversive events? Am Psychol 59:20–28

40. Joinson C (1992) Coping with compassion fatigue. Nursing (Brux) 22:116–120
41. Figley CR (1995) Coping with Secondary Traumatic Stress Disorder in Those Who Treat the Traumatized. Routledge, New York
42. Young JL, Derr DM, Cicchillo VJ, Bressler S (2011) Compassion satisfaction, burnout, and secondary traumatic stress in heart and vascular nurses. Crit Care Nurs Q 34:227–234
43. Elkonin D, van der Vyver L (2011) Positive and negative emotional responses to work-related trauma of intensive care nurses in private health care facilities. Health Sa Gesondheid 16:1–8
44. Huggard P, Dixon R (2011) Tired of caring: the impact of caring on resident doctors. Australas J Disaster Trauma Stud 3:105–112
45. El-bar N, Levy A, Wald HS, Biderman A (2013) Compassion fatigue, burnout and compassion satisfaction among family physicians in the Negev area – a cross-sectional study. Isr J Health Policy Res 2:1–8
46. Sinclair S, Norris JM, McConnell SJ et al (2016) Compassion: a scoping review of the health-care literature. BMC Palliat Care 15:1–16
47. van Mol MMC, Brackel M, Kompanje EJO et al (2016) Joined forces in person-centered care in the intensive care unit: a case report from the Netherlands. J Compassionate Health Care 3:1–7
48. Sabo B (2011) Reflecting on the concept of compassion fatigue. Online J Issues Nurs 16:1–13
49. Kahn WA (1990) Psychological conditions of personal engagement and disengagement at work. Acad Manage J 33:692–724
50. Pastores SM (2016) Burnout syndrome in ICU caregivers: Time to extinguish! Chest 150:1–2

Index

J.-L. Vincent (ed.), *Annual Update in Intensive Care and Emergency Medicine 2017*,
DOI 10.1007/978-3-319-51908-1

W

Y

Printing: Ten Brink, Meppel, The Netherlands
Binding: Ten Brink, Meppel, The Netherlands